Atlas of Critical Care

Atlas of Critical Care

Editors

Yatin Mehta
MD MNAMS FRCA FAMS FIACTA FICCM FTEE
President
Indian Society of Critical Care Medicine
Chairman
Medanta Institute of Critical Care and Anesthesiology
Medanta—The Medicity
Gurugram, Haryana, India

Jeetendra Sharma
MD FICCM
Director and Head
Department of Critical Care
Artemis Hospital
Gurugram, Haryana, India

Forewords

Jean-Louis Vincent
Naresh Trehan
Shirish Prayag

JAYPEE

JAYPEE BROTHERS MEDICAL PUBLISHERS
The Health Sciences Publisher
New Delhi | London | Panama

Jaypee Brothers Medical Publishers (P) Ltd

Headquarters
Jaypee Brothers Medical Publishers (P) Ltd.
4838/24, Ansari Road, Daryaganj
New Delhi 110 002, India
Phone: +91-11-43574357
Fax: +91-11-43574314
E-mail: jaypee@jaypeebrothers.com

Overseas Offices
J.P. Medical Ltd.
83, Victoria Street, London
SW1H 0HW (UK)
Phone: +44-20 3170 8910
Fax: +44(0)20 3008 6180
E-mail: info@jpmedpub.com

Jaypee-Highlights Medical Publishers Inc.
City of Knowledge, Bld. 235, 2nd Floor, Clayton
Panama City, Panama
Phone: +1 507-301-0496
Fax: +1 507-301-0499
E-mail: cservice@jphmedical.com

Jaypee Brothers Medical Publishers (P) Ltd.
Bhotahity, Kathmandu, Nepal
Phone: +977-9741283608
E-mail: kathmandu@jaypeebrothers.com

Website: www.jaypeebrothers.com
Website: www.jaypeedigital.com

Atlas of Critical Care

First Edition: **2019**

ISBN: **978-93-5270-501-6**

Printed at: Ajanta Offset & Packagings Ltd., Faridabad, Haryana

Contributors

Aniruddha Agarwal MD
Senior Resident
Advanced Eye Center, PGIMER, Chandigarh, India
Stanley M Truhlsen Eye Institute
University of Nebraska Medical Center, USA
Ocular Imaging Research and Reading Center (OIRRC)
Menlo Park, CA, USA

Indrajit Agarwal MBBS MD (Medicine) MRCP
Consultant Rheumatologist
Paras Hospitals
Gurugram, Haryana, India

Manju Aggarwal MD DNB (Nephrology) MBA
Chairperson
Department of Nephrology and Kidney Transplantation
Artemis Hospitals
Gurugram, Haryana, India

Dheeraj Arora DNB PDCC MNAMS PGHM
Principle Consultant
Department of Cardiac Anesthesia
Medanta—The Medicity
Gurugram, Haryana, India

Isha Atre DNB
Clinical Associate
PD Hinduja Hospital
Mumbai, Maharashtra, India

Jalpa Bhandari MD
Clinical Associate,
PD Hinduja Hospital
Mumbai, Maharashtra, India

Rahul Bhargava
MD (Medicine) DM (Clinical Hematology, AIIMS)
Fellowship in BMT (Vancouver, Canada)
Director and Head
Department of Hematology, Hemato-Oncology and
Stem Cell Transplant
Fortis Memorial Research Institute
Gurugram, Haryana, India

Shilpushp J Bhosale
MD Fellowship in Pediatric Critical Care (Toronto) DM Critical Care
Assistant Professor
Department of Anesthesiology
Critical Care and Pain
Tata Memorial Hospital
Mumbai, Maharashtra, India

Arunaloke Chakrabarti MD
Professor and In-charge
Center of Advance Research in Medical Mycology
WHO Collaborating Center for Reference and
Research of Fungi of Medical Importance
National Culture Collection of Pathogenic Fungi
Head, Department of Medical Microbiology
Postgraduate Institute of Medical Education and Research
Chandigarh, India

Poulomi Chatterjee MBBS MD DNB EDARM
Associate Consultant
Department of Respiratory Medicine
Medanta—The Medicity
Gurugram, Haryana, India

Dinesh Chaudhary
MBBS MD (Medicine) DM (Cardiology)
PDF (Post-Doctoral Fellowship)
Cardiac Electrophysiology
Associate Professor
Department of Cardiology
Sardar Patel Medical College
Bikaner, Rajasthan, India

Ashim Das MD (Pathology)
Professor
Department of Histopathology
Postgraduate Institute of Medical Education and Research
Chandigarh, India

Shalini Goel MBBS DCP MD SYCM
Consultant
Department of Hematopathology
Division of Laboratory Medicine
Medanta—The Medicity
Gurugram, Haryana, India

Deepak Govil MD EDIC FCCM
Director
Department of Critical Care Medicine
Institute of Critical Care and Anesthesiology
Medanta—The Medicity
Gurugram, Haryana, India

Hardeep Kaur Grewal MBBS PGDCC FNIC
Consultant
Department of Cardiology
Clinical and Preventive Cardiology
Medanta Heart Institute, Medanta—The Medicity
Gurugram, Haryana, India

Amit Gupta MS FACS FCLS FRCS (Glasg.)
Professor
Department of Surgery
Division of Trauma Surgery and Critical Care
Jai Prakash Narayan Apex Trauma Center (JPNATC)
All India Institute of Medical Sciences, New Delhi, India

Mukesh K Gupta
MD (Medicine) FNB (Critical Care Medicine)
Senior Consultant
Department of Critical Care Medicine
Artemis Hospitals
Gurugram, Haryana, India

Rahul Harne DA IDCCM
Consultant
Department of Critical Care Medicine
Institute of Critical Care and Anesthesiology
Medanta—The Medicity
Gurugram, Haryana, India

Dhananjay Jadhav
Senior Technologist
Department of Radiology
Grant Medical Foundation
Ruby Hall Clinic
Pune, Maharashtra, India

Vijay Joshi MD DNB (Nephrology)
Department of Nephrology and
Kidney Transplantation
Artemis Hospitals
Gurugram, Haryana, India

Gaurav Kakkar MBBS (AFMC) FCARCSI CCT (UK)
Senior Consultant
Department of Neuroanesthesia
Medanta Institute of Critical Care and Anesthesiology
Medanta—The Medicity
Gurugram, Haryana, India

RR Kasliwal MBBS MD DM
Chairman
Department of Clinical and Preventive Cardiology
Medanta Heart Institute, Medanta—The Medicity
Gurugram, Haryana, India

Mansi Kaushik MBBS PGDCC FNIC
Consultant
Department of Cardiology
Division of Clinical and Preventive Cardiology
Medanta Heart Institute, Medanta—The Medicity
Gurugram, Haryana, India

GC Khilnani
MD FCCP (USA) FAMS FICCM FICP FNCCP FISDA
Professor and Head
Department of Pulmonary Medicine and Sleep Disorders
All India Institute of Medical Sciences, New Delhi, India
Past President, National College of Chest Physicians
Member, Council of International Governors and Regents
American College of Chest Physicians, USA
Member Executive Council, Indian Chest Society
Chairman, Credential Committee
Indian Society of Critical Care Medicine

Jagadeesh KN MBBS
Associate Consultant
Department of Critical Care Medicine
Institute of Critical Care and Anesthesiology
Medanta—The Medicity
Gurugram, Haryana, India

Lakshme Kottu
FICC (DIP EP Australia) PGDC PGPC Harvard Alumni
Senior Resident
Division of Electrophysiology and Pacing
Medanta Heart Institute, Medanta—The Medicity
Gurugram, Haryana, India

Atin Kumar MD
Professor
Department of Radiology
Jai Prakash Narayan Apex Trauma Center (JPNATC)
All India Institute of Medical Sciences, New Delhi, India

Navin Kumar MBBS MD
Consultant and Head
Department of Clinical Microbiology and Infection Control
Manipal Hospitals
Dwarka, New Delhi, India

Rakesh Kumar DA MD
Professor
Department of Anesthesiology
Maulana Azad Medical College, New Delhi
President, Airway Management Foundation
New Delhi, India

Kaushal Madan MBBS MD DNB DM (Gastro) (AIIMS)
Director
Department of Gastroenterology and Hepatology
Max Smart Super Speciality Hospital
Saket, New Delhi, India

Nirad Mehta MD
Consultant Radiologist
PD Hinduja Hospital
Mumbai, Maharashtra, India

Yatin Mehta
MD MNAMS FRCA FAMS FIACTA FICCM FTEE
President
Indian Society of Critical Care Medicine (ISCCM)
Chairman, Medanta Institute of Critical Care and Anesthesiology
Medanta—The Medicity
Gurugram, Haryana, India

Saurabh Mittal MD DM
Assistant Professor
Department of Pulmonary Medicine and Sleep Disorders
All India Institute of Medical Sciences, New Delhi, India

Sheila Nainan Myatra MD FCCM FICCM
Department of Anesthesiology
Critical Care and Pain
Tata Memorial Hospital
Mumbai, Maharashtra, India
President, All India Difficult Airway Association (AIDAA)
Secretary Elect
Indian Society of Critical Care Medicine (ISCCM)
INICC Secretary for India
International Nosocomial Infection Control Consortium (INICC), Argentina (Headquarters)

Prajeesh M Nambiar MBBS MD DNB FIACTA FICCC FIAE
Consultant
Department of Cardiac Anesthesia and Cardiac Critical Care
Baby Memorial Hospital Pvt Ltd
Calicut, Kerala, India

Avinash Nanivadekar
Director Radiology Services
Grant Medical Foundation, Ruby Hall Clinic
Pune, Maharashtra, India

Raja Babu Panwar
MD (Medicine) DNB (Cardiology)
Vice Chancellor
Rajasthan University of Health Sciences
Jaipur, Rajasthan, India

Tripti Pareek MBBS
Resident Trainee Radiology
Grant Medical Foundation
Ruby Hall Clinic
Pune, Maharashtra, India

Deepika Parmar
MD (Medicine) DNB (Gastroenterology)
Attending Consultant
Institute of Digestive and Hepatobiliary Sciences
Medanta—The Medicity
Gurugram, Haryana, India

Jagat Ram MS FAMS
Director and Professor
Department of Ophthalmology
Advanced Eye Centre, Postgraduate Institute of Medical Education and Research
Chandigarh, India

Amrita Ramaswamy
MD (Medicine) DM (Clinical Hematology)
Associate Consultant
Department of Medical and Hemato-Oncology
Cancer Institute, Medanta—The Medicity
Gurugram, Haryana, India

Vinod Ravindran
MD MSc-Rheumatology (King's College, London, UK)
CCT-Rheumatology (UK) MRCP-Rheumatology (UK) FRCP (Edin)
Consultant Rheumatologist
Center for Rheumatology
Calicut, Kerala, India

KD Rawool
Senior Technologist
Department of Radiology
Grant Medical Foundation
Ruby Hall Clinic
Pune, Maharashtra, India

Camilla Rodrigues MD
Consultant
Department of Microbiology
PD Hinduja National Hospital and
Medical Research Centre
Mumbai, Maharashtra, India

Ritesh Sachdev
MD DNB SCYM FRCPath CESR (CCST Equivalence)
Senior Consultant
Department of Histopathology
Division of Laboratory Medicine
Medanta—The Medicity
Gurugram, Haryana, India

Sham Santhanam MD (Medicine) DM (Rheumatology)
Consultant Rheumatologist
Gleneagles Global Hospitals
Chennai, Tamil Nadu, India

Harsh Sapra MBBS DA Fellowship Neuro Anesthesia (UK)
Director
Department of Neuroanesthesia
Medanta Institute of Critical Care and Anesthesiology
Medanta—The Medicity
Gurugram, Haryana, India

Ashok Seth FRCP FACC FESC MSCAI DSc D Litt
Chairman
Fortis Escorts Heart Institute
New Delhi, India
Chairman, Cardiology Council
Fortis Group of Hospitals

Anand Shah MD
Department of Microbiology
PD Hinduja National Hospital and
Medical Research Centre
Mumbai, Maharashtra, India

Jeetendra Sharma MD FICCM
Director and Head
Department of Critical Care
Artemis Hospitals
Gurugram, Haryana, India

Nivedita Shirol
Resident Trainee Radiology
Grant Medical Foundation
Ruby Hall Clinic
Pune, Maharashtra, India

MR Shivaprakash MD (Microbiology)
Professor
Department of Medical Microbiology
Postgraduate Institute of Medical Education and Research
Chandigarh, India

Balbir Singh
MBBS MD (General Medicine) DM (Cardiology) FACC
Chairman
Division of Electrophysiology and Pacing
Medanta Heart Institute, Medanta—The Medicity
Gurugram, Haryana, India

BP Singh MBBS MD (Med) DNB (Gastro)
Senior Consultant
Department of Gastroenterology and Hepatology
Max Smart Super Speciality Hospital
Saket, New Delhi, India

Kapil Dev Soni MD
Associate Professor
Department of Critical and Intensive Care
Jai Prakash Narayan Apex Trauma Center (JPNATC)
All India Institute of Medical Sciences, New Delhi, India

Nitin Sood
MBBS MD (General Medicine) DNB (General Medicine) MRCP (UK)
MRCPath (Associate Hematology) FRC (Pathology)
CCT (Hemato-Oncology)
Associate Director
Department of Medical and Hemato-Oncology
Cancer Institute, Medanta—The Medicity
Gurugram, Haryana, India

Randhir Sud
MD (Medicine) DM (Gastroenterology)
Chairman
Institute of Digestive and Hepatobiliary Sciences
Medanta—The Medicity, Gurugram, Haryana, India
Awarded Padma Shri by the President of India
Past President, Society of Gastrointestinal Endoscopy of India (SGEI)

KK Talwar
MBBS MD (Medicine) DM (Cardiology) DSc (Hon CAUSA) FAMS FNA FACC
Chairman
Department of Cardiology
Max Healthcare
Max Super Speciality Hospital
Saket, New Delhi, India

Pawan Tiwari MD DM
Assistant Professor
Department of Pulmonary Medicine and Sleep Disorders
All India Institute of Medical Sciences
New Delhi, India

Manish Vinayak MD DM DNB (Cardiology)
Fellow, Interventional Cardiology
Fortis Escorts Heart Institute, New Delhi, India

Sonam Yangzes MS
Senior Resident
Advanced Eye Center, Postgraduate Institute of Medical Education and Research, Chandigarh, India
Stanley M Truhlsen Eye Institute
University of Nebraska Medical Center, USA
Ocular Imaging Research and Reading Center (OIRRC)
Menlo Park, CA, USA

Kapil Zirpe MD FICCM
Director and Head, Department of Neurocritical Care
Grant Medical Foundation, Ruby Hall Clinic
Pune, Maharashtra, India

Foreword

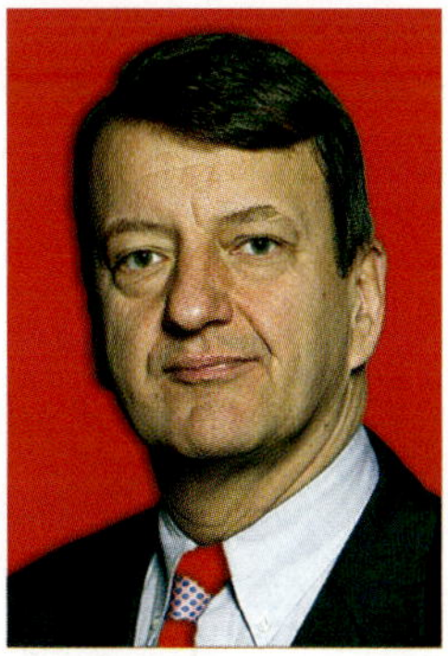

I am honored to have been invited to write the foreword for this *Atlas of Critical Care*, a collection of 26 chapters with 1000 images, the brainchild of Yatin Mehta, President of the Indian Society of Critical Care Medicine.

In today's visual world, images are an increasingly important means of presenting information. Words, however well-written, are limited in their ability to provide accurate descriptions of many of the complex pathways involved in critical care medicine and the interventions employed on our intensive care units. Well-drawn visuals or photographs can provide the reader with a much clearer picture. Indeed, reading long sections of text can be a slow, time-consuming and rather discouraging activity, making it difficult to keep up with the latest data and techniques. Providing the same information in visual form, with short sections of helpful explanatory text where necessary, offers the reader a much more efficient, and pleasurable, learning process.

The *Atlas of Critical Care* meets this need for visual input, providing intensivists and others involved in the management of critically ill patients with some of the latest concepts in a range of important topics, all supported by abundant photos and illustrations.

Yatin Mehta has done much to promote the growth of intensive care medicine in India and is to be congratulated on this new and innovative addition to the current literature in this field.

Jean-Louis Vincent MD PhD
Professor
Department of Intensive Care Medicine
Université Libre de Bruxelles
Consultant
Department of Intensive Care
Erasme University Hospital, Brussels, Belgium
Ex-President
World Federation of Societies of Intensive and
Critical Care Medicine (WFSICCM)

Foreword

It is a pleasure to write the foreword for *Atlas of Critical Care* by Yatin Mehta. As surgeons, we are used to seeing Atlases, but for critical care specialists and students, it is a novel idea.

Visual images always leave a long impression on the mind and their recollection is better. The book has 26 chapters with 1000 images. This is the 3rd book by Yatin Mehta and I am sure that he and his team has done a good job. With critical care services increasing exponentially in India and the atmosphere against high end medicine in public and political circles, this book will certainly help in educating critical care and other specialty doctors regarding this vast and expanding field. I recommend this book to every practicing and aspiring intensivist and to medical libraries.

Naresh Trehan
Chairman, Medanta Heart Institute
MD, Medanta—The Medicity
Gurugram, Haryana, India

Foreword

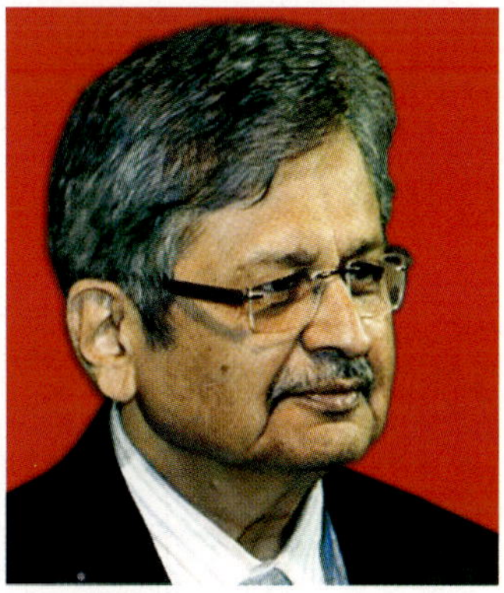

Critical Care Medicine is a very demanding specialty. It is also rapidly developing and evolving. It is an extremely dynamic field of medicine with a very hectic pace. The rapid pace is required not just in the responses of the treating team, but also in the overall outlook of its practitioners to scientific advances in the field. These advances occur continuously as the field of critical care medicine has a huge overlap with other branches of medicine. It is a multiorgan specialty dealing with complex pathophysiological alterations of all the systems. Additionally, the modalities of management include machinery for monitoring, diagnostics and therapeutics. All these factors contribute to make this specialty a very tough one to keep abreast continuously. Thus, practitioners and students of this specialty need to have dynamic tools to keep pace with the expanding volume of available literature in the limited amount of time available. This also makes a case for the modern day methodologies for learning to be very strong and active.

Traditionally, the compilation of the training material was collected in textbooks and the textbooks consisted of chapters of written words. With the decline of attention spans of readers and the available time, the need for pictorial assistance has increased. It is this void in the field of critical care medicine, which has been beautifully filled by this new addition to the increasing number of books. One must compliment Yatin Mehta, the Chief Editor of *Atlas for Critical Care* for the brilliant conceptualization and execution. That this book is finally seeing the light of day in its magnificent content of 26 chapters and 1000 images is a truly remarkable achievement. Despite an exceedingly busy professional life, Yatin Mehta has had time to give us previously two of the important books in critical care. This, his third contribution, is an important landmark in the field of critical care. It is a visual treat and its contents are extremely enriching.

I am very pleased to compliment Yatin Mehta for this enormous contribution to the field of critical care. I am sure that the readers will find this a great treat to watch and read.

Shirish Prayag
MD FCCM
Senior Consultant
Department of Critical Care
Prayag Hospital
Pune, Maharashtra, India

Preface

Critical care is a vast field of medicine with ever expanding horizons involving all medical specialties. In India, the growth of this superspecialty has been exponential in the last couple of decades. Training and education in this field also has become easily available through the Indian Society of Critical Care Medicine (ISCCM), National Board of Examination (NBE) and a few universities having DM in it. With the growth of corporate tertiary care hospitals, the latest technology is also there with us so that our practicing intensivists and aspiring ones are not lacking in expertise, knowledge and skills essential in a modern intensive care unit (ICU).

Since time immemorial, visual impressions are better retained, reproduced and stored in the human mind than written words. This thought led us to conceive this Atlas. Although Atlases are known to surgical and interventional fields, they are nonexistent in critical care medicine. With so many patients with different diseases getting admitted to ICU's undergoing many varied procedures, *Atlas of Critical Care* may be a great addition to the intensivists source of knowledge ultimately resulting in better outcomes.

Yatin Mehta
Jeetendra Sharma

Acknowledgments

Firstly, I would like to thank Jeetendra Sharma, my co-editor, without whose help this endeavor was not possible. I am also grateful to Drs Naresh Trehan, Shirish Prayag and Jean-Louis Vincent not only for writing the Forewords, but also for their constant support and encouragement. This book was not possible without the enthusiasm and help of the Shri Jitendar P Vij (Group Chairman), Mr Ankit Vij (Managing Director), Ms Chetna Malhotra Vohra (Associate Director—Content Strategy) of M/s Jaypee Brothers Medical Publishers (P) Ltd, New Delhi, India and their team. I am thankful to Dr Mukesh Kumar Gupta, Senior Consultant for his help. I am also thankful to Ms Poonam Anand for her assistance. Last but not least the time that I spent on this was stolen from my family time, so I am grateful to my family, particularly my wife for letting me be!

Contents

SECTION 1: AIRWAY MANAGEMENT

1. **Airway Assessment** 3
Shilpushp J Bhosale, Sheila Nainan Myatra
2. **Airway Devices in ICU** 20
Rakesh Kumar

SECTION 2: RESPIRATORY SYSTEM

3. **Bronchoscopic View and Clinical Features** 61
GC Khilnani, Pawan Tiwari, Saurabh Mittal
4. **Respiratory Issues in ICU** 75
Poulomi Chatterjee, Yatin Mehta

SECTION 3: CARDIOLOGY

5. **Echocardiography** 103
RR Kasliwal, Hardeep Kaur Grewal, Mansi Kaushik
6. **Cardiovascular Intervention: Equipment and Procedures** 143
Ashok Seth, Manish Vinayak
7. **Electrocardiography: Heart Blocks** 154
Balbir Singh, Lakshme Kottu
8. **Electrocardiography: Arrhythmias** 165
KK Talwar
9. **Interesting Pictures in Cardiac ICU** 183
Raja Babu Panwar, Dinesh Choudhary
10. **Transesophageal Echocardiography and Aortic Aneurysm** 218
Dheeraj Arora, Jeetendra Sharma, Mukesh K Gupta, Yatin Mehta

SECTION 4: GASTROENTEROLOGY

11. **Endoscopic Images** 239
Randhir Sud, Deepika Parmar
12. **Endoscopic and Radiological Images** 274
BP Singh, Kaushal Madan

SECTION 5: NEUROLOGY

13. **Neuroimaging**......283
Kapil Zirpe, Avinash Nanivadekar, Nivedita Shirol, Tripti Pareek, KD Rawool, Dhananjay Jadhav

14. **Neuromonitoring and Neuroimaging**......335
Harsh Sapra, Gaurav Kakkar

SECTION 6: TRAUMA

15. **Trauma Cases in ICU**......383
Kapil Dev Soni, Atin Kumar, Amit Gupta

SECTION 7: MICROBIOLOGY

16. **Infection and Microbiology**......403
Anand Shah, Camilla Rodrigues

17. **Fungal Infections in Critical Care**......421
Arunaloke Chakrabarti, MR Shivaprakash, Ashim Das

18. **Equipment in Microbiology**......444
Navin Kumar

SECTION 8: MISCELLANEOUS

19. **Nephrology**......455
Manju Aggarwal, Vijay Joshi

20. **Ocular Emergencies: Illustration and Management**......476
Sonam Yangzes, Aniruddha Agarwal, Jagat Ram

21. **Rheumatology**......491
Sham Santhanam, Vinod Ravindran, Indrajit Agarwal

22. **Hemodynamic Monitoring and Equipment in Cardiac ICU**......506
Prajeesh M Nambiar, Yatin Mehta

23. **Hematology**......526
Rahul Bhargava, Amrita Ramaswamy, Nitin Sood, Shalini Goel, Ritesh Sachdev

24. **Lung Ultrasound in ICU**......542
Deepak Govil, Jagadeesh KN, Rahul Harne

25. **Interesting Images in ICU**......557
Jeetendra Sharma, Mukesh K Gupta

26. **Radiology Images in ICU**......585
Nirad Mehta, Jalpa Bhandari, Isha Atre

Index......*631*

SECTION 1

Airway Management

CHAPTER

1

Airway Assessment

Shilpushp J Bhosale, Sheila Nainan Myatra

AIRWAY EVALUATION (FIGS. 1A TO C)

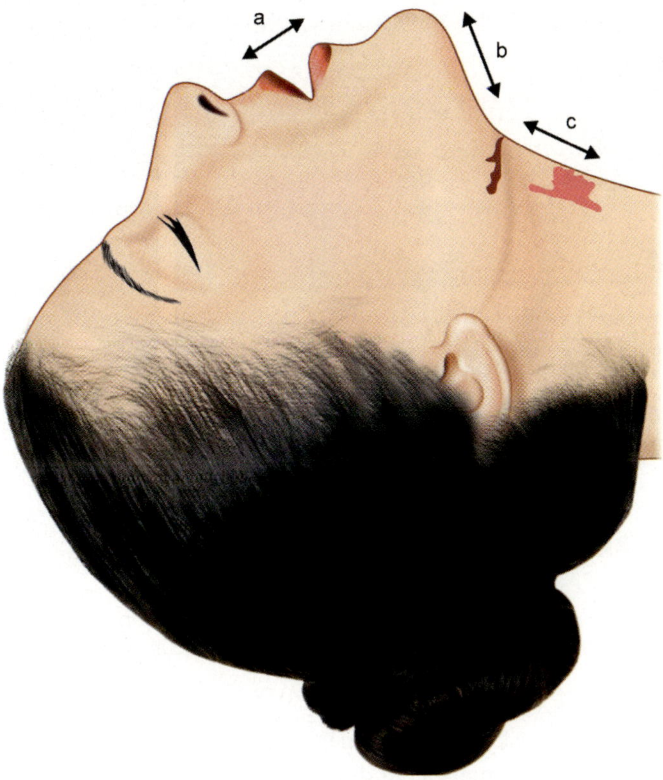

Fig. 1A: (a) Mouth opening three fingers, (b) Mentohyoid three fingers, (c) Thyrohyoid two fingers.

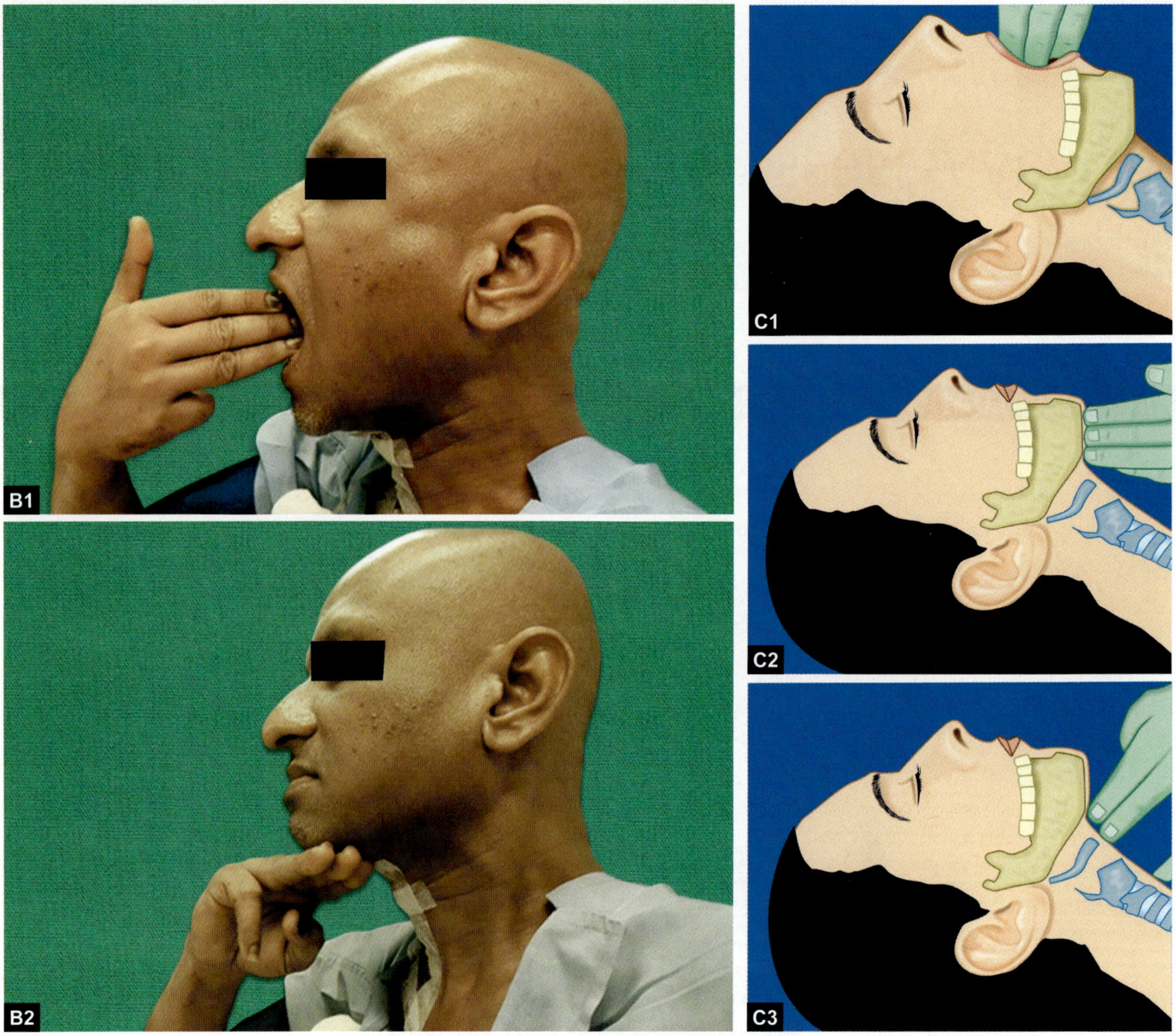

Figs. 1B and C

Figs. 1A to C: 3-3-2 rule for predicting difficult airway.

- Tracheal intubation is one of the most risky procedure in intensive care unit (ICU). Hypoxia, hypotension and cardiac arrest are life endangering complications may occur during endotracheal intubation.
- In nonemergent situation, one can assess airway to predict difficult laryngoscopy and endotracheal intubation by 3-3-2 rule.
- The 3-3-2 rule helps to estimate whether the anatomy of the neck will allow for appropriate opening of the throat and larynx. It serves to roughly estimate if the alignment of the openings for direct visualization of the larynx would be possible with given anatomical findings.
- 3-3-2 rule; first 3—three-finger distance between the upper and lower teeth of the open mouth of a patient indicates the ease of access to the airway through the mouth opening; second 3—three-finger distance anterior tip of the mandible to hyoid bone at the anterior part of the neck provides an estimate of the volume of the submandibular space; third 2—two-finger distance between hyoid to the thyroid notch on the anterior neck identifies the location of the larynx relative to the base of the tongue.

ANATOMY OF THE GLOTTIS AND ENDOTRACHEAL INTUBATION BY DIRECT LARYNGOSCOPY (FIGS. 2A AND B)

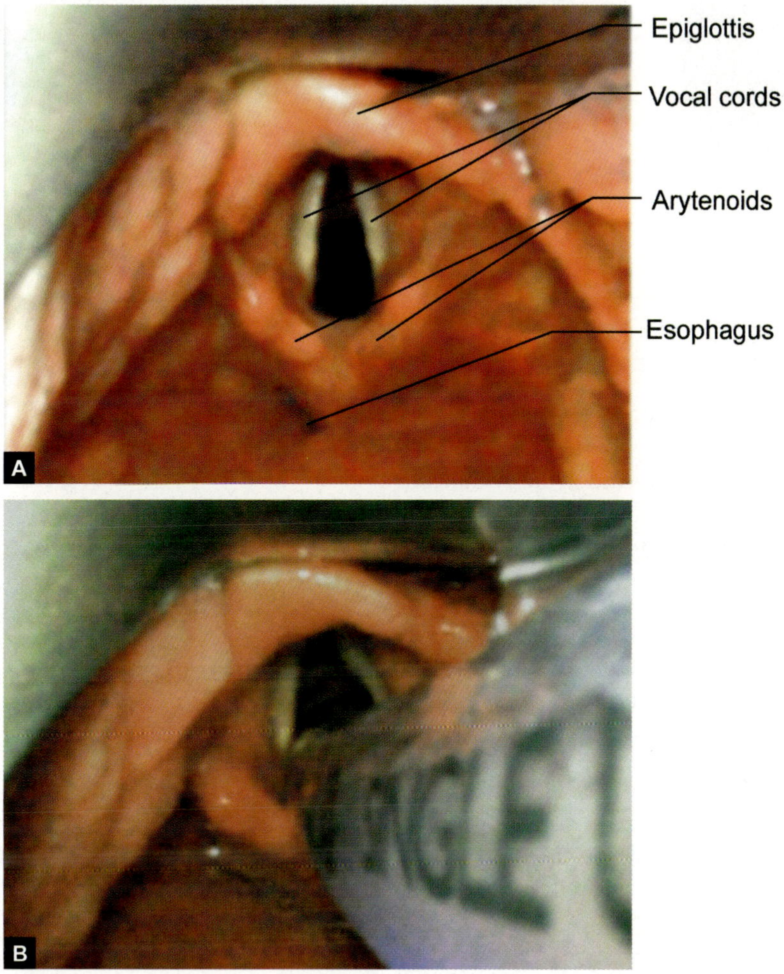

Figs. 2A and B: (A) Before insertion of endotracheal tube; (B) Endotracheal tube being inserted.

- By orotracheal intubation, endotracheal tube passes through vocal cord and stay there for a prolonged period that may results into few complications.
- Throat pain is common complication may be due to focal ischemia, laryngeal mucosal injury or edema.
- Other complications are vocal cord tear, vocal cord paralysis, vocal cord granulation, vocal cord ulcers, and laryngeal stenosis.

AIRWAY ASSESSMENT FOR INTUBATION USING MALLAMPATI SCORE (FIG. 3)

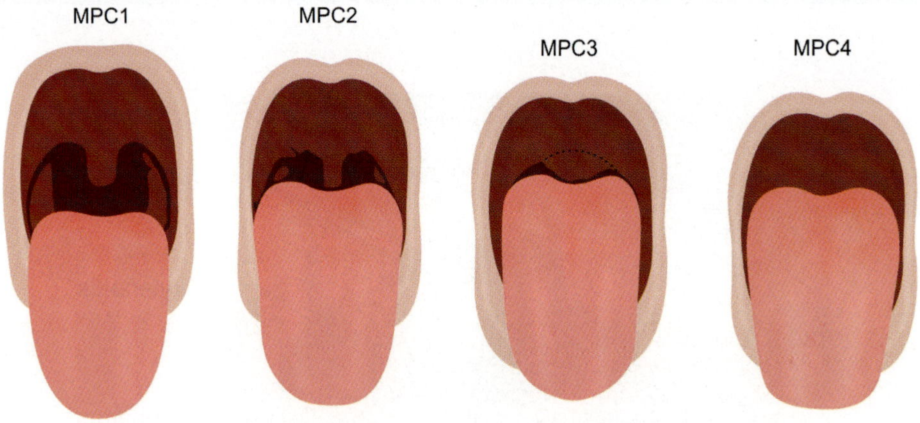

Fig. 3: Modified Mallampati score.

Mallampati Score

- *Class 1*: Faucial pillars, soft palate and uvula visualized.
- *Class 2*: Faucial pillars and soft palate visualized, but uvula masked by the base of the tongue.
- *Class 3*: Only soft palate visualized.

Modified Mallampati Score

- *Class 1*: Soft palate, uvula, fauces, pillars visible—easy predicted intubated.
- *Class 2:* Soft palate, uvula, fauces visible.
- *Class 3:* Soft palate, base of uvula visible.
- *Class 4*: Only hard palate visible—difficult predicted intubation.

PROPER PATIENT POSITIONING FOR INTUBATION (SNIFFING POSITION) (FIG. 4)

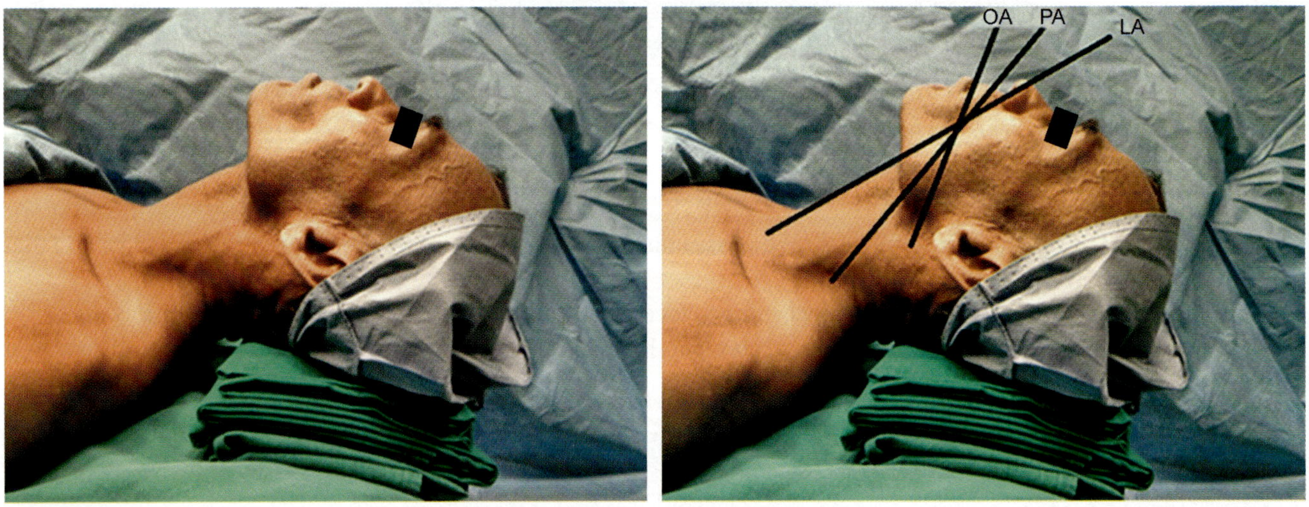

Fig. 4: Position for intubation (sniffing position).

- *Sniffing position*: Flexion at the neck (by placing a pillow/towels below the occiput) and extension *of the head on the atlanto-occipital joint to align the oral axis (OA), the pharyngeal axis (PA) and the laryngeal axis (LA).*

AIRWAY ANATOMY (FIG. 5)

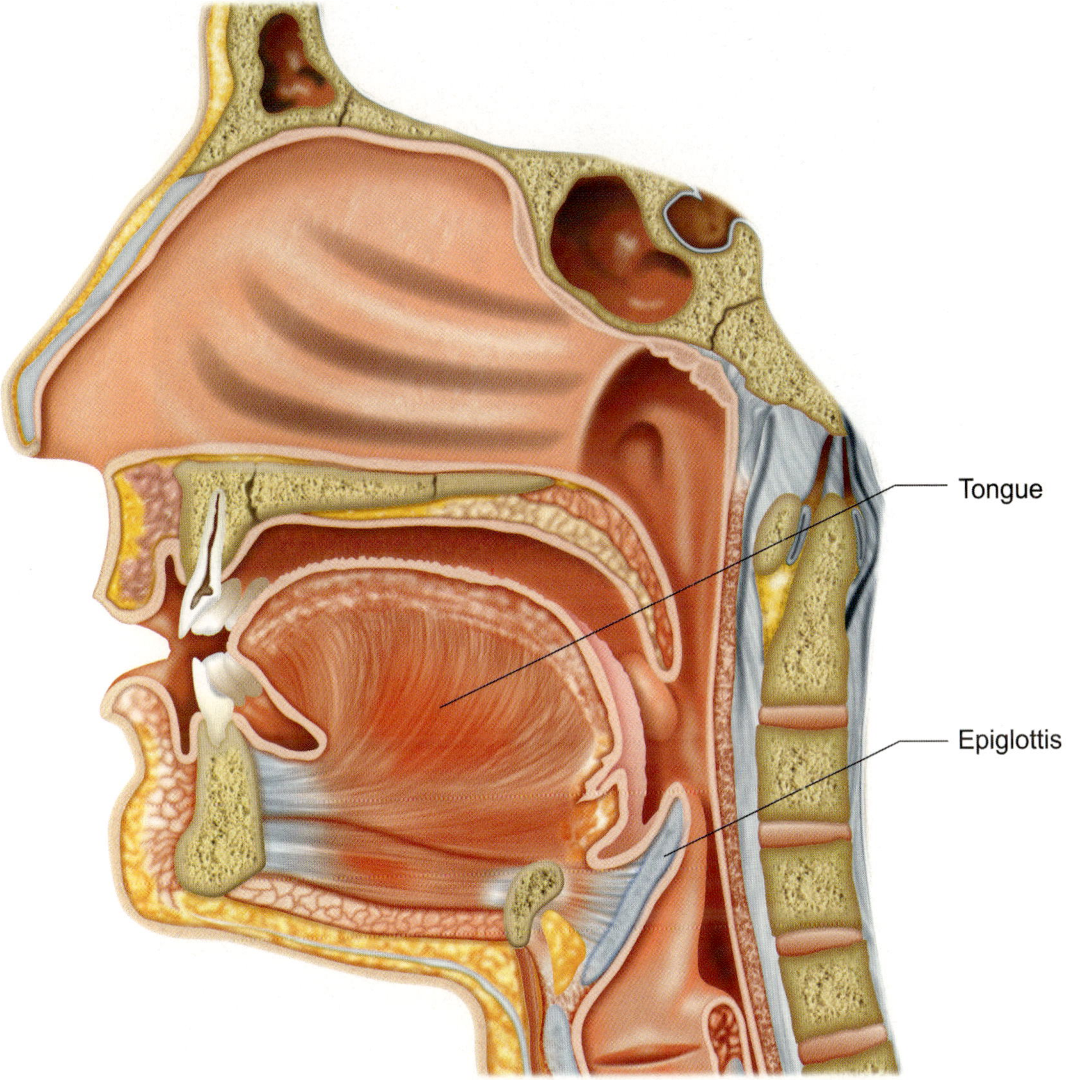

Fig. 5: Sagittal sedation.

RESTRICTED MOUTH OPENING (TRISMUS)—DIFFICULT AIRWAY (FIGS. 6A AND B)

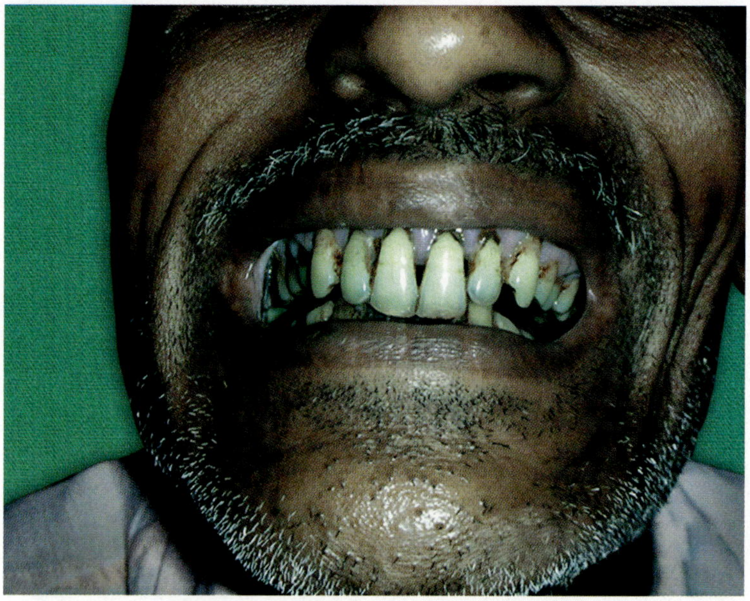

Fig. 6A: Total trismus (no mouth opening).

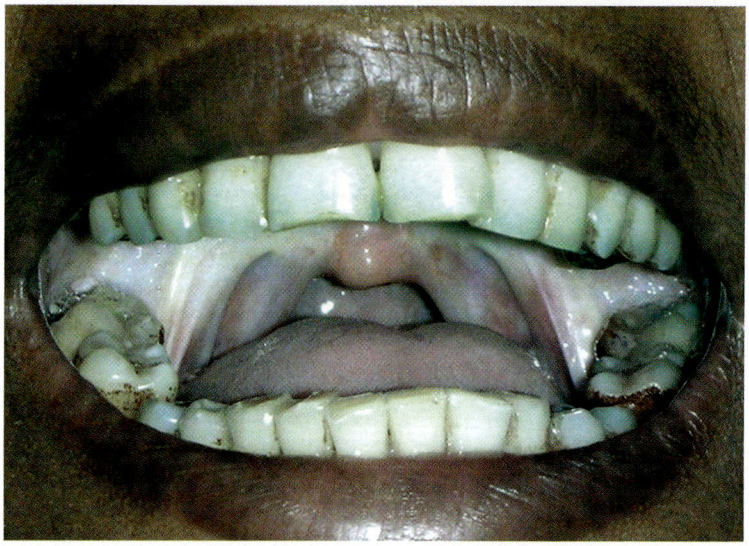

Fig. 6B: Trismus due to intraoral fibrous bands.

- *Common issues*: Tobacco, betel chewing.
- Oral intubation difficult, if required nasal fiberoptic intubation.

MICROGNATHIA (FIGS. 7A AND B)

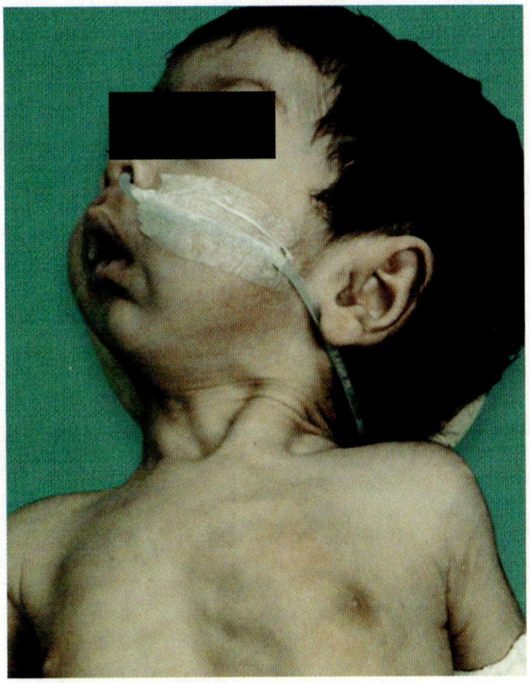

Fig. 7A: Frontal view.

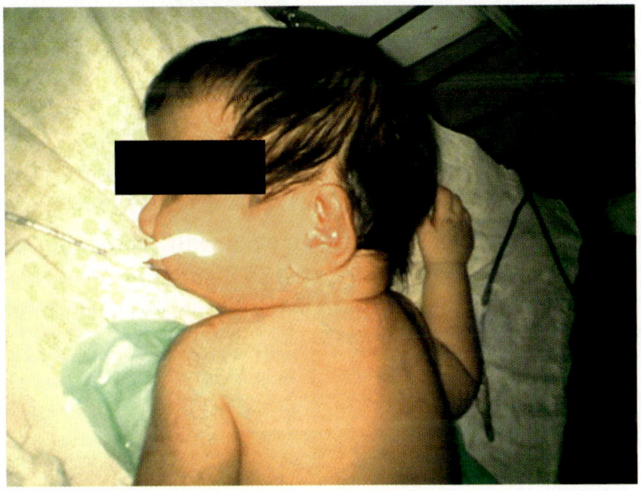

Fig. 7B: Lateral view.

- Child with micrognathia (also called mandibular hypoplasia) showing an undersized jaw.

ANTERIOR EXTRA-THORACIC NECK MASS—DIFFICULT AIRWAY (FIGS. 8A AND B)

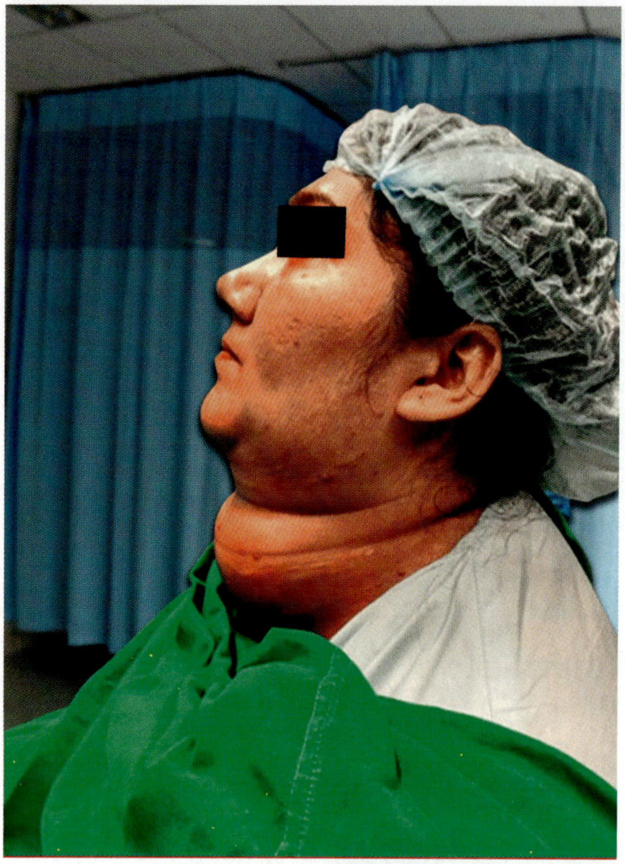

Fig. 8A: Lateral view.

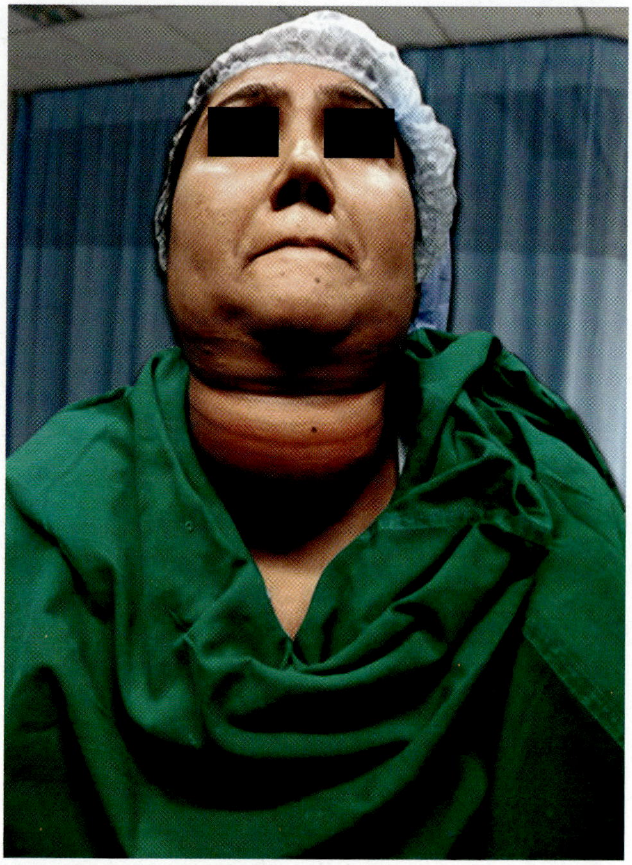

Fig. 8B: Frontal view.

- Large thyroid swelling can lead to complete failure of endotracheal intubation.
- Administration sedation in these patients results into loss of neck muscle tone, and after that due to gravity these tumor masses compress the airway. Ventilation by mask or even with supraglottic devices may not be possible that may lead to disastrous "cannot intubate cannot ventilate (CICV)" situation.
- Awake fiberoptic intubation using loco-sedative technique is advisable in such situation.

ANKYLOSING SPONDYLITIS—DIFFICULT AIRWAY (FIGS. 9A TO D)

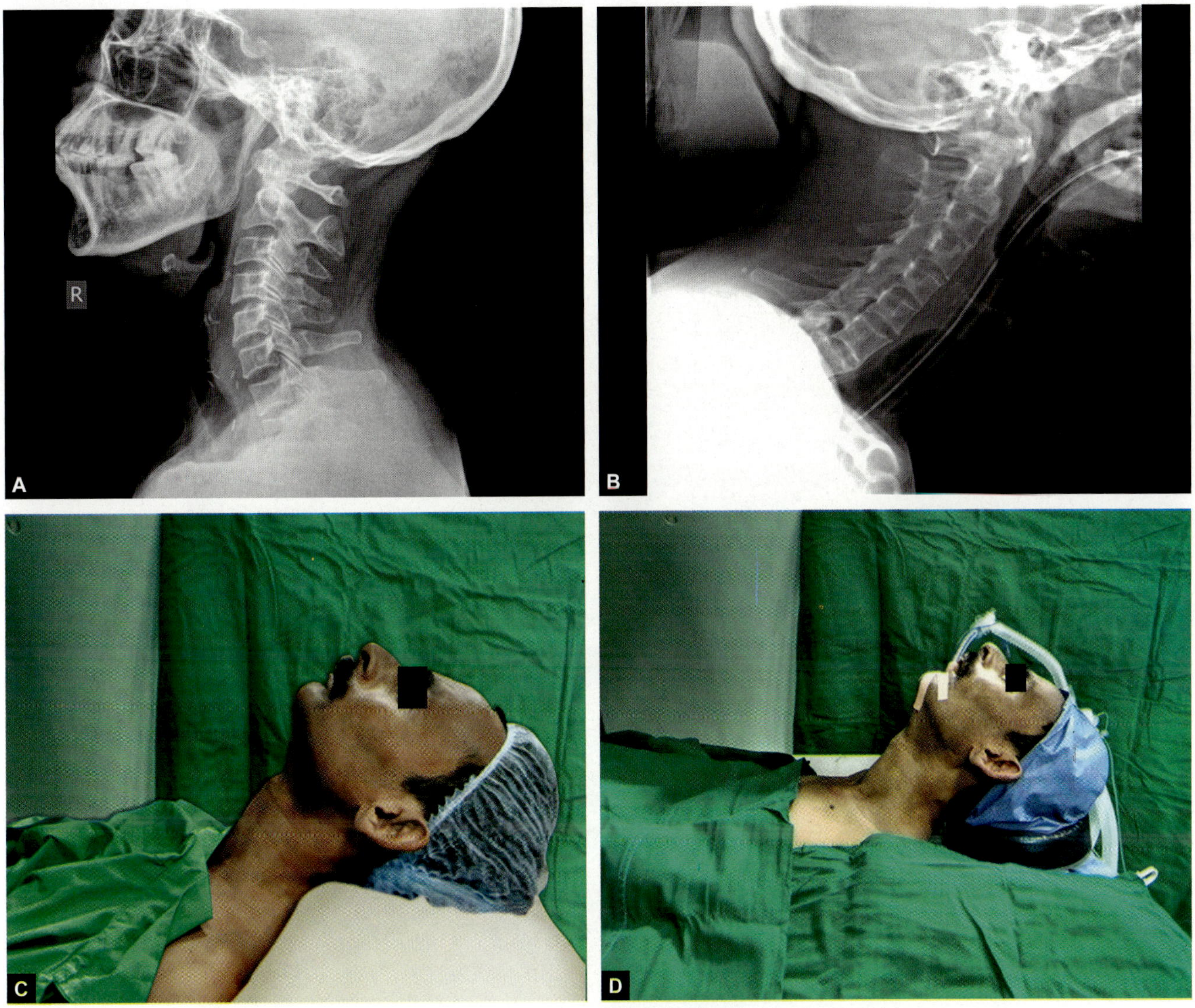

Figs. 9A to D: (A and C) Before intubation; (B and D) After intubation.

- Ankylosing spondylitis is an inflammatory disease, which over time can cause the vertebrae in the spine to fuse (bamboo spine) that results into stiff spine. This fusing makes the spine less flexible and can result in a hunched-forward posture.
- Stiff neck and lack of movements at neck make oral intubation challenging. Awake intubation with fiberoptic bronchoscopy is safe in nonemergent situation. However, in emergency airway, expert is required with cart sometime require surgical access of airway by tracheostomy or cricothyrotomy.

SHORT NECK—DIFFICULT AIRWAY (FIGS. 10A AND B)

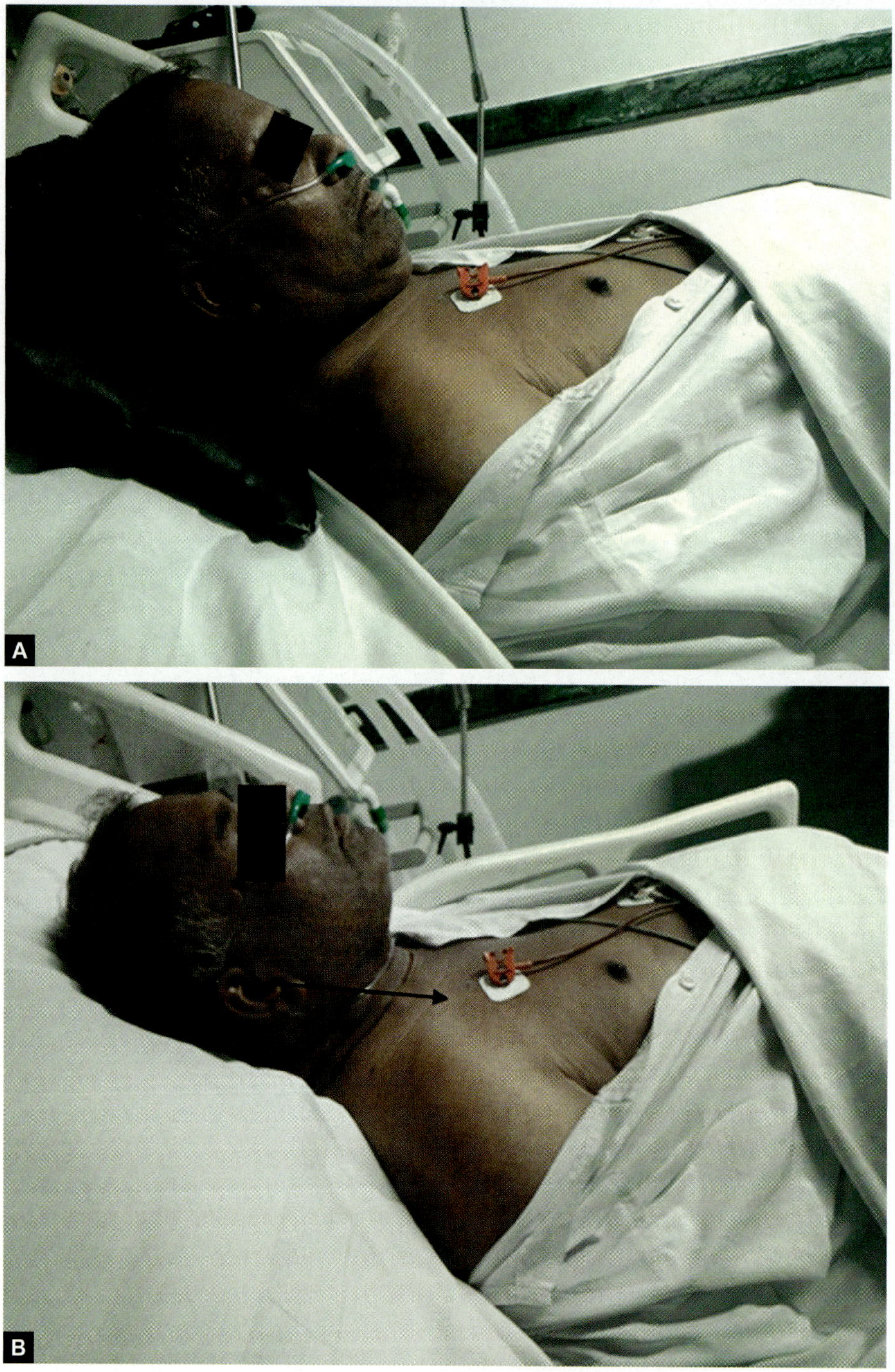

Figs. 10A and B: (A) Short neck; (B) Appropriate position for intubation where tragus aligned to manubrium sterni (showed as black arrow).

MORBIDLY OBESE PATIENT—DIFFICULT AIRWAY (FIG. 11)

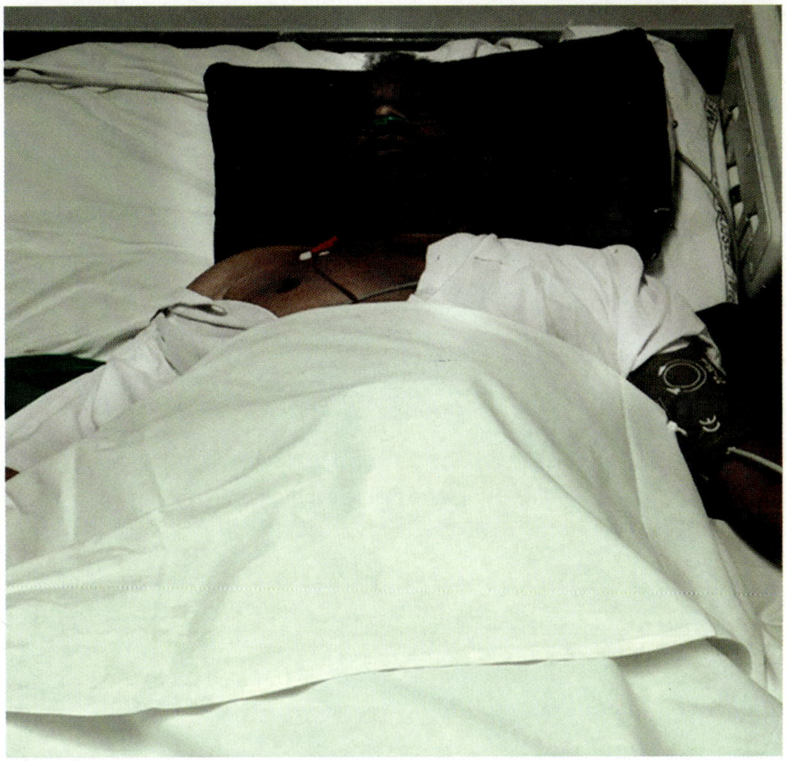

Fig. 11: Morbidly obese patient.

PIERRE ROBIN SYNDROME (FIG. 12)

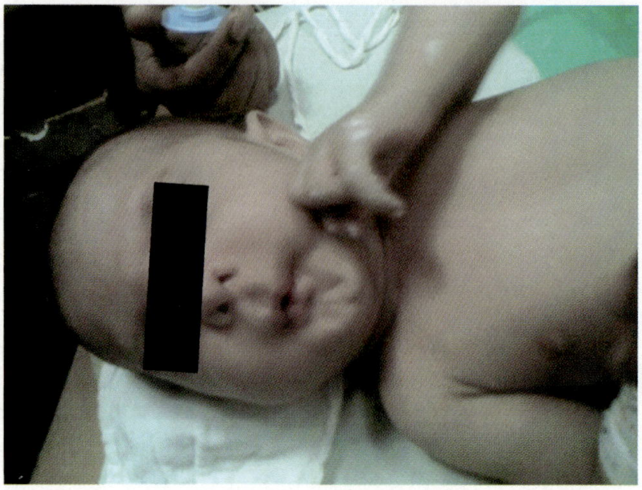

Fig. 12: Pierre Robin syndrome.

- Cleft palate.
- Retrognathia.
- Glossoptosis.

TREACHER COLLINS SYNDROME (FIG. 13)

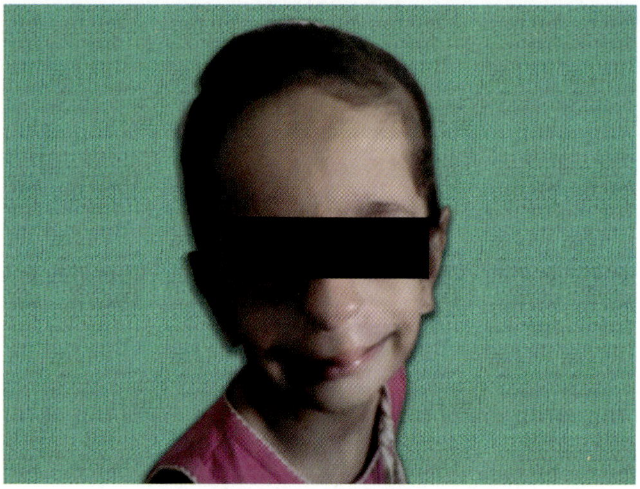

Fig. 13: Treacher Collins syndrome.

- Cleft palate.
- Micrognathia.

RETROGNATHIA (FIG. 14)

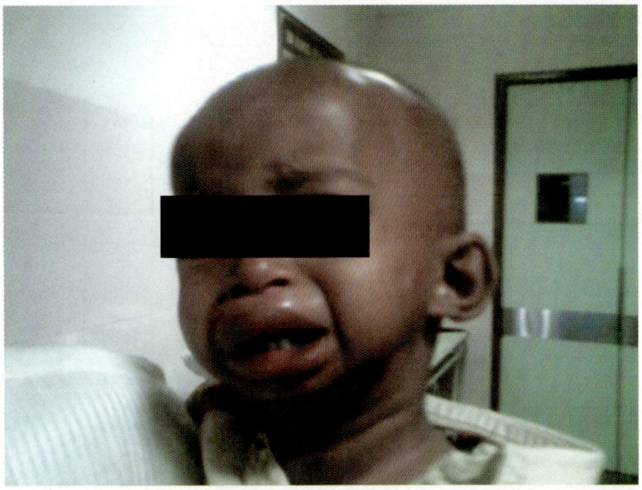

Fig. 14: Retrognathia.

CRANIOSYNOSTOSIS (FIG. 15)

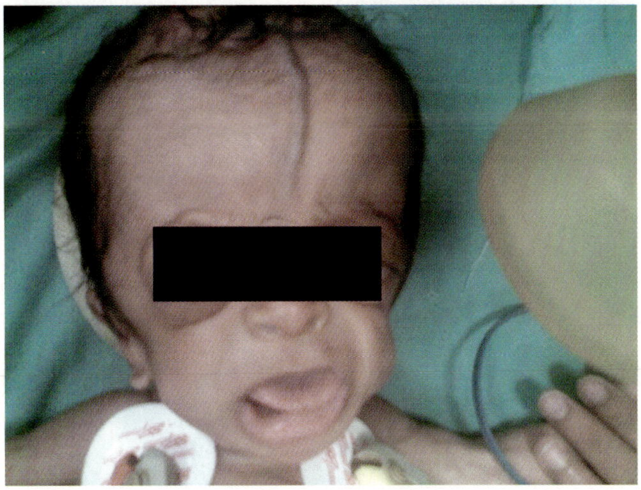

Fig. 15: Craniosynostosis.

CLEFT LIP/PALATE (FIG. 16)

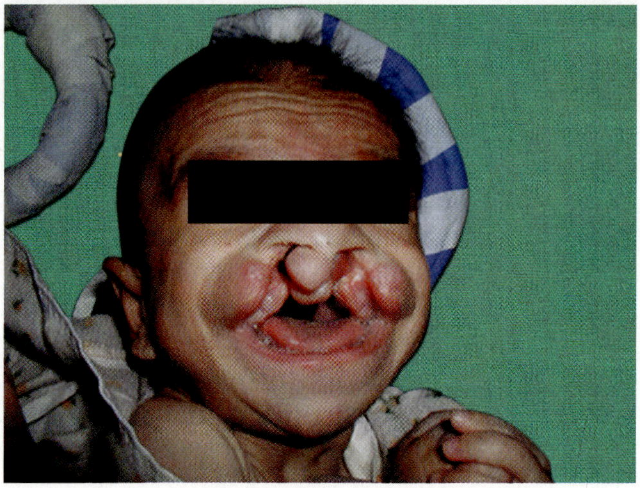

Fig. 16: Cleft lip/Palate.

CERVICAL MENINGOMYELOCELE (FIG. 17)

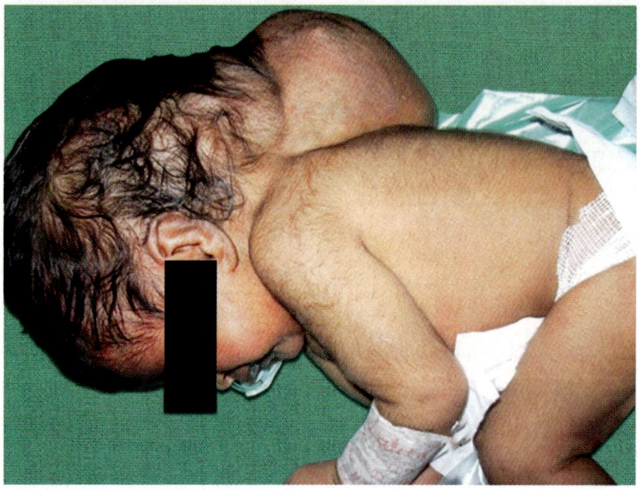

Fig. 17: Cervical meningomyelocele.

X-RAY NECK (ANTEROPOSTERIOR AND LATERAL VIEW) (FIGS. 18A AND B)

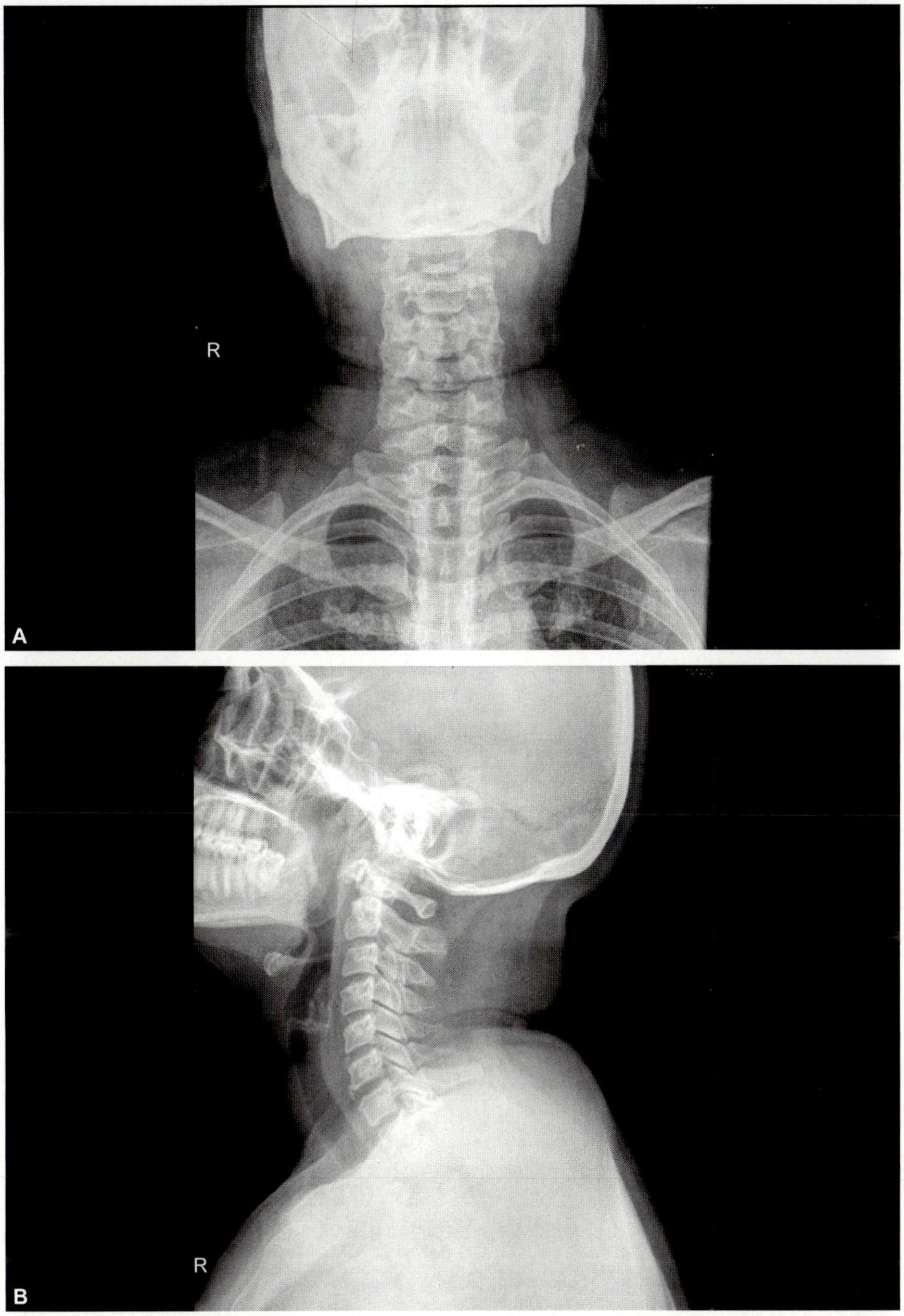

Figs. 18A and B: X-ray neck (anteroposterior and lateral view).

CHEST X-RAY—POSITION OF ENDOTRACHEAL TUBE (CORRECT AND MALPOSITIONED) (FIGS. 19A AND B)

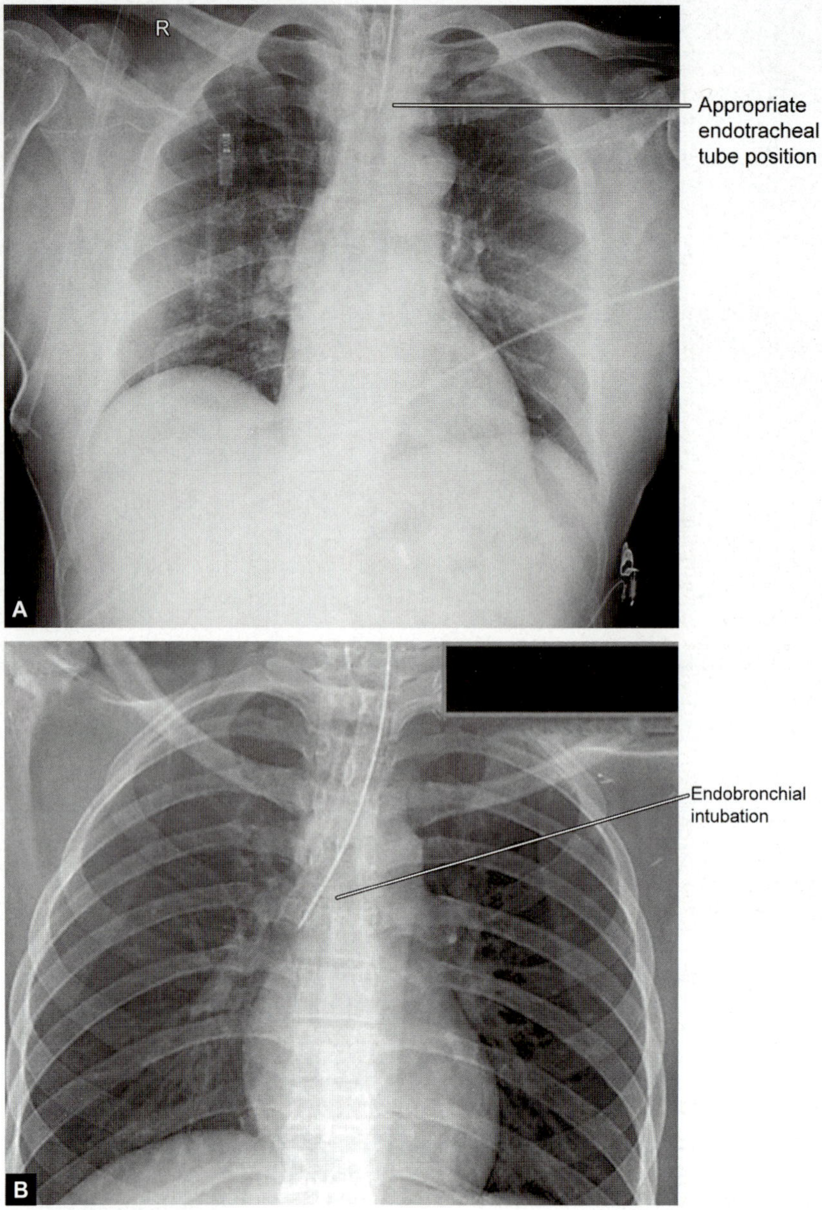

Figs. 19A and B: Chest X-ray—position of endotracheal tube (correct and malpositioned).

- Acceptable position of tip of endotracheal tube (ETT) is about 5–7 cm from carina, but it markedly varies with neck position and rotation and hence, the inclusion of the mandible is a helpful indicator.
- In neutral position—the lower border of the mandible should be projected over C5/C6; and tip of ETT 5 cm (± 2 cm) above carina.
- In flexed position—the lower border of the mandible should be projected around T1; and tip of ETT 3 cm (± 2 cm) above carina.
- In extended position—the lower border of the mandible should be projected over C3/C4; and tip of ETT 7 cm (± 2 cm) above carina.

CT SCAN OF THE THORAX SHOWING ENDOTRACHEAL TUBE IN CORRECT POSITION (FIG. 20)

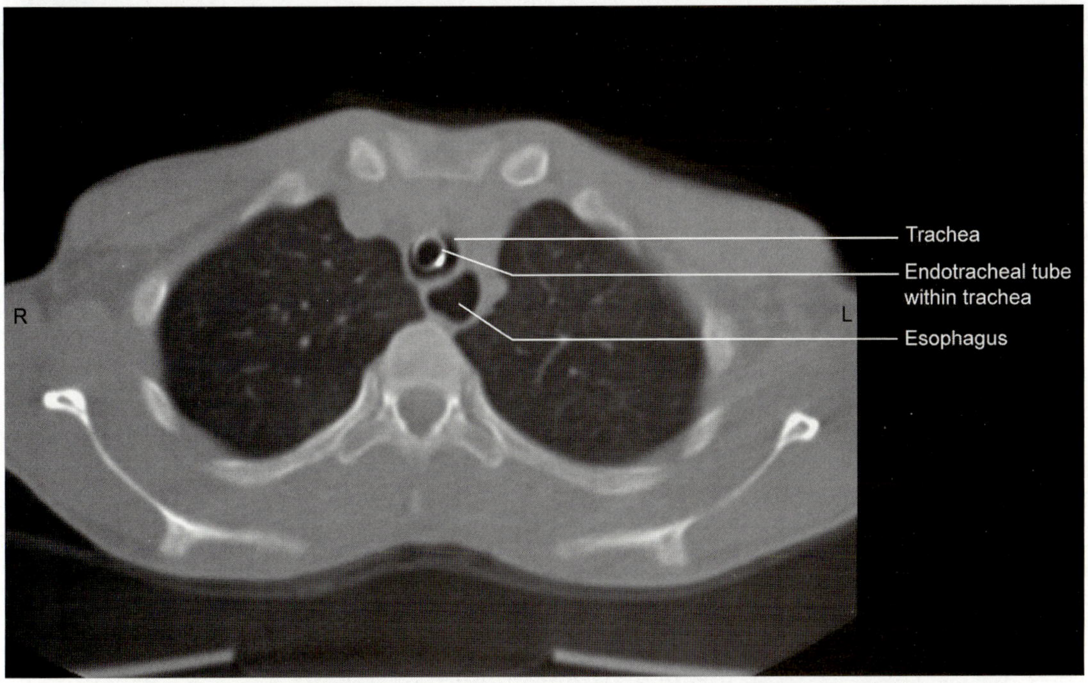

Fig. 20: Endotracheal tube is visible in the trachea.

CT SCAN OF THE CHEST SHOWING ENDOTRACHEAL TUBE MALPOSITIONED (FIG. 21)

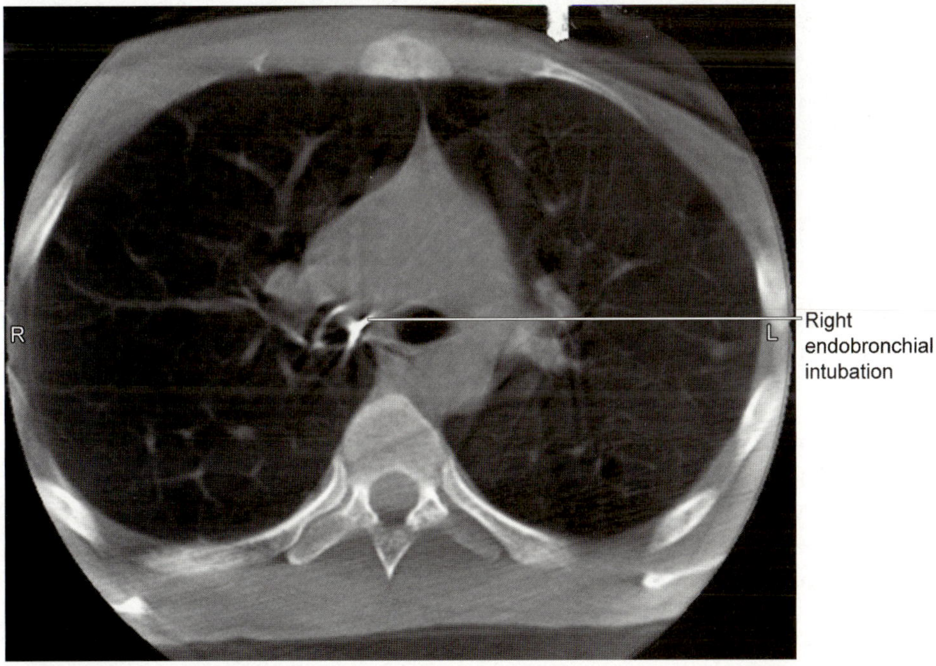

Fig. 21: CT scan of the chest showing endotracheal tube (ETT) malpositioned.

CHAPTER 2

Airway Devices in ICU

Rakesh Kumar

BAG AND MASK (FIG. 1)

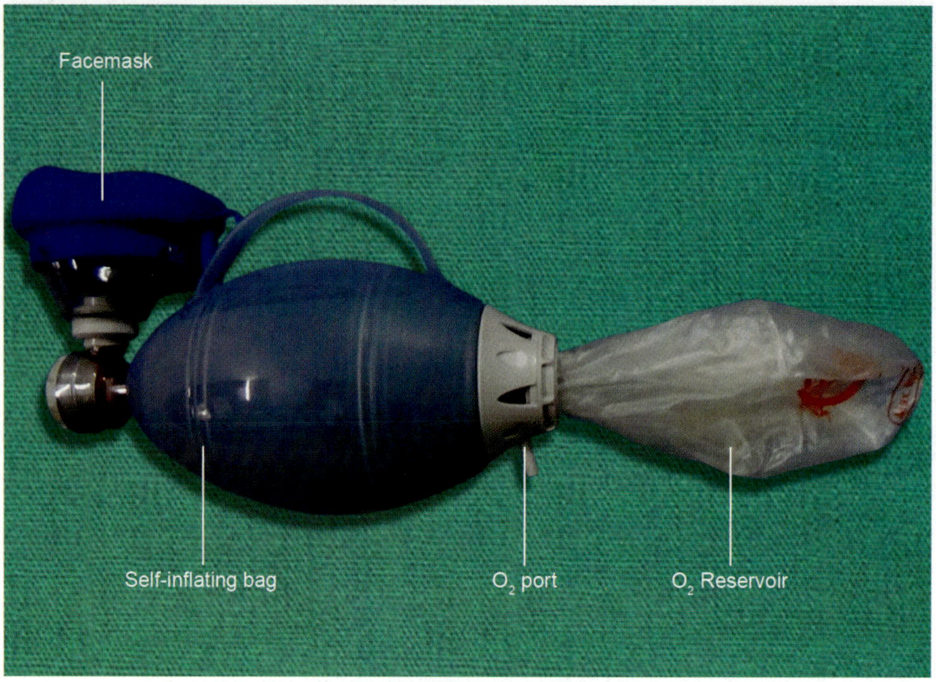

Fig. 1: Ambu bag mask.

- Mask ventilation is commonly carried out in an intensive care unit (ICU) while awaiting intubation or supraglottic airway device (SAD) insertion.

OROPHARYNGEAL AIRWAY (OPA) (FIGS. 2A AND B)

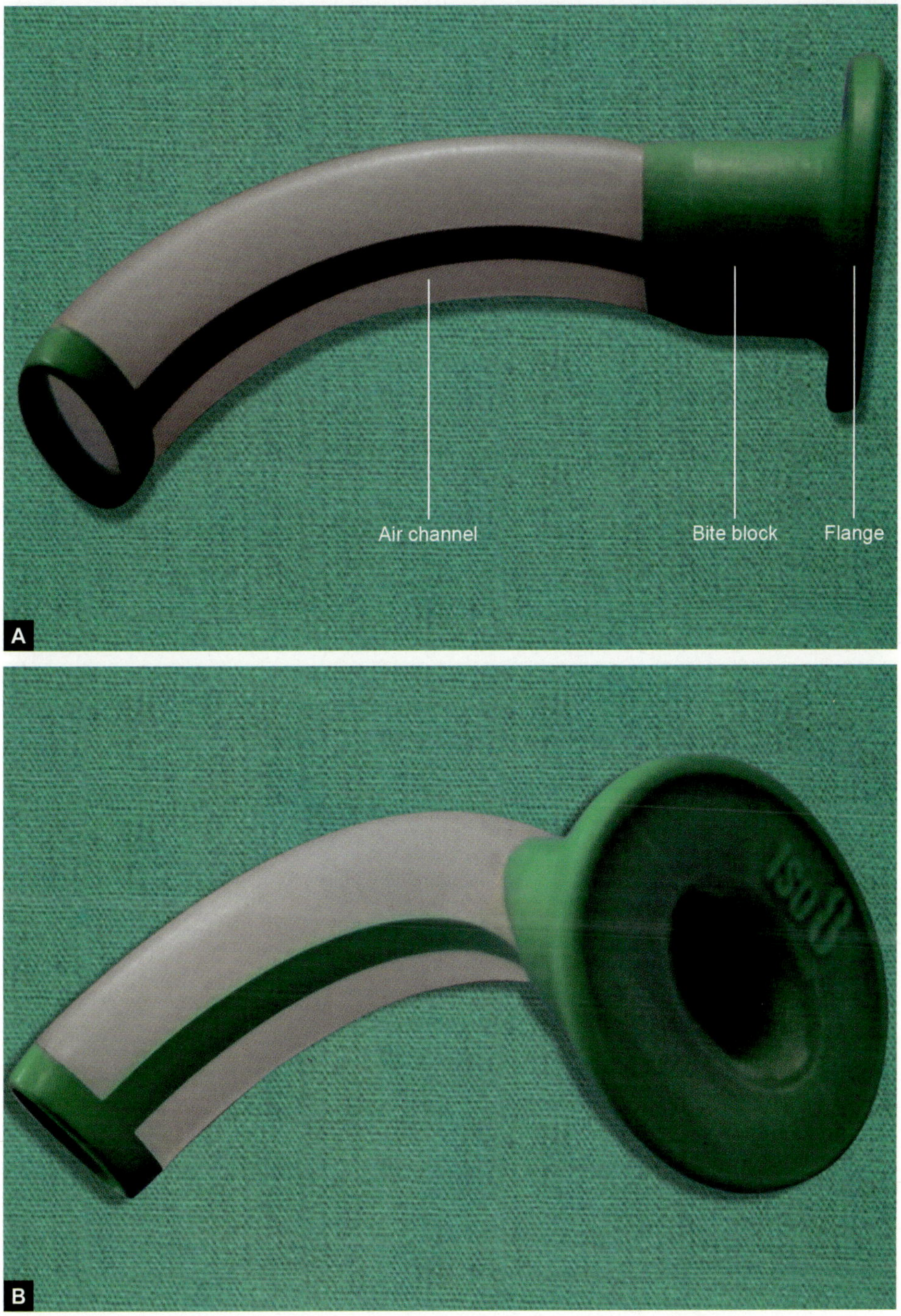

Figs. 2A and B: Different positions of oropharyngeal airway.

- These adjuncts are needed to optimize the mask ventilation.

NASOPHARYNGEAL AIRWAY (NPA) (FIGS. 3A AND B)

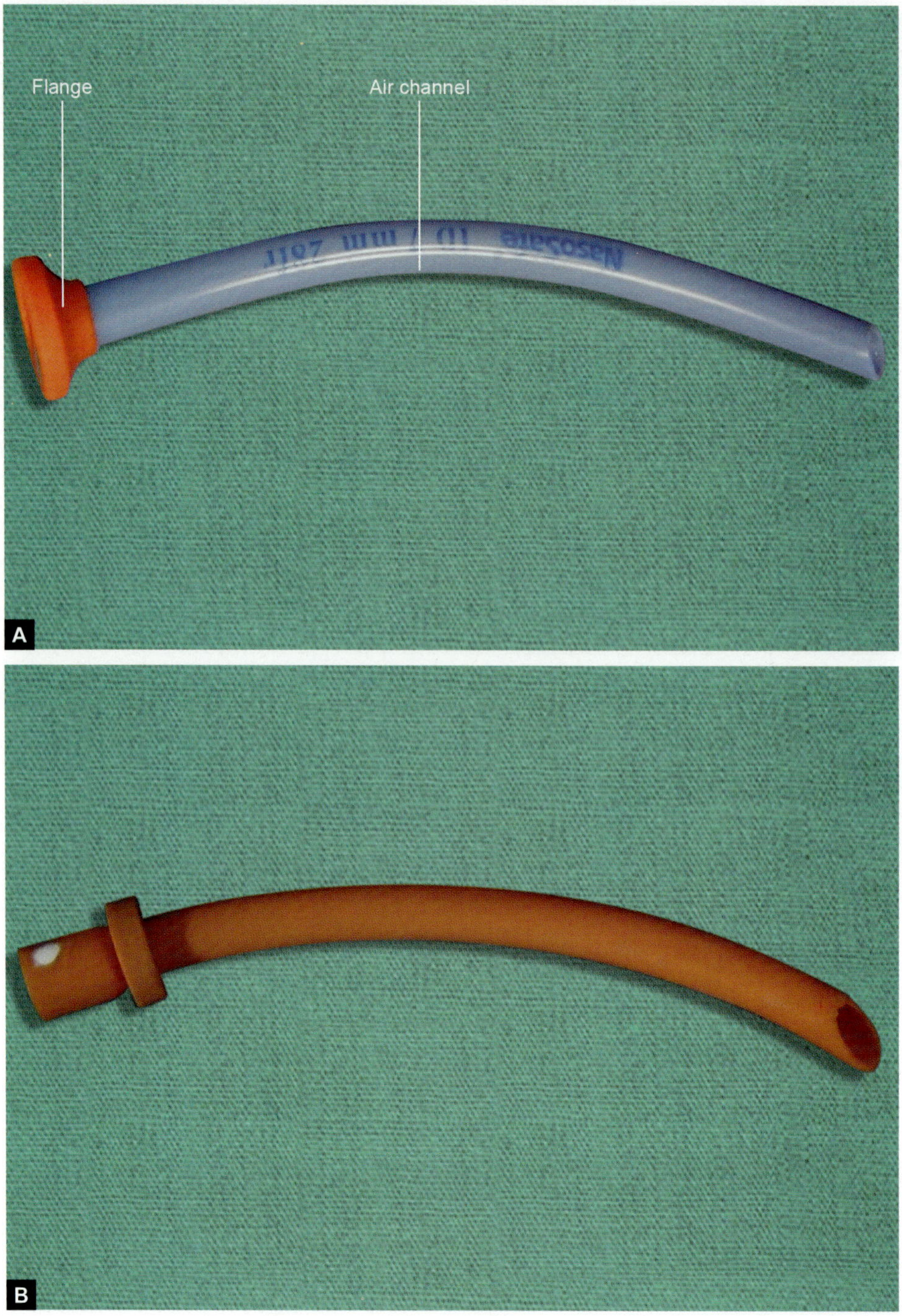

Figs. 3A and B: Different positions of Ambu AuraOnce. Nasopharyngeal airways easy to tolerate, inserted through nostrils after lubricating.

- These adjuncts are needed to optimize the mask ventilation (Figs. 3A and B).

MAGILL FORCEPS (FIG. 4)

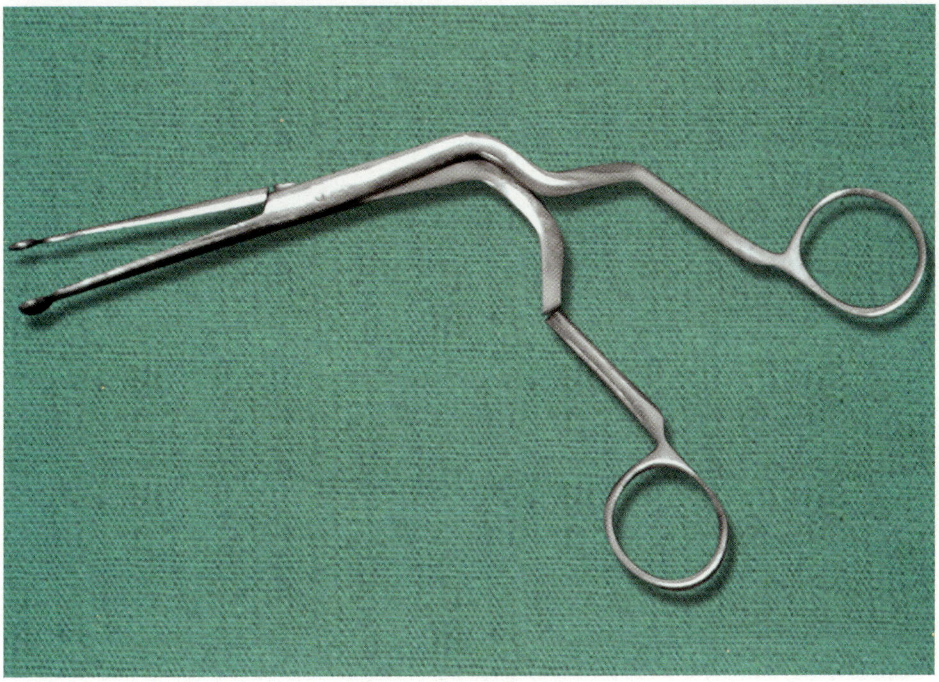

Fig. 4: Magill forceps.

- Magill forceps helps manipulating the endotracheal tube (ETT) during nasal intubation.
- It also helps in throat packing and foreign body removal.

LARYNGOSCOPE (FIG. 5)

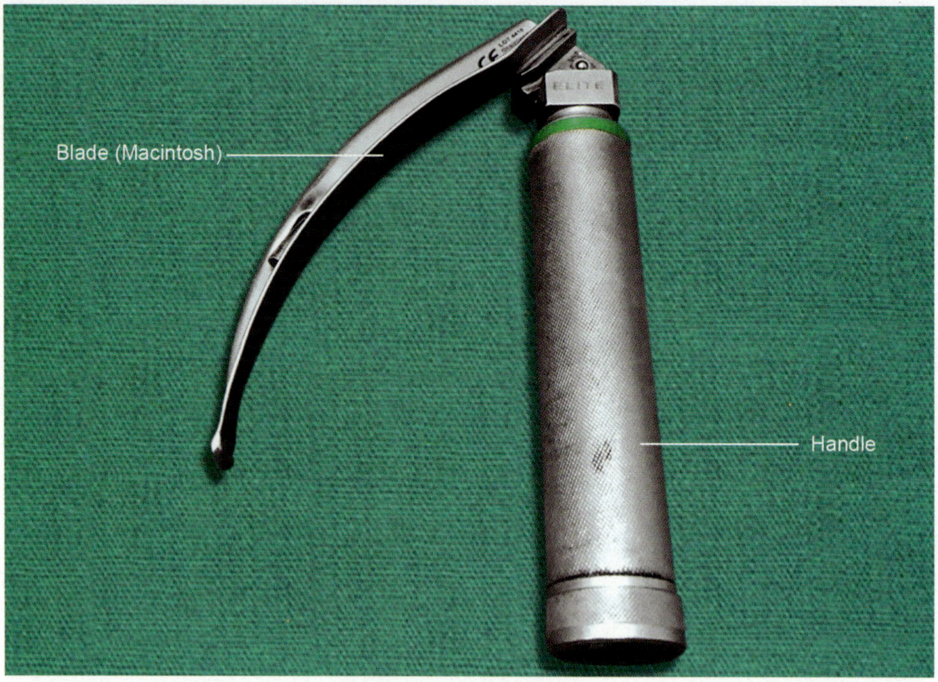

Fig. 5: Laryngoscope.

- Laryngoscope is used for direct view of laryngeal inlet by operator's eye.
- This curved blade is Macintosh blade.
- Handle houses the battery.

CUFFED POLYVINYL CHLORIDE ENDOTRACHEAL TUBE (FIGS. 6A AND B)

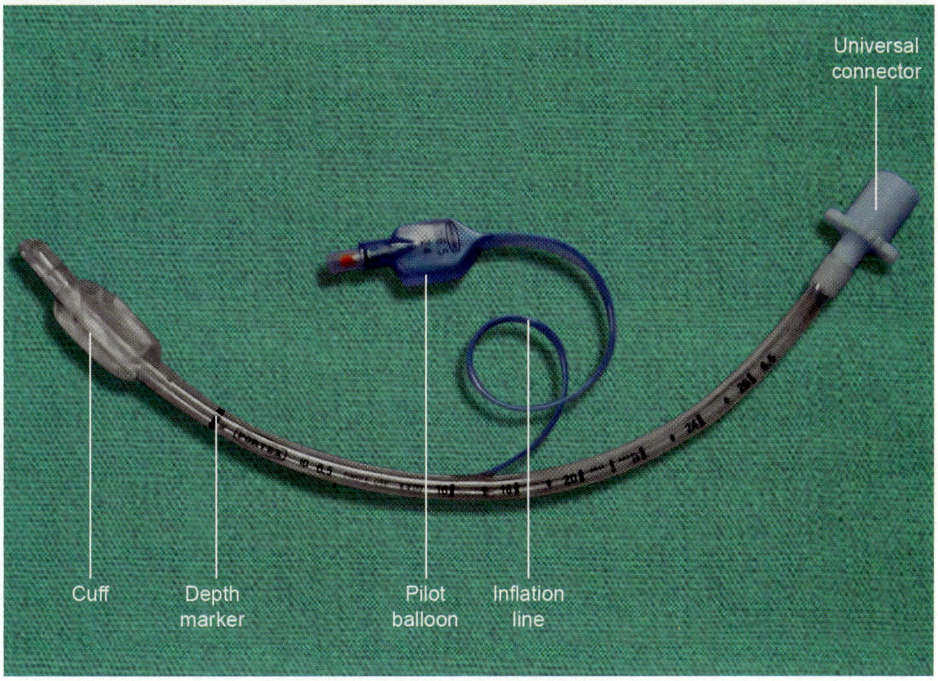

Fig. 6A: Cuffed PVC endotracheal tube.

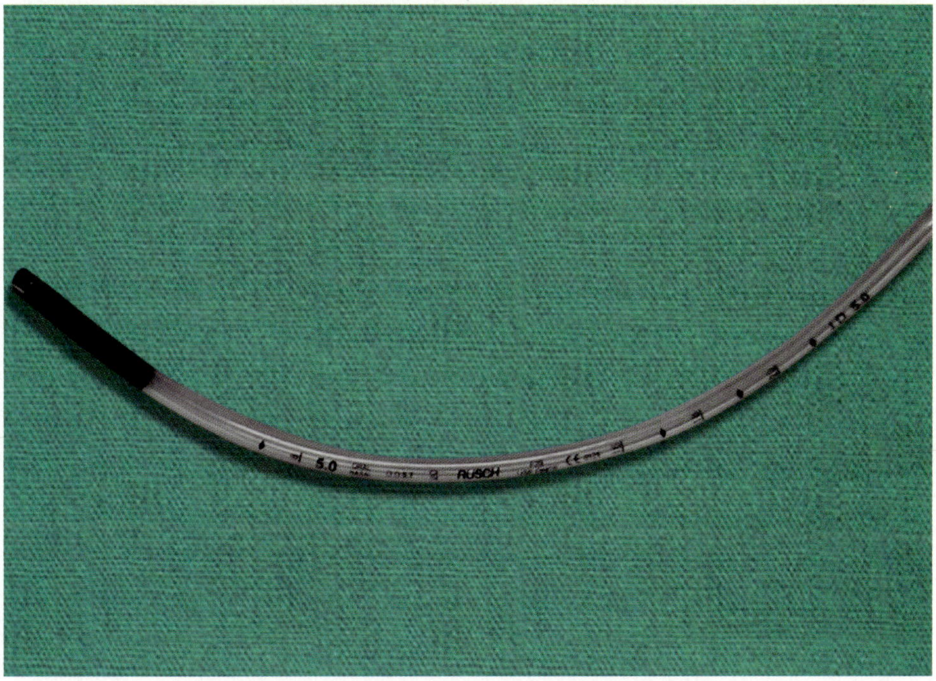

Fig. 6B: Pediatric endotracheal tube (non-cuffed).

- The cuffed polyvinyl chloride (PVC) ETT and pediatric ETT are shown in above figures.

ARMORED (REINFORCED/FLEXOMETALLIC) ETT (FIGS. 7A AND B)

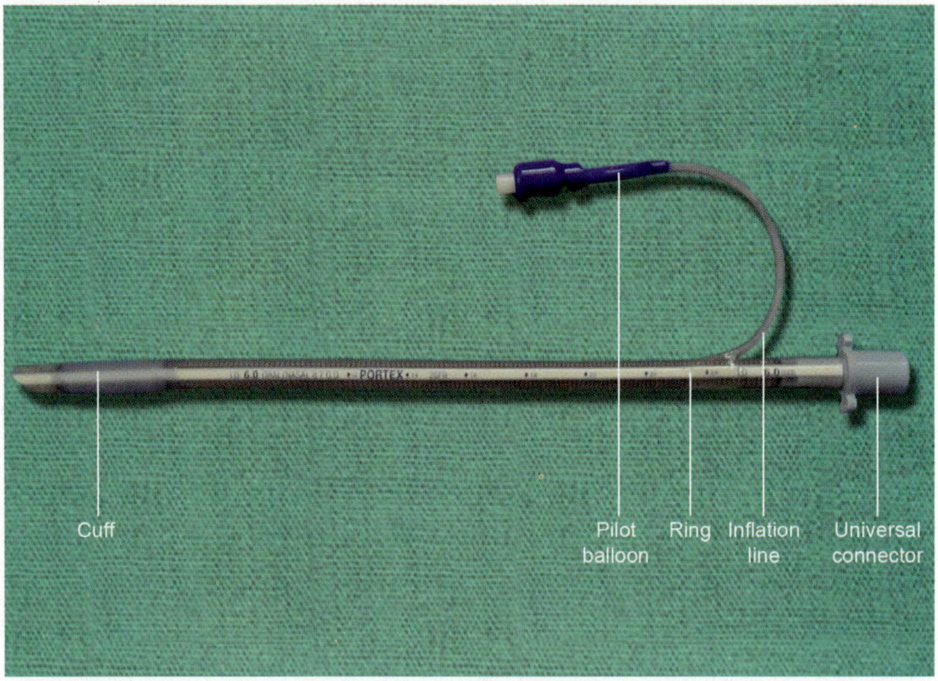

Fig. 7A: Reinforced ETT.

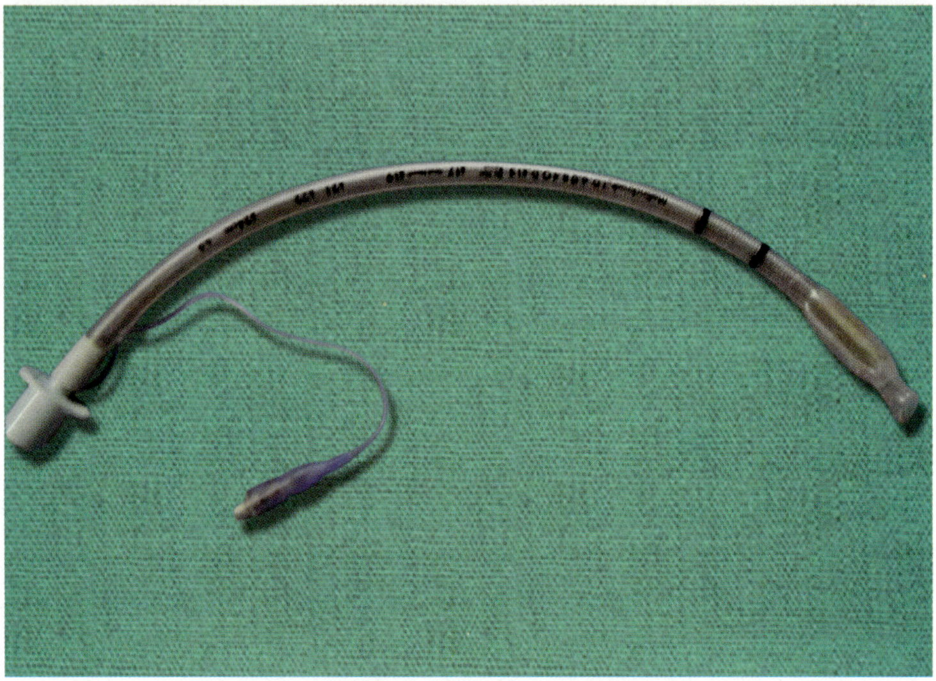

Fig. 7B: Different model of reinforced ETT.

- Reinforced by metal or plastic rings in the wall of the ETT.
- Makes it nonkinkable on bending.

PREFORMED ENDOTRACHEAL TUBE (FIGS. 8A AND B)

Ring-Adair-Elwyn (RAE) (North Pole) ETT (Fig. 8A)

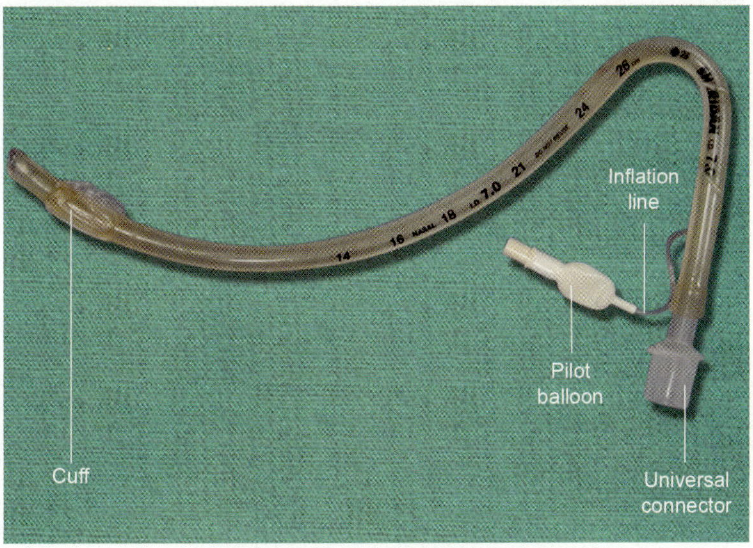

Fig. 8A: RAE North pole ETT (Nasal).

RAE (South Pole) ETT (Fig. 8B)

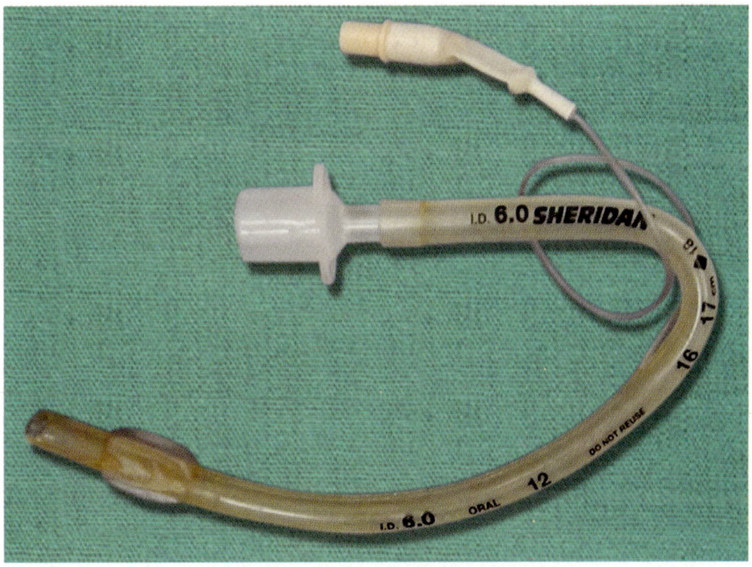

Fig. 8B: RAE South pole ETT (Oral).

- RAE-North pole ETT keeps it toward the head end and makes access to mouth and neck easier.
- RAE-South pole ETT keeps it bent toward the foot end and makes access to nose and head easier.
- Many times patient's after shifted to ICU, intubated with these tubes after head and neck surgery and extubated later.
- If patient remain longer with RAE tube, it has to be cut at preformed bend to ease the suctioning of endotracheal tube.

ENDOTRACHEAL TUBE WITH SUBGLOTTIC SUCTION (FIG. 9)

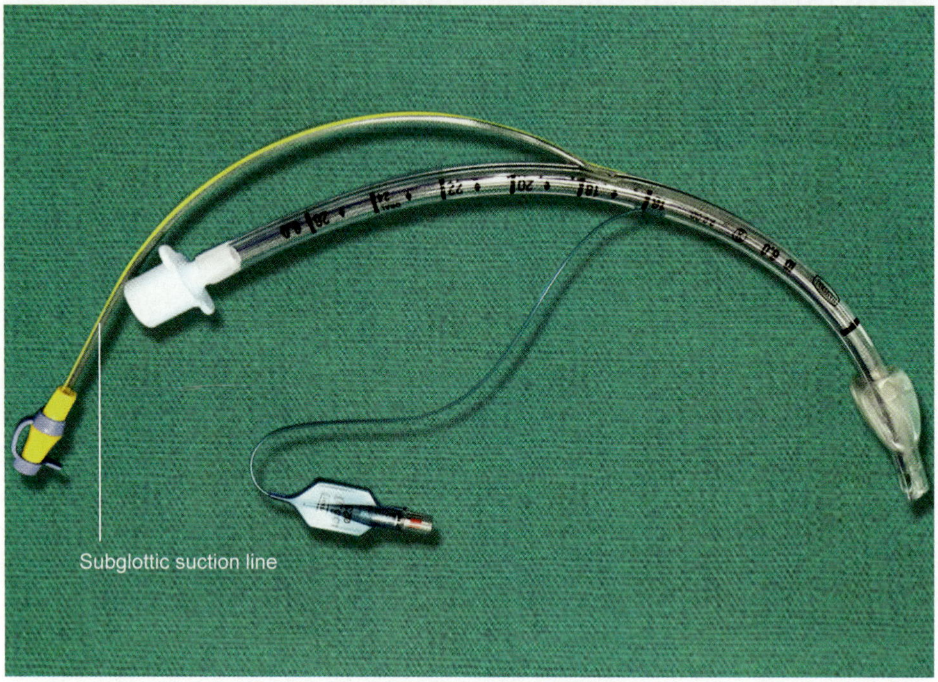

Fig. 9: ETT with subglottic suction.

- Useful in cases where there is possibility of significant amount of liquid (secretion, blood, pus, etc.) above the cuff.
- Through subglottic suction port subglottic secretions are removed by using a syringe or utilization of wall suction that helps in reducing the incidence of ventilator-associated pneumonia (VAP).

DOUBLE-LUMEN TUBE (FIGS. 10A TO D)

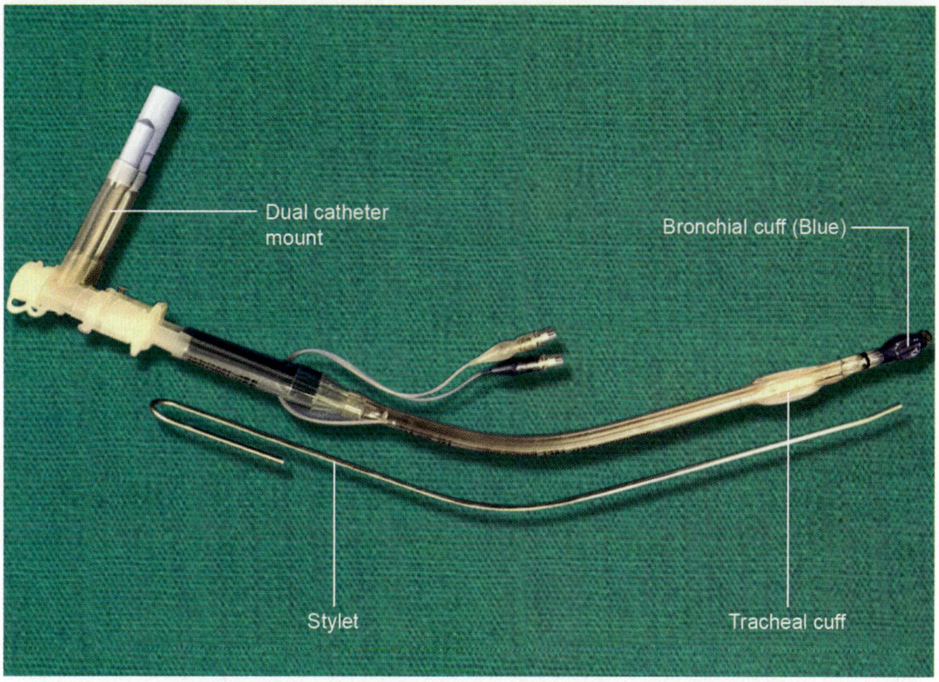

Fig. 10A: Anterior position of left-sided double-lumen tube (DLT).

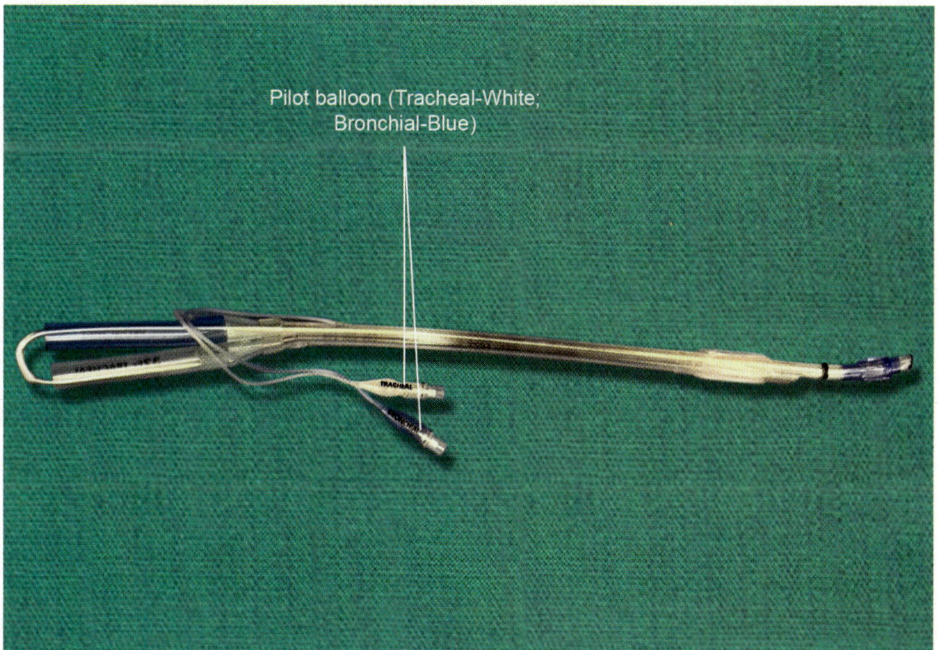

Fig. 10B: Posterior position of left-sided DLT.

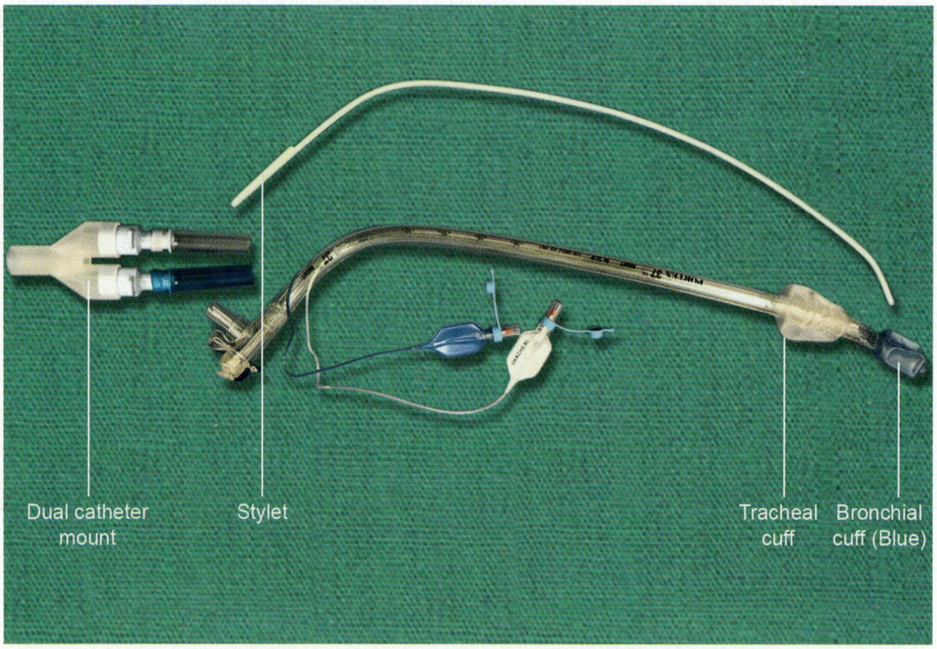

Fig. 10C: Anterior position of right-sided DLT.

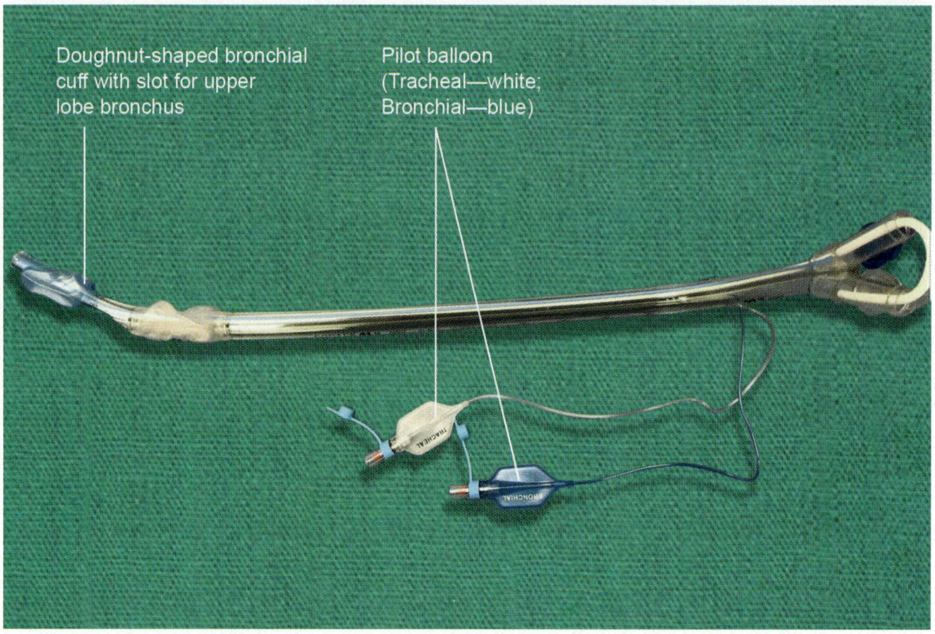

Fig. 10D: Posterior position of right-sided DLT.

- Double-lumen tubes (DLTs) may be "left" or "right" depending on bronchus they are designed to intubate.
- Left DLT is commonly used for independent lung ventilation.
- Right-sided tubes have a slit to be positioned to facilitate ventilation of right upper lobe (RUL) but are more difficult to position, so left DLTs are more commonly used.
- Appropriate size for males 39–41 Fr and for females 37–39 Fr.
- *Common indications of independent lung ventilation in ICU*: Massive hemoptysis, copious secretions in bronchiectasis or lung abscess, bronchopleural fistula, bronchopleural cutaneous fistula, unilateral bronchospasm and pneumonectomy.

UNIVENT TUBE (FIG. 11)

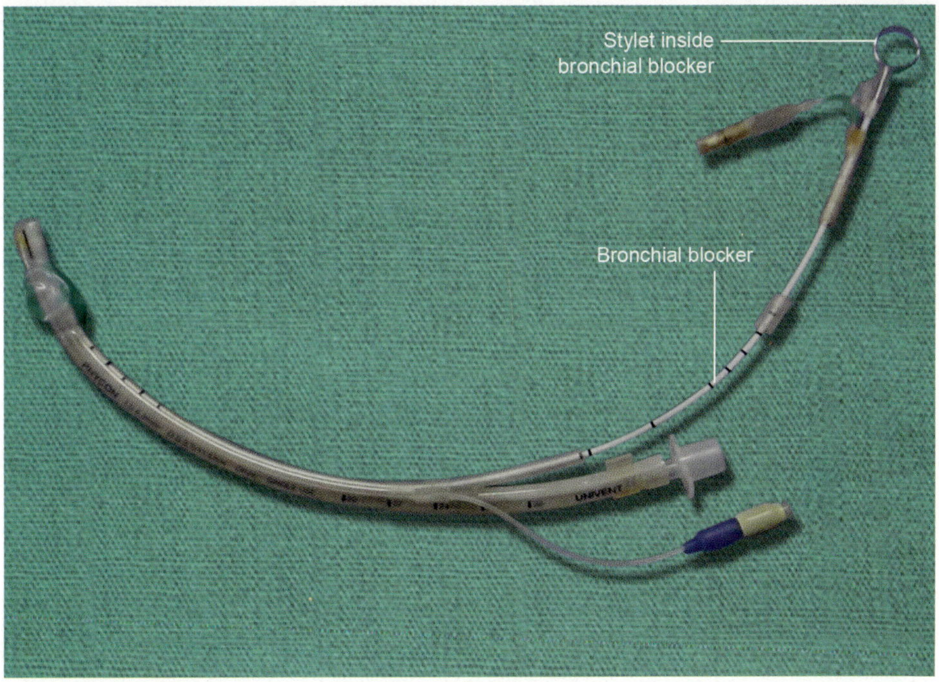

Fig. 11: Univent tube.

- Achieves one-lung ventilation in difficult airway cases where DLT introduction may take longer.

BRONCHOSCOPIC VIEW OF LARYNGEAL INLET (FIG. 12)

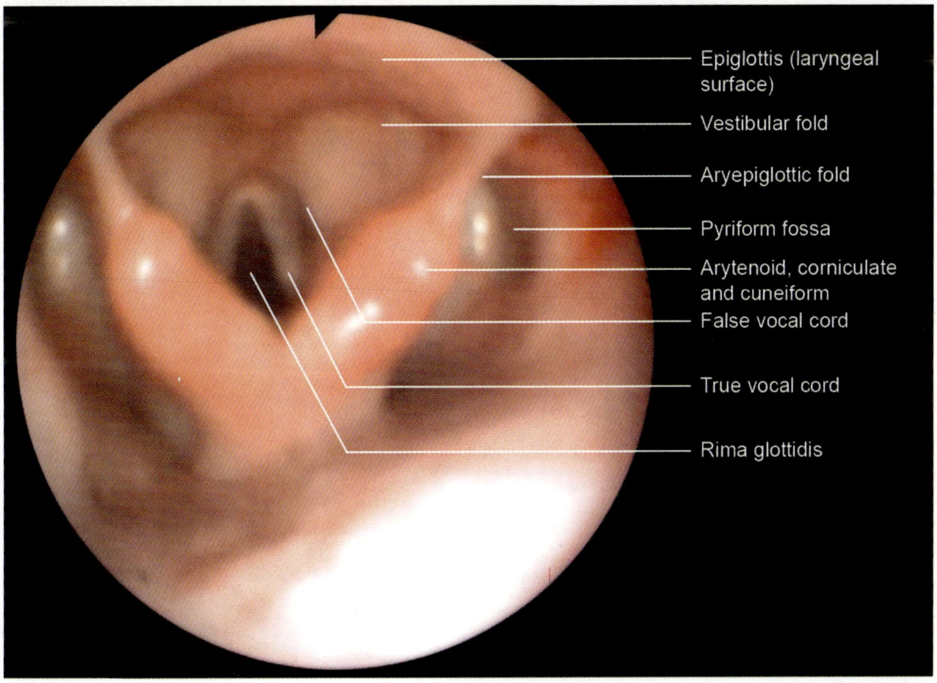

Fig. 12: Laryngeal inlet.

STYLETS (FIGS. 13A AND B)

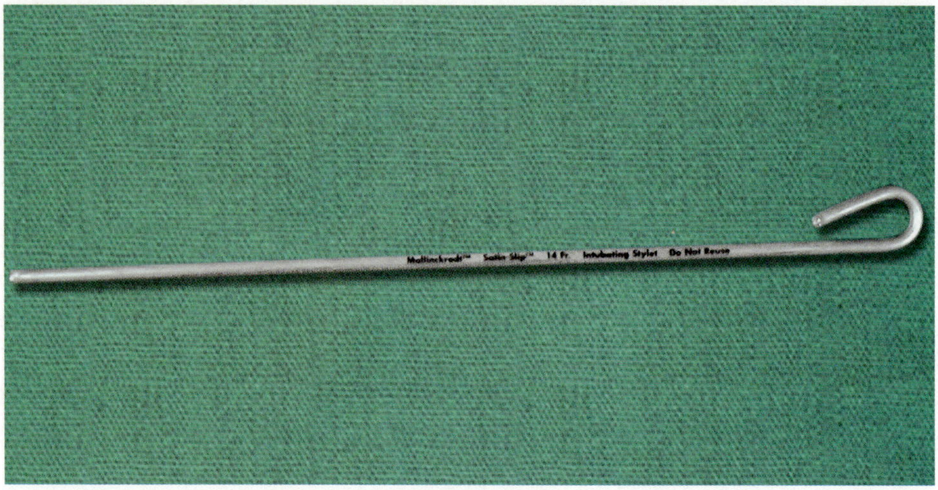

Fig. 13A: Stylet.

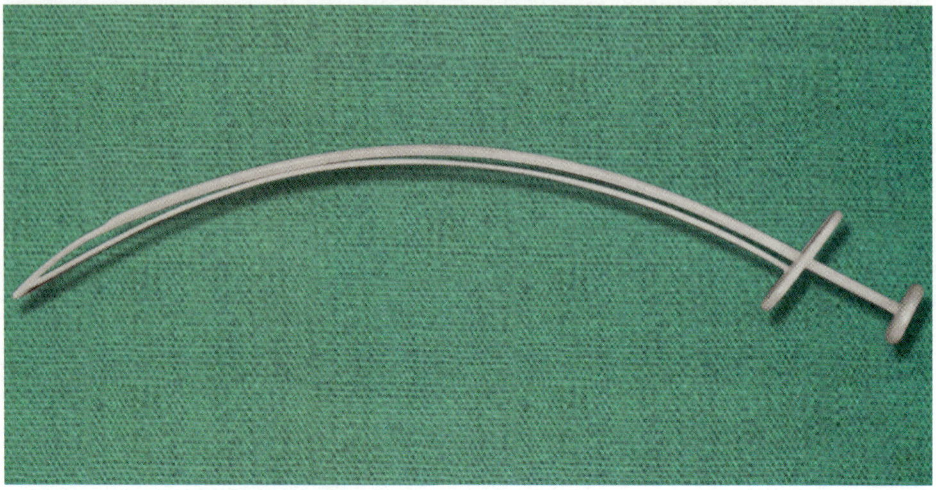

Fig. 13B: Adjustable stylet.

- Stylets are used to give the desired bend to the ETTs.

TRACHEAL TUBE INTRODUCER (BOUGIE) (FIG. 14)

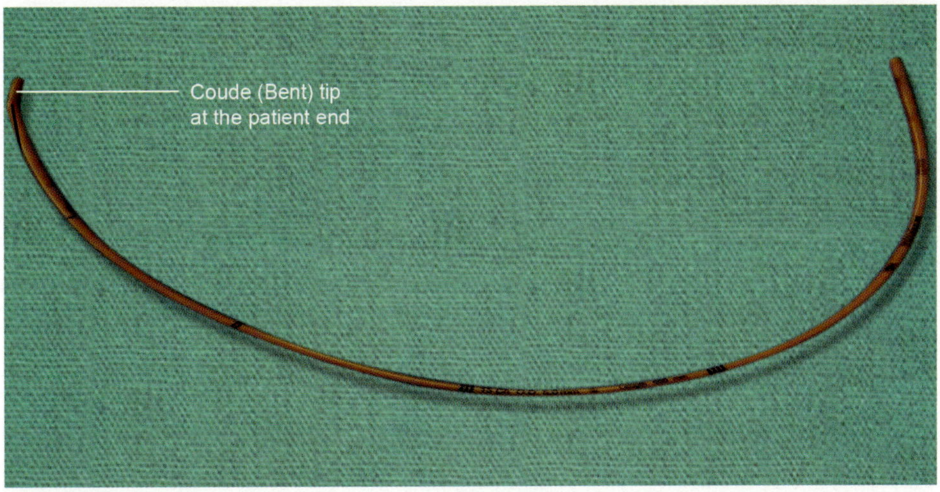

Fig. 14: Bougie.

- Tracheal tube introducer allows the operator to enter an almost nonvisualized glottis by traveling "behind" epiglottis because of its bent tip.
- Once inside, the bougie becomes the conduit to guide the ETT into trachea.

McCOY LARYNGOSCOPE (FIG. 15)

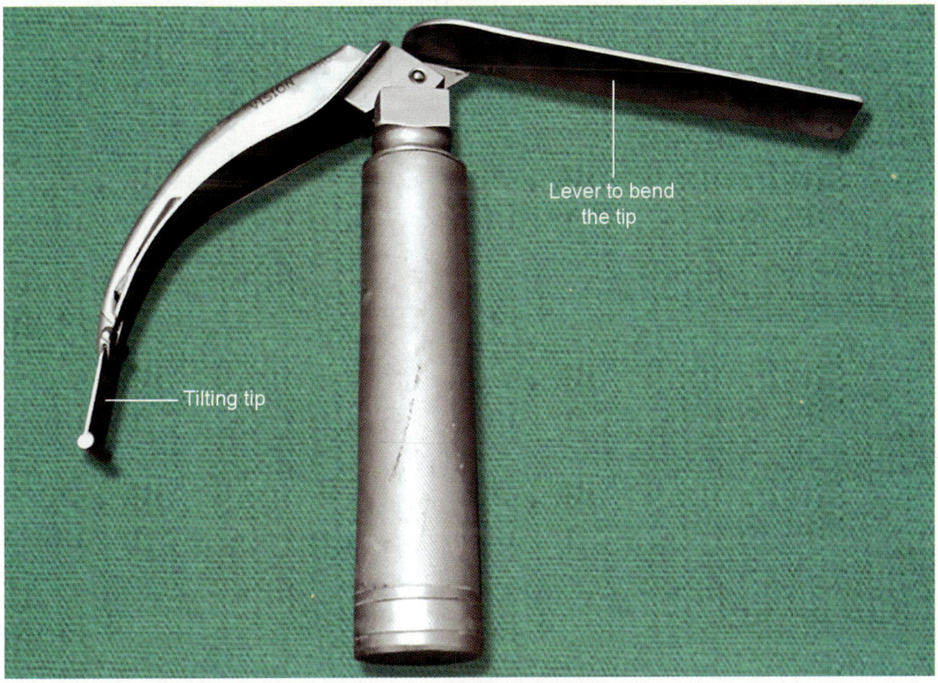

Fig. 15: McCoy laryngoscope.

- The lever of McCoy blade bends the tip of its blade up thereby lifting the epiglottis out of the way of glottis during direct laryngoscopy.

VIDEOLARYNGOSCOPE—AMBU KING VISION (FIGS. 16A AND B)

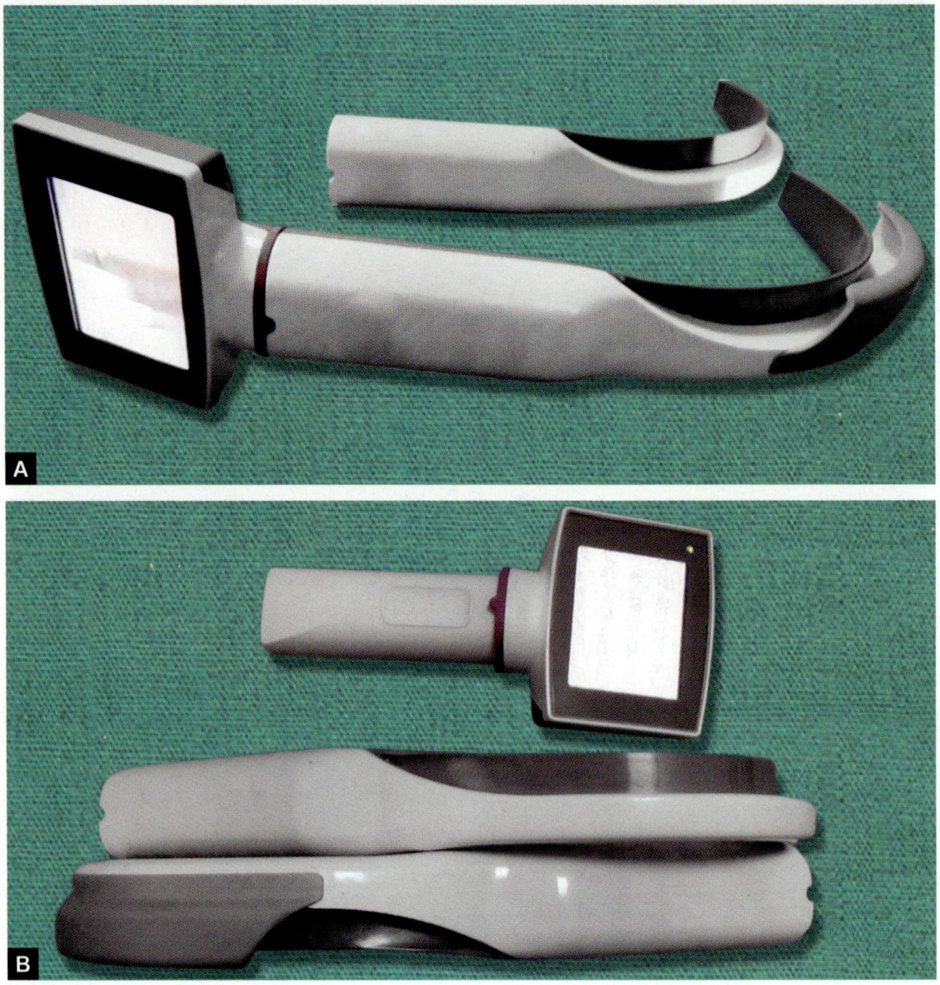

Figs. 16A and B: Videolaryngoscope—Ambu King Vision.

VIDEOLARYNGOSCOPE—C-MAC (MACINTOSH AND D-BLADES) (FIG. 17)

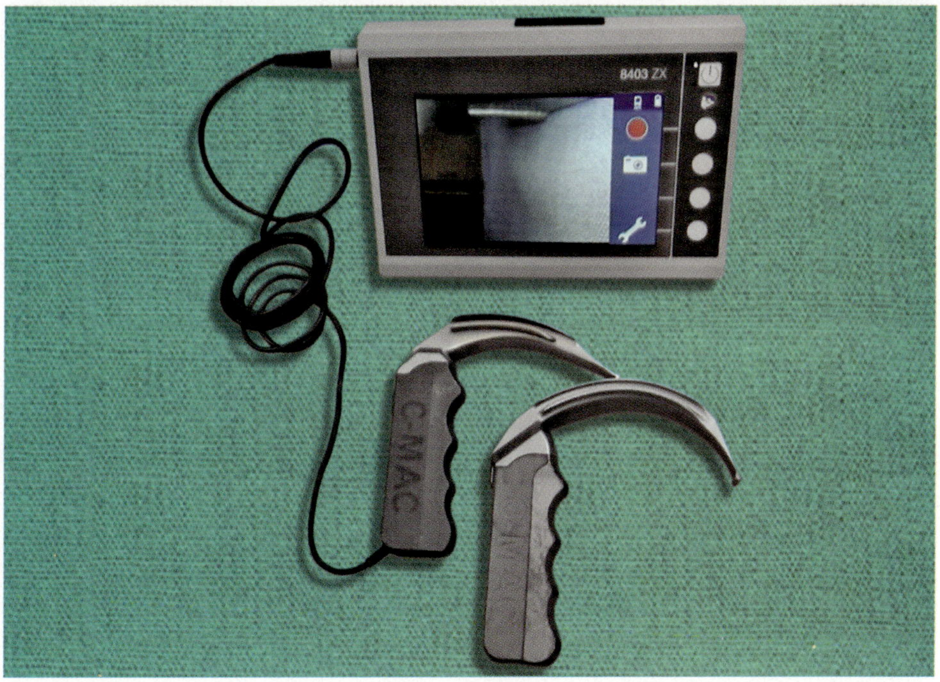

Fig. 17: Videolaryngoscope—C-Mac.

VIDEOLARYNGOSCOPE—McGRATH (FIGS. 18A AND B)

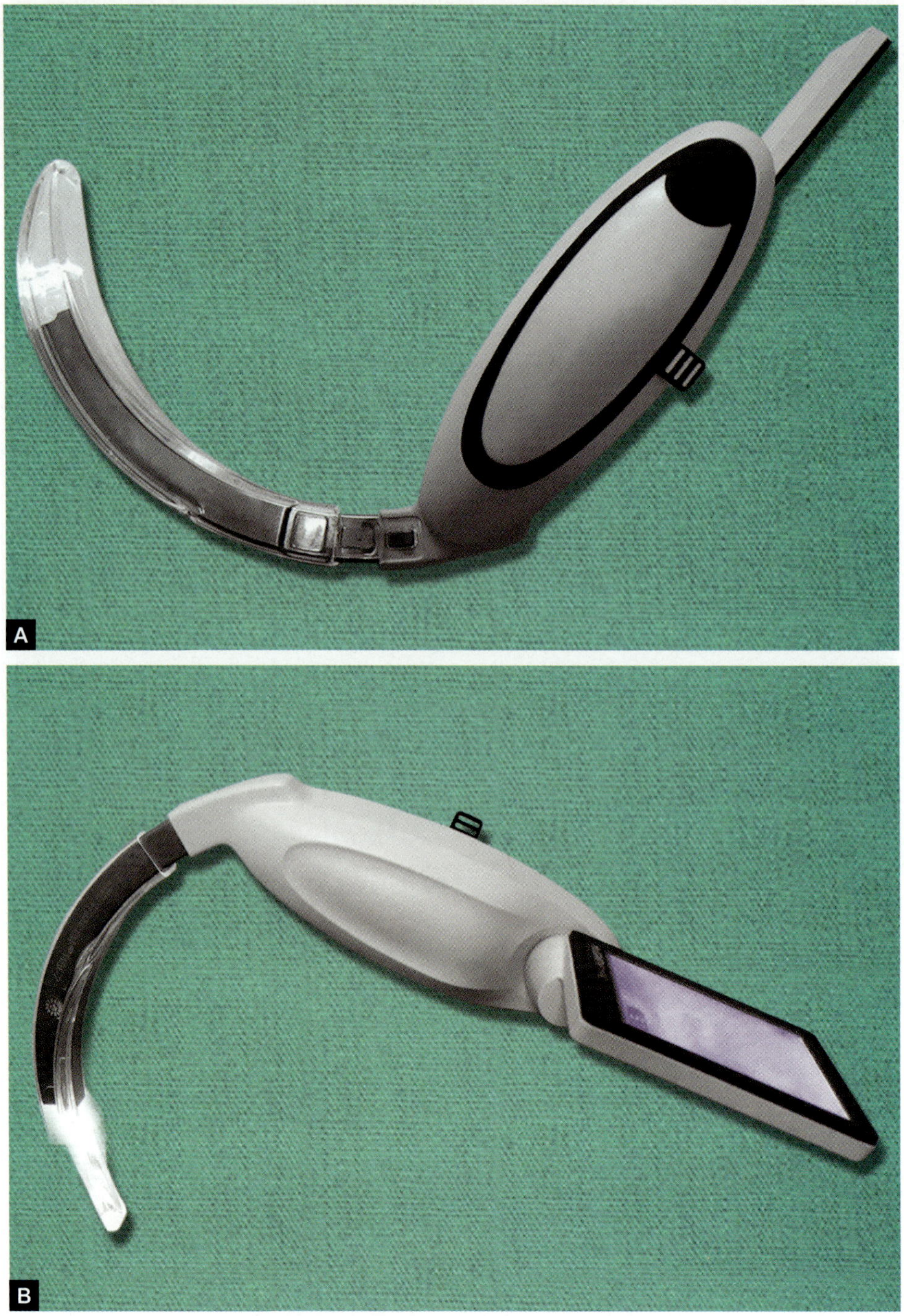

Figs. 18A and B: Videolaryngoscope—McGrath.

- Videolaryngoscopes provide indirect view of the laryngeal inlet.
- The camera placed near the tip of the blade allows the operator to see "around the bend".
- Monitors may be in-built (King Vision, McGrath) or separate (C-Mac).
- These are used in difficult intubations.

FLEXIBLE VIDEOENDOSCOPE (FIBERSCOPE)—AMBU A3 SCOPE (FIGS. 19A AND B)

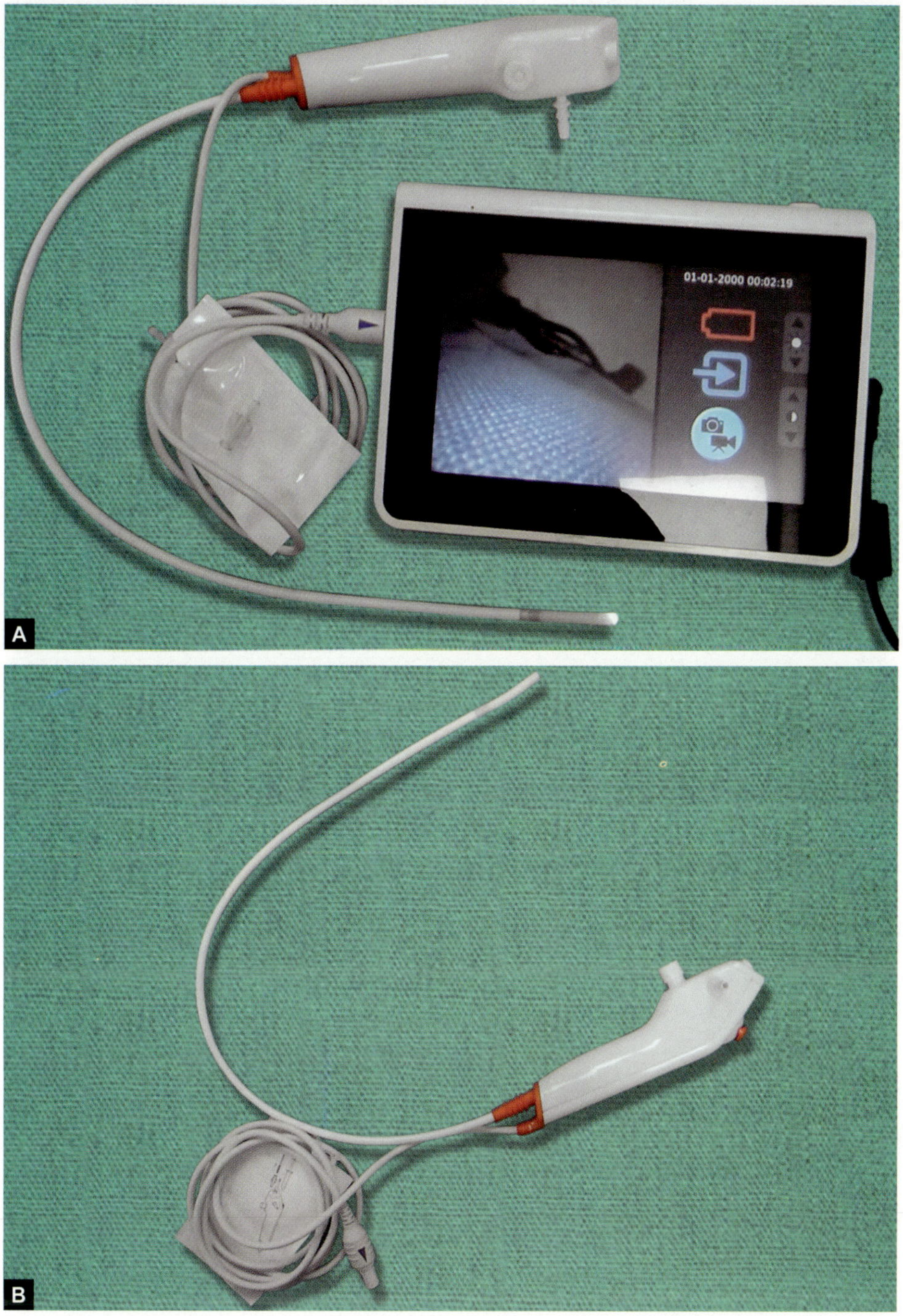

Figs. 19A and B: (A) Fiberscope—Ambu A3 scope; (B) Part of Ambu A3 scope.

FLEXIBLE VIDEOENDOSCOPE (FIBERSCOPE)—FIVE (FIGS. 20A AND B)

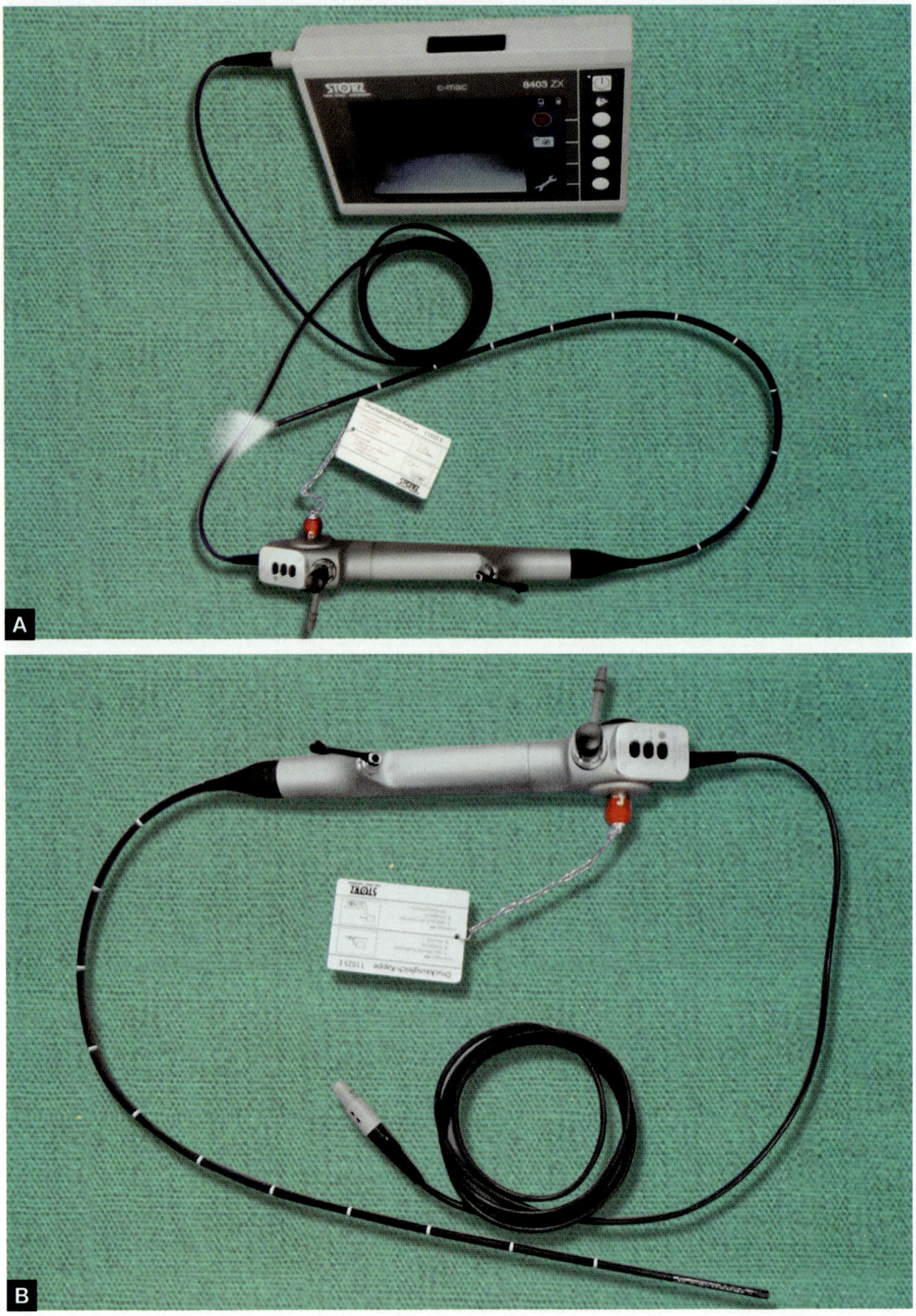

Figs. 20A and B: (A) Flexible videoendoscope—Karl Storz; (B) Part of the same.

- Flexible fiberscopes also provide indirect view of the laryngeal inlet.
- These are excellent devices to intubate the trachea by either oral or nasal route for anticipated difficult airway situations.
- Ambu A3 scope is a single use device while its monitor is reused.
- Flexible intubating videoendoscope (FIVE, Karl Storz) and its monitor are reusable devices.
- These are used in difficult intubations.

BRONCHOSCOPY AIRWAY FOR ORAL FIBERSCOPY—ACCESSORIES TO AID FLEXIBLE FIBERSCOPY (FIG. 21)

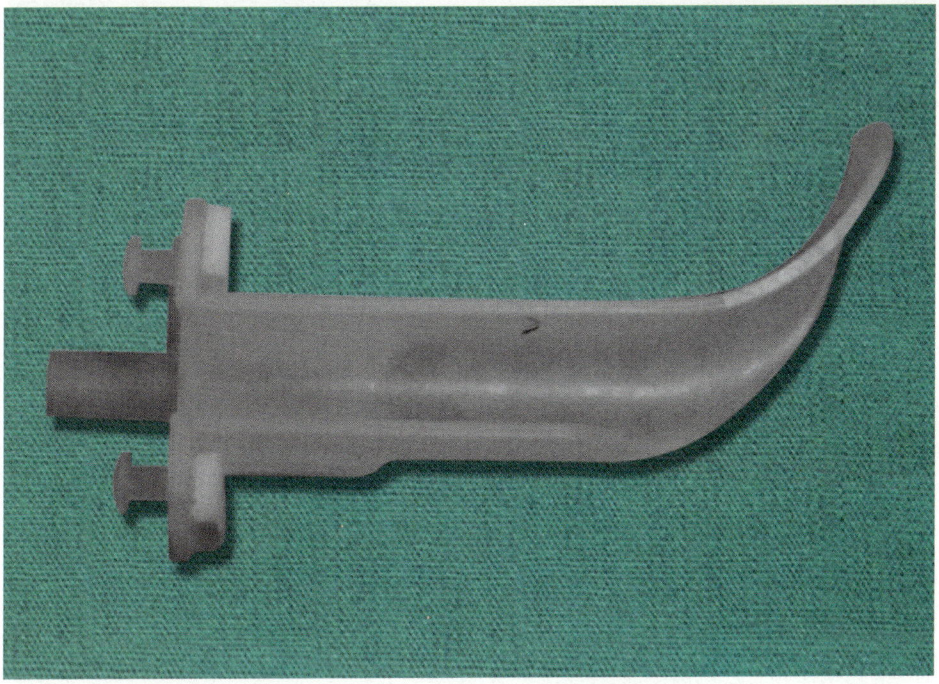

Fig. 21: Bronchoscopy airway—oral fiberscopy.

BRONCHOSCOPY MASKS—ACCESSORIES TO AID FLEXIBLE FIBERSCOPY (FIGS. 22A AND B)

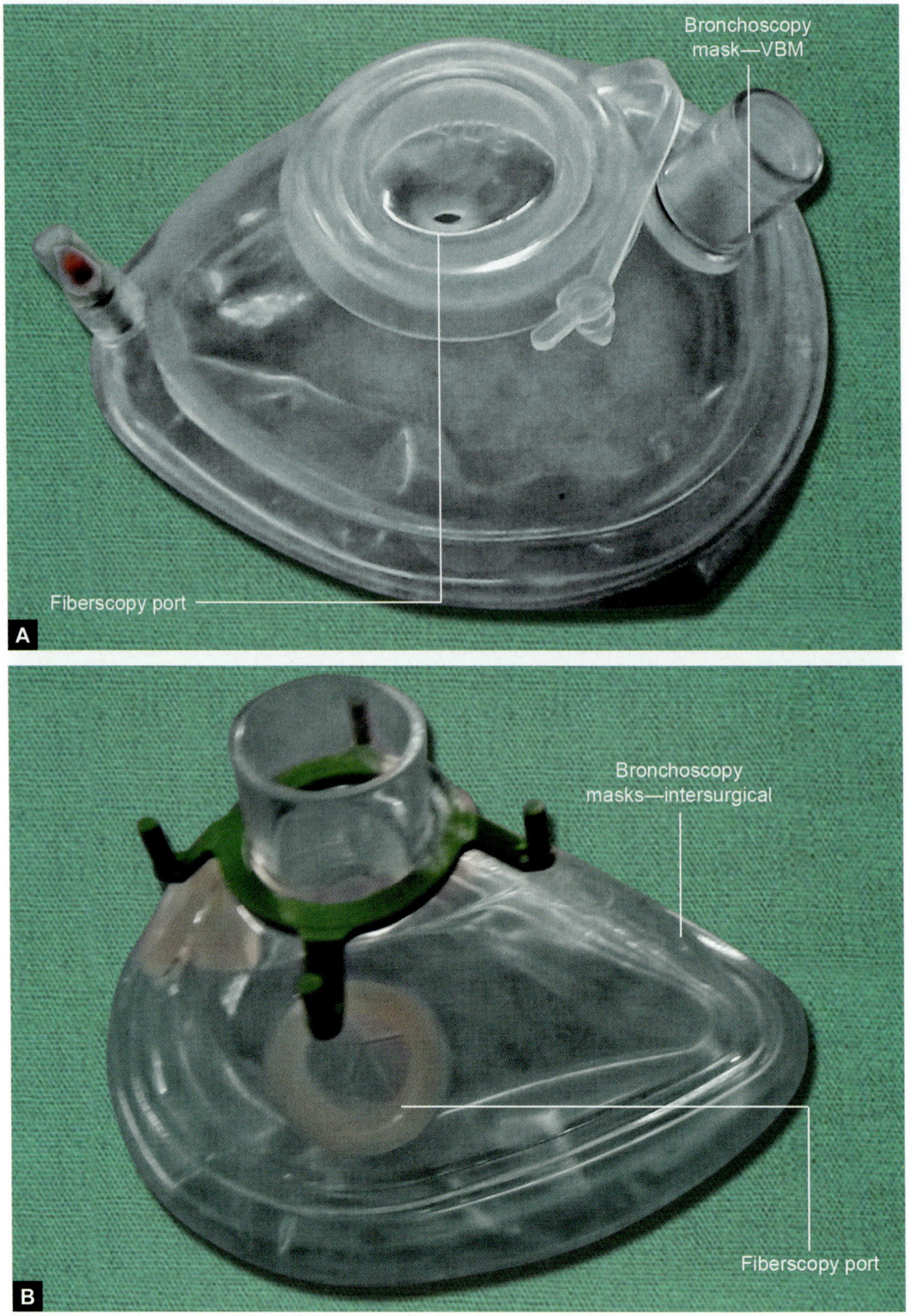

Figs. 22A and B: Bronchoscopy masks. (A) Manufactured by VBM; (B) Manufactured by intersurgical.

- Transparent masks help in detecting vomit/secretions while oxygenating/ventilating.

AMBU AURA-I LARYNGEAL MASK AIRWAY (FIGS. 23A AND B)

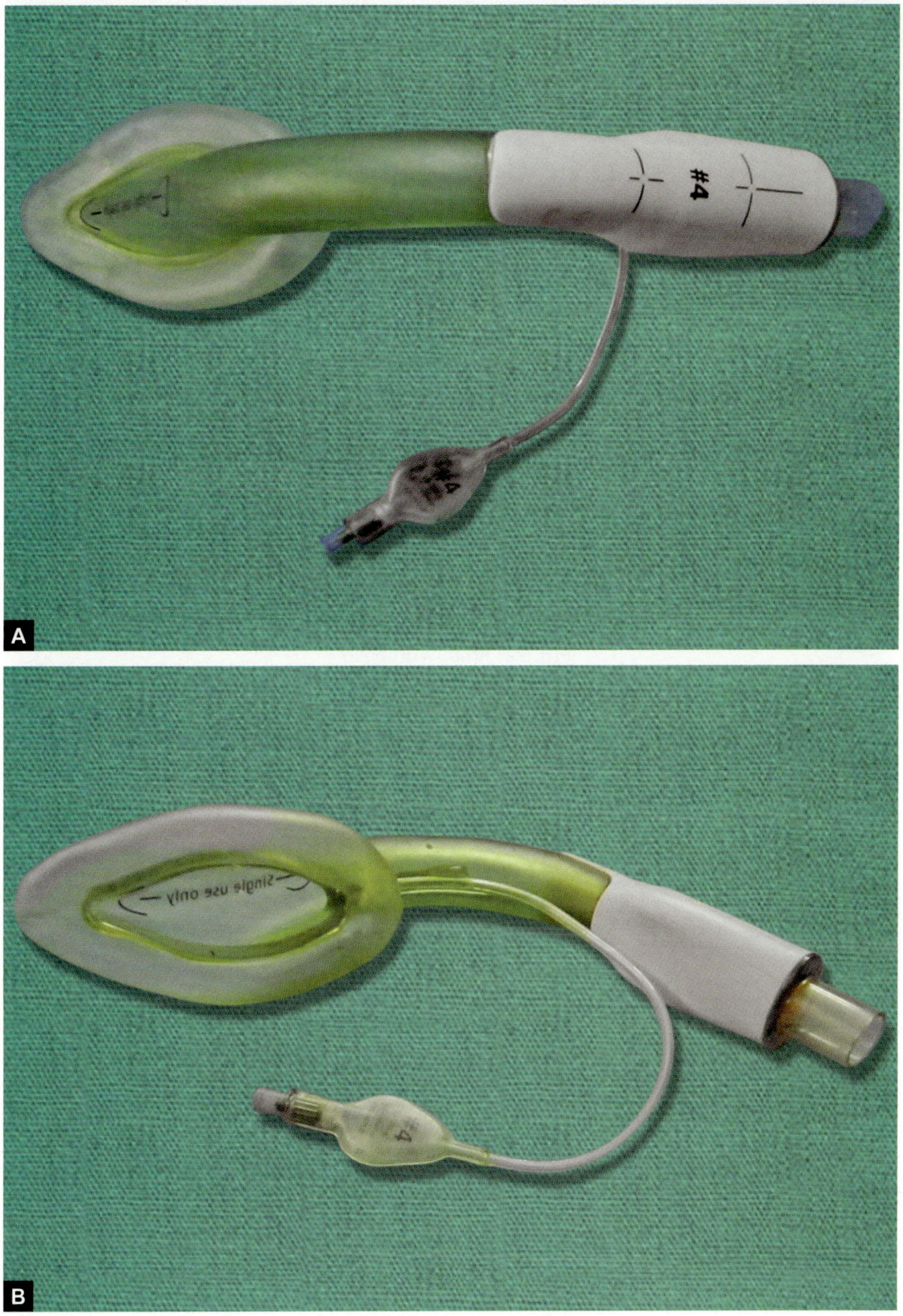

Figs. 23A and B: Ambu Aura-I.

- These are supraglottic devices used for mechanical ventilation without actually inserting ETT. Can be used for difficult airways.

AMBU AURAGAIN (FIG. 24)

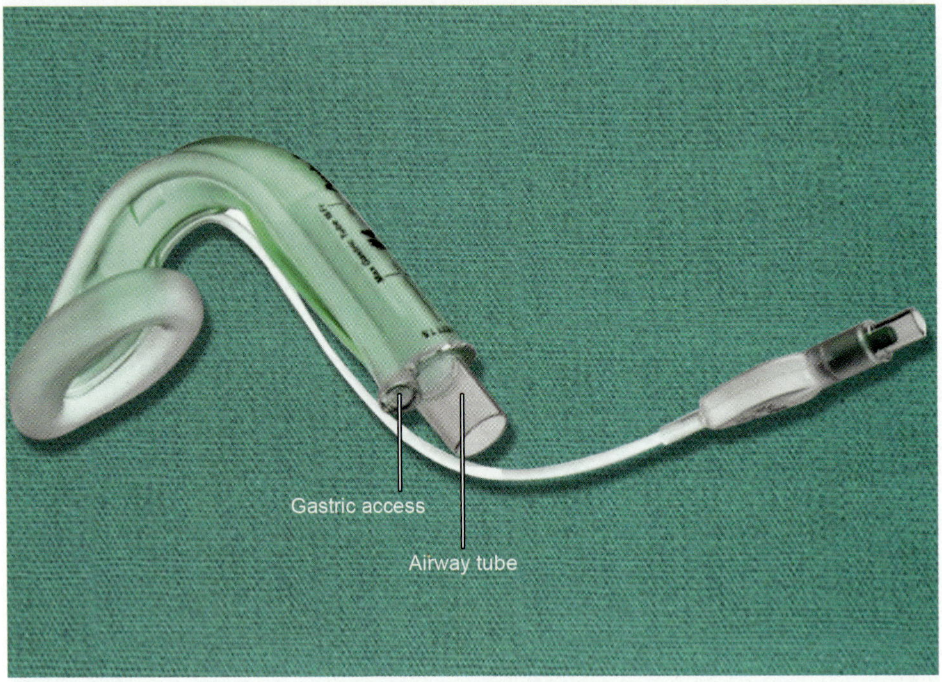

Fig. 24: Ambu AuraGain.

- It has facility for gastric access and intubation.

I-GEL (FIGS. 25A AND B)

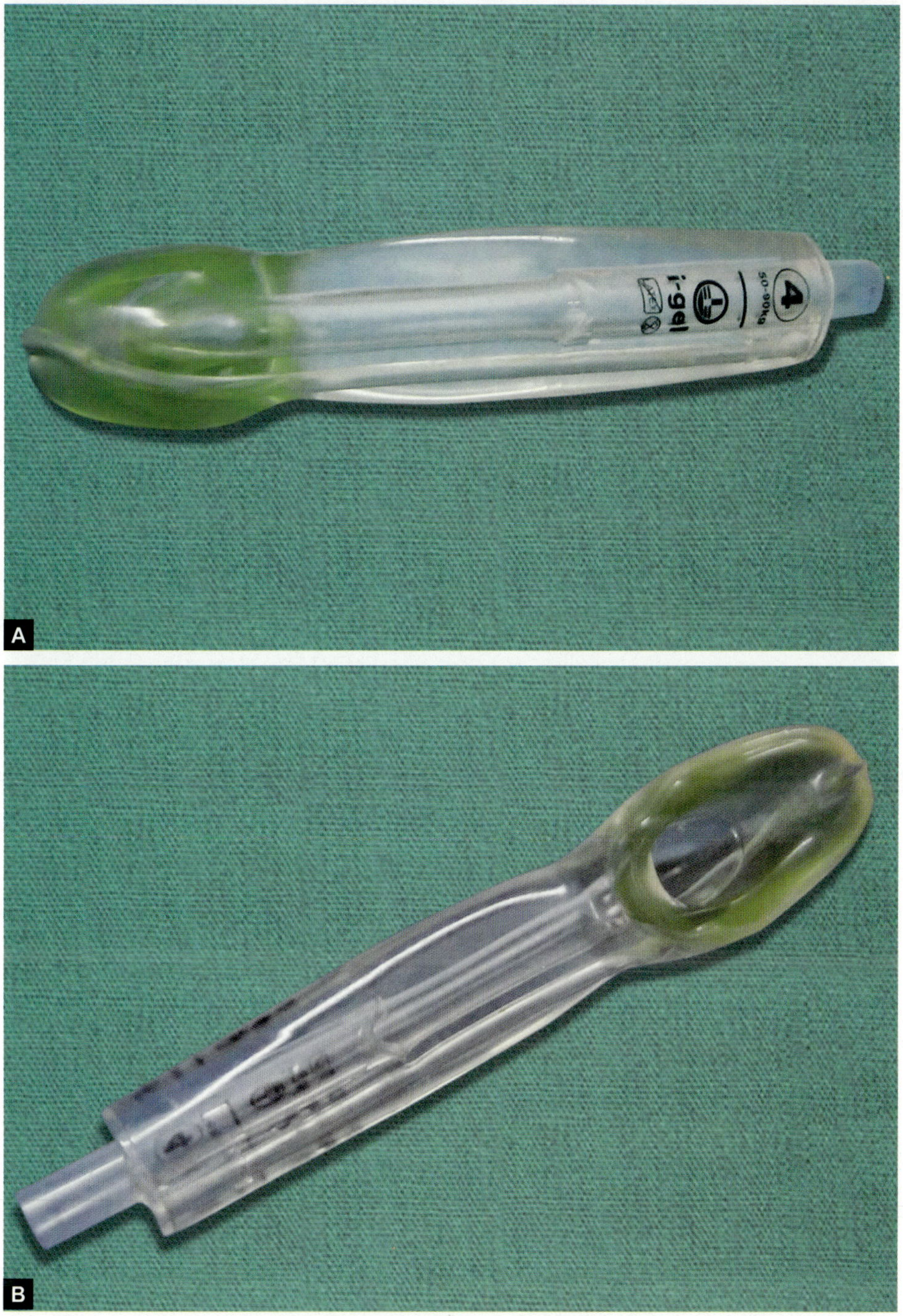

Figs. 25A and B: Different positions of i-gel.

INTUBATING LARYNGEAL TUBE SUCTION (FIG. 26)

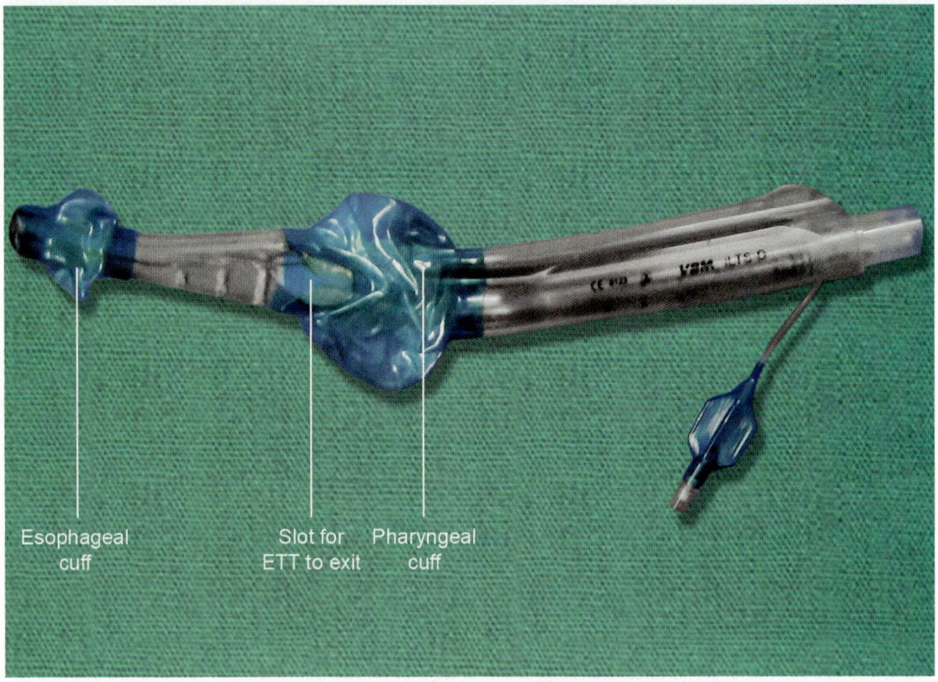

Fig. 26: Intubating laryngeal tube suction (ILTS).

INTUBATING LARYNGEAL MASK AIRWAY (FIG. 27)

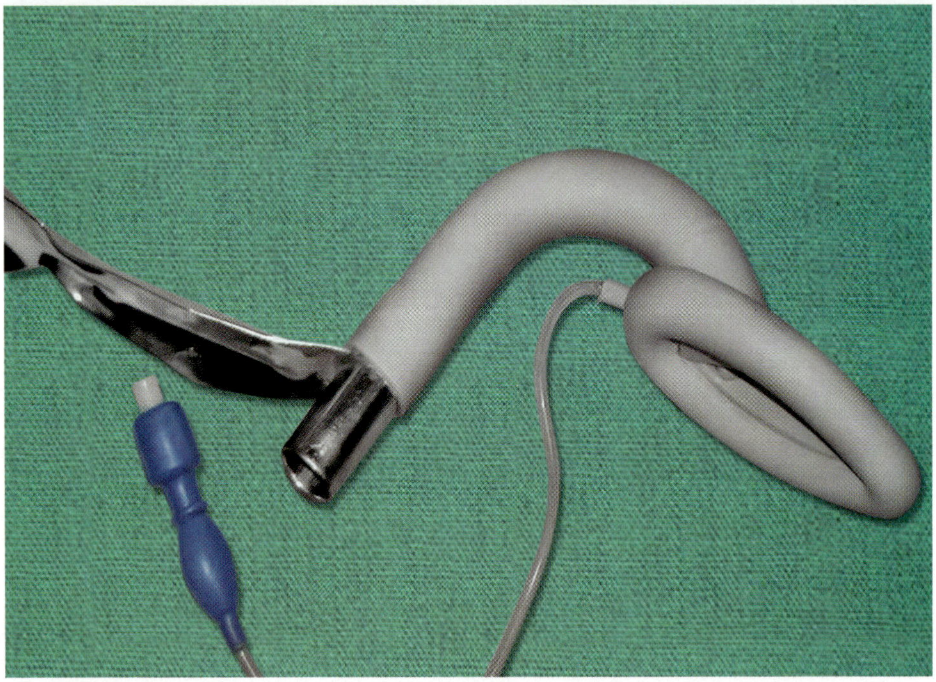

Fig. 27: Intubating laryngeal mask airway (ILMA). ETT can be inserted blindly through it.

AMBU AURAONCE (FIGS. 28A AND B)

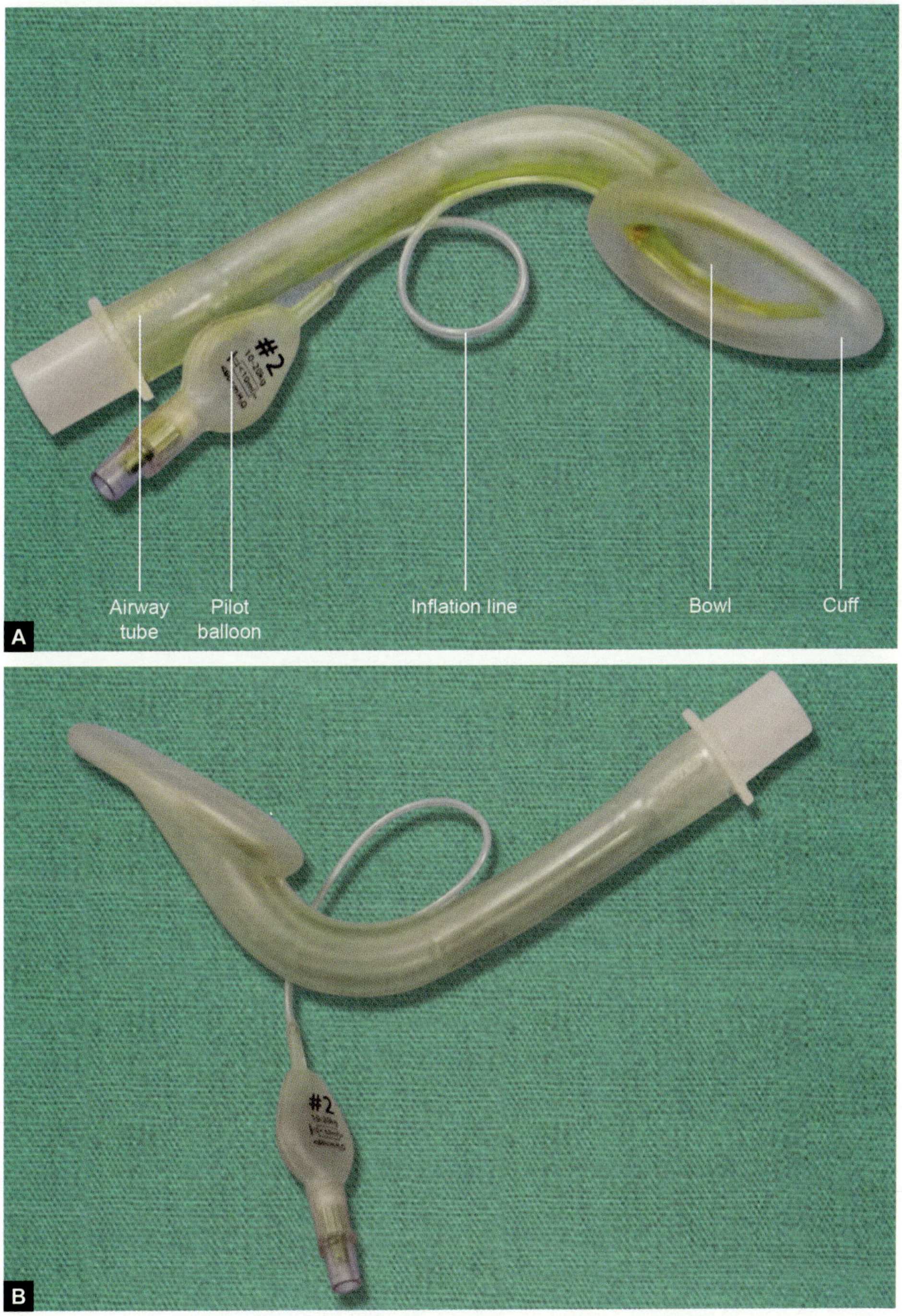

Figs. 28A and B: Different positions of Ambu AuraOnce.

LARYNGEAL TUBE SUCTION (FIG. 29)

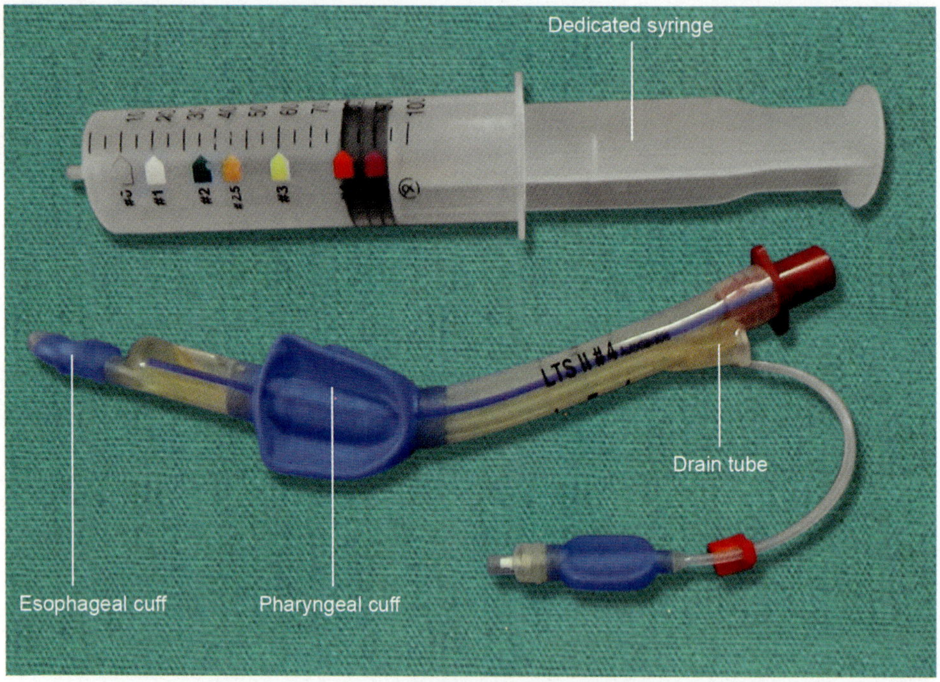

Fig. 29: Laryngeal tube suction (LTS).

LARYNGEAL MASK AIRWAY—PROSEAL (FIG. 30)

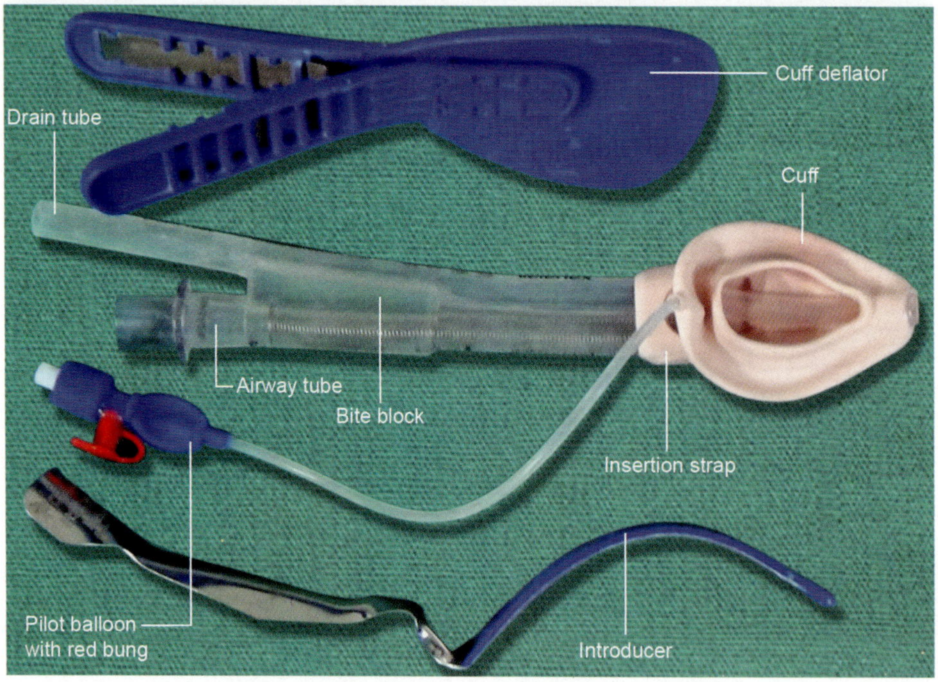

Fig. 30: Laryngeal mask airway (LMA)—ProSeal.

LARYNGEAL MASK AIRWAY—CLASSIC (FIGS. 31A AND B)

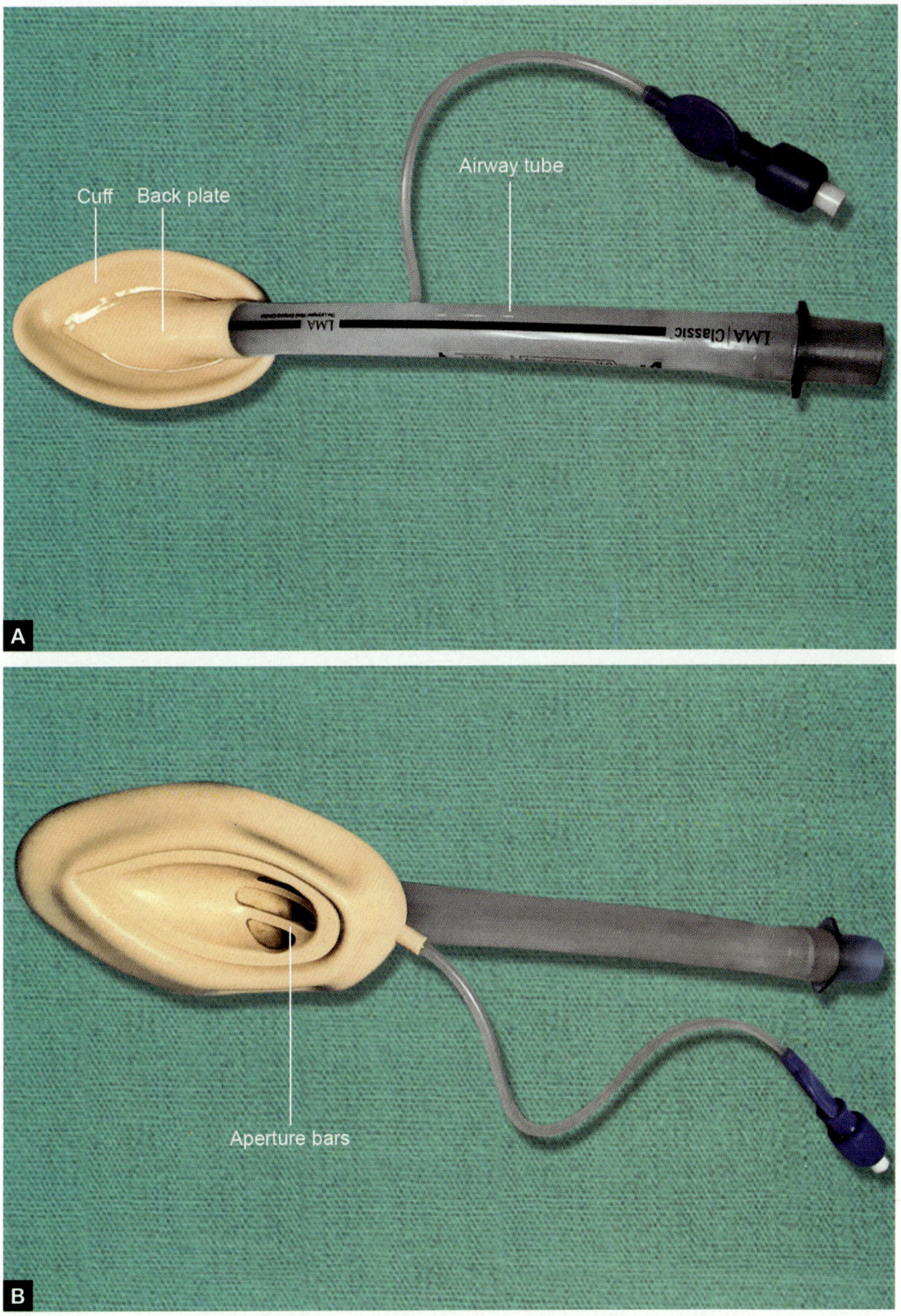

Figs. 31A and B: Laryngeal mask airway (LMA)—classic.

LARYNGEAL MASK AIRWAY—SUPREME (FIGS. 32A TO C)

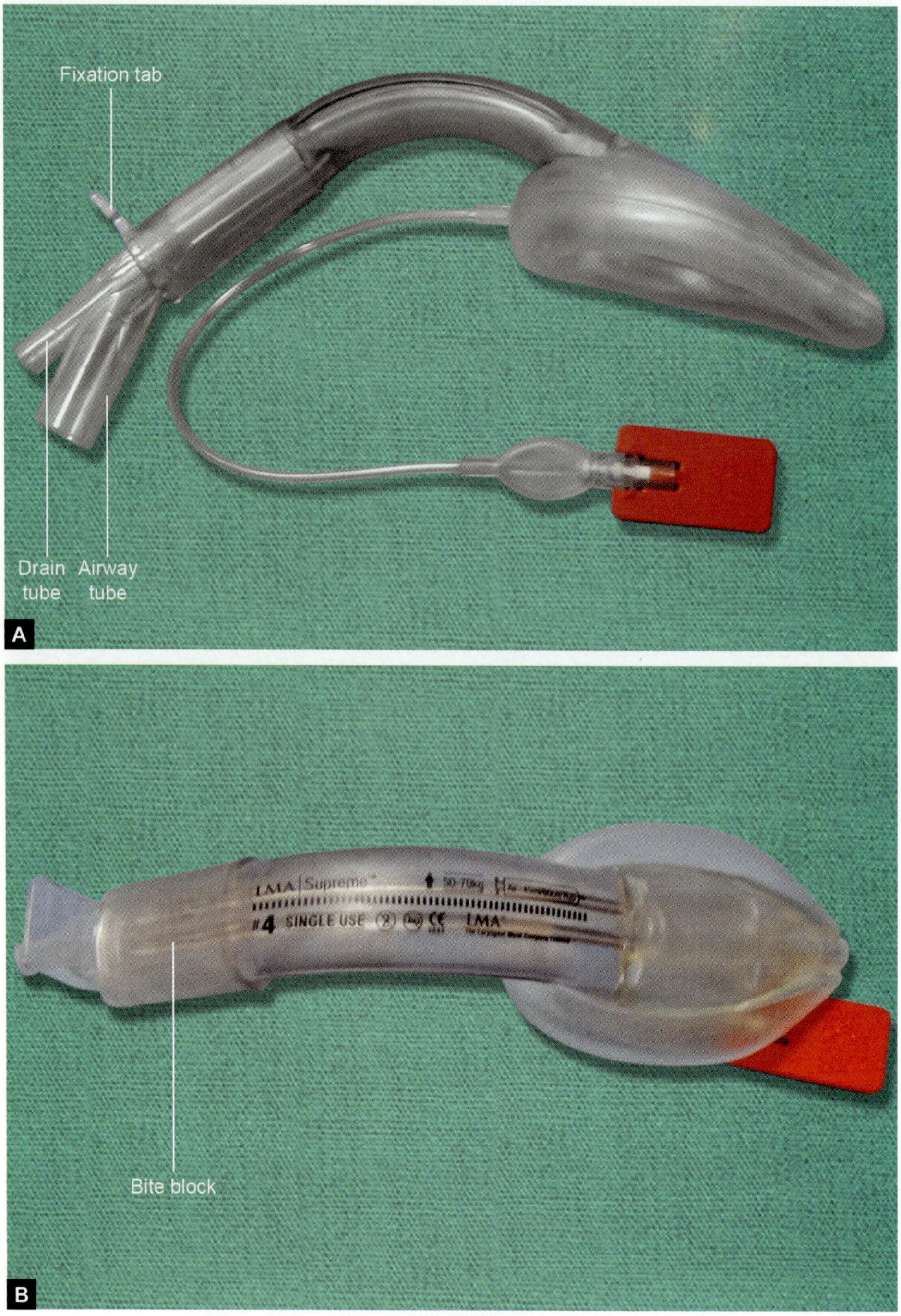

Figs. 32A and B

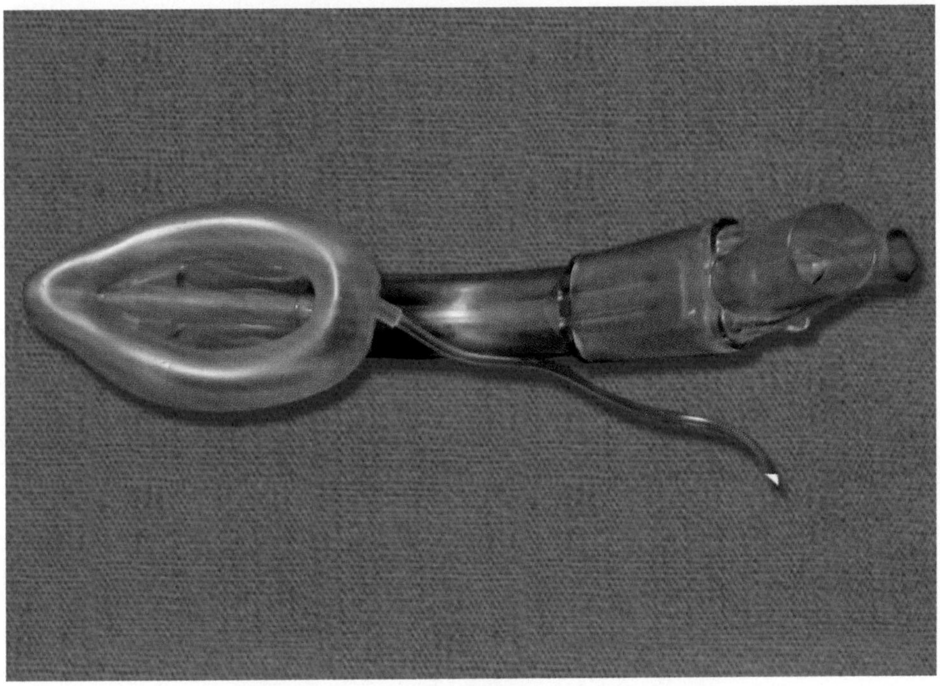

Fig. 32C

Figs. 32A to C: Laryngeal mask airway (LMA)—Supreme.

- Supraglottic airway devices (SADs) can be used to provide ventilation in ICU where endotracheal tube placement is not possible.
- Intubating SADs (Ambu AuraGain, Ambu Aura-I, i-gel, iLTS, ILMA) tide over the immediate crisis of failure to intubate.
- These also provide perfect conduit to introduce ETT fiberscopically through them without losing the airway at any time.
- Some other adjuncts can substitute for difficult mask ventilation. These are—SADs (nonintubating—LTS, ProSeal, Supreme, Classic-LMA, Ambu AuraOnce; intubating already shown).

HIGH FLOW NASAL OXYGEN CANNULA (HFNC) (FIG. 33)

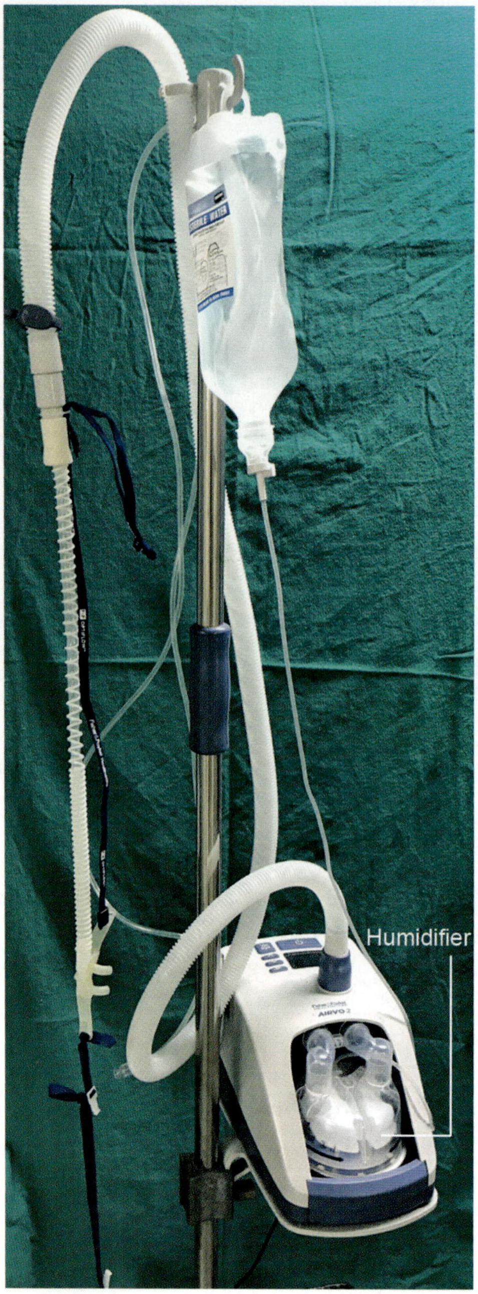

Fig. 33: High flow oxygen therapy (HFOT).

- Provides high flow (up to 60 L) of humidified O_2 with up to 4 cm continuous positive airway pressure (CPAP) (up to 100% which is regulatable) which is comfortable to the patient. Can be used while intubating or during bronchoscopy.

PERCUTANEOUS TRACHEOSTOMY SET (FIG. 34)

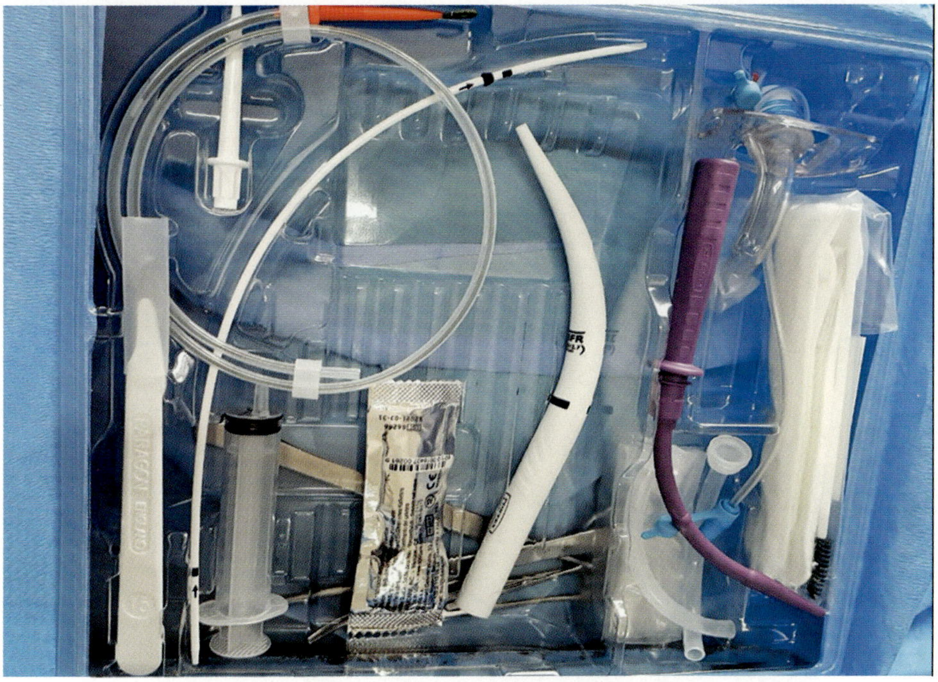

Fig. 34: Percutaneous tracheostomy (PCT)—single dilator technique.

Commonly used techniques for percutaneous tracheostomy:

- Single dilator technique.
- Blue Rhino single dilator technique.
- Ciaglia (graduated dilator) technique.
- Griggs (forceps) technique.
- PercTwist—tracheal stoma is created by a screw like device.

Indications

- Upper airway obstruction (due to trauma, burn, tumor, corrosive poisoning, obstructive sleep apnea, etc).
- Inability to protect the airway from aspiration (due stroke, head injury postneurosurgery, etc).
- Conduit for pulmonary toilet.
- Weaning facilitation from prolonged mechanical ventilation.

MINI-TRACHEOSTOMY SET (FIG. 35)

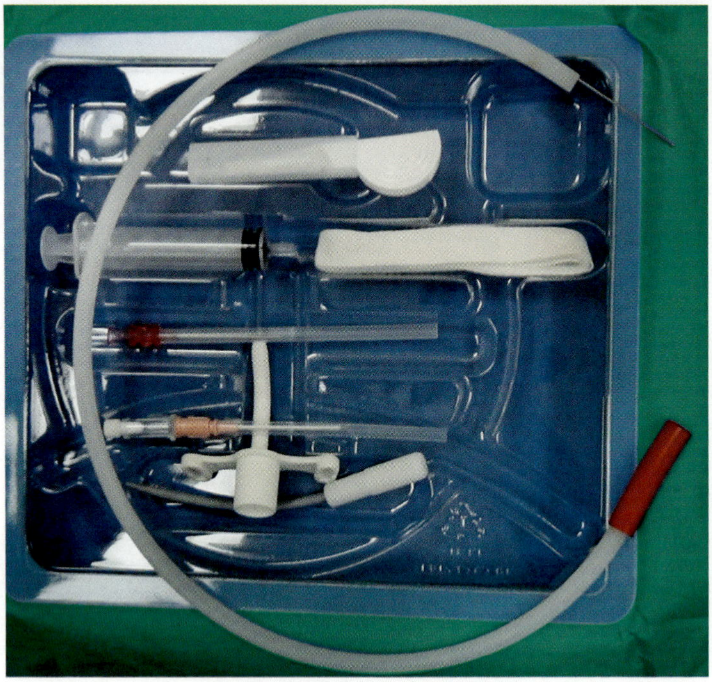

Fig. 35: Mini-tracheostomy set.

- Mini-tracheostomy is a technique to place a small (4 mm internal diameter) uncuffed tube percutaneously.
- It is usually inserted through cricothyroid membrane.
- Mini-tracheostomy is primarily meant for pulmonary toileting by tracheal suction through mini-tracheostomy tube.
- It does not protect airway from aspiration.

TRACHEOSTOMY TUBE (FIGS. 36A AND B)

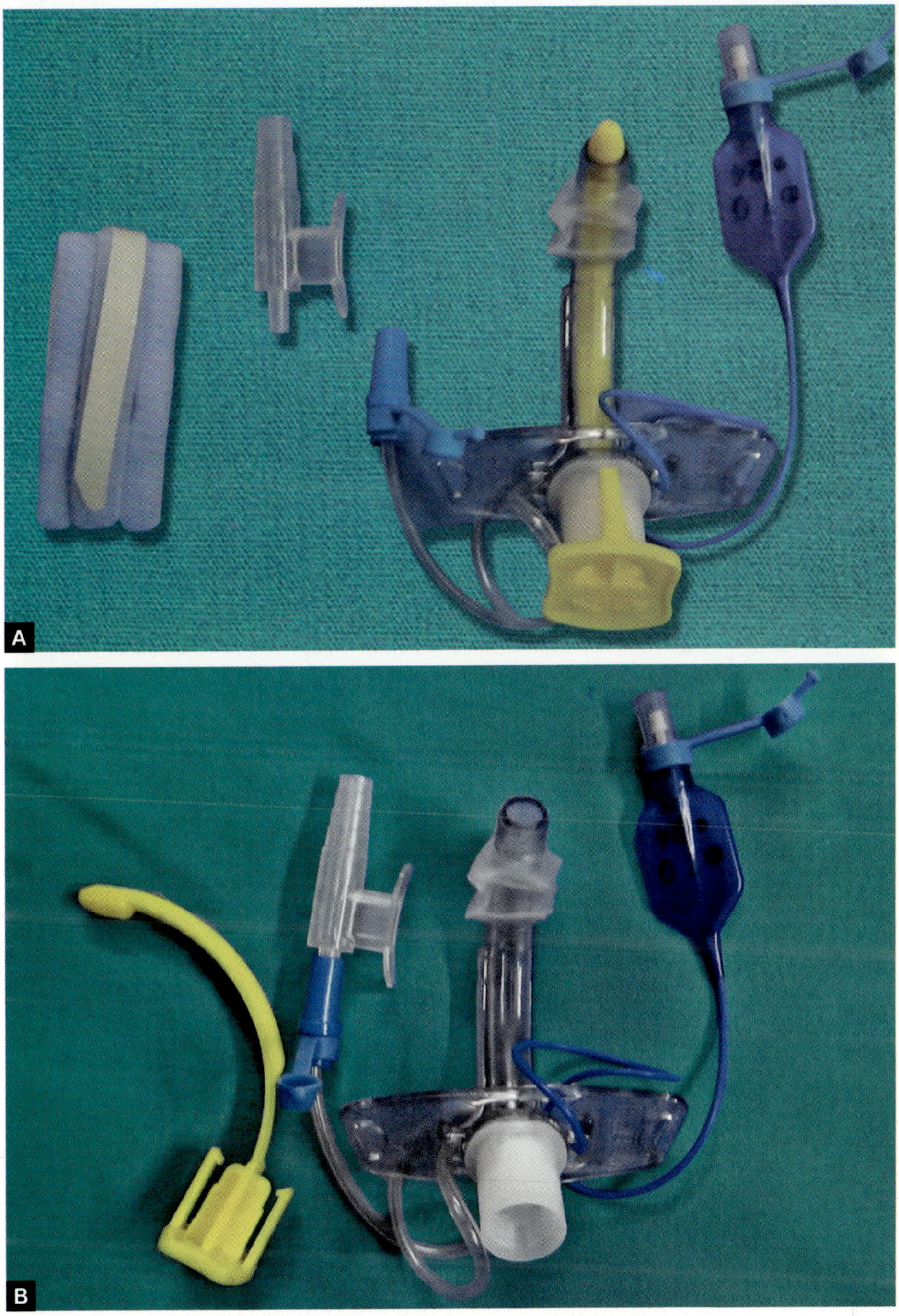

Figs. 36A and B: Different sets of tracheostomy tube.

T-PIECE (FIG. 37)

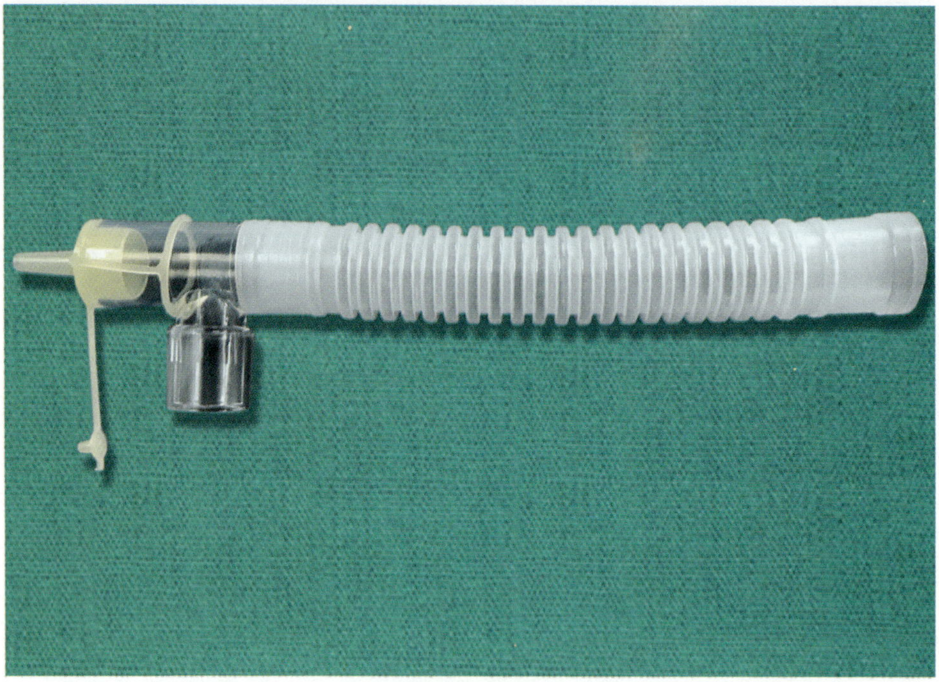

Fig. 37: T-piece.

- T-piece is used for oxygen supplementation through endotraheal tube and tracheostomy. It is also frequently used for spontaneous breathing trial during weaning from ventilation.
- T-piece provides precise FiO_2 and adequate humidification.

AIRWAY EXCHANGE CATHETER (FIG. 38)

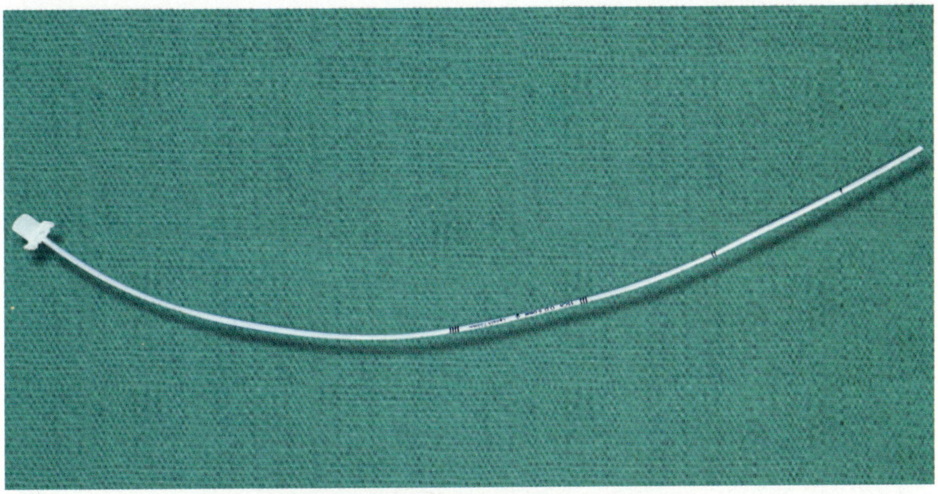

Fig. 38: Airway exchange catheter (AEC).

HEAT AND MOISTURE EXCHANGE (HME) CATHETER WITH FILTER (FIG. 39)

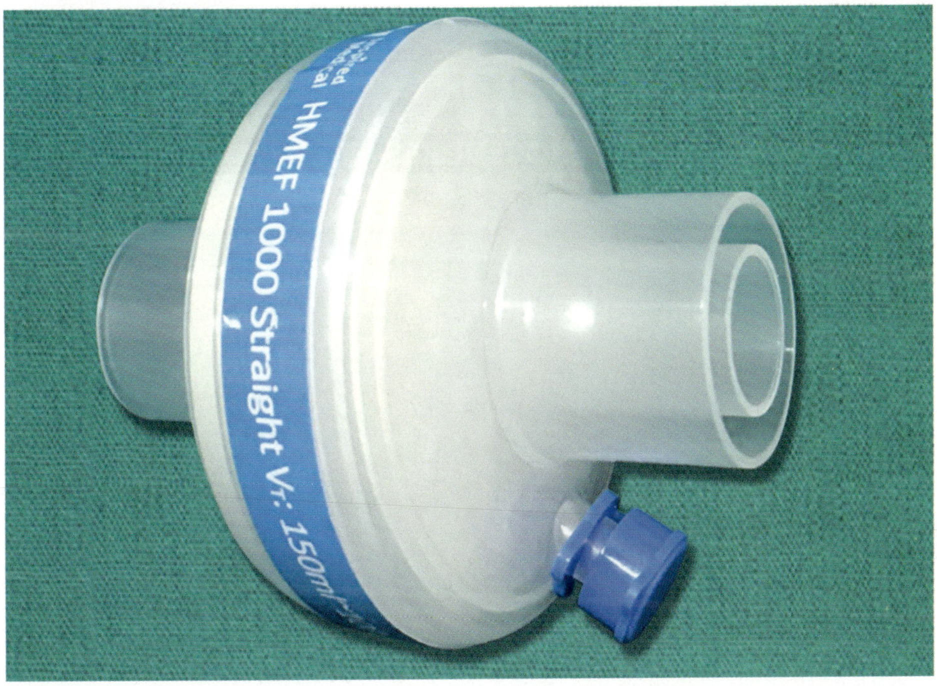

Fig. 39: Heat and moisture exchange filter (HMEF).

- Providing humidification.
- Can be a bacterial/viral filter.
- Generally changed every 24 hours.

SWEDISH NOSE (FIG. 40)

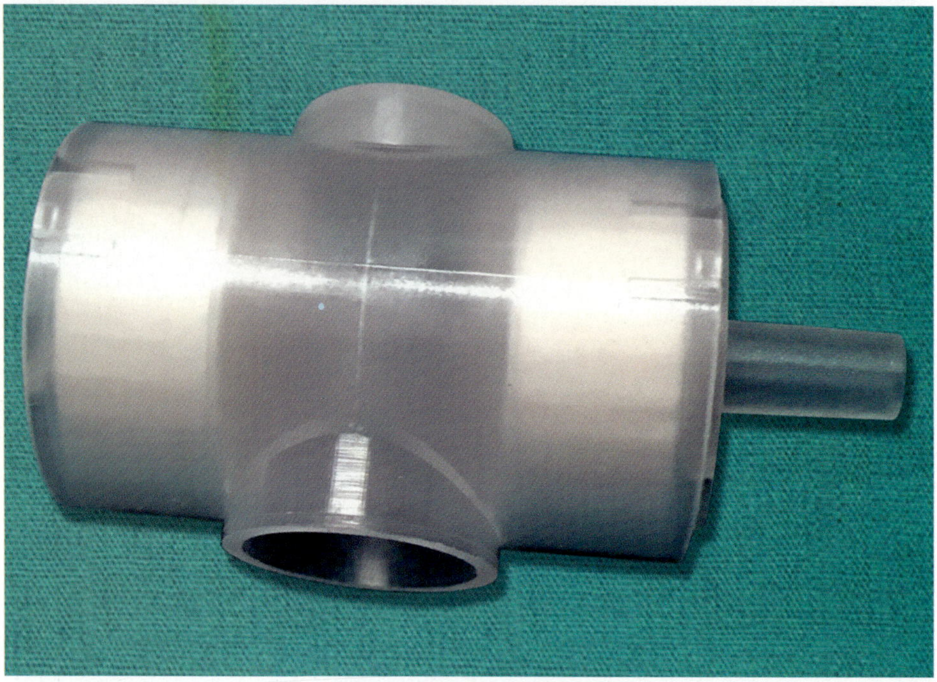

Fig. 40: "Swedish" nose.

- Used once patient is weaned off the ventilator with a tracheostomy.

CATHETER MOUNT WITH PORT FOR PROCEDURES (FIG. 41)

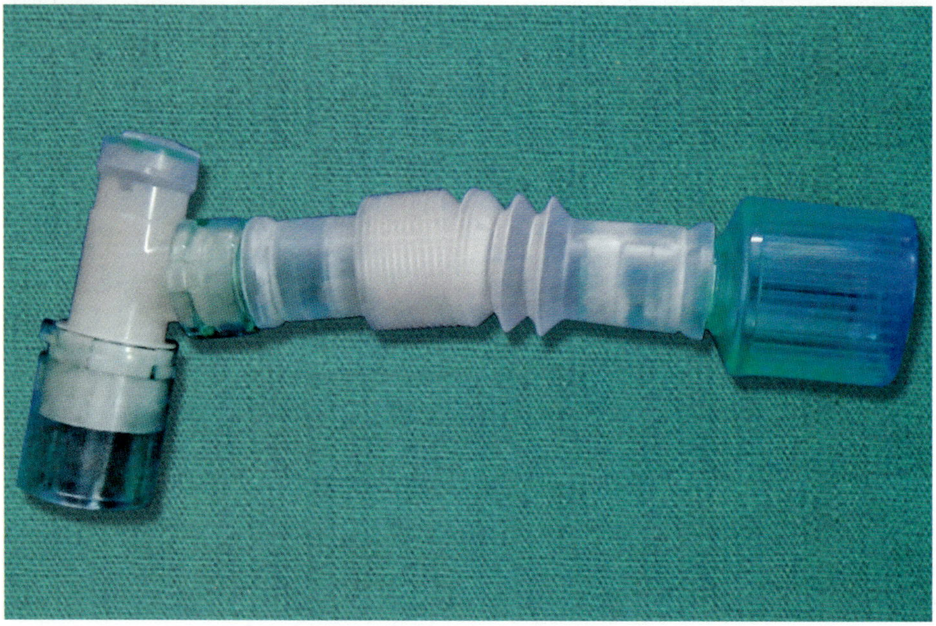

Fig. 41: Catheter mount with port.

BAIN CIRCUIT (FIG. 42)

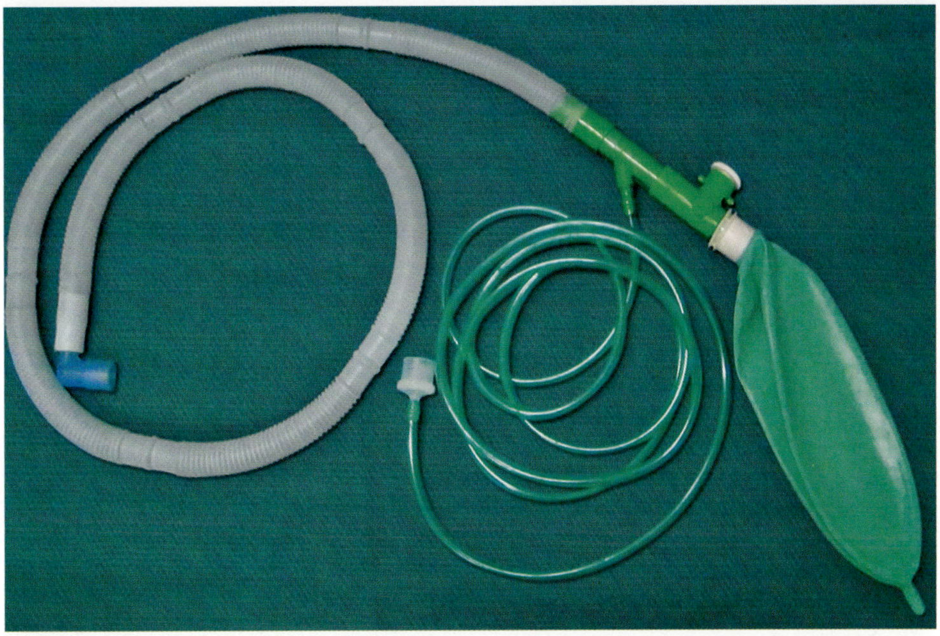

Fig. 42: Bain circuit.

VENTILATOR CIRCUIT (FIG. 43)

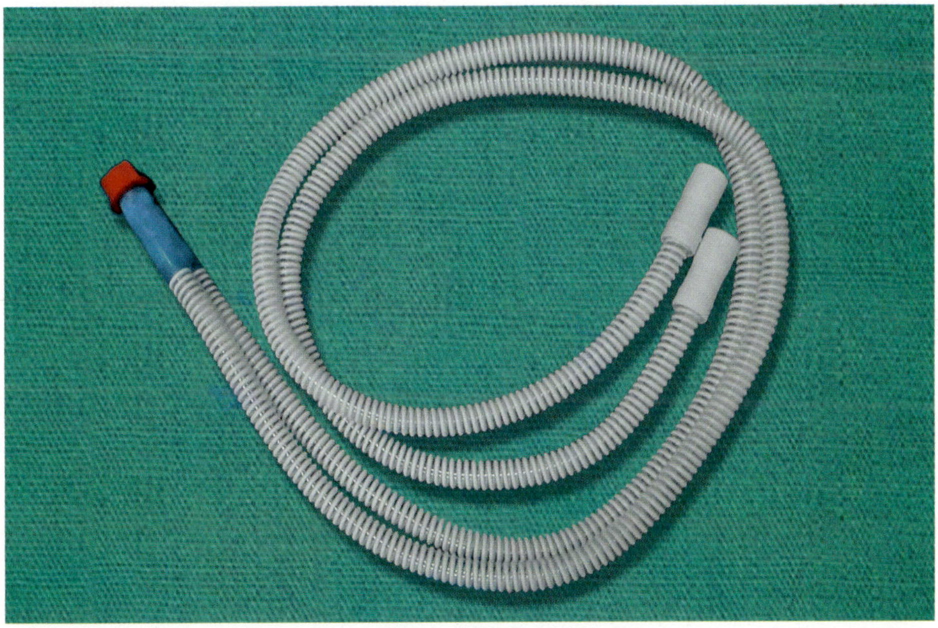

Fig. 43: Ventilator circuit.

MAPLESON-C CIRCUIT (FIG. 44)

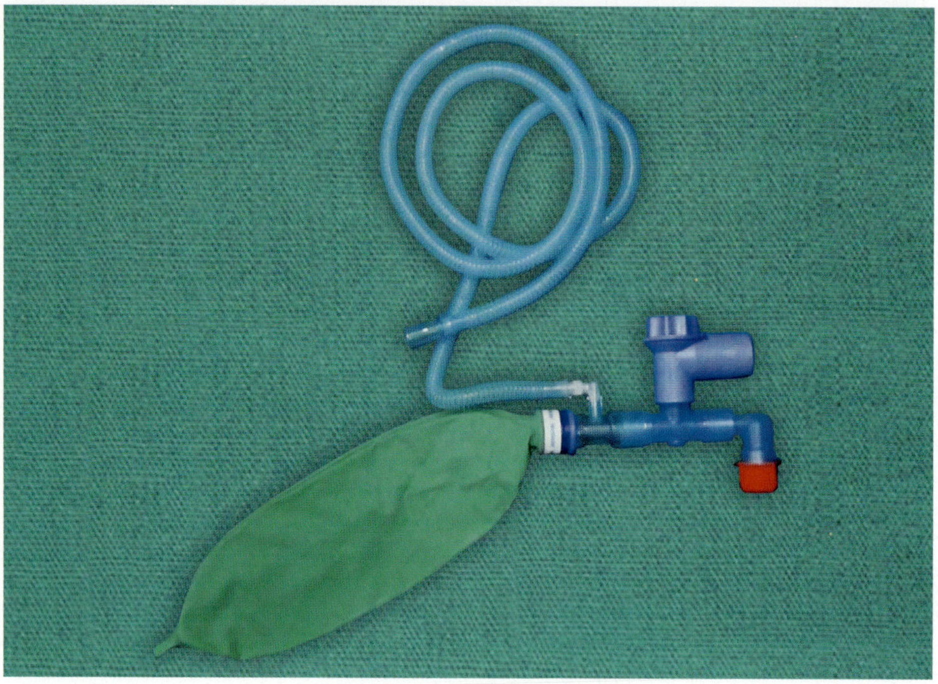

Fig. 44: Mapleson-C circuit.

SECTION 2

Respiratory System

CHAPTER

3

Bronchoscopic View and Clinical Features

GC Khilnani, Pawan Tiwari, Saurabh Mittal

BRONCHOSCOPIC VIEW OF NORMAL ANATOMY (FIGS. 1 TO 20)

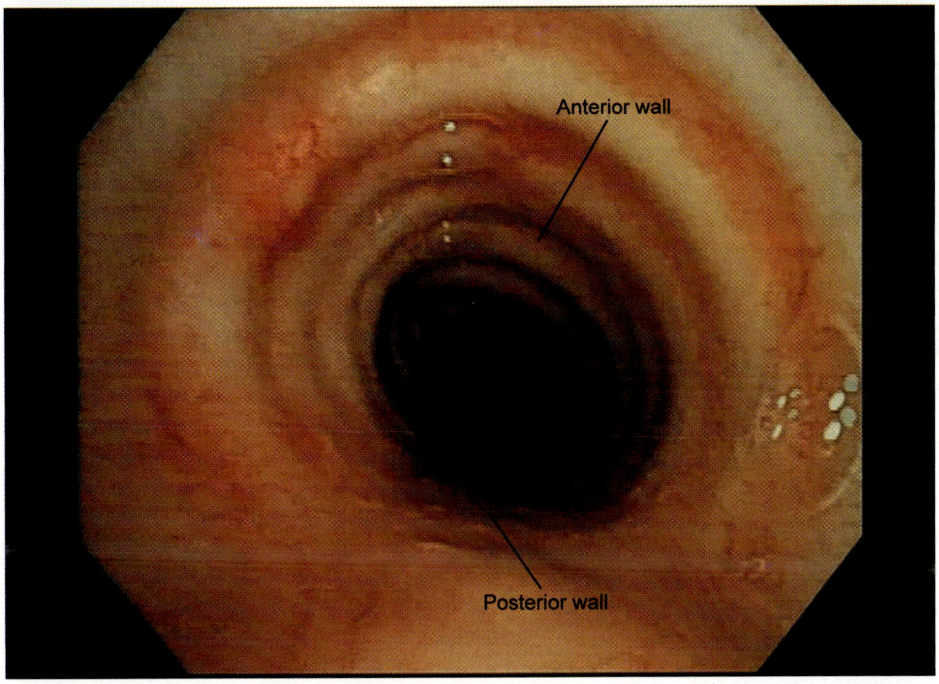

Fig. 1: Normal trachea.

- C-shaped cartilaginous rings in anterolateral wall.
- Membranous posterior wall.

Lower Trachea showing Carina, Left and Right Main Bronchi (Fig. 2)

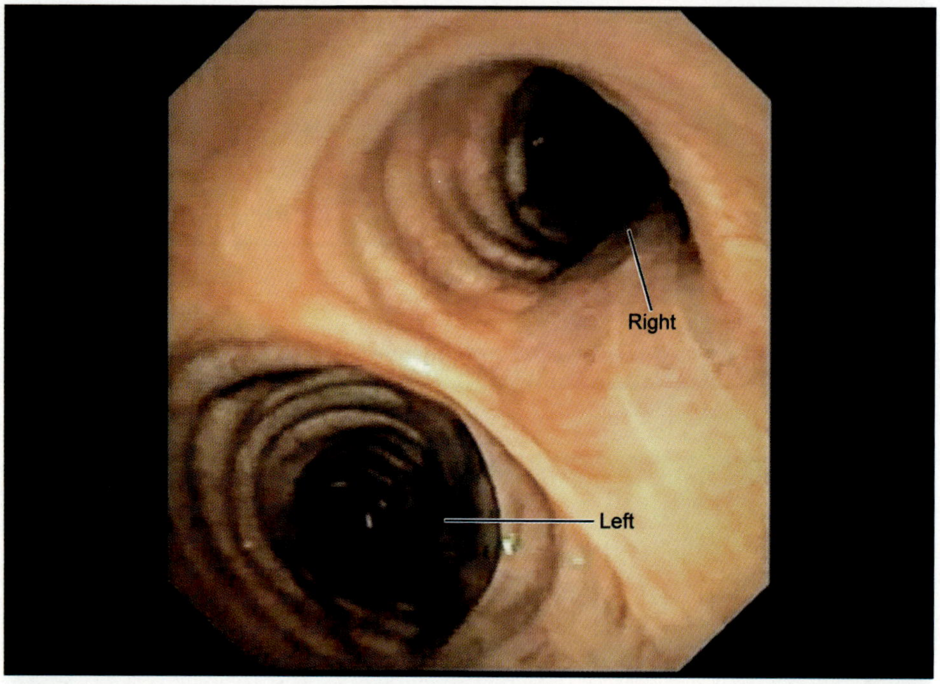

Fig. 2: Carina and both main bronchi.

Right Upper Lobe Bronchus dividing into Anterior, Apical and Lateral Segments (Fig. 3)

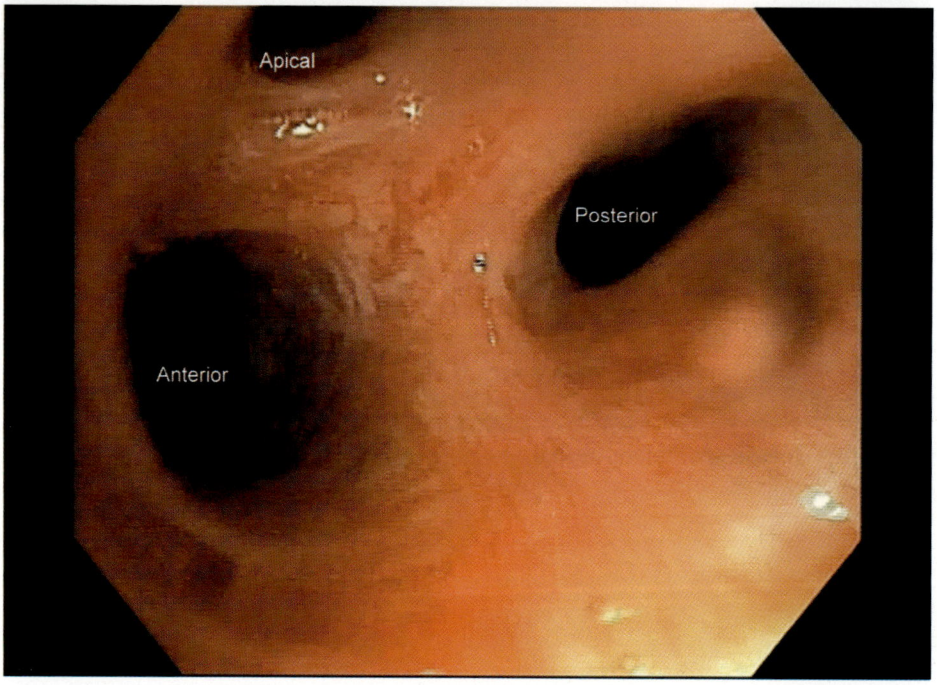

Fig. 3: Normal right upper lobe bronchus with anterior, apical and posterior segmental openings.

Lower Bronchus Intermedius showing Right Middle Lobe Bronchus, Right Lower Lobe Bronchus and Right Lower Lobe Apical Segment Bronchus (Fig. 4)

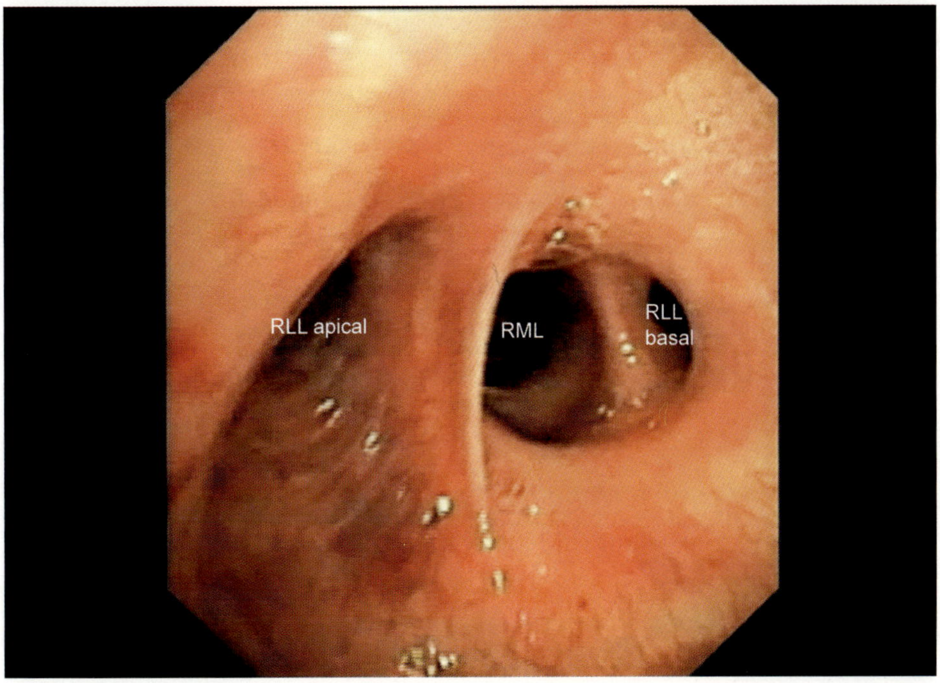

Fig. 4: Bronchus intermedius with RML RLL apical and RLL basal segments. (RML: Right middle lobe; RLL: Right lower lobe)

Right Middle Lobe Bronchus showing Medial and Lateral Segments (Fig. 5)

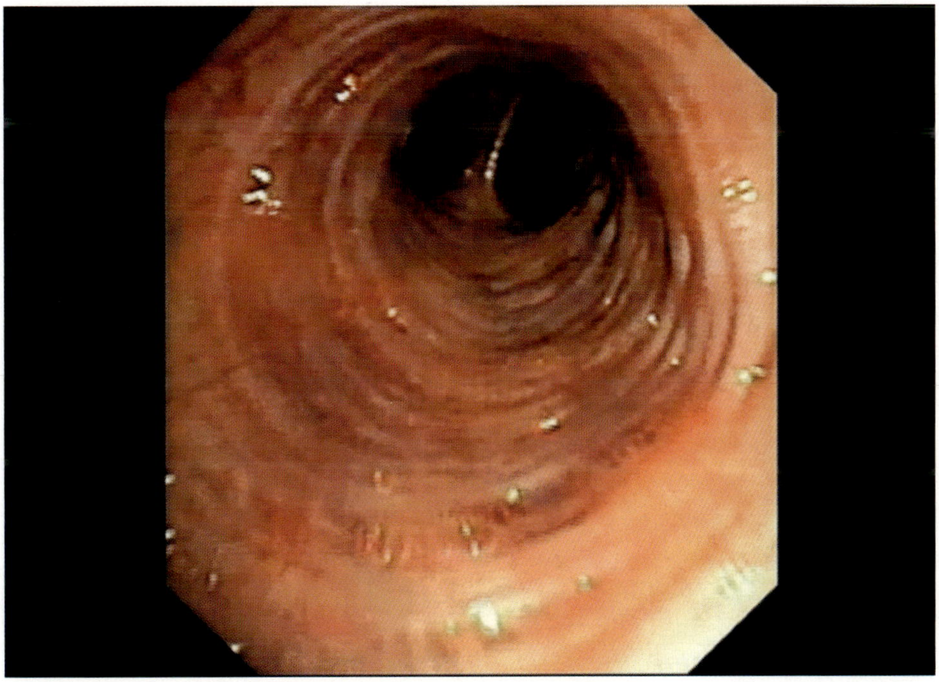

Fig. 5: Right middle lobe (RML) with segmental bronchi.

Right Lower Lobe Basal Segments with Anterior, Lateral and Posterior Basal Segmental Openings (Fig. 6)

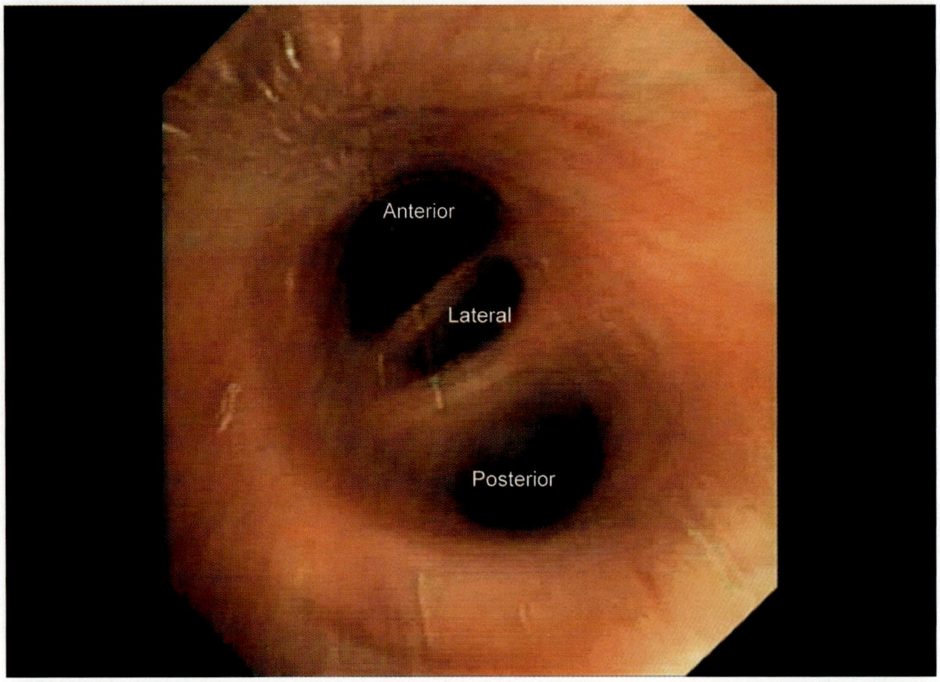

Fig. 6: Right lower lobe (RLL) with anterior, lateral and posterior (ALP) basal segmental openings.

Distal Left Main Bronchus dividing into Left Upper and Lower Lobe Bronchi (Fig. 7)

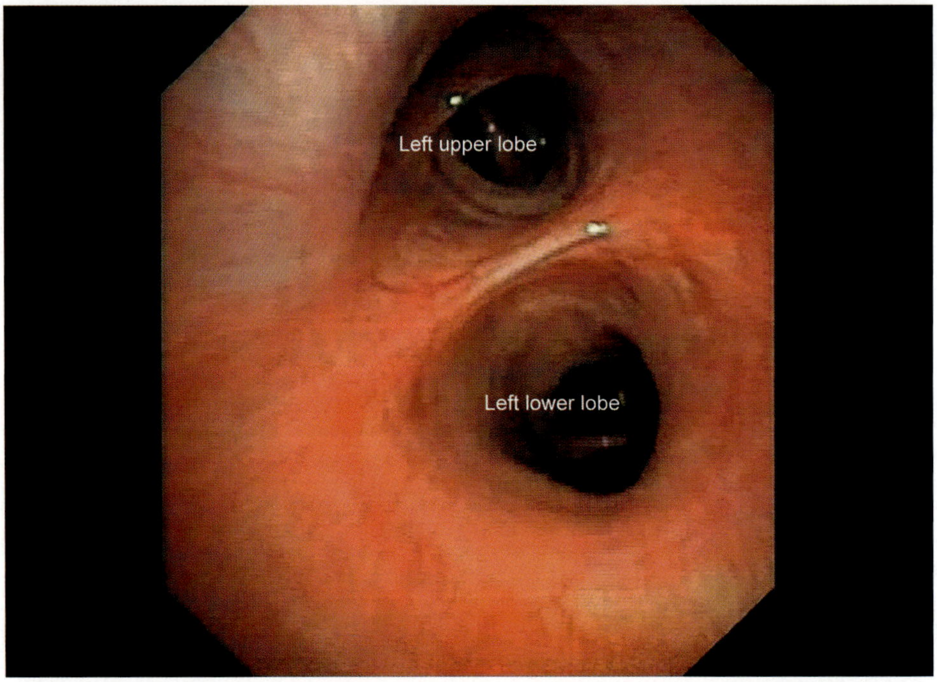

Fig. 7: Distal left main bronchus (LMB) with upper and lower lobe bronchus.

Left Lower Lobe Bronchus with Left Lower Lobe Apical Segment and Left Lower Lobe Basal Segments (Fig. 8)

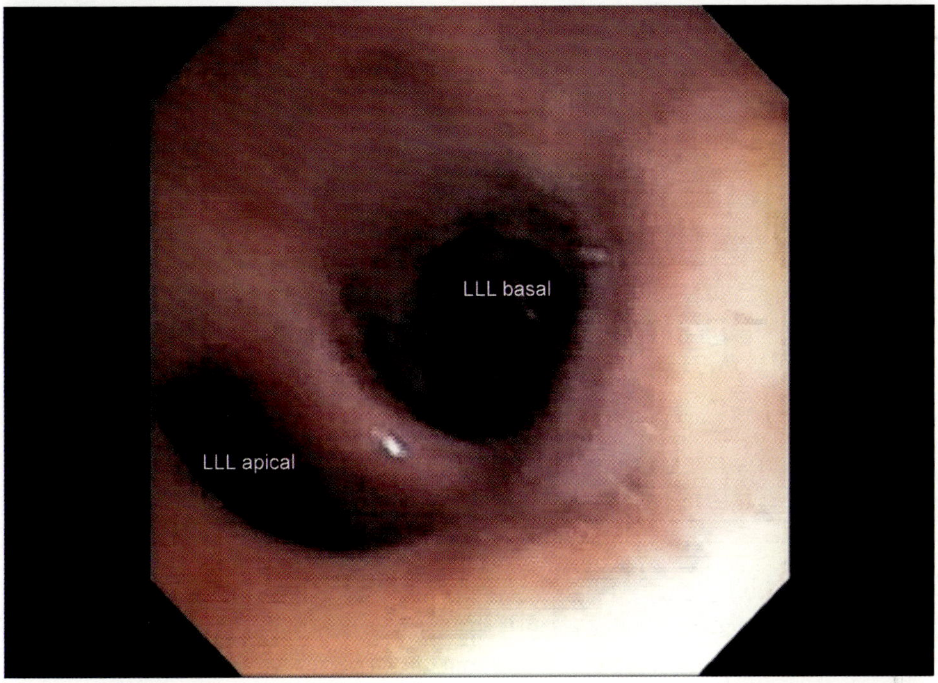

Fig. 8: Left lower lobe (LLL) bronchus with LLL apical and basal segments.

Left Lower Lobe Basal Segments: Anterior, Lateral and Posterior (Fig. 9)

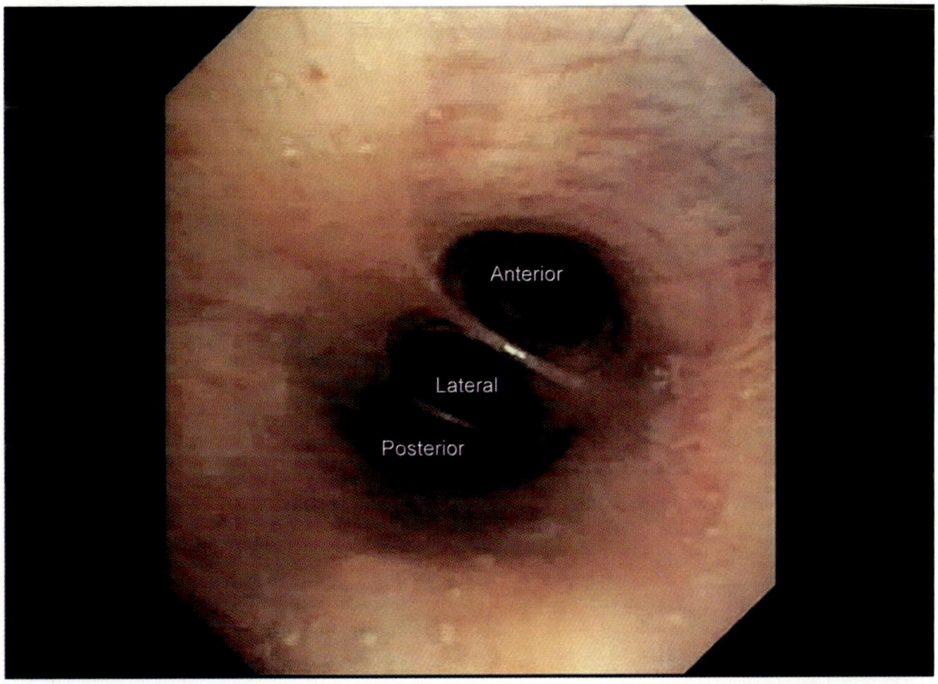

Fig. 9: Left lower lobe (LLL) basal segments anterior, lateral and posterior (ALP).

Left Main Bronchus Mucous Plug in a Patient with Left Lung Collapse (Fig. 10)

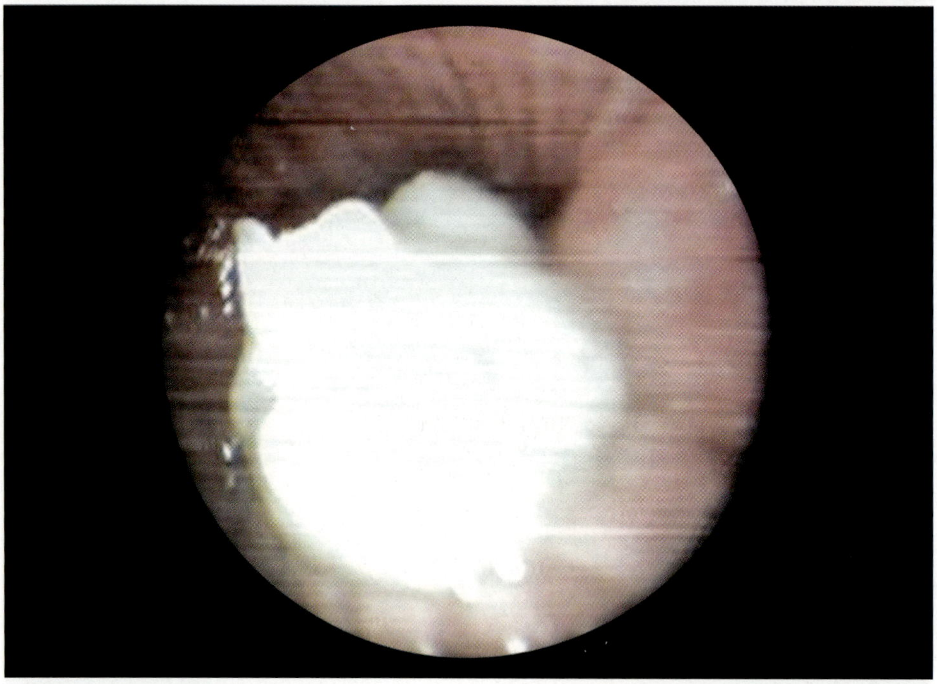

Fig. 10: Left main bronchus (LMB) thick mucous plug.

Endobronchial Mass Completely Occluding Right Main Bronchus (Fig. 11)

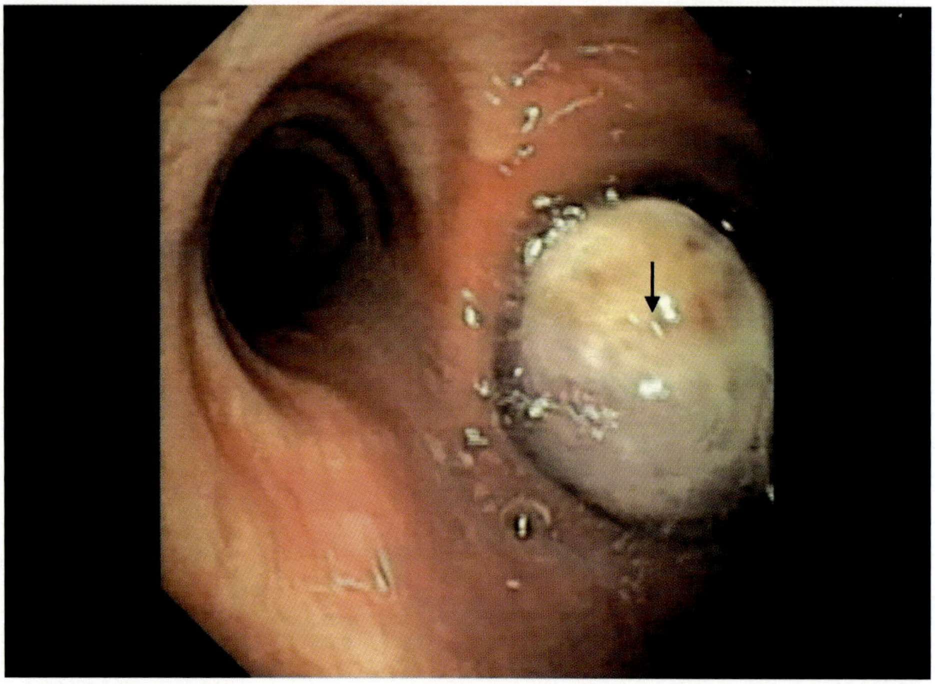

Fig. 11: Endobronchial mass in right main bronchus.

Extrinsic Compression of Posterior Tracheal Wall in a Patient with Esophageal Carcinoma (Fig. 12)

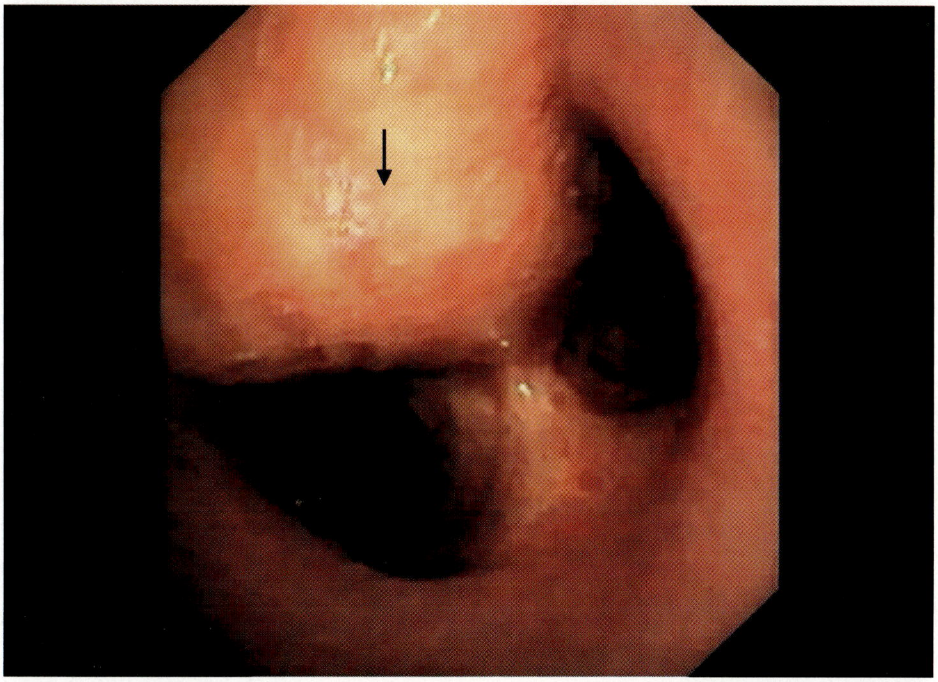

Fig. 12: Posterior tracheal compression (Carcinoma: esophagus).

Right Lower Lobe Basal Segment with Sharp Foreign Body (Board Pin) (Fig. 13)

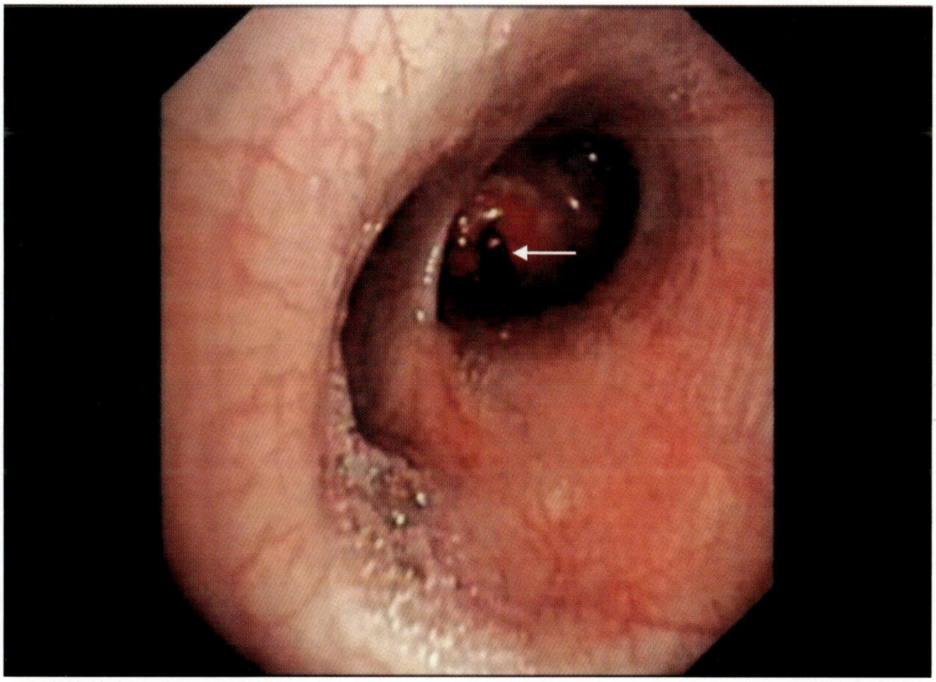

Fig. 13: Foreign body (Pin).

Tracheoesophageal Fistula Near Carina in a Patient with Carcinoma Esophagus (Fig. 14)

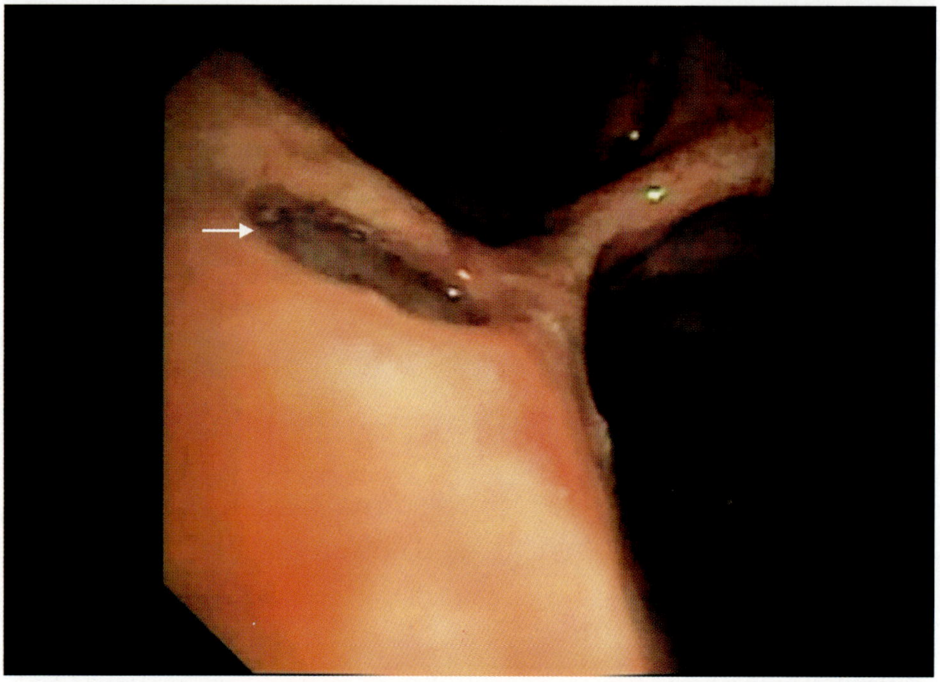

Fig. 14: Tracheoesophageal fistula.

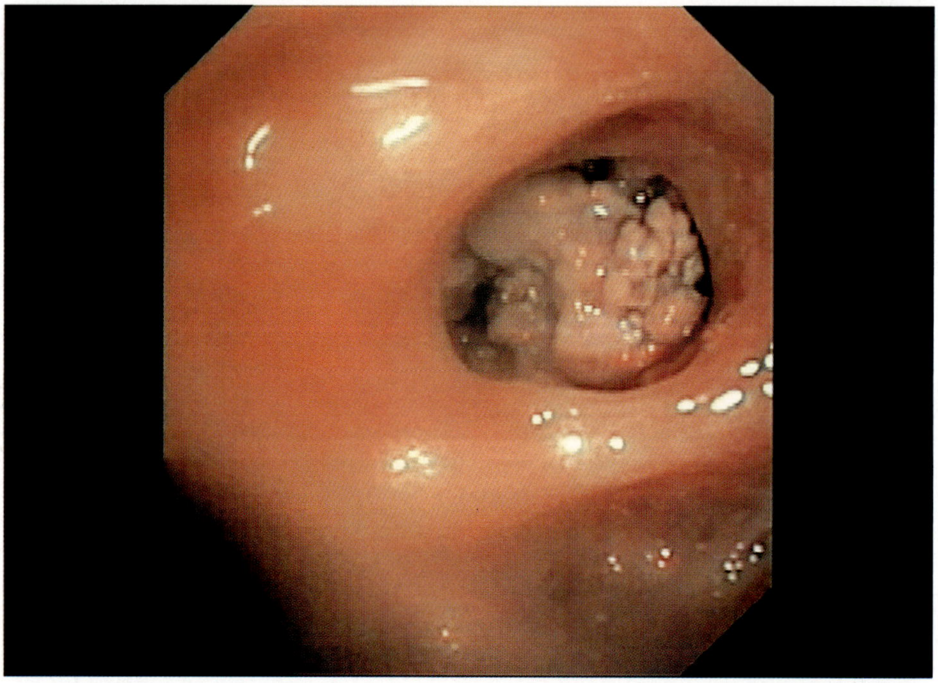

Fig. 15: Left upper lobe anteroinferior segment cavity with aspergilloma.

Bronchoscopic View of Blue Rhinotracheal Dilator during Percutaneous Tracheostomy (Fig. 16)

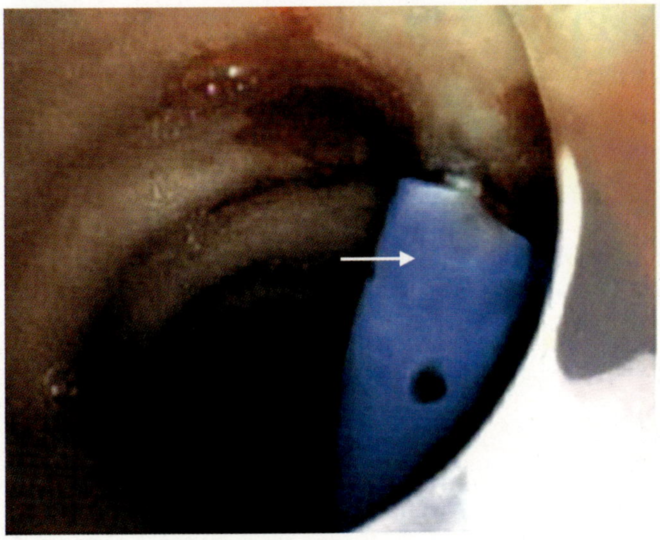

Fig. 16: Tracheostomy dilator bronchoscopic view.

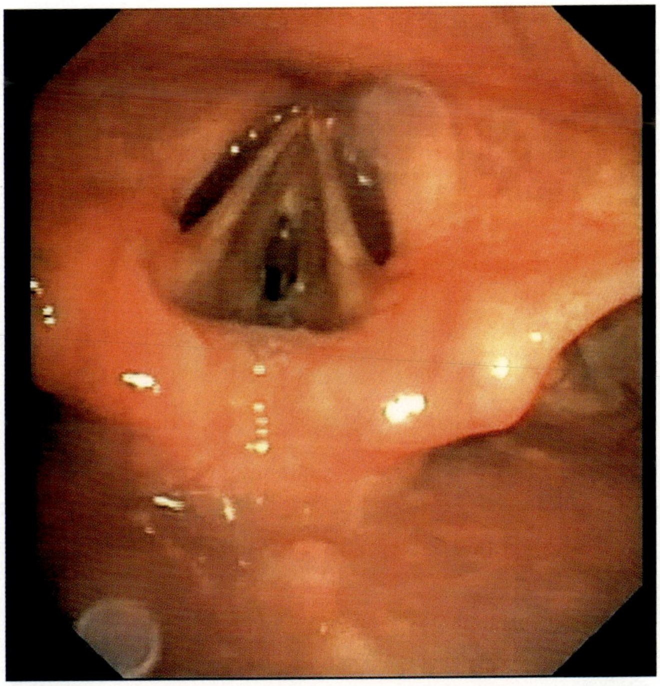

Fig. 17: Subglottic tracheal stenosis.

Endobronchial Mass with Necrotic Surface and Active Bleeding (Fig. 18)

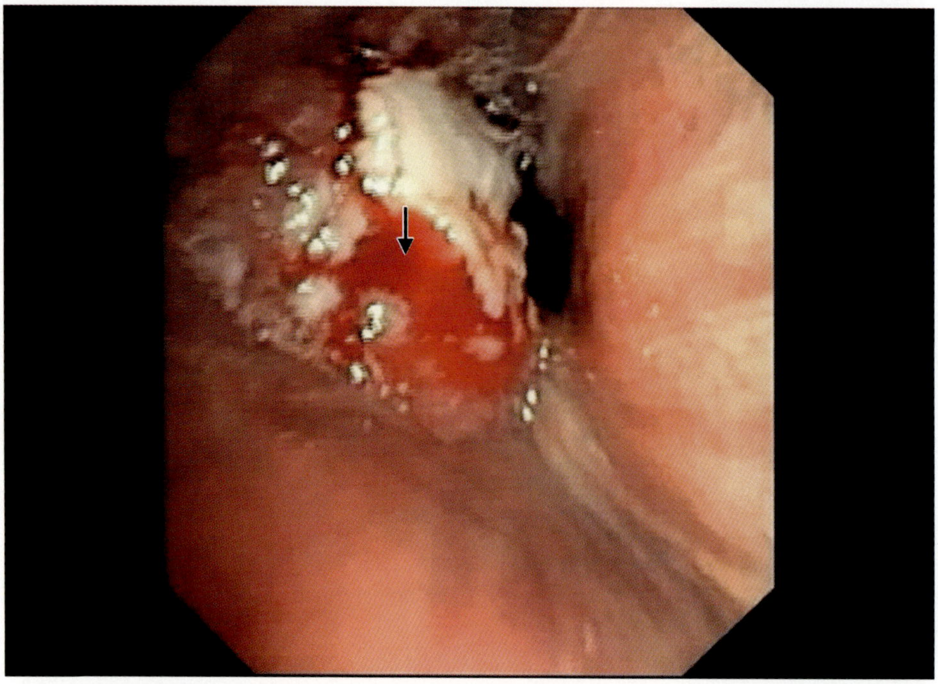

Fig. 18: Endobronchial lesion with active bleeding preargon photocoagulation.

Covered Self-expanding Metallic Tracheal Stent *in situ* in a Patient with Tracheal Carcinoma (Fig. 19)

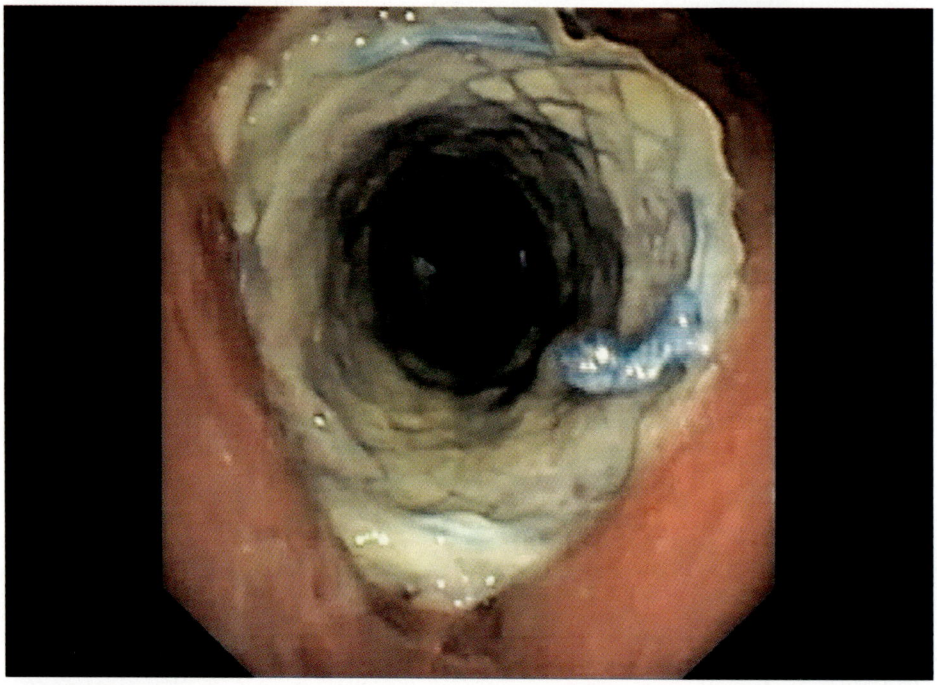

Fig. 19: Tracheal self-expanding metallic tracheal stent (SEMS) postdeployment proximal view.

Tracheal Silicon Stent *in situ* with Proximal Granulation Tissue in a Patient with Postintubation Tracheal Stenosis (Fig. 20)

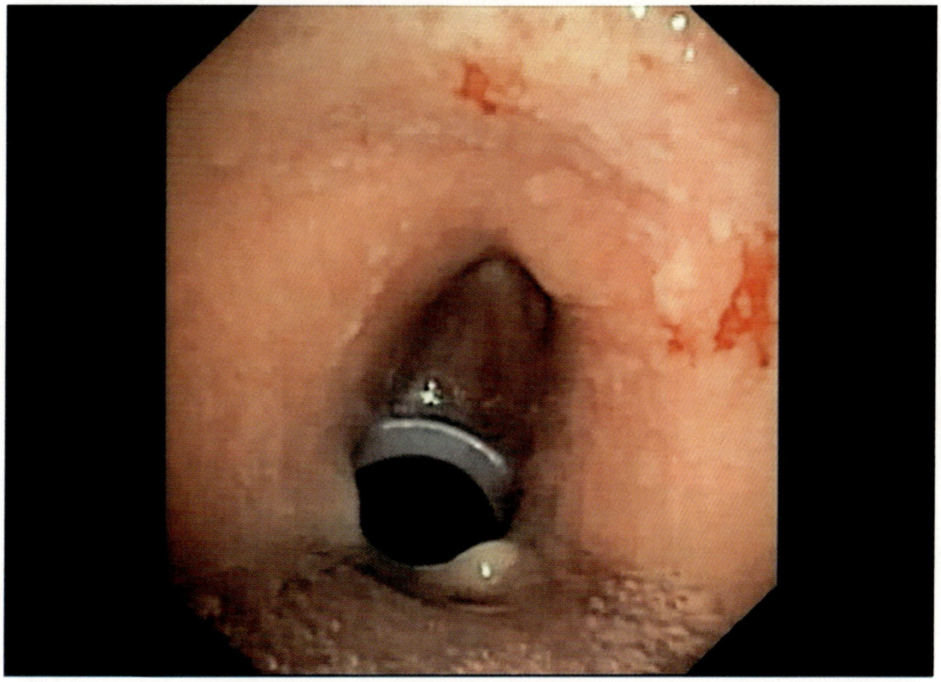

Fig. 20: Tracheal silicon stent with proximal granulation.

CLINICAL FEATURES (FIGS. 21 TO 24)

Obstructive Sleep Apnea Syndrome (Fig. 21)

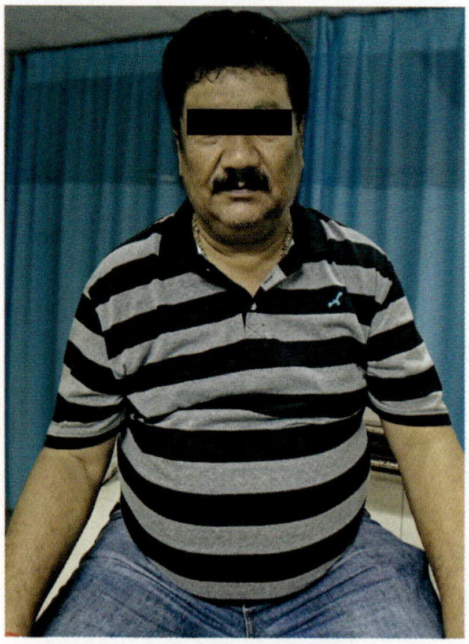

Fig. 21: Appearance in obstructive sleep apnea (OSA).

Clinical appearance in a patient of obstructive sleep apnea (OSA) syndrome:

- Truncal obesity.
- High waist hip ratio.
- Fat deposition around neck.
- Patient had snoring disturbing bed partner, excessive daytime somnolence and witnessed choking spells.

Kyphoscoliosis (Fig. 22)

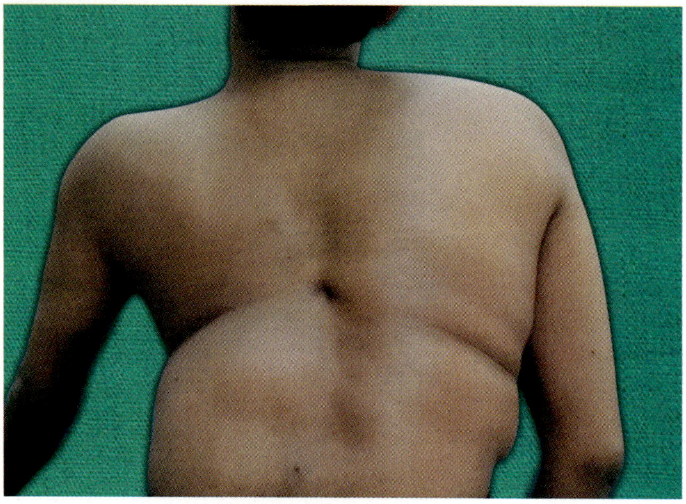

Fig. 22: Kyphoscoliosis posterior view.

- Posterior view showing abnormal lateral curvature of the spine.
- Abnormal skin folds along with dimpling of skin.
- Kyphotic deformity visible at mid-dorsal spine.
- Leads to restrictive ventilatory defect on spirometry.

Pigeon Chest (Pectus Carinatum) (Figs. 23A and B)

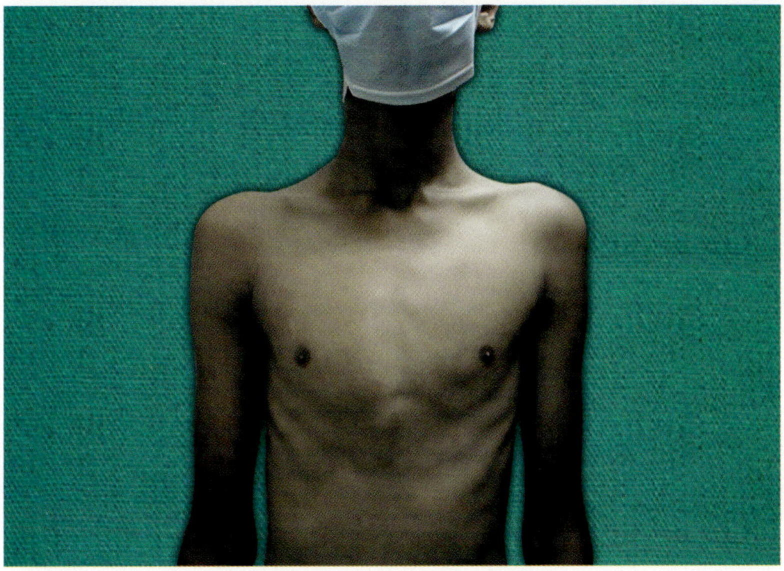

Fig. 23A: Pigeon chest anterior view.

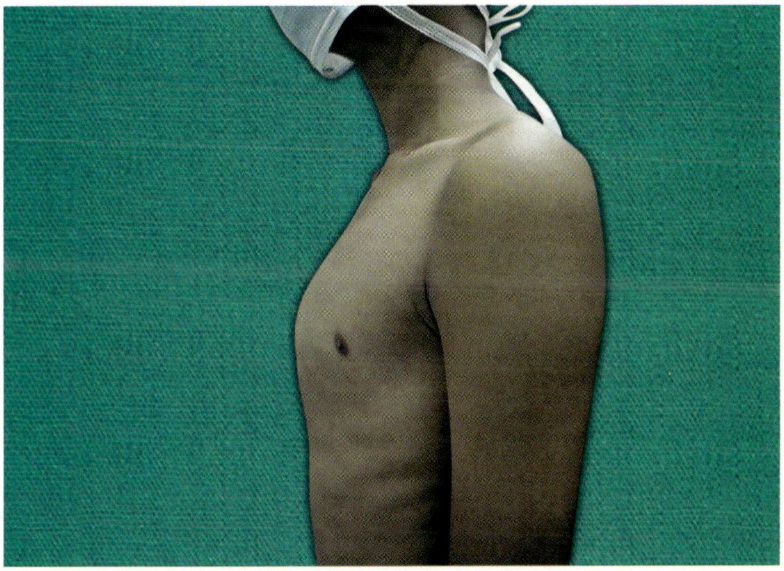

Fig. 23B: Pigeon chest lateral view.

- Congenital deformity.
- Forward protrusion of lower end of sternum.
- Usually asymptomatic.
- Treatment required for cosmetic purposes.

Prominent Accessory Muscles of Respiration (Fig. 24)

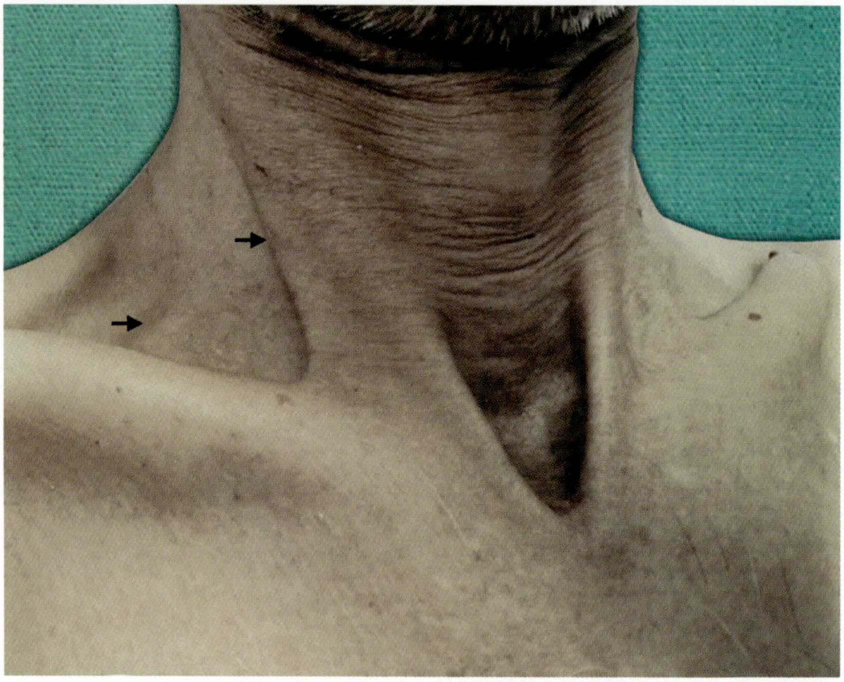

Fig. 24: Use of accessory muscles of respiration.

- Prominent sternocleidomastoid and scalene muscles.
- Suggest respiratory distress.

CHAPTER 4

Respiratory Issues in ICU

Poulomi Chatterjee, Yatin Mehta

CLINICAL SIGNS

Digital Clubbing (Figs. 1A and B)

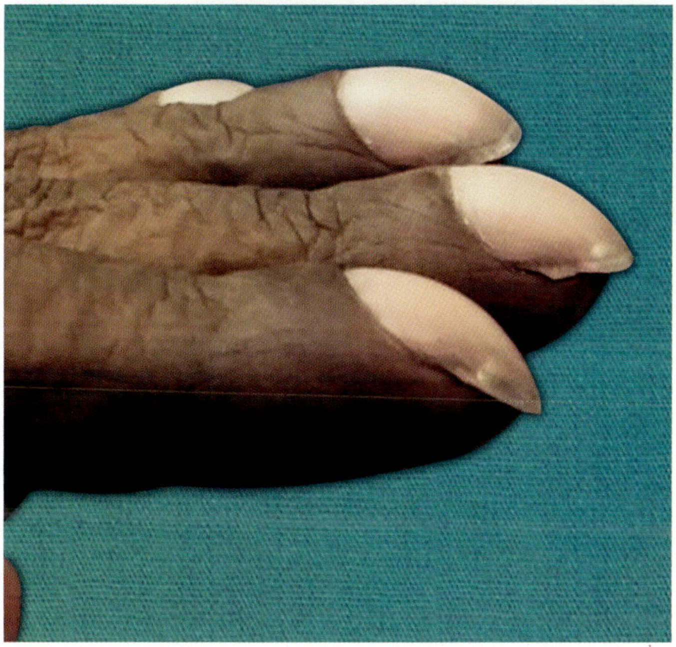

Fig. 1A: Patient with lung cancer with Grade 3 clubbing.

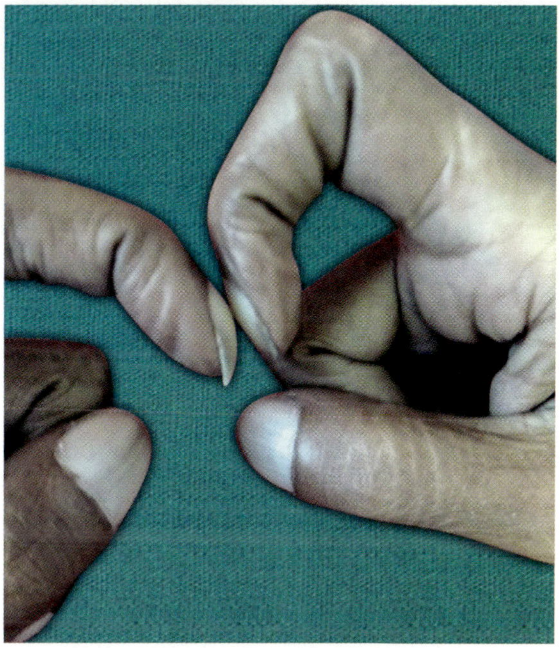

Fig. 1B: Schamroth's test—obliteration of the Schamroth's window—the earliest sign of clubbing.

It is the obliteration of the angle between the nail bed and cuticula (Lovibond's angle) (normal value 160°).

Many etiologies may be associated:

- C—Cardiac—congenital heart disease (cyanotic).
- L—Interstitial lung disease
  - Bronchiectasis
  - Suppurative lung disease—empyema, cystic fibrosis.
- U—Ulcerative colitis, Crohn's disease.
- B—Biliary cirrhosis and malabsorption.
- Idiopathic.
- N—Neoplastic disease—carcinoma, lymphoma.
- G—Graves' disease.

Most commonly associated with chronic hypoxemia.

Pedal Edema (Fig. 2)

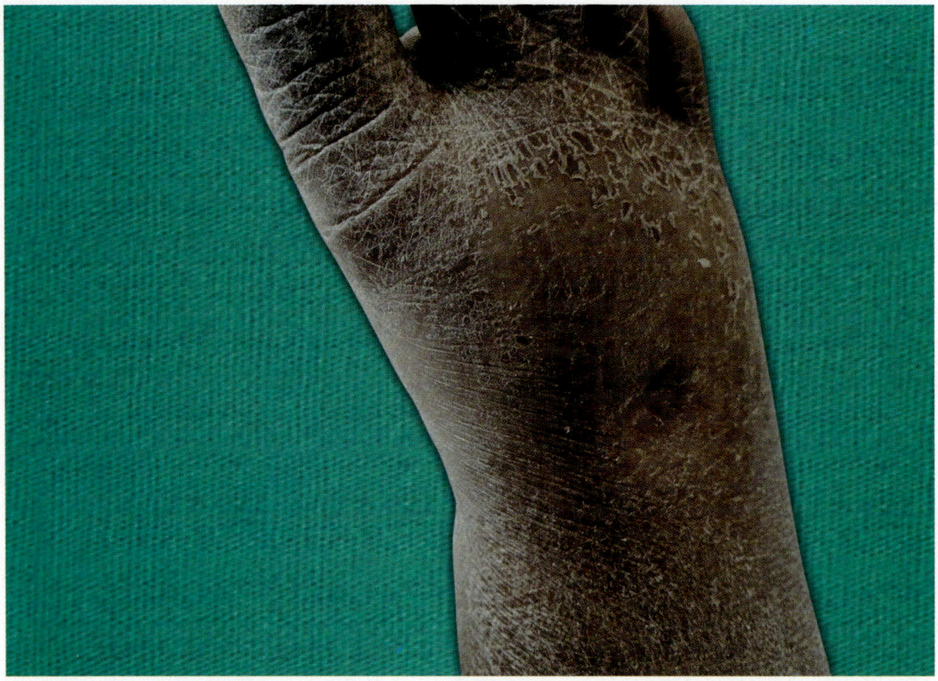

Fig. 2: Patient with severe hypoalbuminemia with pitting pedal edema.

- Accumulation of fluid in the subcutaneous tissue of the feet.
- Most commonly associated with increased venous capillary pressure—right ventricular (RV) dysfunction [i.e. secondary to chronic obstructive pulmonary disease (COPD)], kidney dysfunction, decreased oncotic pressure—hypoalbuminemia, deep venous thrombosis (DVT)—unilateral.
- Diuresis is the most common treatment.

OXYGEN DELIVERY DEVICES (FIGS. 3 TO 7)

- Indicated in both hypoxic and hypercapnic respiratory failure.
- Postoperative case.
- Postacute myocardial infarction.

Nasal Prongs (Fig. 3)

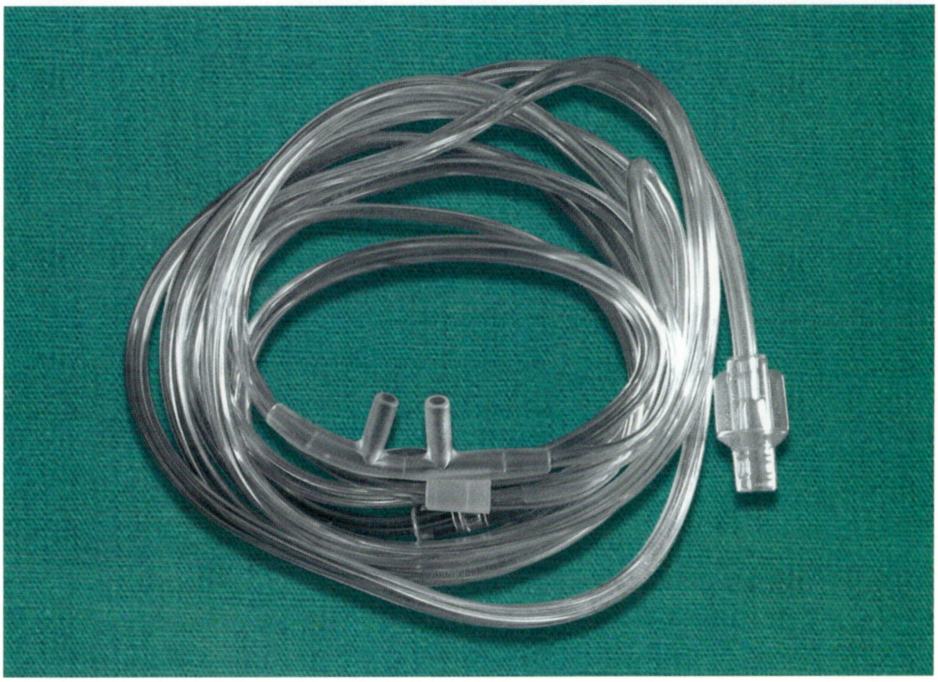

Fig. 3: Nasal prongs.

- FiO_2 is variable depends upon respiratory rate depth of inspiration and oxygen flow to device.
- Flow to nasal prongs varies between 1 L/min and 6 L/min oxygen).
- No reservoir in the device.

Face Mask (Fig. 4)

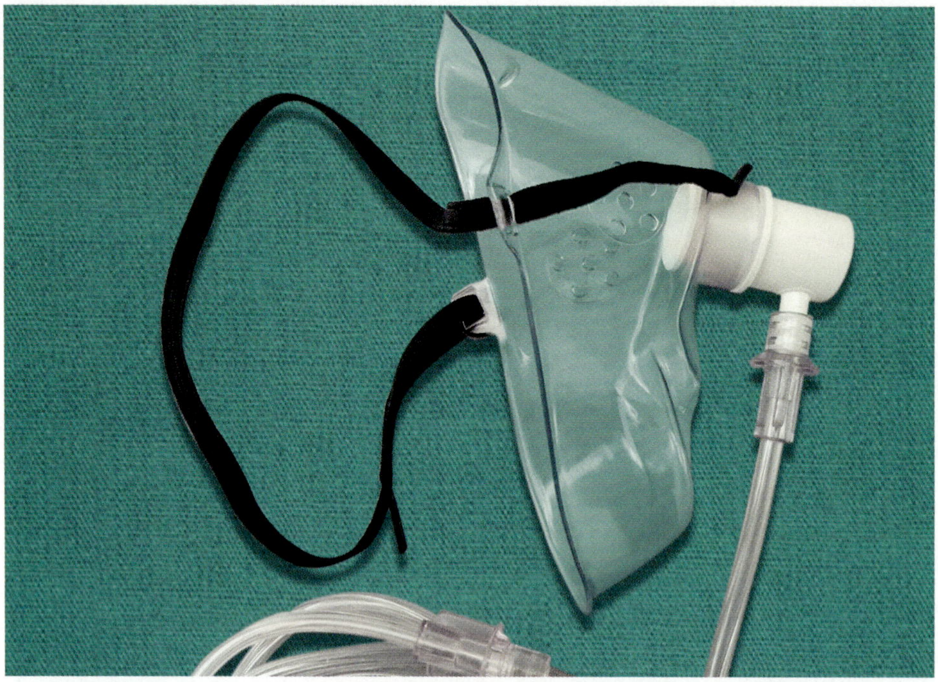

Fig. 4: Simple face mask.

- FiO_2 is variable depends upon respiratory rate depth of inspiration and oxygen flow to device.
- Flow to face mask varies between 6 L/min and 10 L/min of oxygen.
- Maximum FiO_2 - 0.6.

Reservoir Face Mask (Figs. 5A and B)

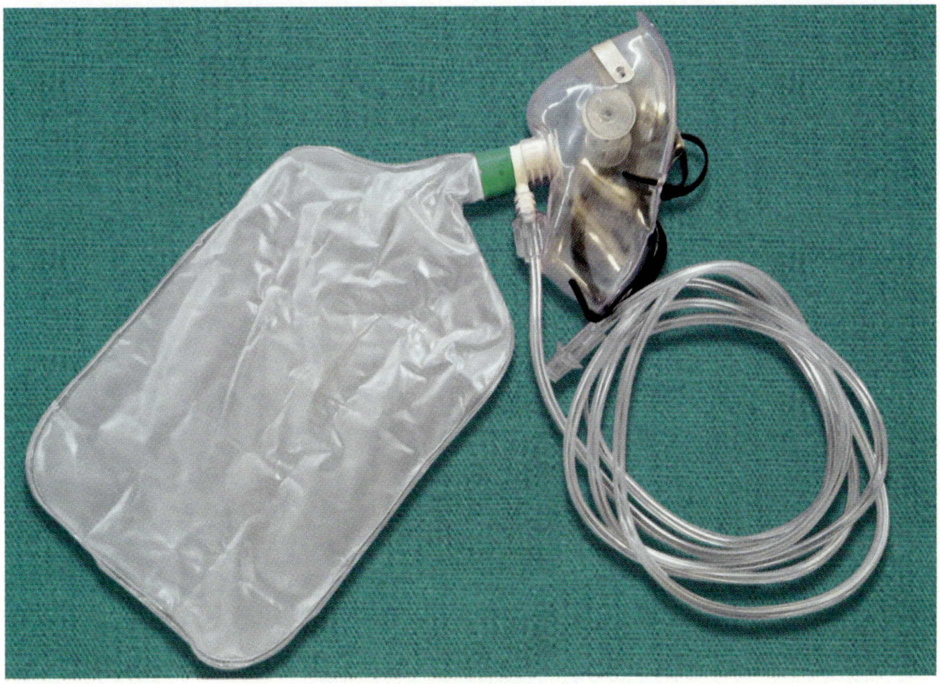

Fig. 5A: Reservoir face mask—minimum flow rate required is 12–15 L/min, generates an FiO_2 between 75% and 85%.

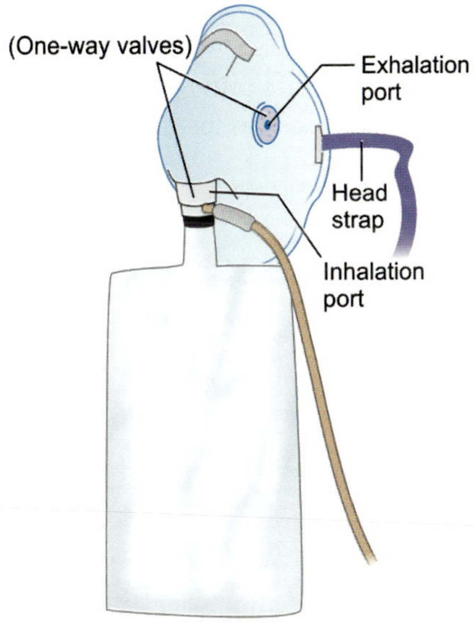

Fig. 5B: Illustrated mechanism of reservoir face mask.

- FiO_2 is variable depends upon amount of mixing of air through leakage around mask.
- During inspiration, patient inhale oxygen of reservoir bag through one-way inspiratory valve.
- During expiration, patient exhale through expiratory valve present on the mask and inspiratory valve will be closed.
- Reservoir face mask also known as non-rebreather mask (NRB).

Venturi Mask (Fig. 6)

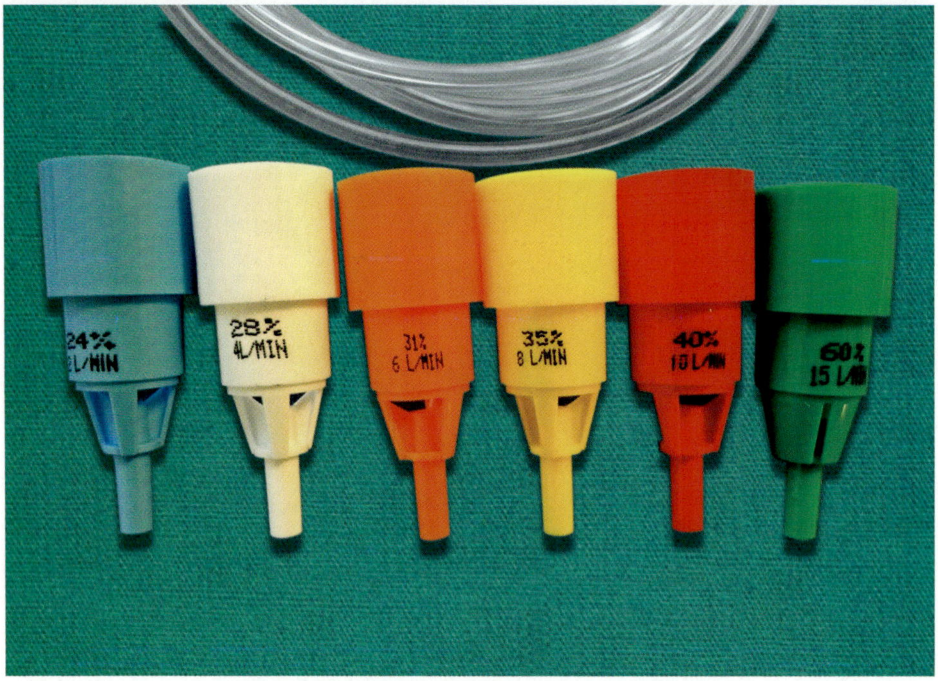

Fig. 6: Venturi mask—with different colored systems.

- Delivers oxygen at fixed FiO_2. Based on the Bernoulli's principle.
- Provides FiO_2 ranging from 26% to 60%—available as per fixed color codes.
- It is fixed oxygen concentration delivery devices.

High Flow Nasal Cannula (Figs. 7A and B)

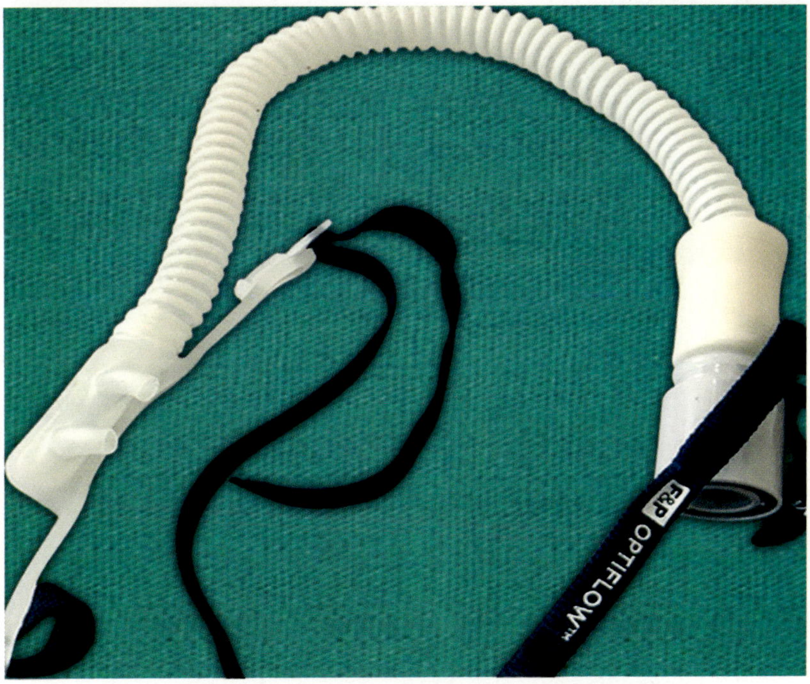

Fig. 7A: Nasal cannula of the high flow nasal cannula system.

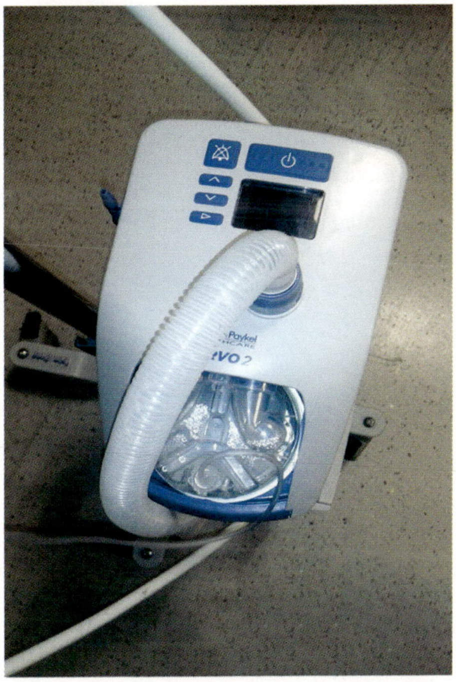

Fig. 7B: Humidifier device of the HFNC system.

- Delivers oxygen at fixed FiO_2. Based on the Bernoulli's principle.
- Provides FiO_2 ranging from 26% to 60%—available as per fixed color codes.
- It is fixed oxygen concentration delivery devices.

Noninvasive Ventilation Device (Fig. 8)

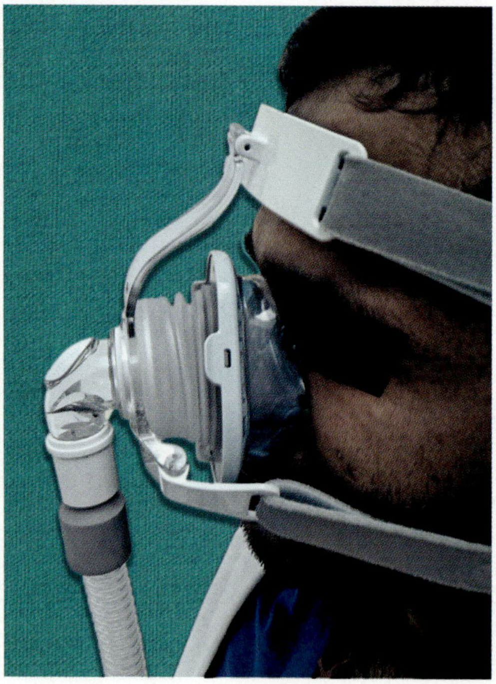

Fig. 8: Nasal mask with noninvasive ventilation (NIV) in addition to oxygenation also provides positive end-expiratory pressure (PEEP).

- Provides oxygen at a fixed FiO_2.
- In addition it can also help in ventilation—in weaning and in avoidance of ventilation.
- *Indications*: Type II respiratory failure, e.g. chronic obstructive pulmonary disease (COPD). Type I respiratory failure, e.g. postoperative hypoxemia, mild acute respiratory distress syndrome (ARDS), heart failure.
- It is fixed oxygen concentration delivery devices.

INTERCOSTAL CHEST DRAIN (FIGS. 9A TO C)

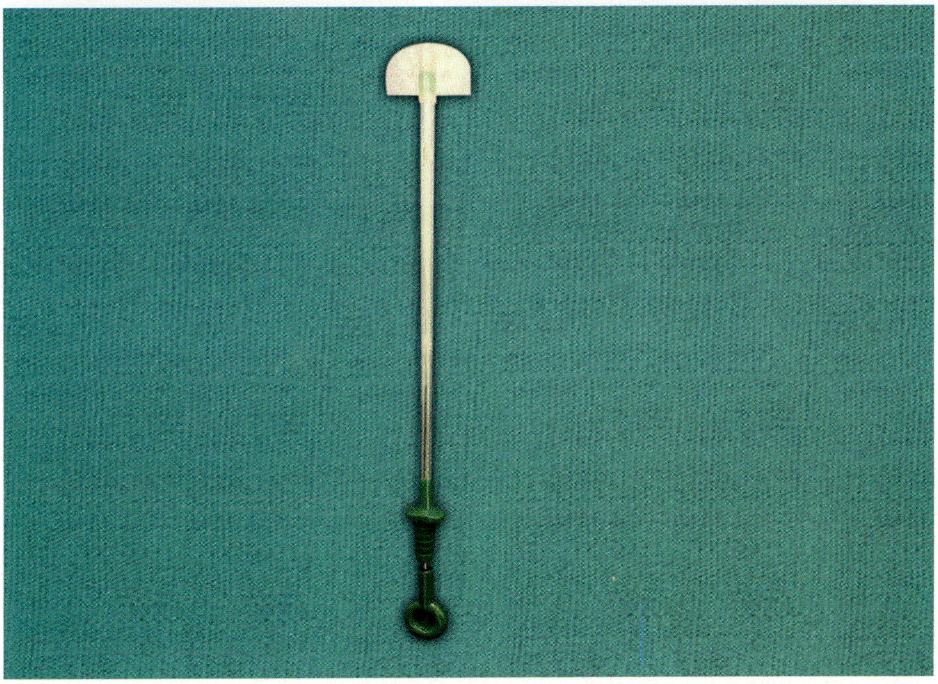

Fig. 9A: Intercostal chest drain with trocar.

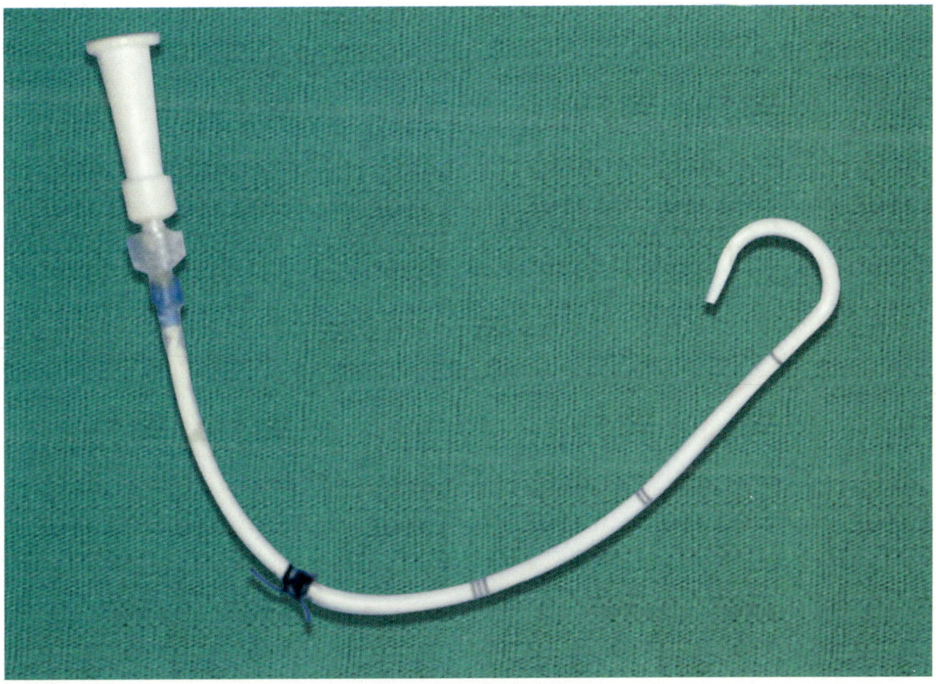

Fig. 9B: Pig tail catheter.

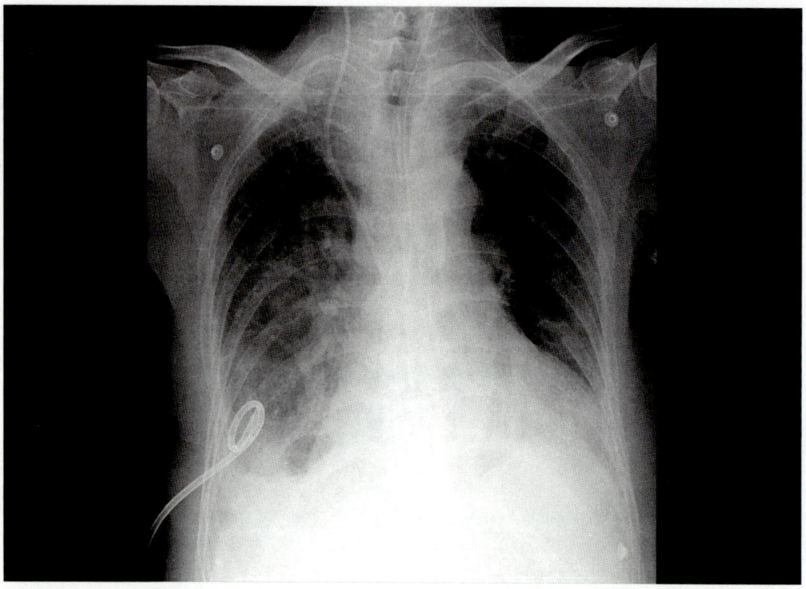

Fig. 9C: Pig tail *in situ* for right-sided pleural effusion.

- Used to drain intrapleural air, fluid, blood, and chyle.
- Contraindicated in—coagulopathy.
- Except in tension pneumothorax and hemothorax, small bore tubes (12–16 Fr) are preferred.

PULMONARY REHABILITATION DEVICE (FIGS. 10 TO 12)

Incentive Spirometry (Fig. 10)

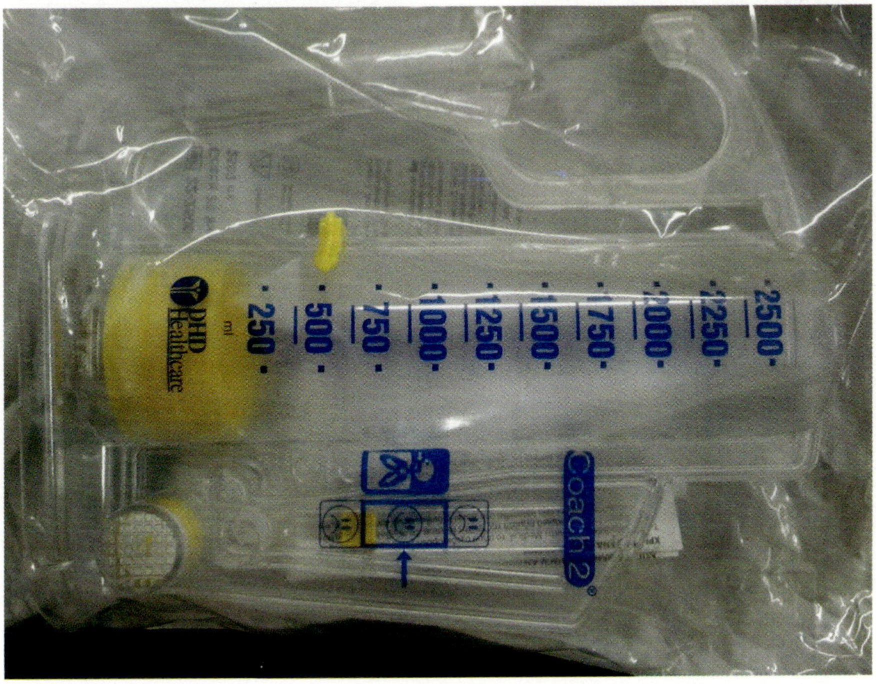

Fig. 10: Incentive spirometry—with objective estimate of tidal volume generated.

- Incentive spirometry is commonly used post-surgery and/or bedridden patients to prevent lung atelectasis.
- During breath-holding spell, a greater number of alveoli are popped open, thereby improving oxygenation.
- It is also used in type-II respiratory failure to washout to CO_2.

Acapella (Fig. 11)

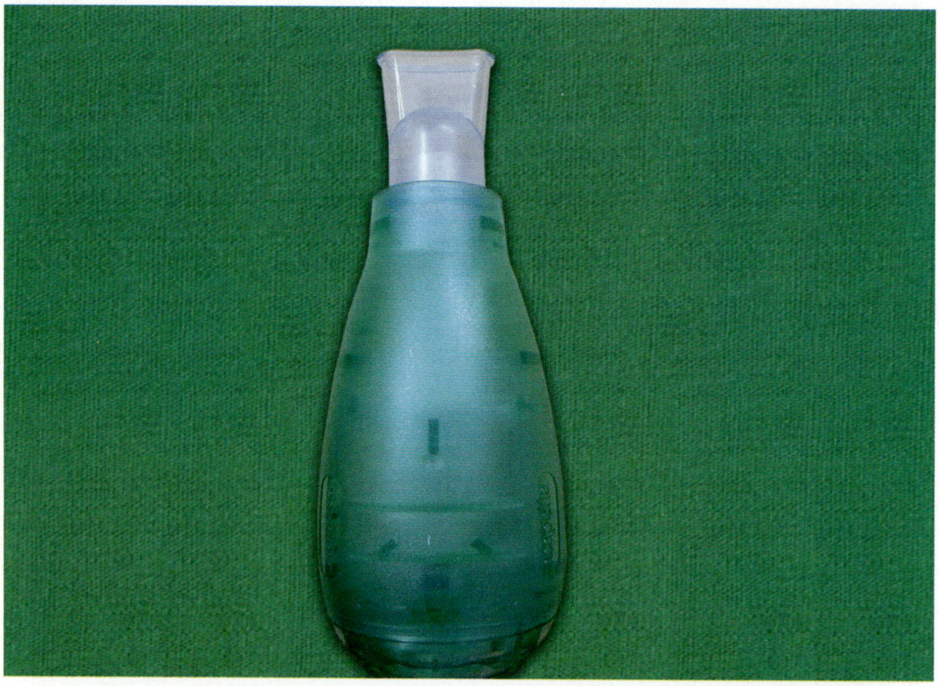

Fig. 11: Acapella device—expiratory device for expectoration of secretions.

- Acapella combines both the benefit of positive expiratory pressure and airway vibrations, thereby mobilizing the secretions.
- It can be used by the patient in any position.
- It is also useful in chronic suppurative lung diseases like bronchiectasis and COPD.

Finger Pulse Oximetry (Fig. 12)

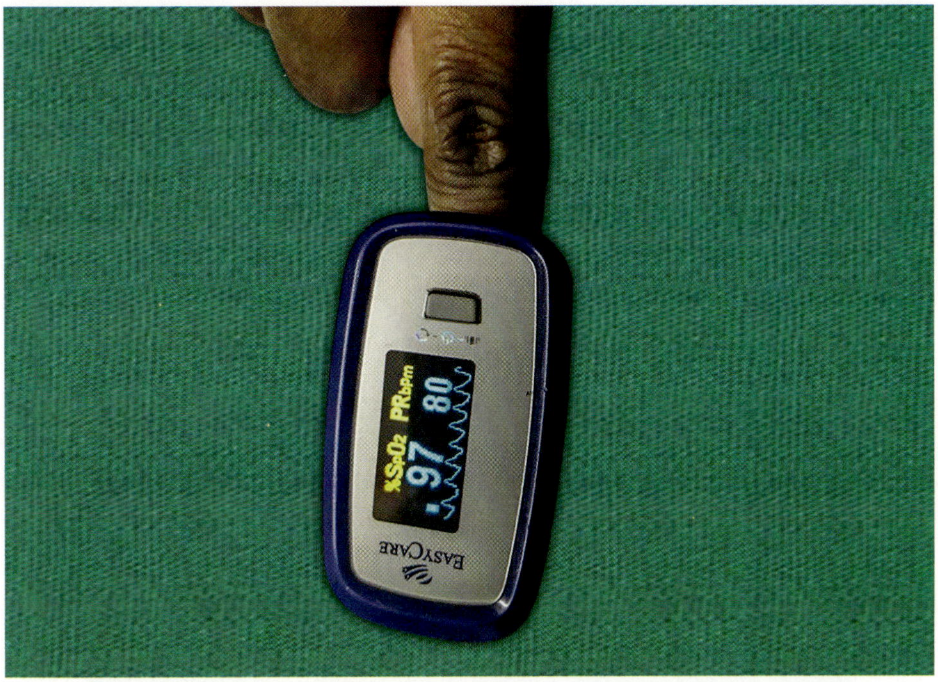

Fig. 12: Finger pulse oximeter.

- Monitors peripheral oxygen saturation of blood noninvasively.
- Generally a thin part of the body, finger tip or earlobe is used.
- It measures the difference in the wavelength of the transmitted light between the red and infrared beams, representing the oxy- and deoxyhemoglobin (900 nm and 940 nm respectively).
- Not useful in peripheral vasoconstriction—shock and methemoglobinemia.

INTERVENTION DEVICES (FIGS. 13 TO 15)

Flexible Bronchoscope (Figs. 13A and B)

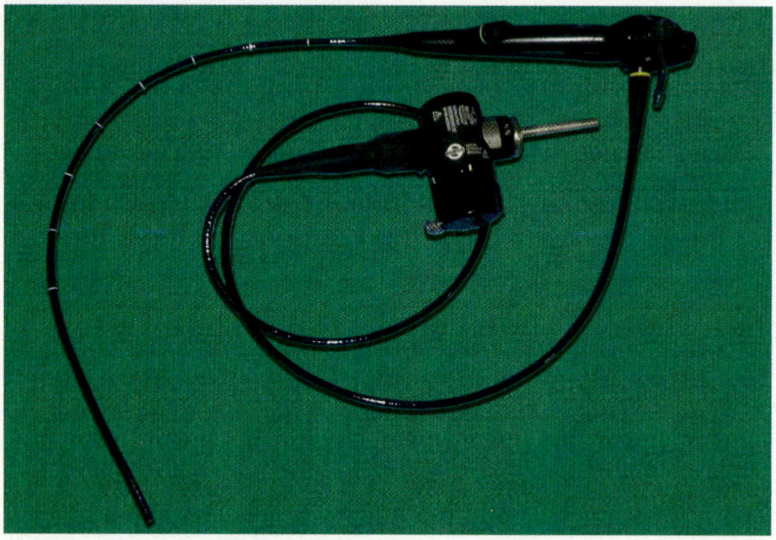

Fig. 13A: Fiberoptic bronchoscope.

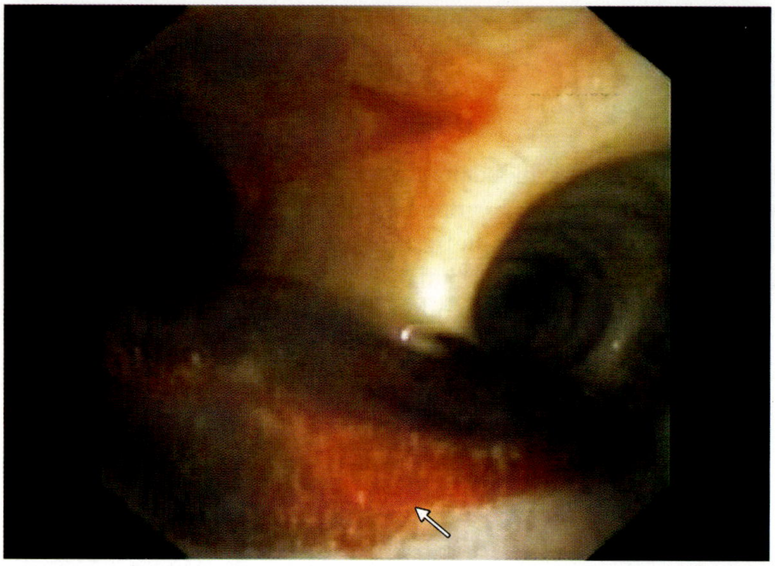

Fig. 13B: Bronchoscopic image of active left lung bleed with spillage to right—at the level of carina.

- Flexible bronchoscope is a pipe like instrument with fiberoptic cables and a light source at the tip for visualization of the airway.
- It can be navigated to the level of subsegmental bronchi.
- Therapeutic uses include clearing a collapsed lobe, to remove blood clot and for guidance of percutaneous tracheostomy.
- *Diagnostic*: To take biopsies from endobronchial mass.
- Contraindicated in case of coagulopathy, drowsy patient with an unsecured airway, high oxygen requirement and uncontrolled hypertension.

Fogarty Catheter (Fig. 14)

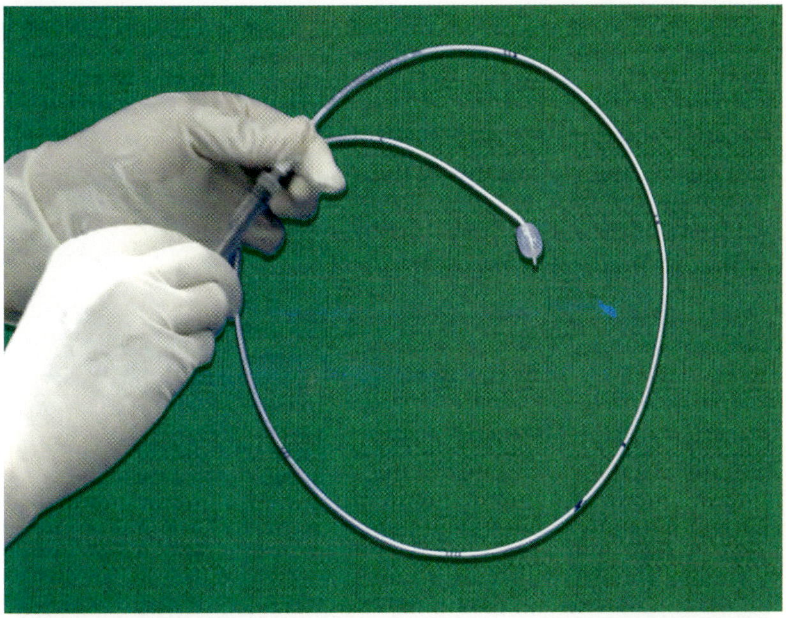

Fig. 14: Fogarty catheter with inflated balloon.

- Fogarty catheter is used for mechanical tamponade of a bleeding focus visualized by a bronchoscope.
- It has a 3 mL balloon and the catheter can be inserted through the bronchoscope.

Double Lumen Endotracheal Tube (Fig. 15)

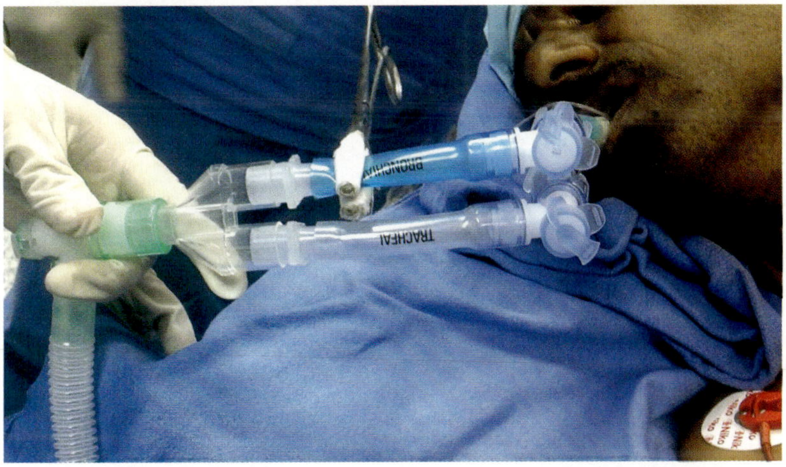

Fig. 15: Double lumen tube *in situ*, the bronchial lumen is clamped.

- Used to isolate a single lung. The lung undergoing the procedure is nondependent.
- It has two lumens one would stay in the trachea and the other in the main stem bronchi of the nondependent lung.
- Indicated in case of massive hemoptysis to isolate the lung where bleeding has occurred.
- Also in surgeries like lobectomy, pneumonectomy, bullectomy, pleural decortication.
- Also for differential lung ventilation.

RADIOLOGY IMAGES (FIGS. 16 TO 24)

Pneumonia (Figs. 16A and B)

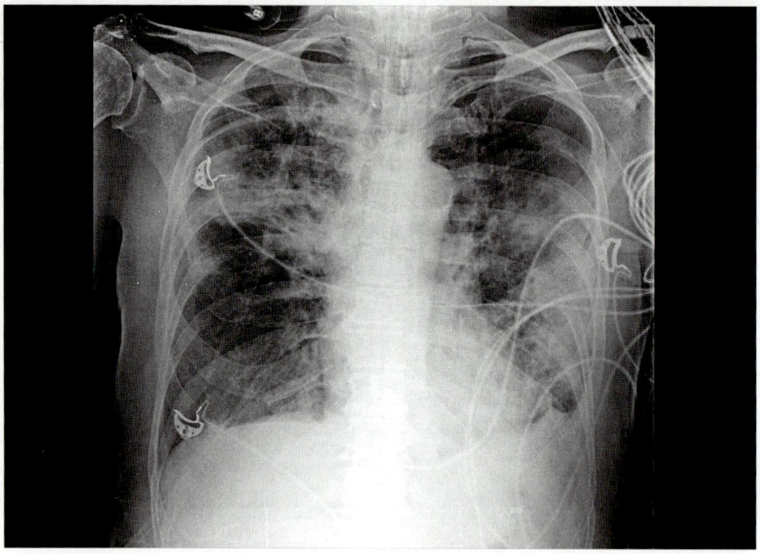

Fig. 16A: Pneumonia (X-ray).

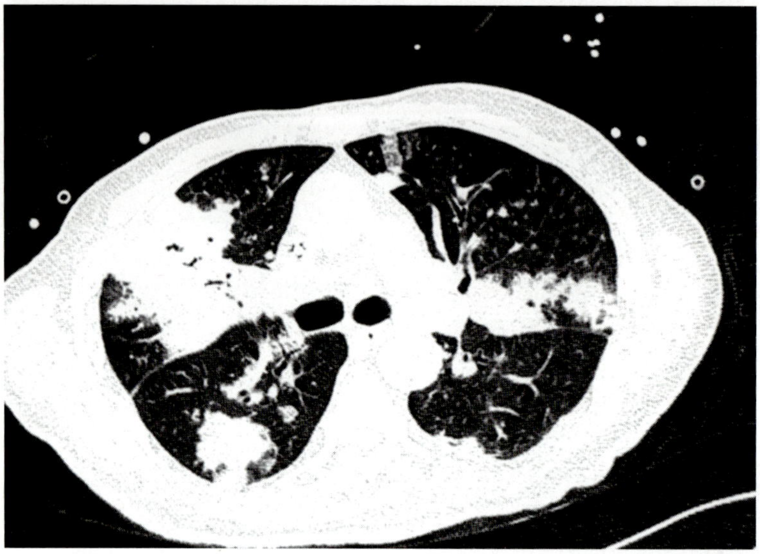

Fig. 16B: Pneumonia (CT).

- Portable chest X-ray suggestive of patchy consolidation in right middle zone, left middle and lower zone, suggestive of bronchopneumonia.
- CT thorax of the above patient, suggestive of bilateral patchy areas of consolidation—bilateral upper and right lower lobe, air bronchogram also seen.

Bronchiectasis (CT) (Figs. 17A and B)

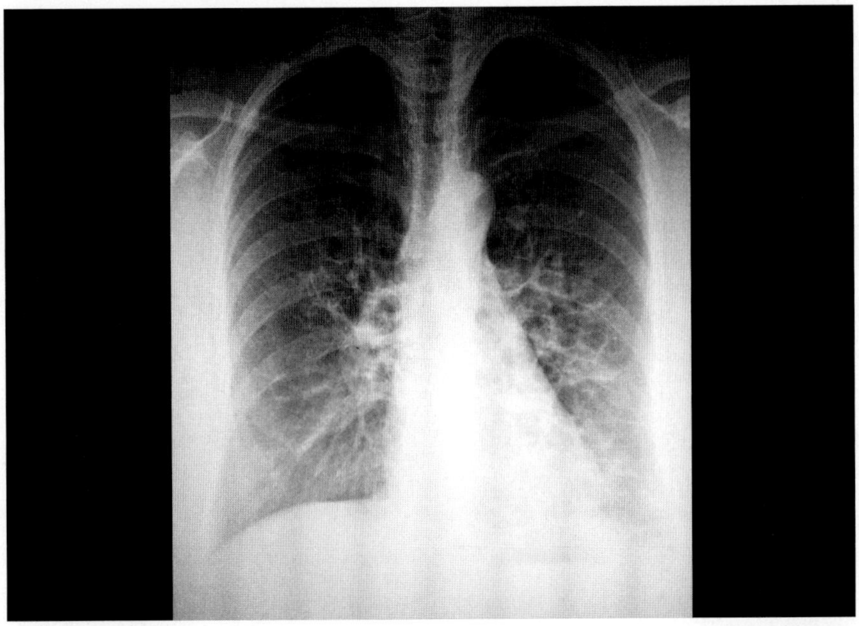

Fig. 17A: Bronchiectasis (Chest X-ray).

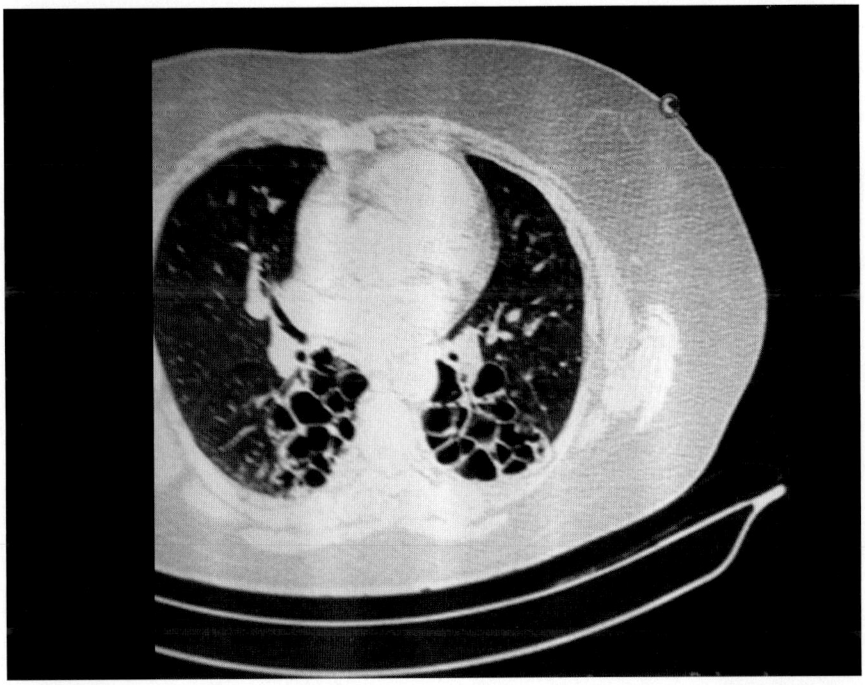

Fig. 17B: Bronchiectasis (Chest CT scan).

- Chest X-ray posteroanterior (PA) view suggestive of cystic lesions in bilateral mid and lower zones. Patient was admitted with massive hemoptysis.
- Contrast enhanced CT of the same patient suggestive of bilateral lower lobe cystic changes suggestive of cystic bronchiectasis.

Interstitial Lung Disease (Figs. 18A to D)

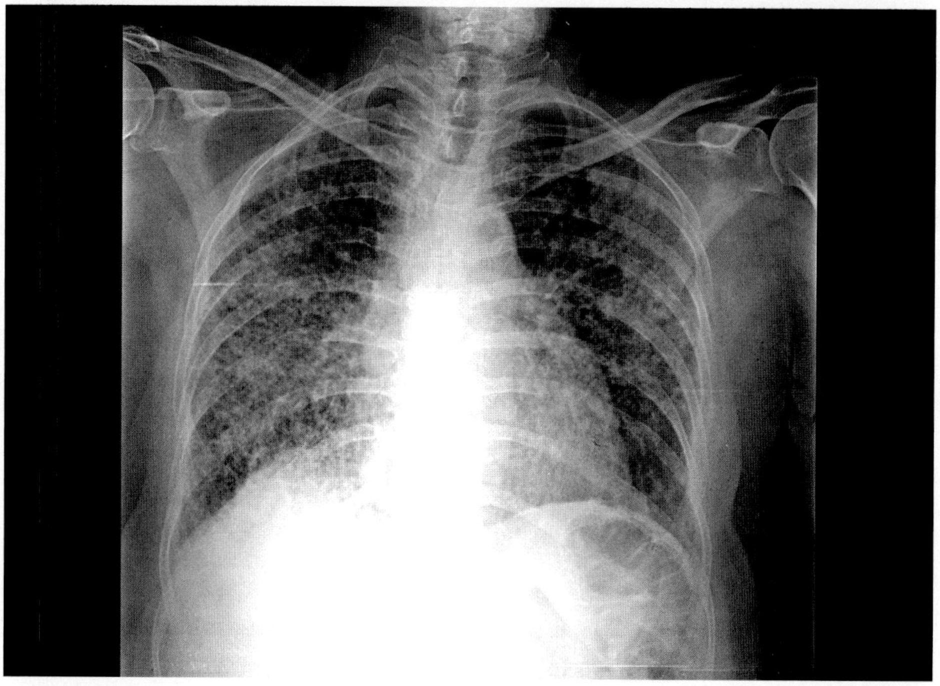

Fig. 18A: Chest X-ray PA view suggestive of bilateral diffuse reticular shadows in all zones.

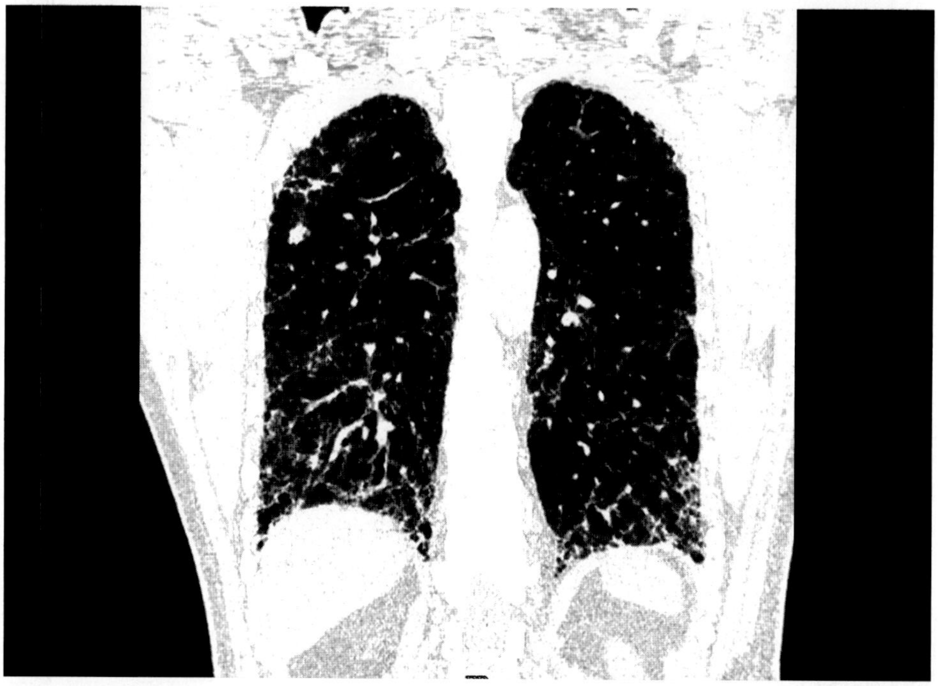

Fig. 18B: High resolution CT suggestive of lower lobe predominant, subpleural, interlobular septal thickening with traction bronchiectasis and honeycombing, suggestive of idiopathic pulmonary fibrosis. Patient was admitted with severe hypoxemia in ICU.

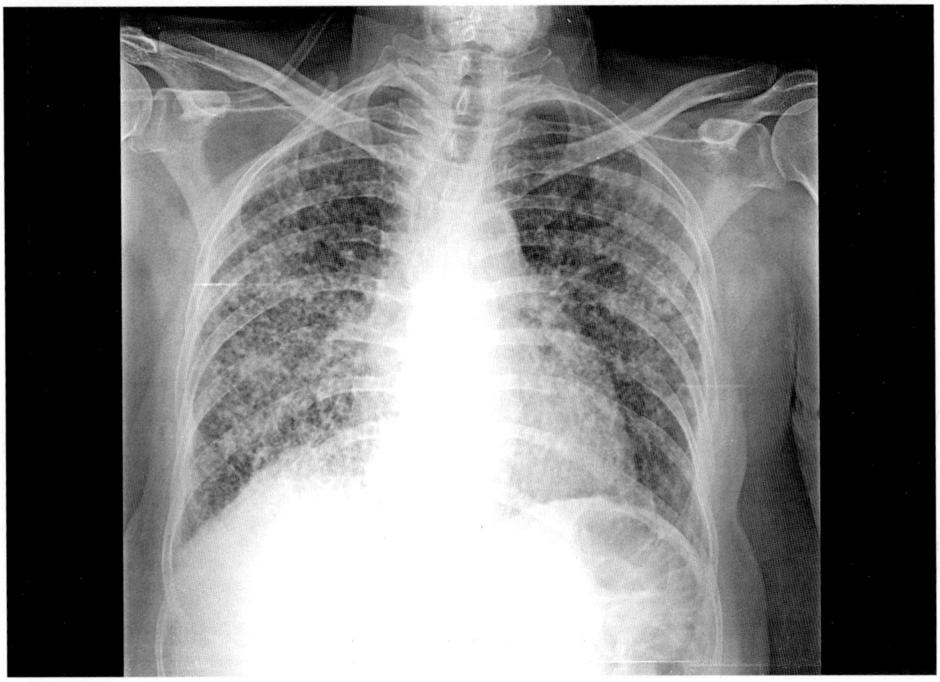

Fig. 18C: Chest X-ray PA view suggestive of bilateral diffuse reticulonodular opacities in all zones, patient had type 1 respiratory failure with history to exposure to poultry.

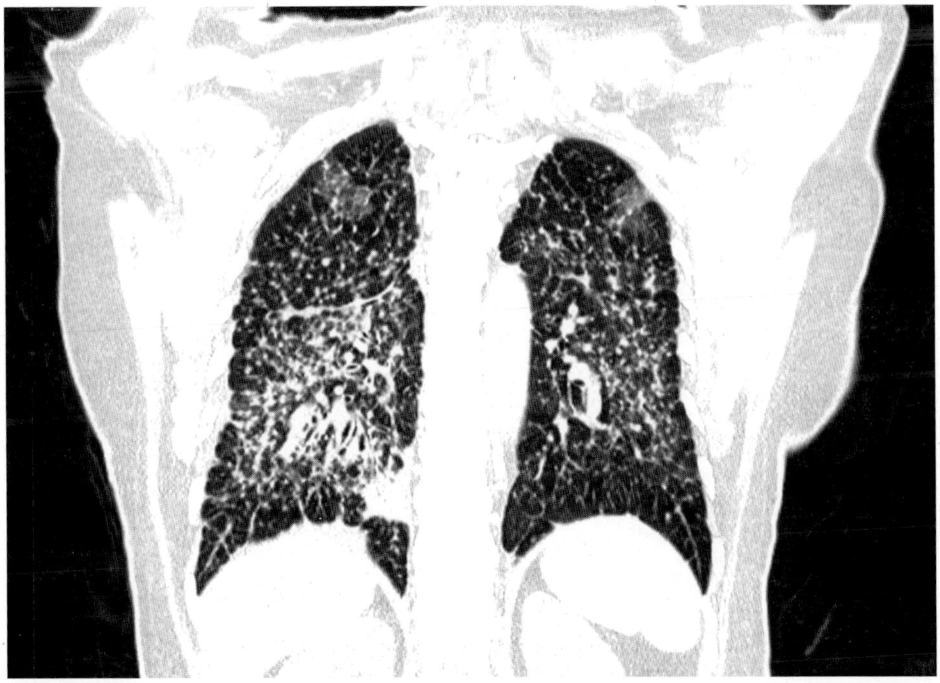

Fig. 18D: High resolution CT thorax of the patient with bilateral diffuse interlobular septal thickening and areas of ground-glass opacities, suggestive of interstitial lung disease (ILD)—most probably hypersensitivity pneumonitis.

Acute Respiratory Distress Syndrome (Figs. 19A and B)

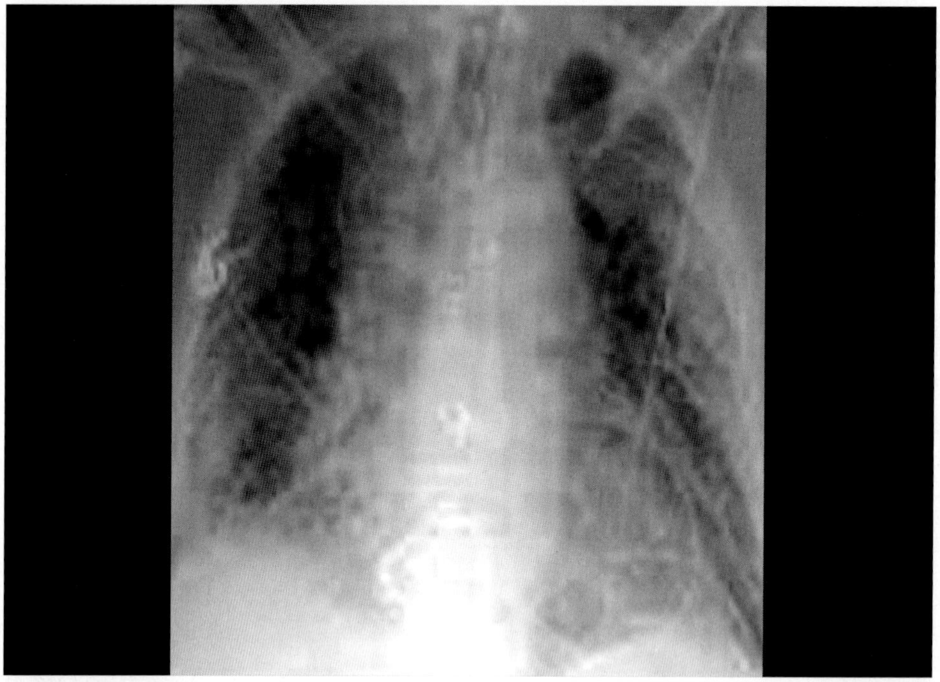

Fig. 19A: Chest X-ray portable suggestive of bilateral diffuse reticulonodular shadow with H1N1 positivity.

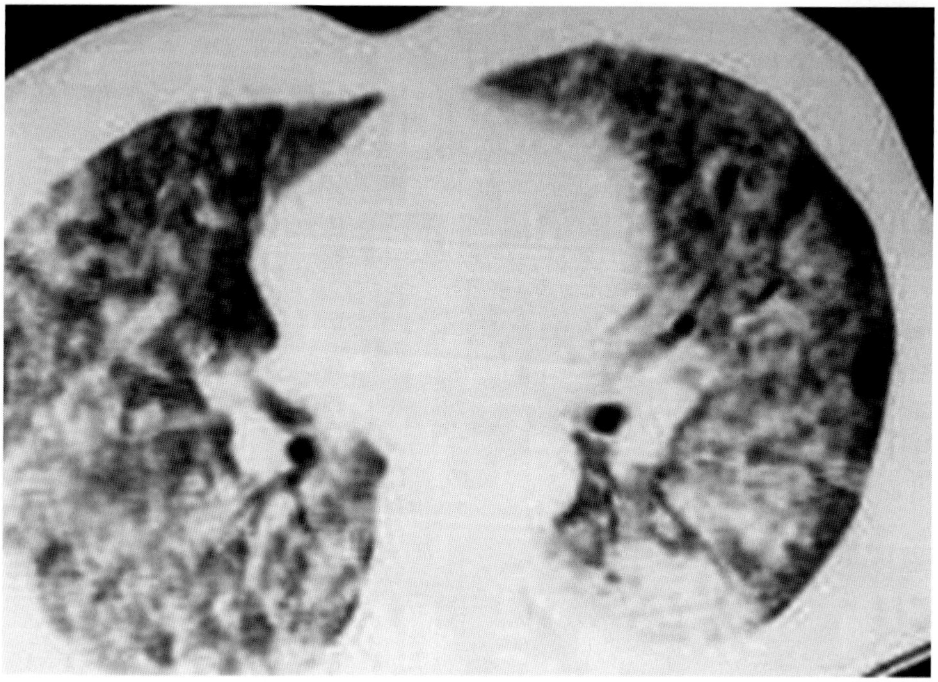

Fig. 19B: High resolution computed tomography (HRCT) thorax of the same patient suggestive of bilateral diffuse patchy opacities, with severe hypoxemia suggestive of acute respiratory distress syndrome (ARDS).

Pneumothorax (Figs. 20A and B)

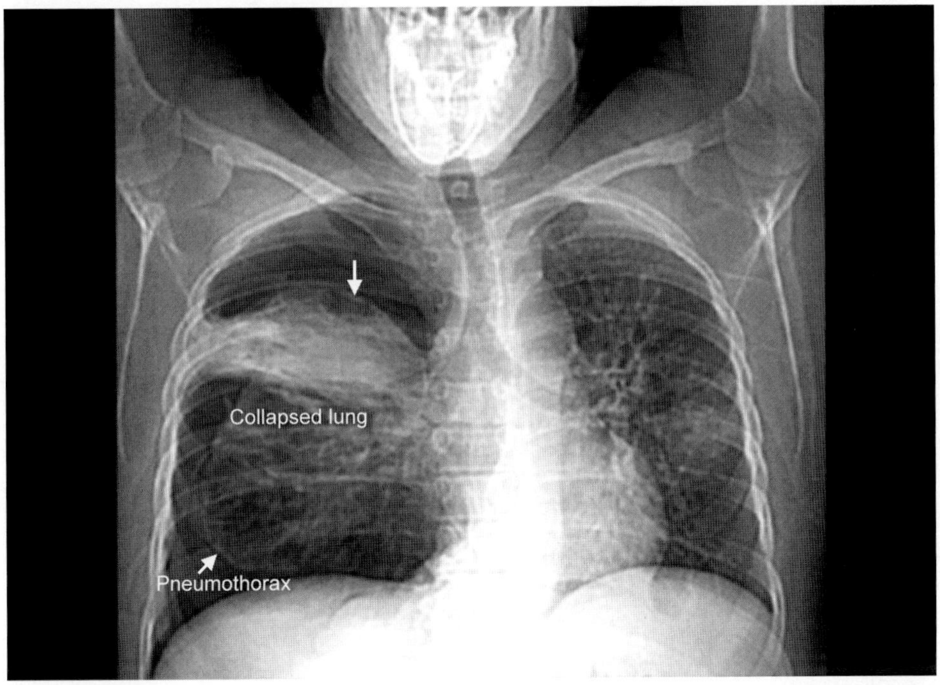

Fig. 20A: Portable chest X-ray of a patient with right-sided tension pneumothorax.

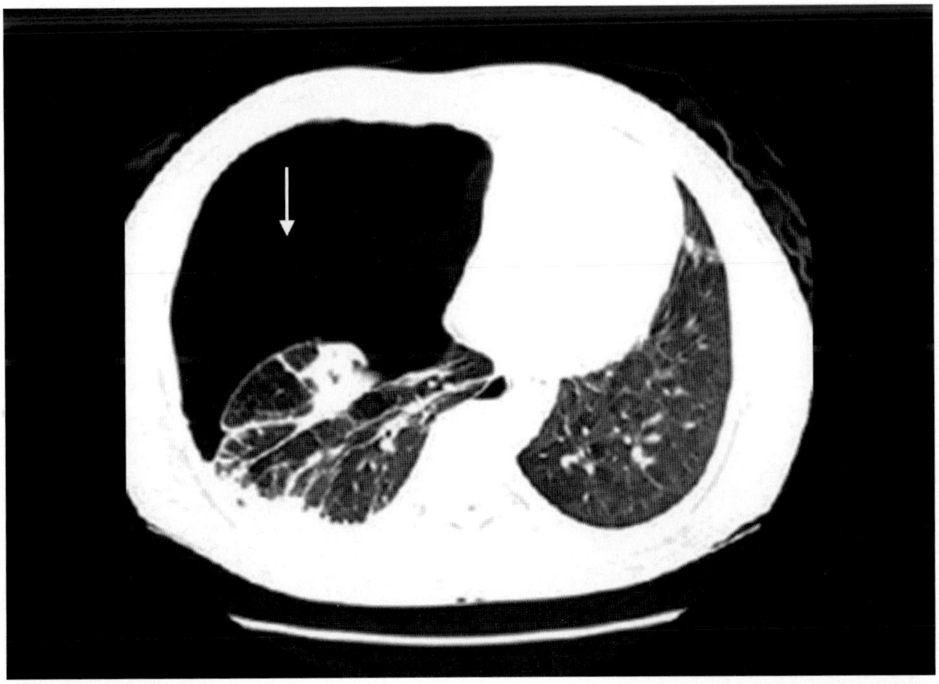

Fig. 20B: High resolution computed tomography (HRCT) thorax suggestive of right-sided tension pneumothorax with shift of mediastinum to opposite side.

Pleural Effusion (Figs. 21A to C)

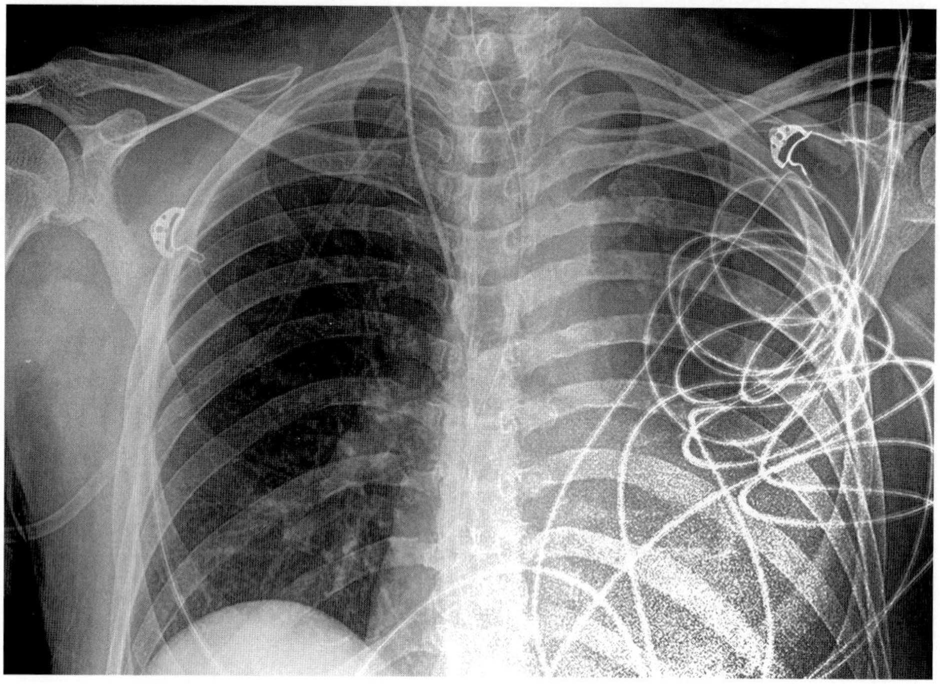

Fig. 21A: Chest X-ray PA view suggestive of left-sided pleural effusion.

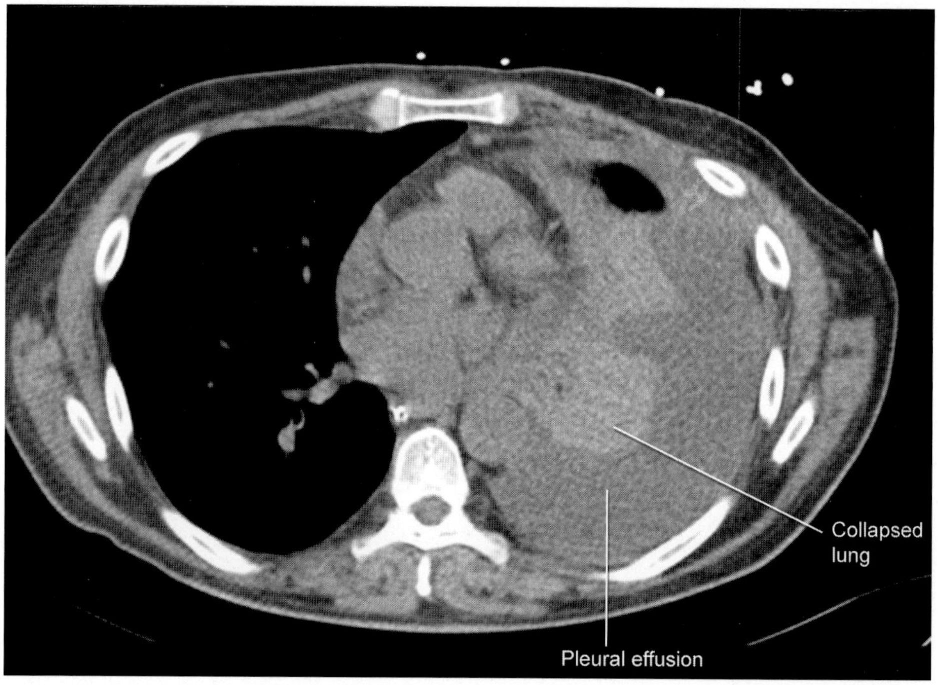

Fig. 21B: Contrast-enhanced computed tomography (CECT) thorax of the same patient suggestive of left-sided pleural effusion with underlying lung collapse.

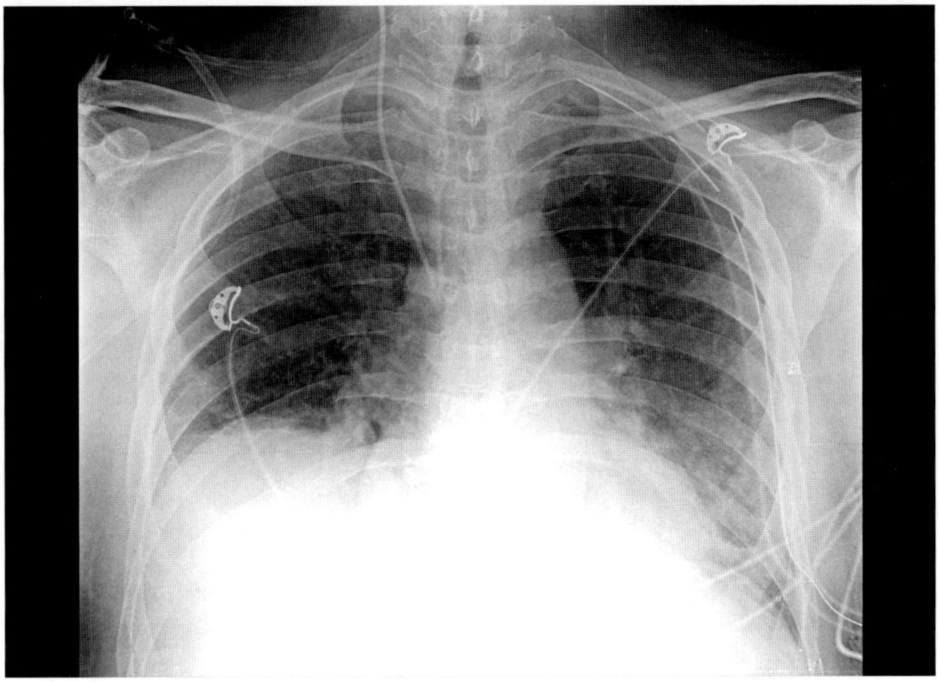

Fig. 21C: Chest X-ray PA view postintercostal chest drain of the same patient.

Subcutaneous Emphysema (Figs. 22A and B)

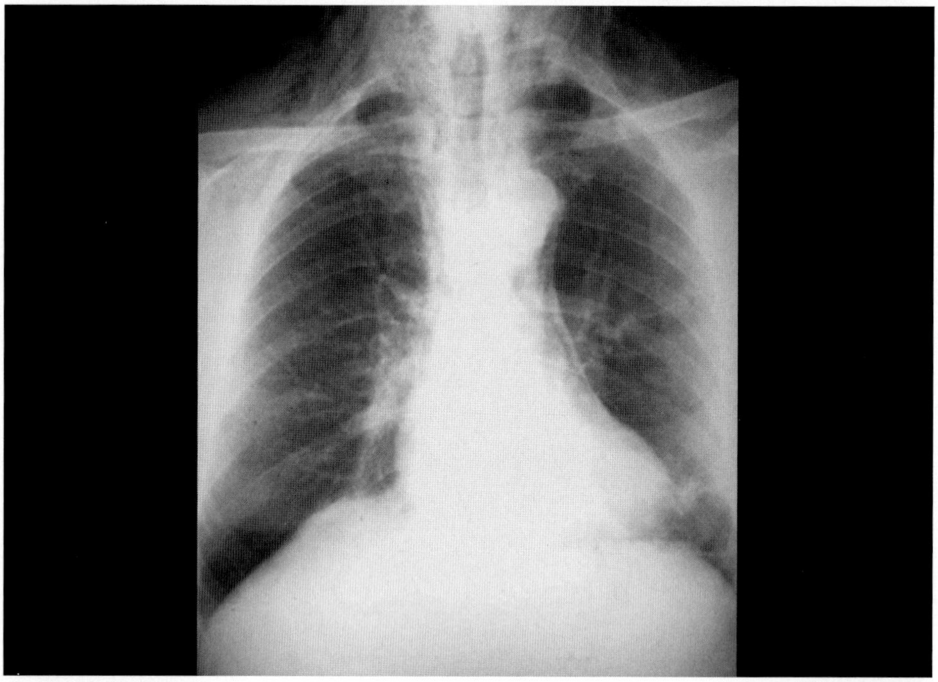

Fig. 22A: Chest X-ray PA view of bilateral subcutaneous emphysema around the neck, no pneumothorax noted.

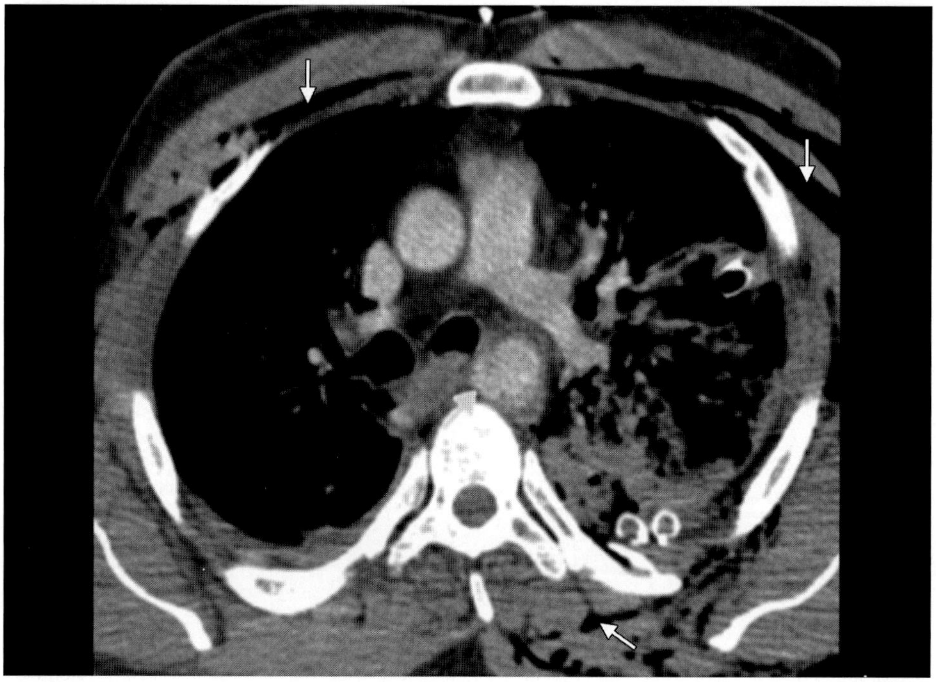

Fig. 22B: High resolution computed tomography (HRCT) thorax suggestive of bilateral subcutaneous emphysema.

Pulmonary Embolism (Figs. 23A and B)

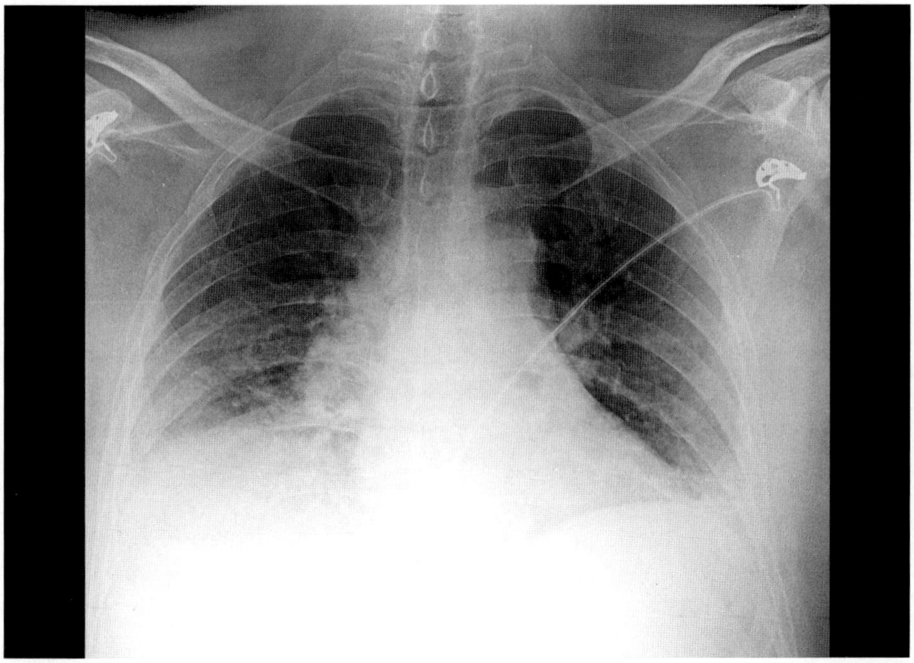

Fig. 23A: Chest X-ray PA view suggestive of right mid and lower zone haziness suggestive of pleural effusion. Patient presented with right-sided pleuritic chest pain after fracture of right tibia.

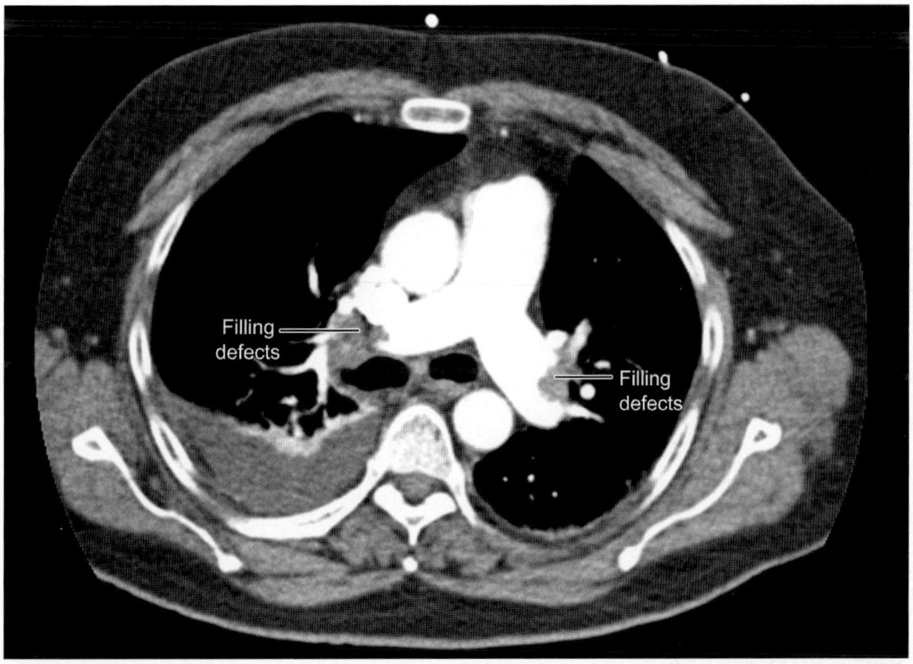

Fig. 23B: Contrast-enhanced computed tomography (CECT) thorax suggestive of bilateral filling defects in bilateral lower lobar branches of the pulmonary artery, with right-sided pleural effusion, responsible for the right-sided pleuritic chest pain.

Pulmonary Edema (Figs. 24A and B)

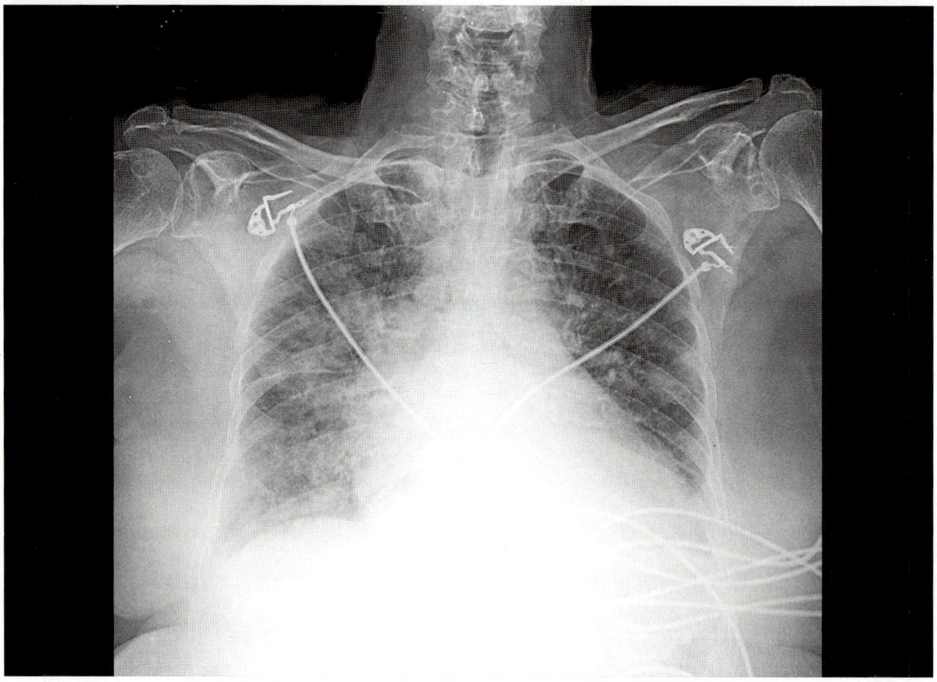

Fig. 24A: Chest X-ray PA view suggestive of cardiomegaly bilateral perihilar haze, suggestive of pulmonary edema.

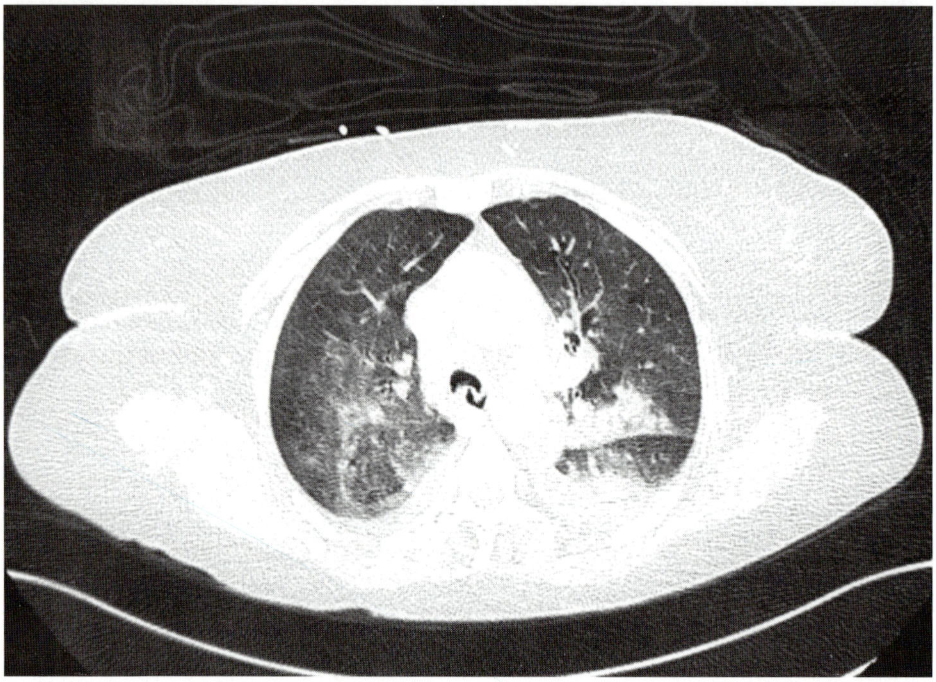

Fig. 24B: High resolution computed tomography (HRCT) thorax suggestive of bilateral perihilar ground-glass haze with left lower lobe consolidation and perifissural consolidation, suggestive of pulmonary edema. Patient improved on Lasix infusion.

SECTION 3

Cardiology

Echocardiography

CHAPTER 5

RR Kasliwal, Hardeep Kaur Grewal, Mansi Kaushik

MITRAL REGURGITATION (FIGS. 1 AND 2)

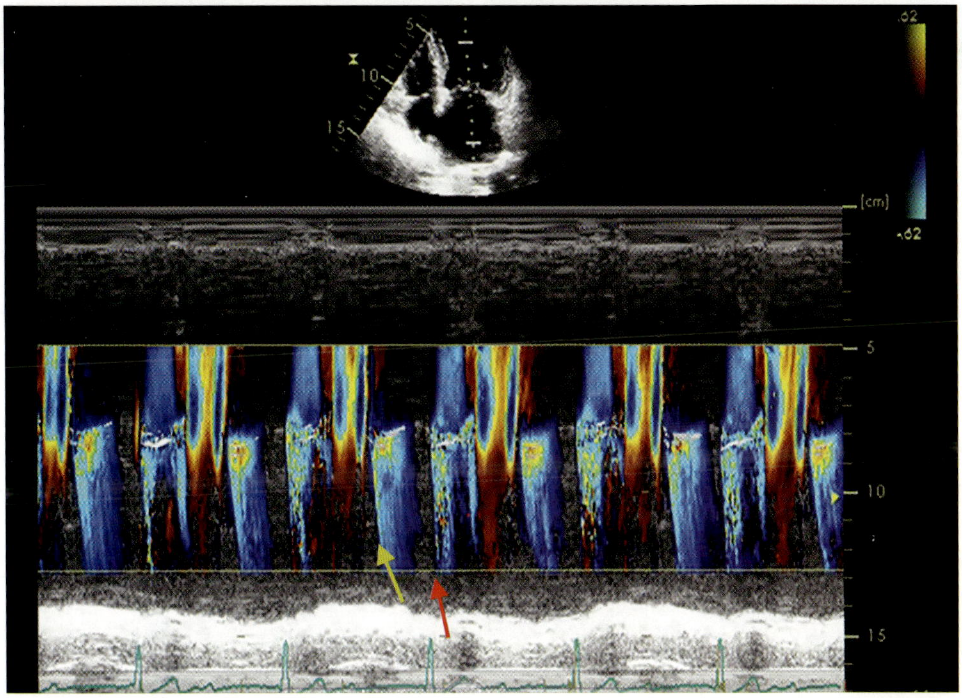

Fig. 1: Color M-mode showing initially systolic murmur (red arrow) and then diastolic murmur (yellow arrow) after diastolic filling.

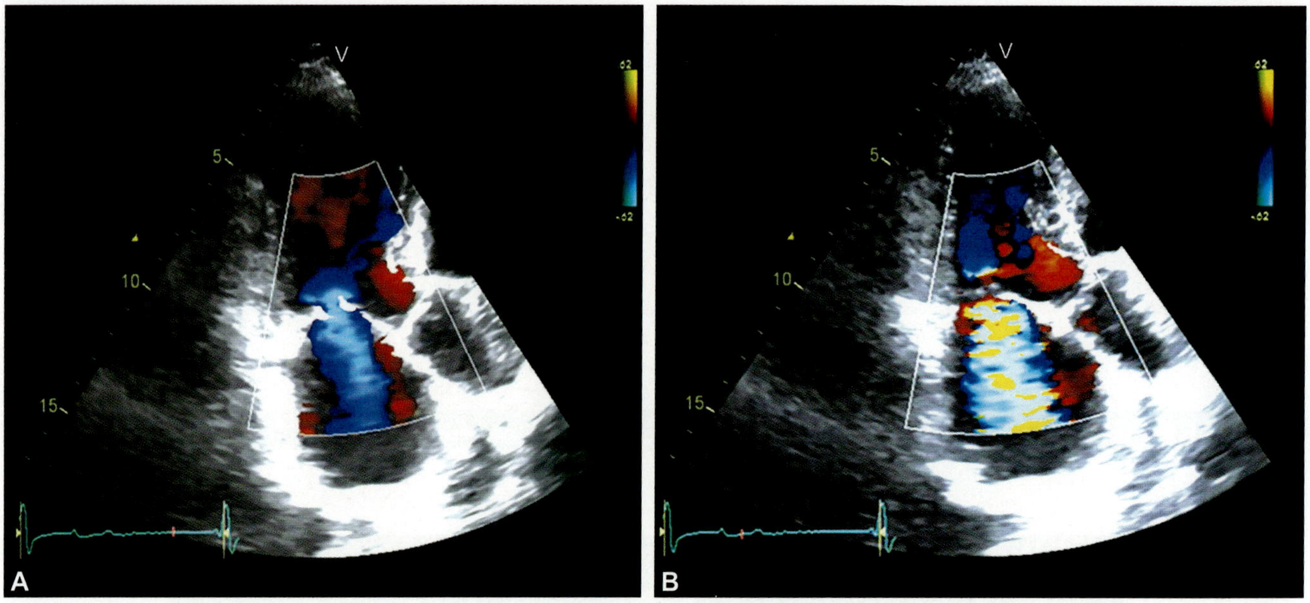

Figs. 2A and B: Diastolic (A) and systolic (B) mitral regurgitation in same patient. Please note red cursor on ECG for cardiac timing cycle.

- Mitral regurgitation (MR) usually occurs in systole during left ventricular (LV) contraction. If LV pressure exceeds the mean left atrial (LA) pressure at any point during diastole, i.e. reversal in atrioventricular (AV) gradient, diastolic MR can occur.
- It usually occurs in later part of diastole as it takes a time lapse to reverse atrioventricular gradient.
- Diastolic MR has been reported in patients with severe aortic regurgitation (AR) (mainly in acute AR or chronic AR with decompensated LV), AV block, cardiomyopathies (with significantly elevated LV diastolic pressures), and in patients with long filling periods in atrial tachyarrhythmias.
- Careful analysis of electrocardiography (ECG) gated echocardiography images is very important in order to delineate systolic and diastolic MR, and their timing in systole and diastole.

CARDIAC AMYLOIDOSIS (FIG. 3)

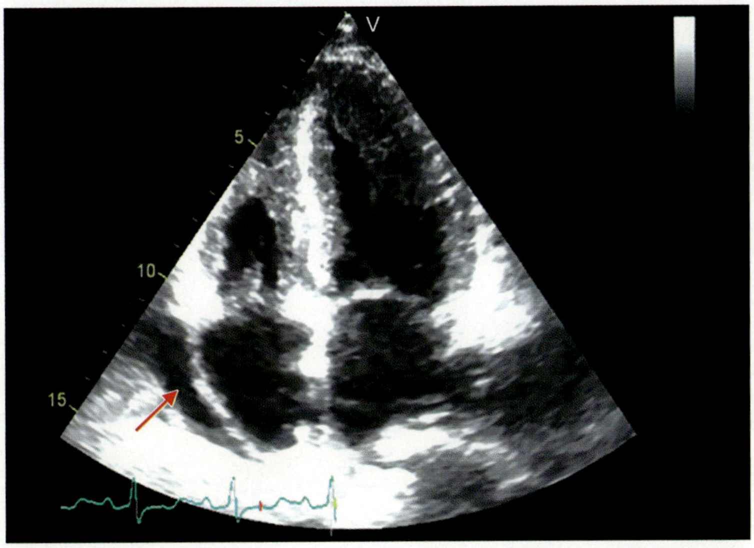

Fig. 3: Significantly increased ventricular wall thickness in a patient of cardiac amyloidosis. Mild pericardial effusion (arrow) seen along right atrial wall, on transthoracic echocardiography (TTE).

- Cardiac amyloidosis (CA) is a condition where there is the deposition of the amyloid protein in the cardiac muscle.
- CA causes ventricular and valvular thickening, classical granular myocardial texture, biatrial enlargement, restrictive diastolic filling pattern, with normal to mildly reduced systolic function.
- Primary (AL) amyloidosis, transthyretin amyloidosis (ATTR) and senile systemic amyloidosis (SSA) commonly involve the myocardium.
- Echocardiography is recommended in all patients with suspected amyloidosis.

SEPTAL BOUNCE (FIG. 4)

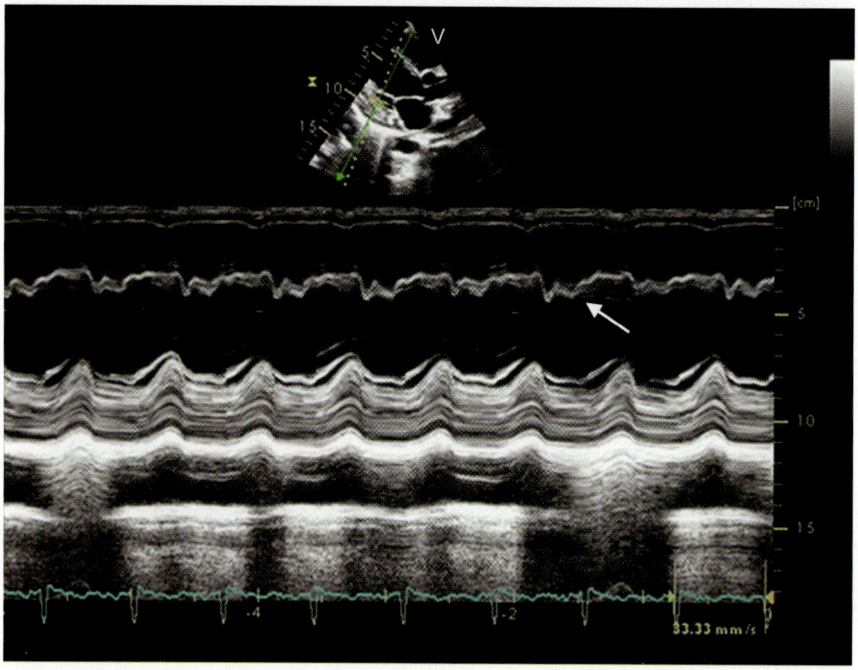

Fig. 4: Paradoxical bouncing motion of the interventricular septum initially toward and then away from the left ventricle during early diastole also known as *septal bounce* (arrow) seen on M-mode, seen in patients of chronic constrictive pericarditis.

- Septal bounce, typically seen in constrictive pericarditis, indicates the phenomena of ventricular interdependence.
- This phenomenon occurs due to reduced ventricular compliance secondary to fixed pericardial volume.
- Because right ventricular filling begins slightly earlier than left ventricular filling, the change in pressure in right ventricle results in paradoxical leftward motion of the interventricular septum.
- The septal bounce is accentuated during inspiration due to increased venous return to the right ventricle with opposite effect during expiration.
- Echocardiography demonstrates exaggerated ventricular interdependence which is manifested by paradoxical interventricular septal movement during diastole with initial septal movement towards and then away from the left ventricle.

LEFT ATRIAL APPENDAGE (FIG. 5)

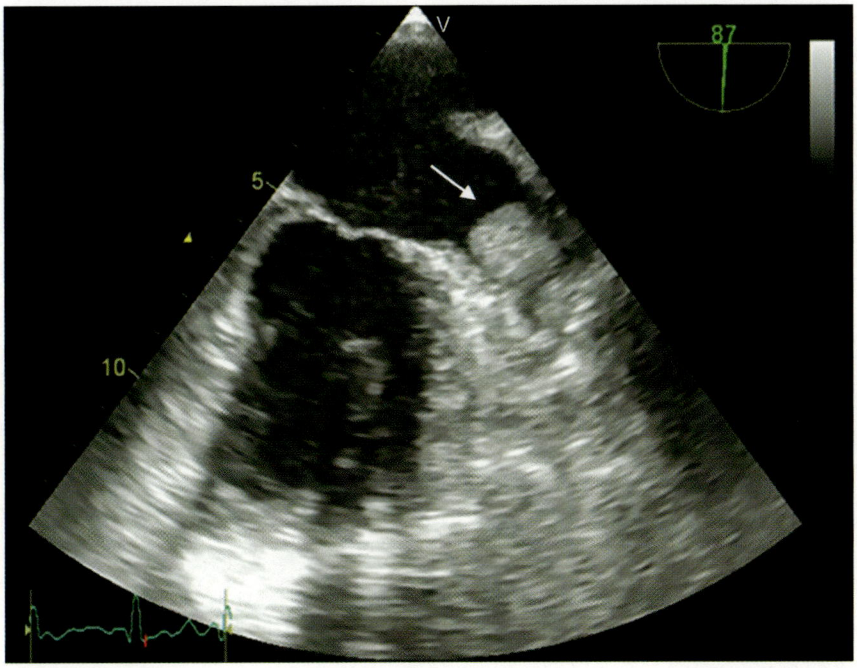

Fig. 5: Clot (arrow) seen in left atrial appendage on transesophageal echocardiography (TEE).

- Left atrial appendage (LAA) is a finger like out pouching from the main body of left atrium (LA) and it is the most common site for cardiac thrombus.
- LAA clots are most commonly seen in patients with atrial fibrillation and flutter.
- During atrial arrhythmias, LAA loses contractility resulting in decreased flow velocities with stagnation of blood in LAA leading to clot formation.
- Transthoracic views are usually not adequate to detect LAA clots.
- Transesophageal echocardiography (TEE) has high accuracy to detect LAA clot with some studies reporting sensitivity and specificity of TEE to be as high as 100% and 99% respectively.
- A meticulous scanning of the LAA from multiple imaging planes should be done to avoid any misdiagnosis.

RIGHT ATRIAL APPENDAGE (FIG. 6)

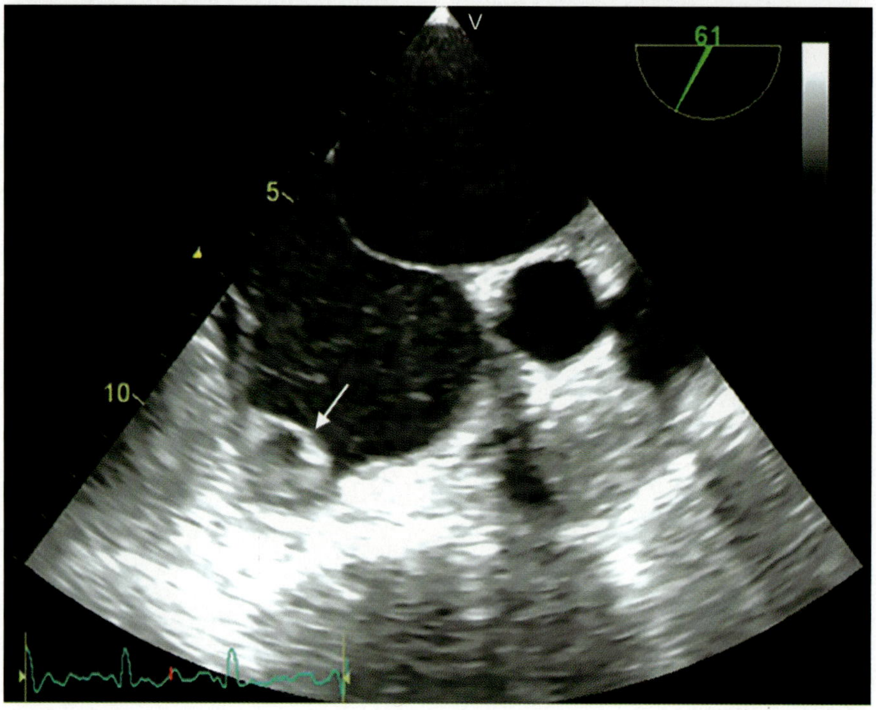

Fig. 6: Clot (arrow) seen in right atrial appendage with evidence of central thrombolysis (on TEE).

- Right atrial appendage (RAA) has a wide neck and broad base with a more simple and conical shape unlike left atrial appendage which is a deeper structure with narrow neck and multiple recesses.
- Due to these anatomical differences, clot formation in RAA is less common than LAA.
- Constant superior vena cava (SVC) flow which is abutting the RAA also protects against clot formation.
- In routine transesophageal echocardiographic evaluation for atrial fibrillation (AF), examination is generally limited to LA and LAA.
- Although relatively rare when compared with the left side, RAA thrombus also has the potential of embolism and should be screened.
- RAA clot should be specifically looked for in chronic AF and any severe right heart failure.

MITRAL STENOSIS (FIGS. 7A TO C)

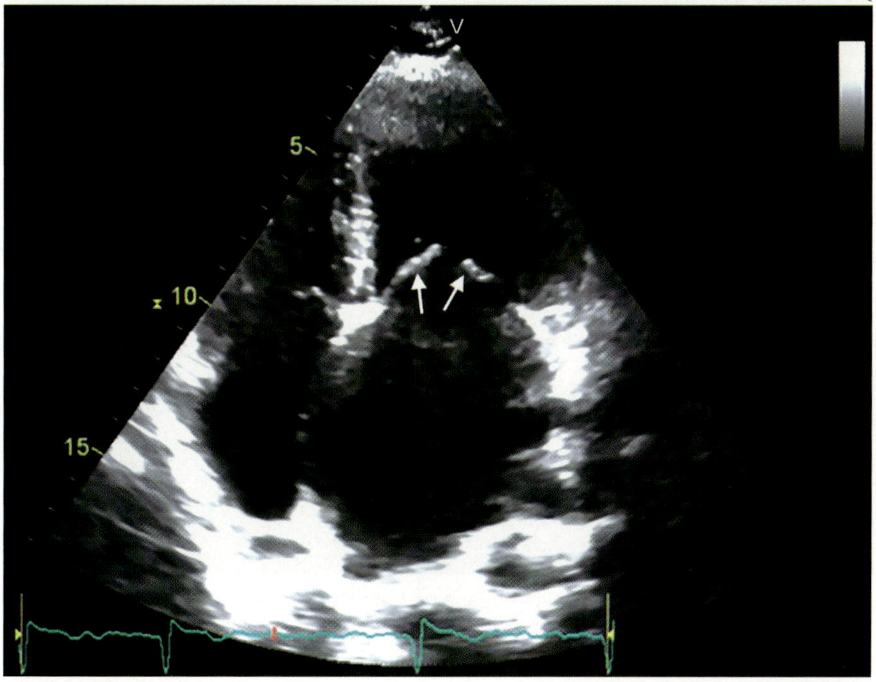

Fig. 7A: Thickened mitral valve leaflets (arrows) with restricted valve opening, in a patient of chronic rheumatic heart disease (apical four-chamber view).

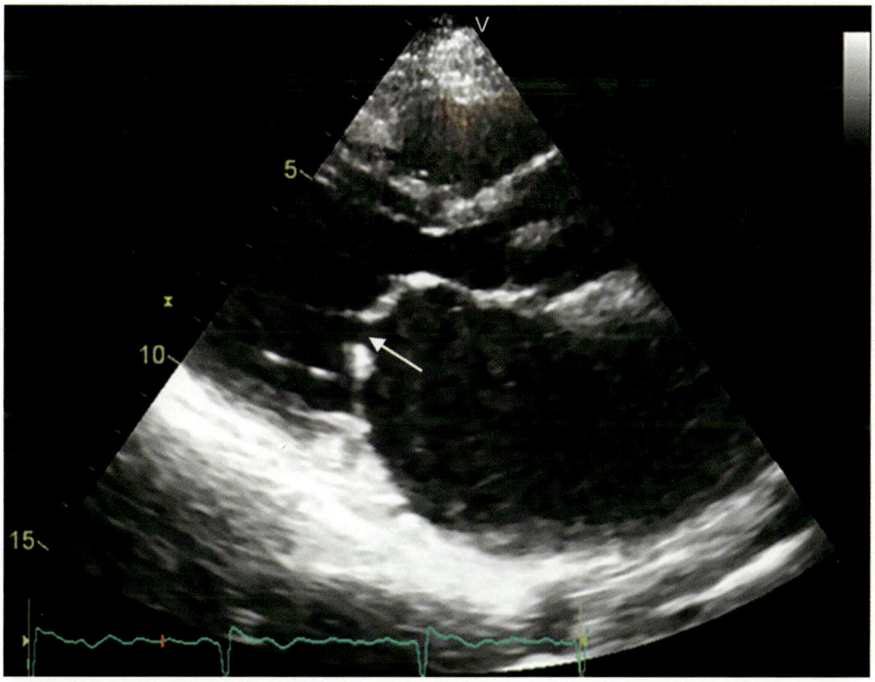

Fig. 7B: Thickened mitral valve leaflets with characteristic hockey stick (arrow) appearance of anterior mitral leaflet in diastole with restricted valve opening, suggestive of rheumatic etiology (parasternal long-axis view).

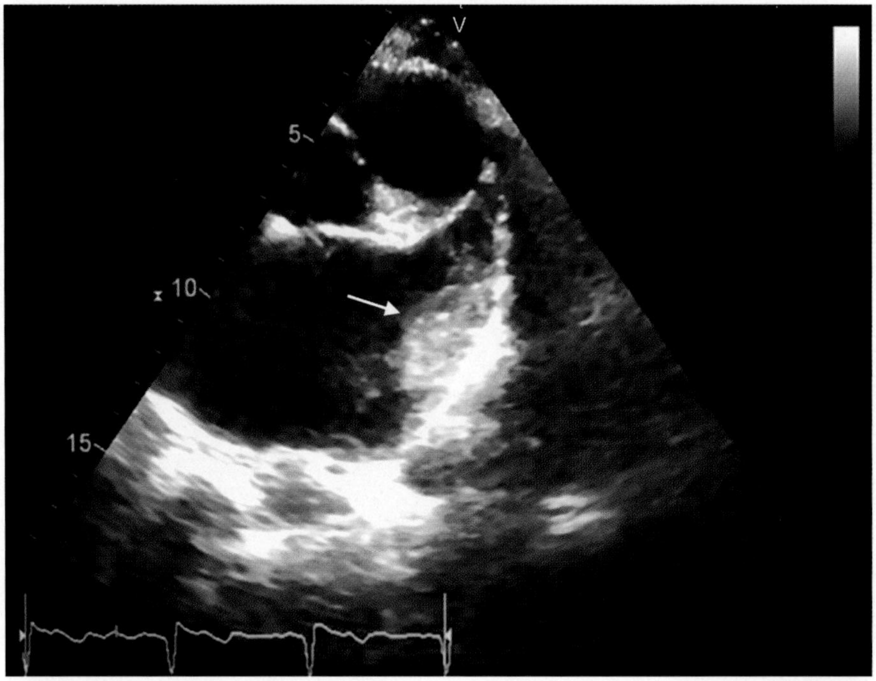

Fig. 7C: Clot seen in left atrial appendage on transthoracic echocardiography (TTE).

- Most common cause of mitral stenosis (MS) is rheumatic heart disease (RHD) characterized by mitral commissural fusion; thickened, restricted mitral valve leaflets; and thickening, fibrosis and shortening of the chordae tendineae.
- Stenotic mitral valve causes an obstruction to the flow of blood into the left ventricle, creating a pressure gradient across the mitral valve and eventually leading to increased left atrial (LA) pressures and LA dilatation.
- Echocardiography is the modality to assess MS severity by parameters like mitral valve orifice area planimetry, mitral valve area (MVA) calculation by pressure half time (PHT) and transmitral gradients.
- On transthoracic echocardiography (TTE), left atrial appendage (LAA) can be seen in the apical two-chamber view and in parasternal short axis view at the level of great vessels.
- However, the ability of TTE to identify or exclude LA or LAA thrombi is limited due to poor visualization of the LAA. Despite the inadequacy of TTE, careful transthoracic evaluation should always be done to look for LAA clot in suspected cases as detection of clot on TTE can obviate the need of TEE.

LOEFFLER ENDOCARDITIS (FIGS. 8A AND B)

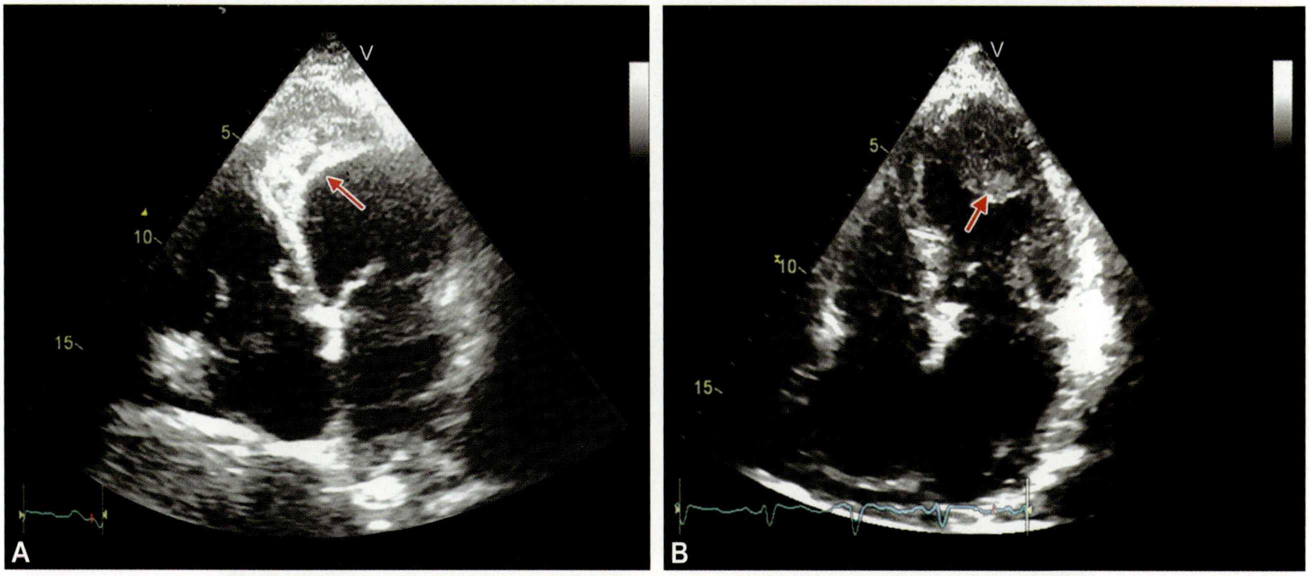

Figs. 8A and B: Loeffler's endocarditis: Usually associated with eosinophilic states. Eosinophilia results in endocardial damage and myocardial infiltration, leading to formation of thrombi (red arrows in images) in ventricular cavity. Seen in two different patients (A and B).

- Loeffler endocarditis is a rare type of restrictive cardiomyopathy which involves abnormal endomyocardial infiltration of eosinophils, with subsequent tissue damage from eosinophilic degranulation, leading to thrombus formation and fibrosis.
- This entity is characterized by initial inflammatory and necrotic stage followed by thrombotic stage and finally leading to stage of fibrosis.
- Echocardiography allows detection of endomyocardial thickening and intraventricular thrombus. Apical thrombus in the presence of normal apical contraction is one of the main clues in suspected Loeffler's endomyocarditis.
- Eosinophilic states that may underlie Loeffler's endocarditis include primary eosinophilias like chronic eosinophilic leukemia, the hypereosinophilic syndrome and clonal hypereosinophilia and secondary causes like allergic and autoimmune diseases; parasitic infestations; malignant and premalignant hematologic disorders associated with hypereosinophilia.

MIDESOPHAGEAL BICAVAL (FIGS. 9A AND B)

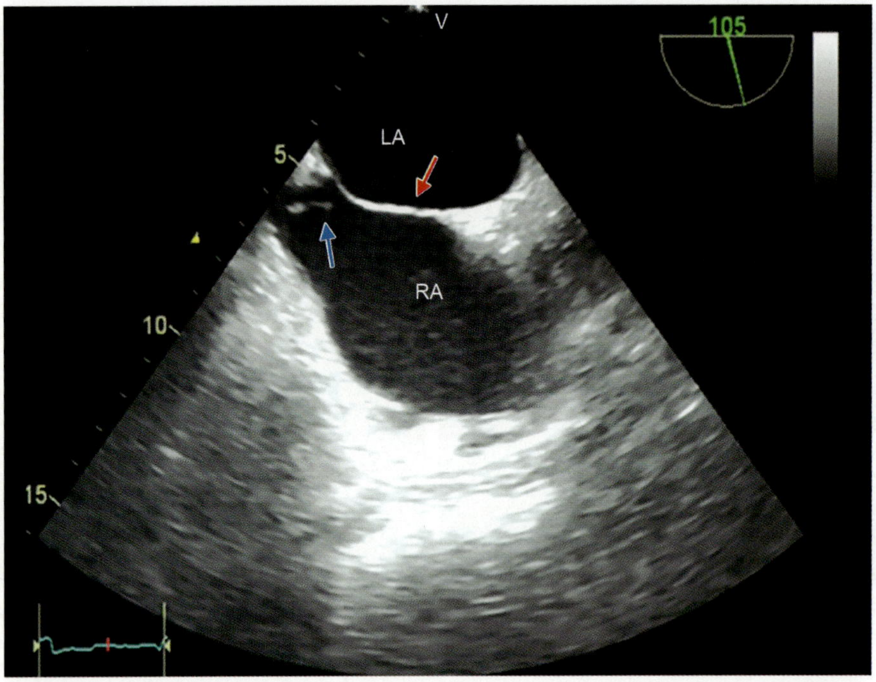

Fig. 9A: Modified bicaval transesophageal view showing interatrial septum (red arrow) and Eustachian valve (blue arrow).

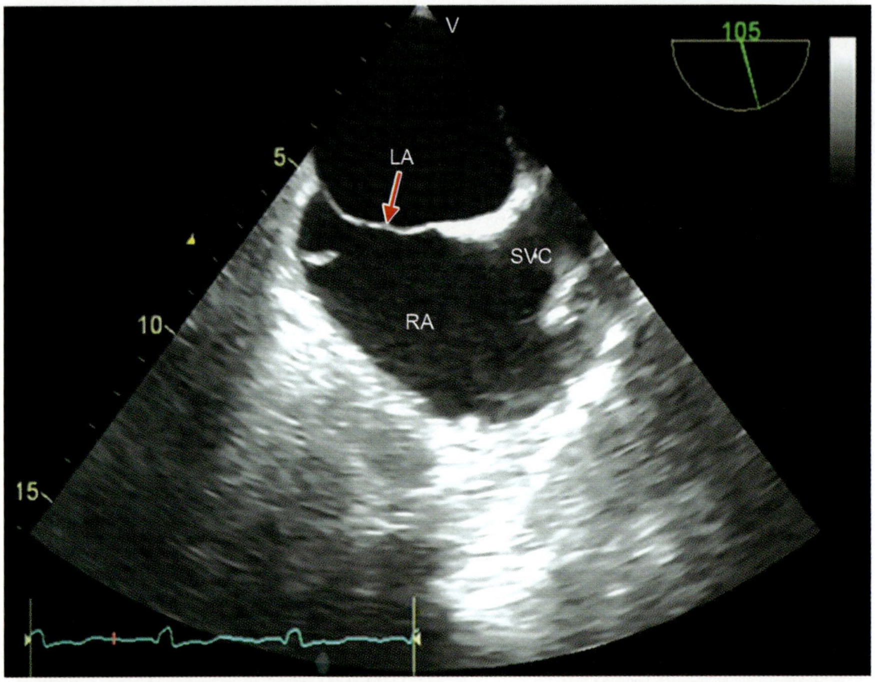

Fig. 9B: Bicaval transesophageal view showing interatrial septum (red arrow) and opening of superior vena cava (SVC).

- In midesophageal bicaval view, interatrial septal morphology, Eustachian valve, inferior vena cava and superior vena cava inflow are well imaged.
- Further turning the probe clockwise with slight withdrawal enables imaging of the right pulmonary veins.

HYPERTROPHIC CARDIOMYOPATHY (FIG. 10)

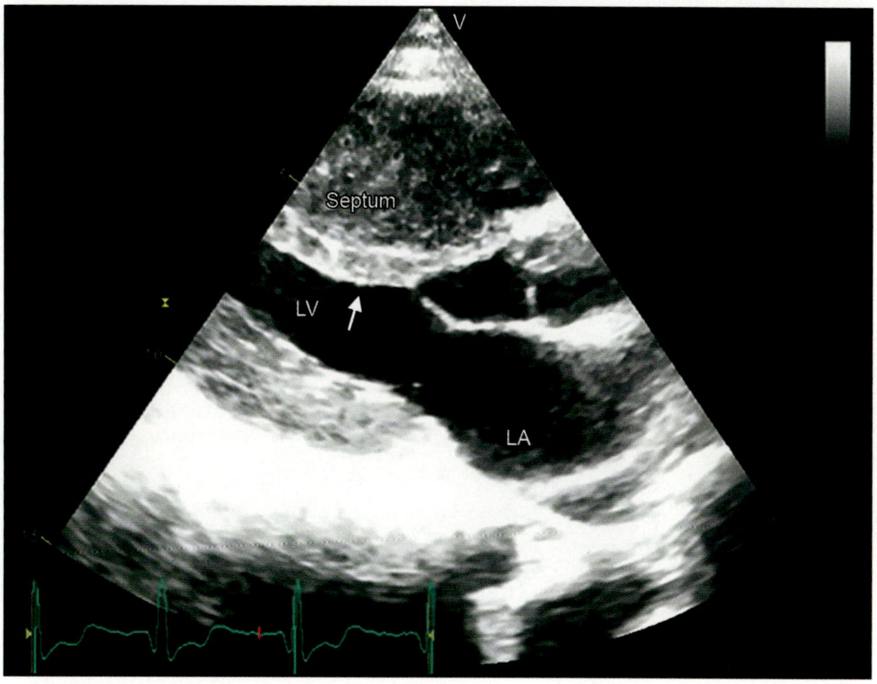

Fig. 10: Asymmetrical septal hypertrophy (arrow) in hypertrophic cardiomyopathy.

- Hypertrophic cardiomyopathy (HCM) is a genetic disorder, characterized by left ventricular (LV) hypertrophy, defined by an end-diastolic ventricular septal thickness of ≥ 13 mm, in the absence of secondary causes.
- It is commonly asymmetrical with significant hypertrophy of the basal interventricular septum. Occasionally the hypertrophy is restricted to apex, mid-ventricle and posterior wall of LV.
- Approximately one-third of patients have LV outflow tract obstruction at rest, one-third have provocable left ventricular outflow tract (LVOT) obstruction and one-third have no resting and provocable obstruction.
- The histological features of HCM include myocyte hypertrophy and disarray, as well as interstitial fibrosis.
- HCM is the most common cause of sudden cardiac death (SCD) in adolescents and young adults, particularly in competitive athletes.
- Echocardiography has pivotal role in the diagnosis, choosing the appropriate therapeutic strategy and in prognostic assessment of this disease.

TISSUE DOPPLER IMAGING (FIG. 11)

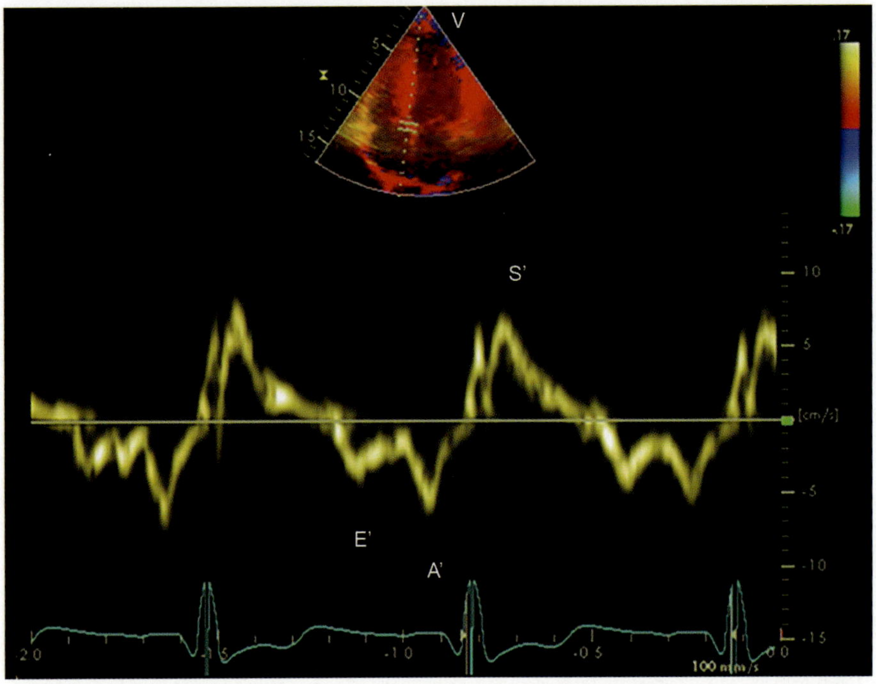

Fig. 11: Tissue Doppler waveforms at medial mitral annulus, i.e. tissue systolic velocity (S') and tissue diastolic velocities (E' and A').

- Tissue Doppler imaging (TDI) is an echocardiographic technique that uses Doppler principles to measure the low velocity high amplitude signals of myocardial motion.
- TDI can be performed in pulsed-wave and color modes.
- Pulsed-wave TDI is used to measure peak myocardial velocities and is particularly well suited to the measurement of long-axis ventricular motion.
- To measure longitudinal myocardial velocities, the sample volume is placed in the ventricular myocardium immediately adjacent to the mitral annulus.
- Three waveforms are produced as shown in the figure: S', systolic myocardial velocity above the baseline as the annulus descends toward the apex and is a measure of longitudinal systolic function; E', early diastolic myocardial relaxation velocity below the baseline as the annulus ascends away from the apex; A', myocardial velocity associated with atrial contraction.
- The ratio of mitral inflow E and Doppler E', i.e. E/E' ratio can be used to estimate LV filling pressures: E/lateral E'>10 or E/septal E'>15 indicates elevated LV end-diastolic pressure, and E/E'<8 is indicates normal LV end-diastolic pressure.

SPECKLE TRACKING ECHOCARDIOGRAPHY (FIG. 12)

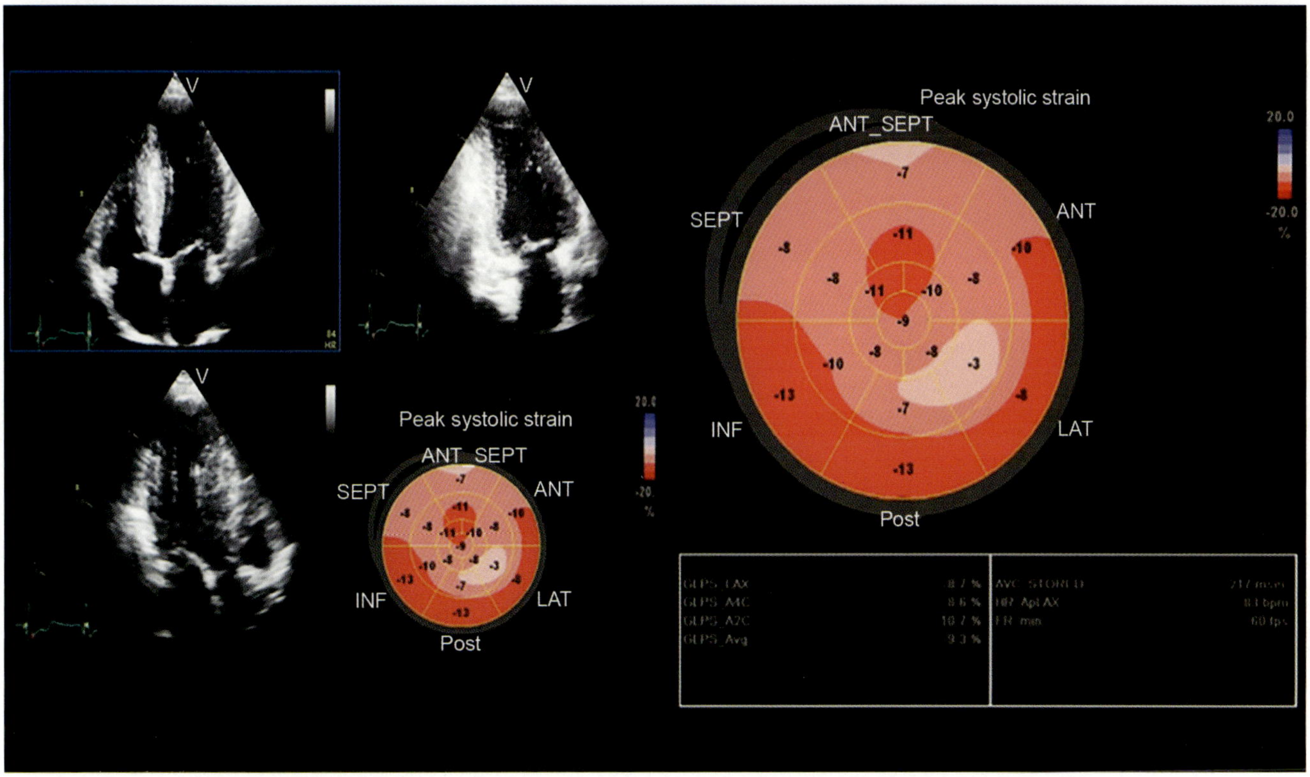

Fig. 12: Bull's eye plot of peak systolic longitudinal strain by speckle tracking echocardiography.

- Speckle tracking echocardiography (STE) is a technique to quantify myocardial deformation.
- The best evaluated strain parameter is global longitudinal strain (GLS).
- GLS has been found to more sensitive than left ventricular ejection fraction (LVEF) as a measure of systolic function and may be used to identify sub-clinical LV dysfunction.
- GLS is now recommended as routine measurement in patients undergoing chemotherapy to detect reduction in LV function prior to fall in LVEF.
- The longitudinal strain bull's eye plot derived from 2D speckle tracking imaging provides an overview of the global and regional left ventricular myocardial function in a single diagram.
- The bull's eye mapping is clinically feasible and the plot patterns could provide clues to the etiology of cardiomyopathies.
- The bull's eye plot can be configured to display either 18 or 17 segments.
- Each myocardial segment is displayed in an intuitively color-coded polar map (red-pink-blue) based on the magnitude of longitudinal strain.
- The inner ring represents the apex of the LV, the middle ring represents the mid-segments and the outer ring represents the basal segments.
- Bright red denotes normal strain values (<–16%), light red denotes reduced value (–16 to –11%), light pink (–10 to –6%) and pale pink (–5 to 0%) denotes severely reduced values, and blue denotes a positive value suggesting paradoxical systolic expansion.
- In a healthy subject, uniformly red pattern of the bull's eye plot represents a normal range in strain values.

TRANSGASTRIC TWO-CHAMBER VIEW (FIG. 13)

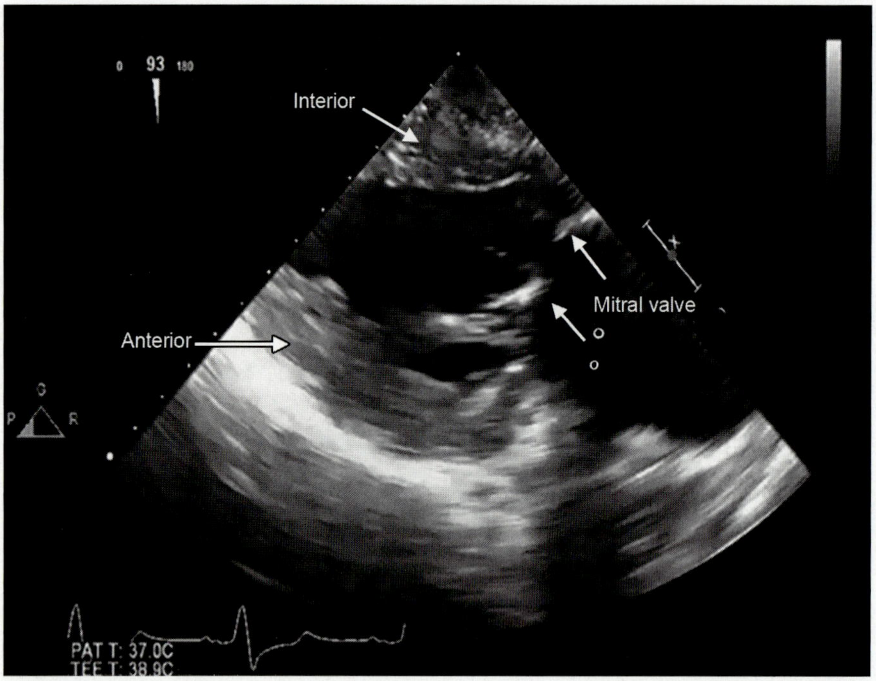

Fig. 13: Transgastric two-chamber view on TEE demonstrating anterior and inferior walls of left ventricular (LV).

- In transgastric two-chamber view, the inferior and anterior walls of the left ventricle, papillary muscles, chordae and mitral valve can be imaged.

ATRIAL SEPTAL DEFECT (FIGS. 14A TO D)

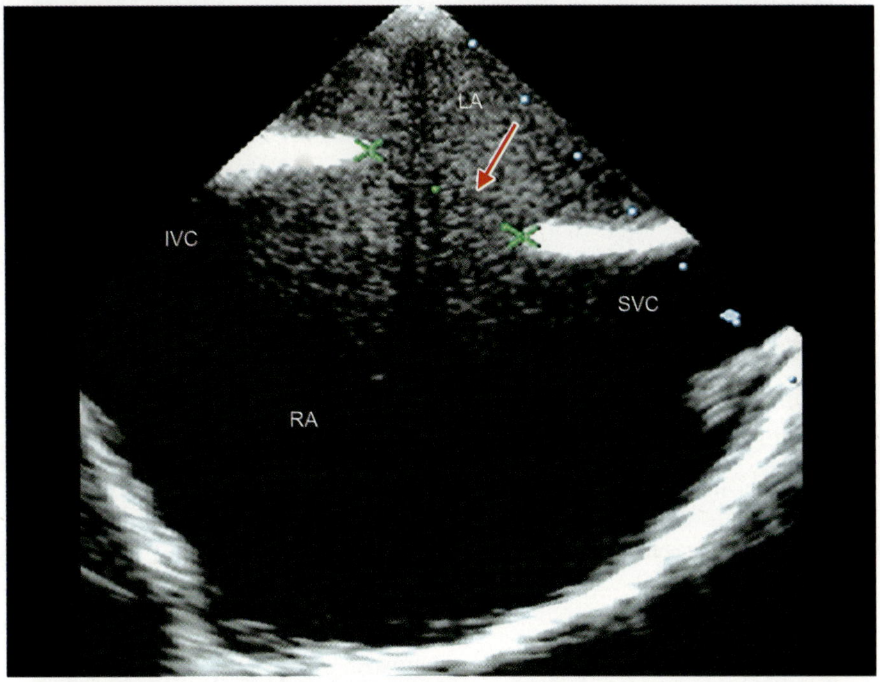

Fig. 14A: Superior vena cava (SVC) and inferior vena cava (IVC) rims of ostium secundum atrial septal defect (ASD) (red arrow) on TEE (bicaval view).

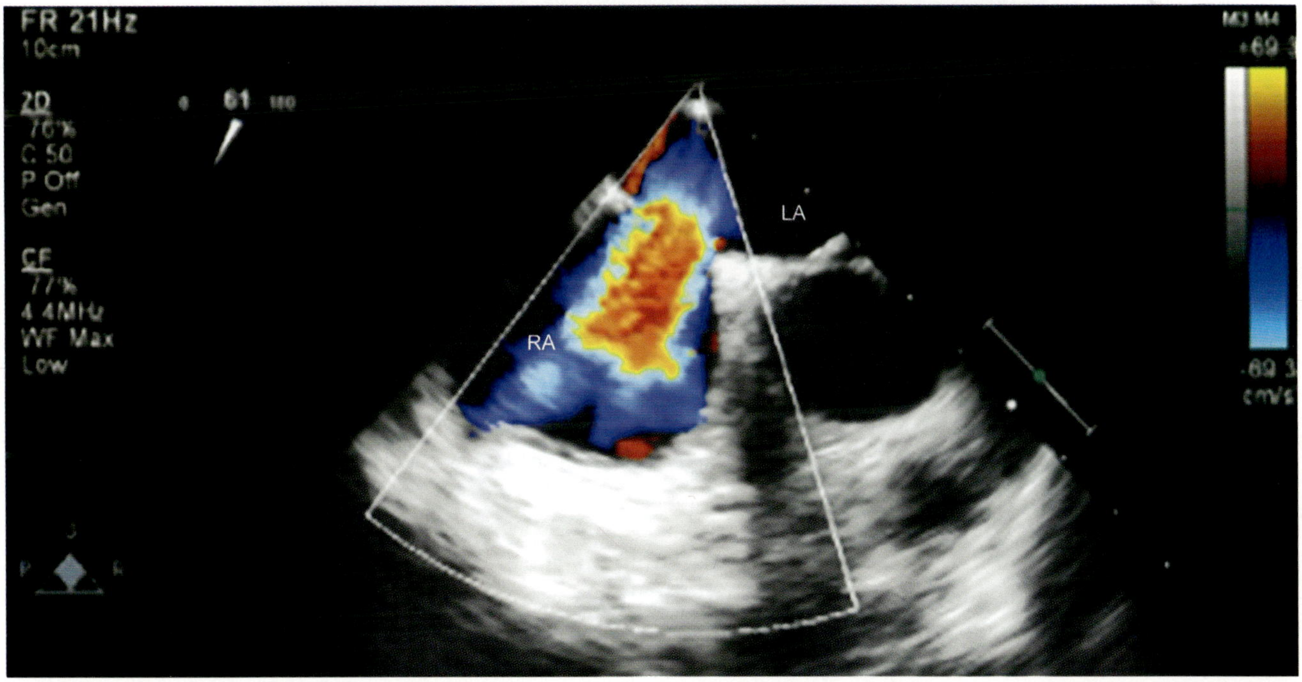

Fig. 14B: Ostium secundum atrial septal defect (ASD) with left to right shunt.

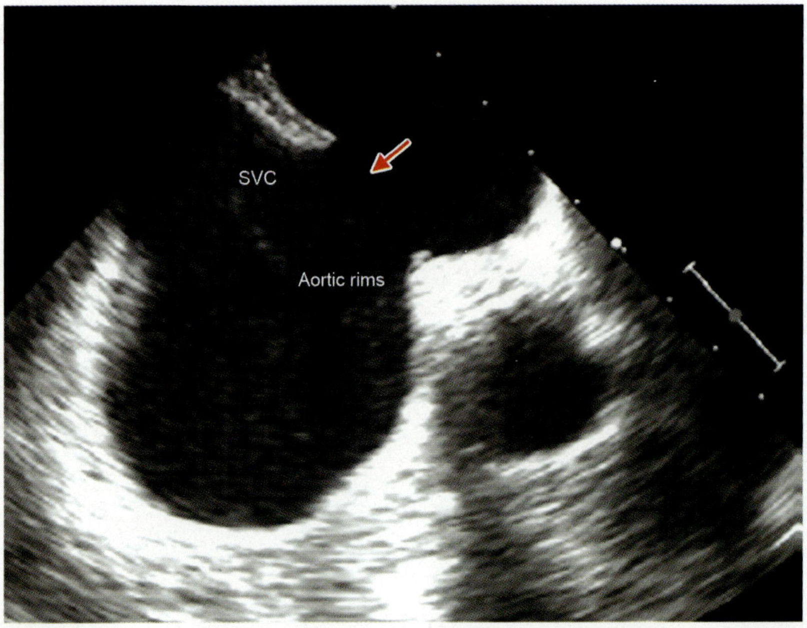

Fig. 14C: Superior vena cava (SVC) and aortic rims of ostium secundum ASD (red arrow) on TEE in basal transverse view. Aortic rim is deficient.

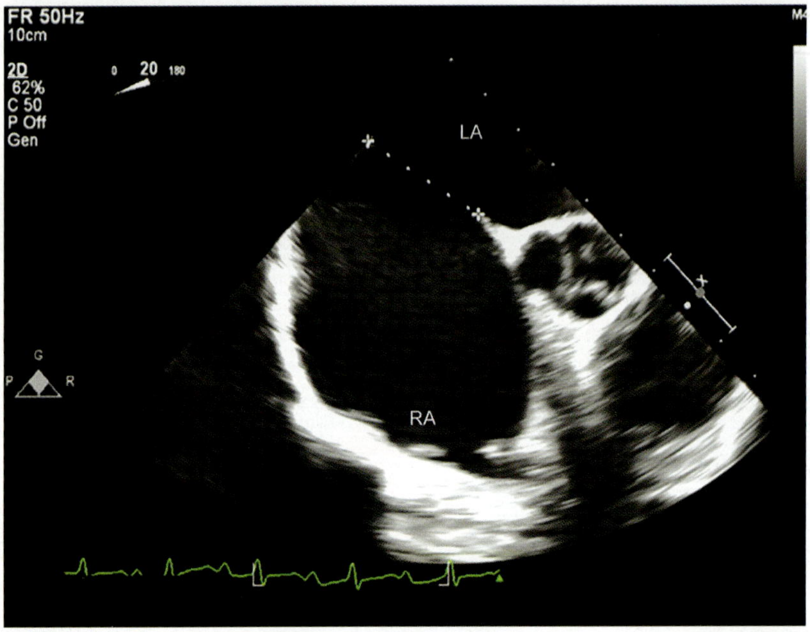

Fig. 14D: Midtransesophageal short-axis view in a 22-year-old patient. Large ostium secundum ASD is visualized.

- The ostium secundum atrial septal defect is the most common type of atrial septal defect.
- Transthoracic echocardiography is the most preferred initial diagnostic modality for the detection and diagnosis of ASD.
- However, TEE is required to further characterize the atrial septal abnormalities and to assess for the suitability for transcatheter closure, because the TTE image quality is usually not sufficient for comprehensive evaluation of the IAS.
- There are six rims for ASD—aortic (superoanterior), mitral (AV valve or inferoanterior), SVC (superoposterior), IVC (inferoposterior), posterior (atrial free wall) and coronary sinus rim.

SINUS VENOSUS ATRIAL SEPTAL DEFECTS (FIG. 15)

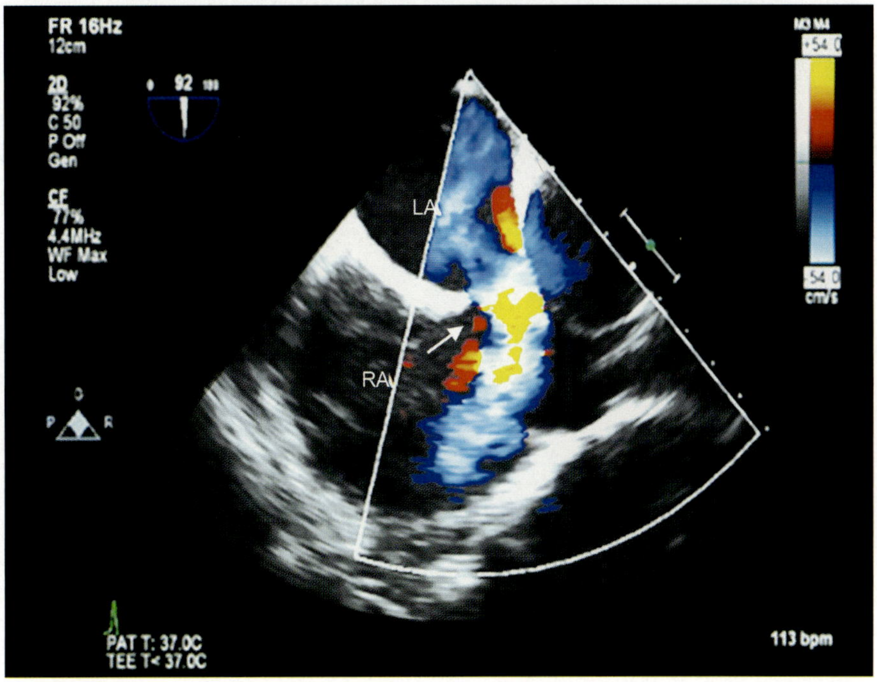

Fig. 15: Superior vena cava (SVC) type of sinus venosus atrial septal defect (ASD) (arrow) with left to right shunt.

- Sinus venosus atrial septal defects (SVASD) are less common than ostium secundum ASDs and are not true ASDs.
- In this defect, interatrial communication is caused by a partial or complete deficiency of the common wall between the superior vena cava (SVC) and the right-sided pulmonary veins, usually associated with anomalous pulmonary venous connection (APVC) of some or all of the pulmonary veins, which produces additional left-to-right shunting.
- In most cases of sinus venosus defects of the SVC type, the right upper pulmonary vein is connected normally but drains anomalously to the RA.
- However, in some cases, the right pulmonary vein or veins will be abnormally connected to the SVC superior to the RA.
- Sinus venosus defects cannot be closed by device and typically require surgical closure (baffling of the right pulmonary veins to the LA by way of an ASD patch).
- Reimplantation of the SVC (Warden procedure) is may be required if the right pulmonary veins are directly connected to the SVC.

PERICARDIAL EFFUSION (FIG. 16)

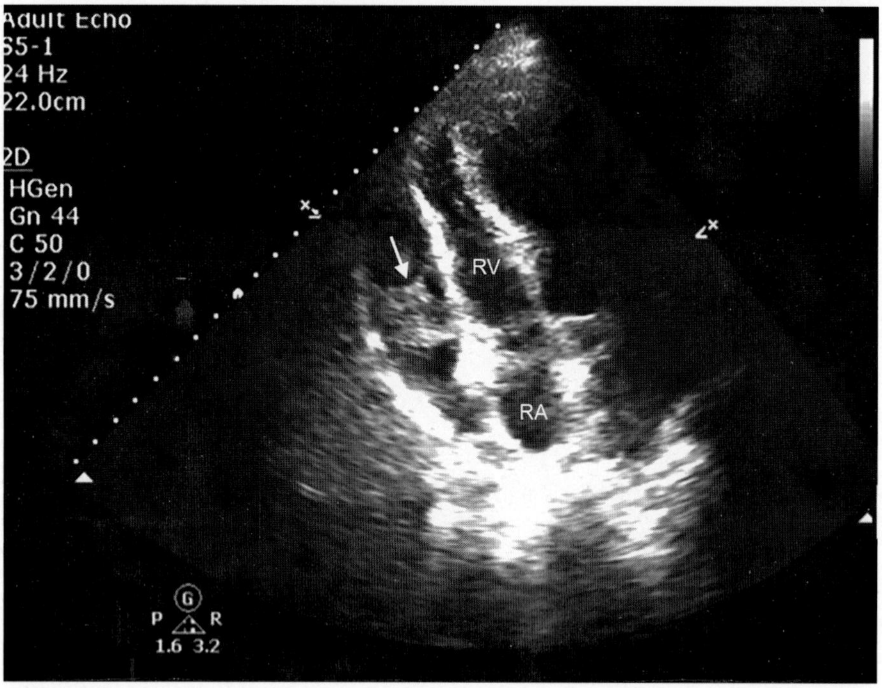

Fig. 16: Pericardial effusion seen along right ventricle (RV) and right atrium (RA) with evidence of clot (arrow) in pericardial space. Echocardiography was done on postoperative day 1 of coronary artery bypass graft (CABG). There were features of cardiac tamponade also, seen as RA and RV collapse.

- Pericardial effusion is a commonly encountered complication of adult cardiac surgery.
- During postoperative period, the pressure–volume relationship of the pericardium is such that rapid accumulation of only small volumes may lead to significant localized increases in intrapericardial pressure.
- Patients following cardiac surgery are less likely to present with classical echocardiographic and clinical features of tamponade because of various factors like localized effusions, underlying cardiac pathology, and positive pressure ventilation used.
- Therefore, one cannot rely on classical echocardiographic features of tamponade to diagnose a hemodynamically significant pericardial collection in cardiac surgical patients and very high index of clinical suspicion should be kept and unconventional transthoracic echo views should be used to thoroughly assess for pericardial effusion or clot in the pericardial space.
- The threshold for doing TEE in postoperative period should be kept low if the transthoracic echo window is poor.

AORTIC REGURGITATION (FIG. 17)

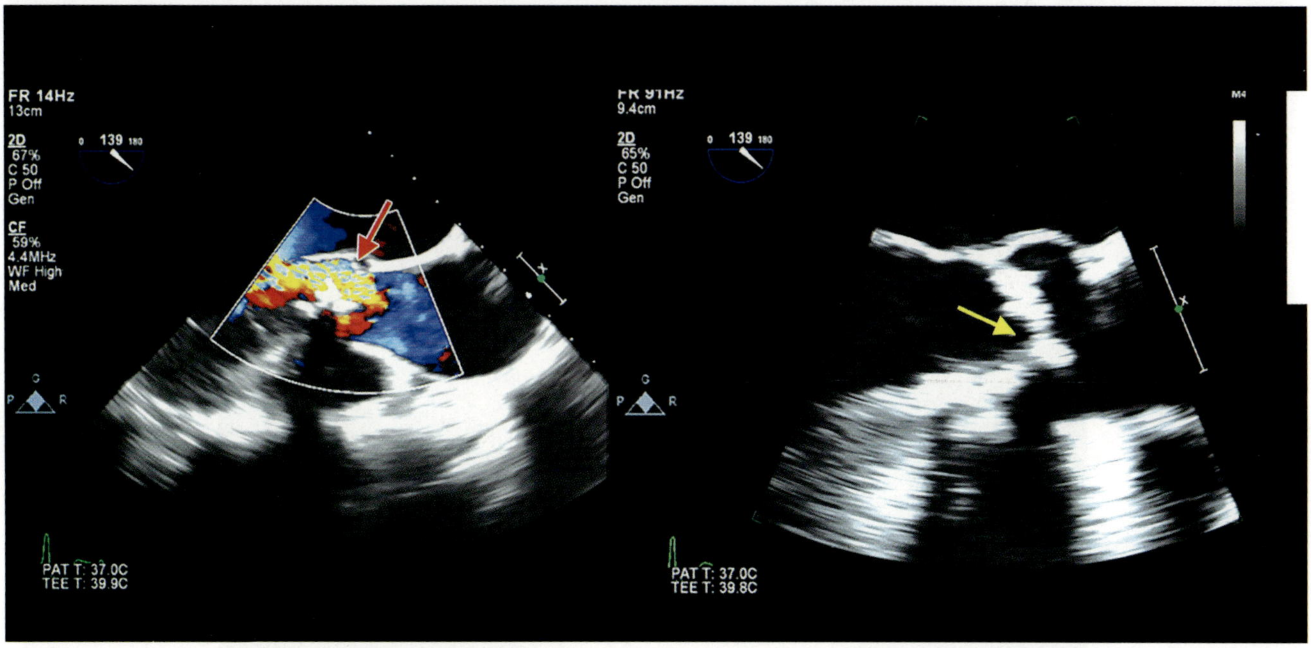

Fig. 17: Thickened aortic cusps (yellow arrow) with severe aortic regurgitation (red arrow) seen in midesophageal long-axis view on TEE.

- Aortic regurgitation (AR) results from the aortic leaflets pathology and/or the aortic root dilatation. Modification of Carpentier classification has been used to classify types of AR.
- **Type I**—normal leaflet motion and is subcategorized based on the pathology involving aortic root or valve. **Type Ia**—when AR is in the presence of sinotubular junction enlargement and dilatation of the ascending aorta, **Type Ib**—AR resulting from dilatation of the sinuses of Valsalva and the sinotubular junction, **Type Ic**—when there is dilatation of the annulus, and **Type Id** results from cusp perforation or fenestration without a primary functional aortic annular lesion.
- **Type II** is associated with excessive leaflet motion from leaflet prolapse.
- **Type III** is seen in congenitally abnormal valves, degenerative calcification, or any other cause of thickening/fibrosis or calcification of the valve leaflets resulting in restricted leaflet movement. AR severity is assessed by various quantitative and semi-quantitative methods such as ratio of jet width to left ventricular outflow tract (LVOT), ratio of jet area to LVOT area, vena contracta, proximal flow convergence, flow reversal in proximal descending aorta, density of regurgitant jet and AR jet deceleration rate.

EFFUSIVE-CONSTRICTIVE PERICARDITIS (FIG. 18)

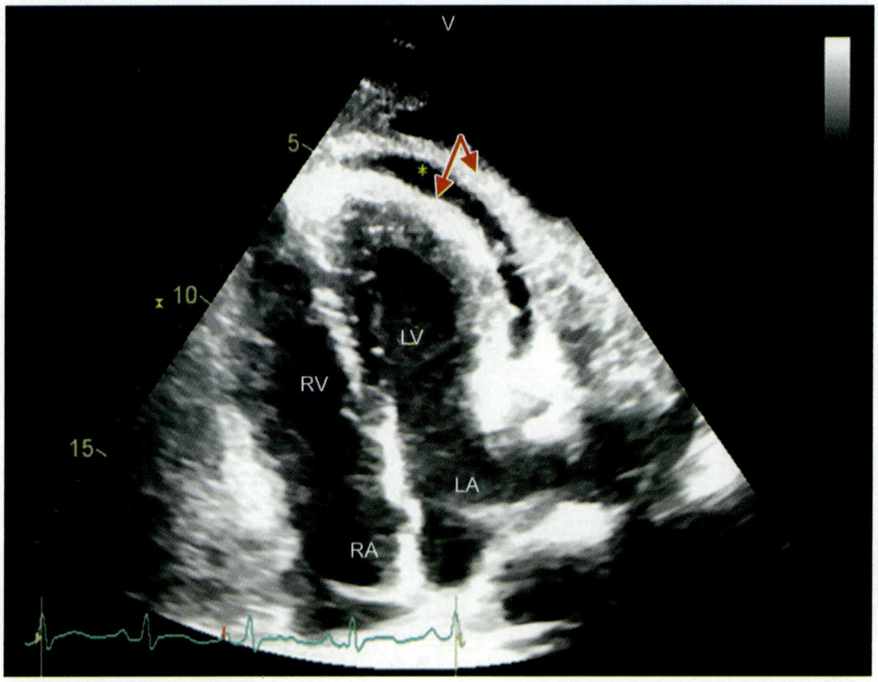

Fig. 18: Thickened visceral and parietal pericardium (arrows) with pericardial effusion (asterisk) along anterolateral wall of left ventricle (LV) in a patient of effusive-constrictive pericarditis.

- Effusive-constrictive pericarditis (ECP) is a disorder on the continuum between effusive and constrictive pericarditis.
- It is due to pericardial inflammation causing constriction in the presence of pericardial effusion. The etiology is similar to that of constrictive pericarditis, though the condition is more often seen in tuberculous pericarditis.
- The accurate diagnosis is made by invasive methods by measuring simultaneous intrapericardial and right atrial pressures with pericardiocentesis.
- Echo-based Doppler methods can assess residual hemodynamic findings of constriction following pericardiocentesis.
- Identifying patients with ECP requires a high index of clinical suspicion. These patients are sometimes identified when the atrial pressures remain elevated after pericardiocentesis.

BICUSPID AORTIC VALVE (FIG. 19)

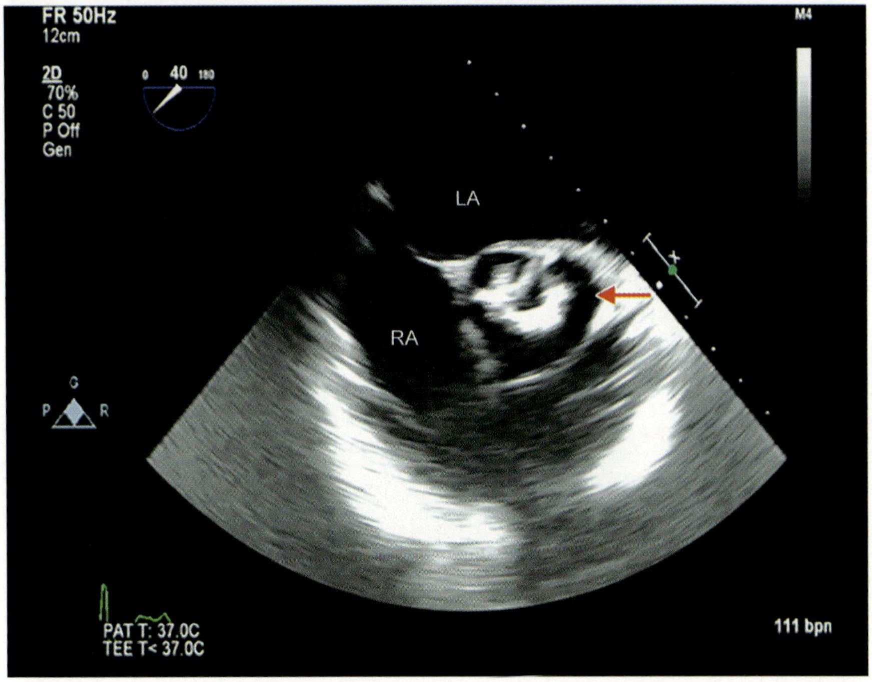

Fig. 19: Midesophageal aortic valve short-axis view on TEE showing thickened bicuspid aortic valve with fish mouth appearance.

- Bicuspid aortic valve (BAV) is the most common congenital cardiac abnormality, affecting almost 1–2% of the general population.
- The BAV is composed of two abnormal leaflets, usually unequal in size and can be complicated with aortic stenosis, aortic regurgitation and endocarditis.
- BAV can also have associated aortopathy which may lead to aortic aneurysm, dissection and rupture. Twenty percent of patients with BAV have another major complication, i.e. coarctation of aorta.

FLAIL MITRAL LEAFLET (FIGS. 20A TO D)

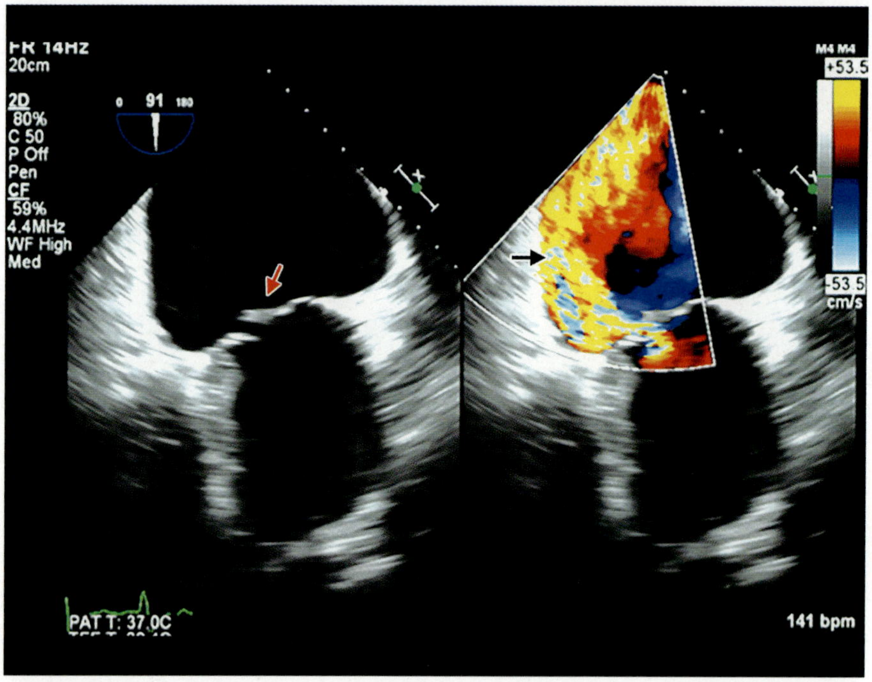

Fig. 20A: Midesophageal long-axis TEE view showing flail anterior mitral leaflet (AML) (red arrow) resulting in posteriorly directed jet of severe mitral regurgitation (black arrow).

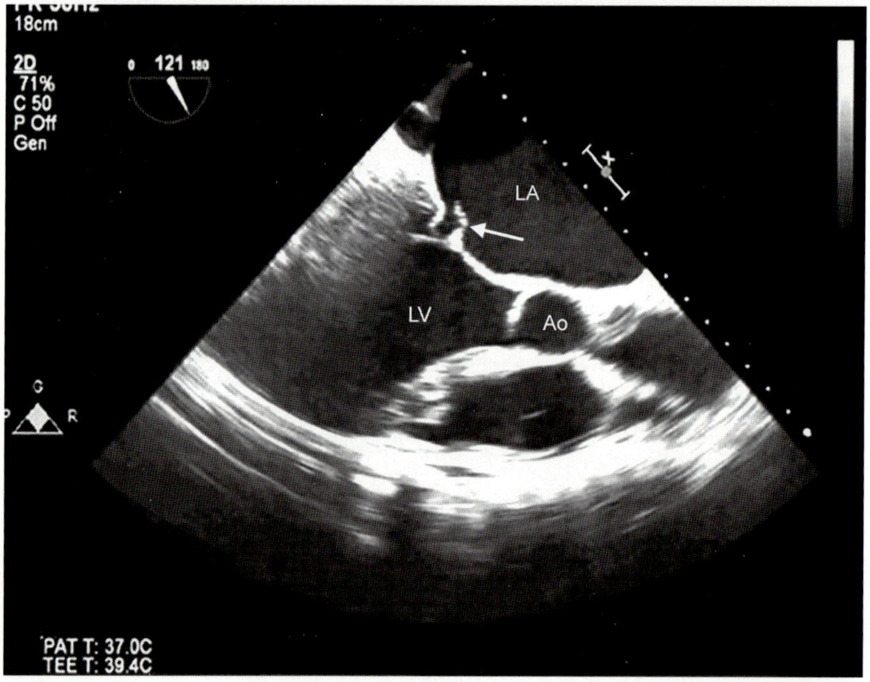

Fig. 20B: Midesophageal long-axis TEE view: flail A3 scallop of anterior mitral leaflet (AML) (arrow).

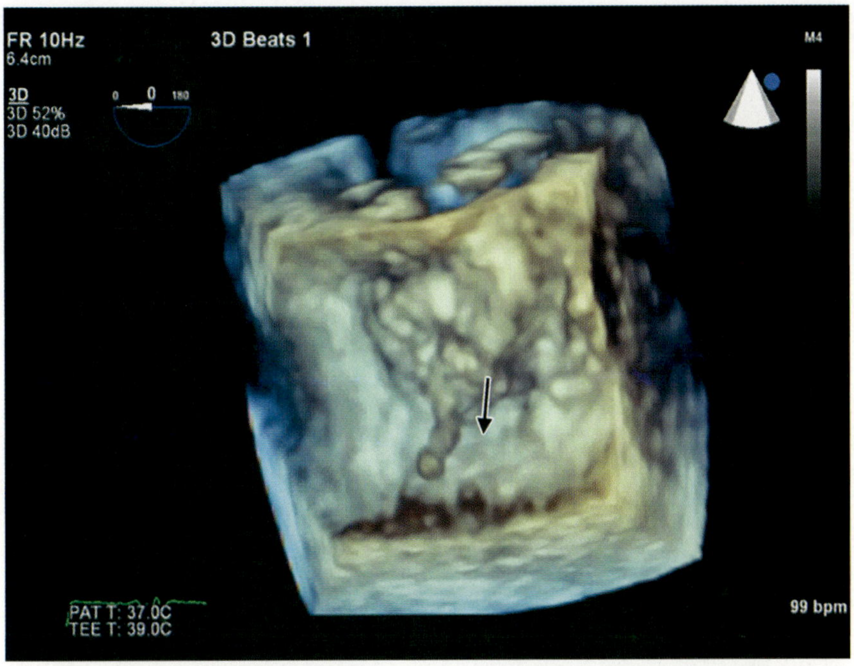

Fig. 20C: Transesophageal 3D image showing flail A2 scallop. Ruptured chorda is seen attached to the flail segment.

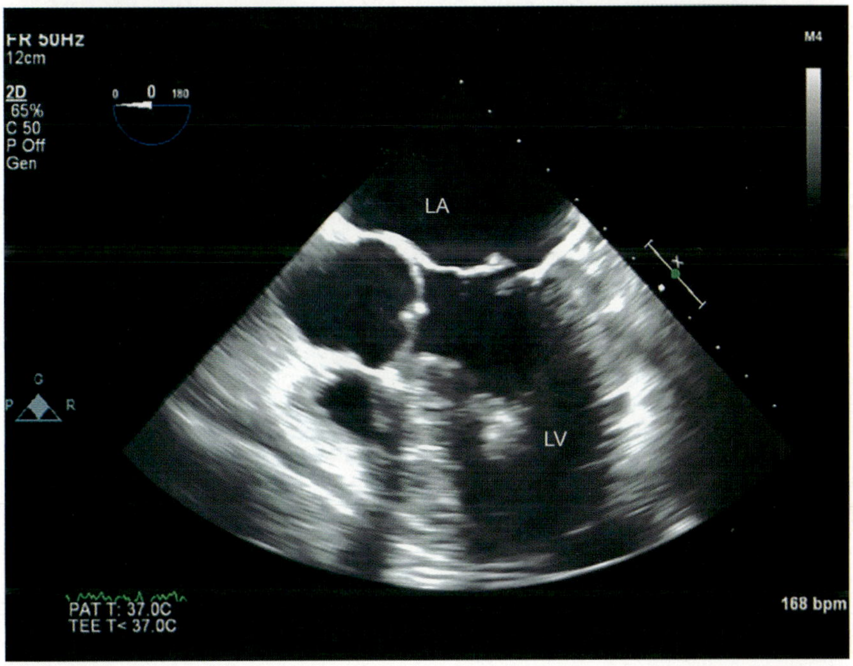

Fig. 20D: Transesophageal view demonstrating flail anterior mitral leaflet (AML) with non-coaptation.

- Most common causes of flail mitral leaflet are chordal rupture, myxomatous degeneration, infective endocarditis and papillary muscle rupture.
- Flail mitral leaflets usually lead to severe mitral regurgitation and unlike mitral valve prolapse, tip of flail leaflet points towards left atrium and away from apex in systole.
- Transesophageal echo is an extremely useful modality in assessing the mitral valve morphology and to identify the involved scallop of mitral valve.
- Management—surgical repair.

SINUS OF VALSALVA ANEURYSMS (FIGS. 21A AND B)

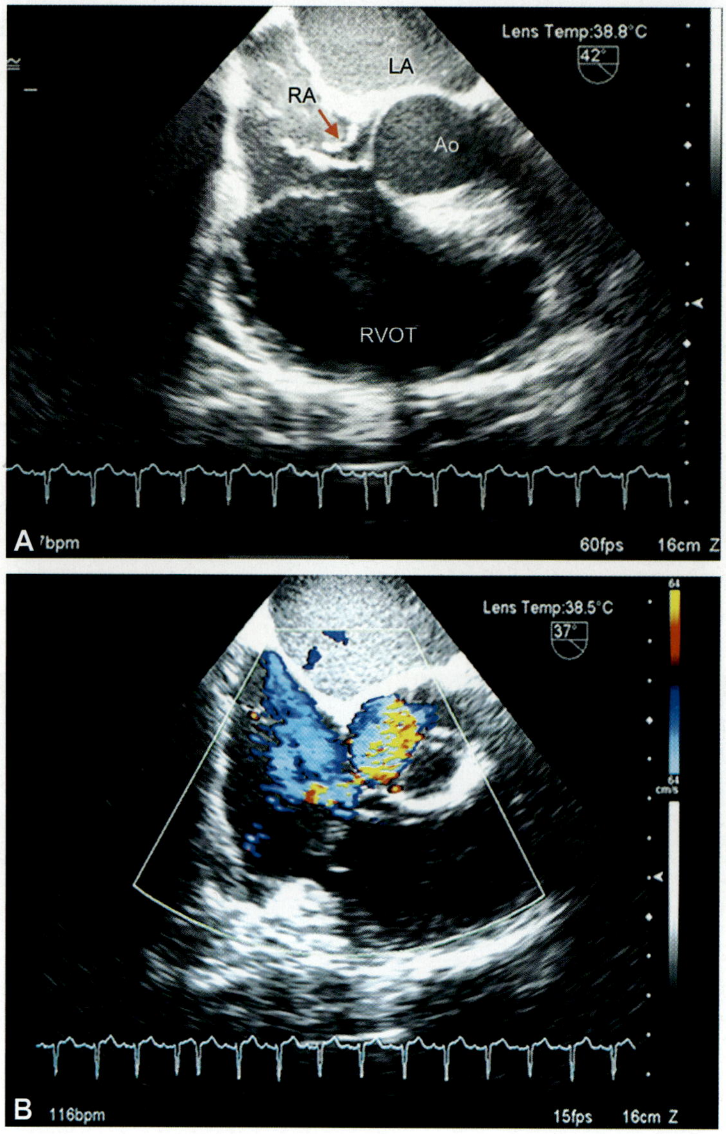

Figs. 21A and B: Midesophageal aortic valve short-axis view on TEE showing ruptured noncoronary sinus of Valsalva (RSOV) (red arrow) to right atrium (RA).

- Aneurysm of sinus of Valsalva can be congenital or acquired.
- Congenital lack of continuity in the media, between the aorta and annulus fibrosus of the aortic valve, may result in aneurysm formation.
- Acquired aneurysms are seen in association with Marfan syndrome, infective endocarditis, syphilis, trauma, atherosclerosis, and collagen vascular disorders.
- Majority of sinus of Valsalva aneurysms (SVA) arise from right coronary sinus and rupture in right ventricle and those arising from noncoronary sinus rupture into right atrium.
- Left aortic sinus aneurysm commonly ruptures into left atrium or left ventricle or pulmonary artery.
- His Echocardiography remains the most commonly used diagnostic modality for ruptured sinus of Valsalva.
- The gold standard diagnostic test is cardiac catheterization with aortography. Other imaging techniques include MRI and CT angiography.

BICUSPID AORTIC VALVE (FIG. 22)

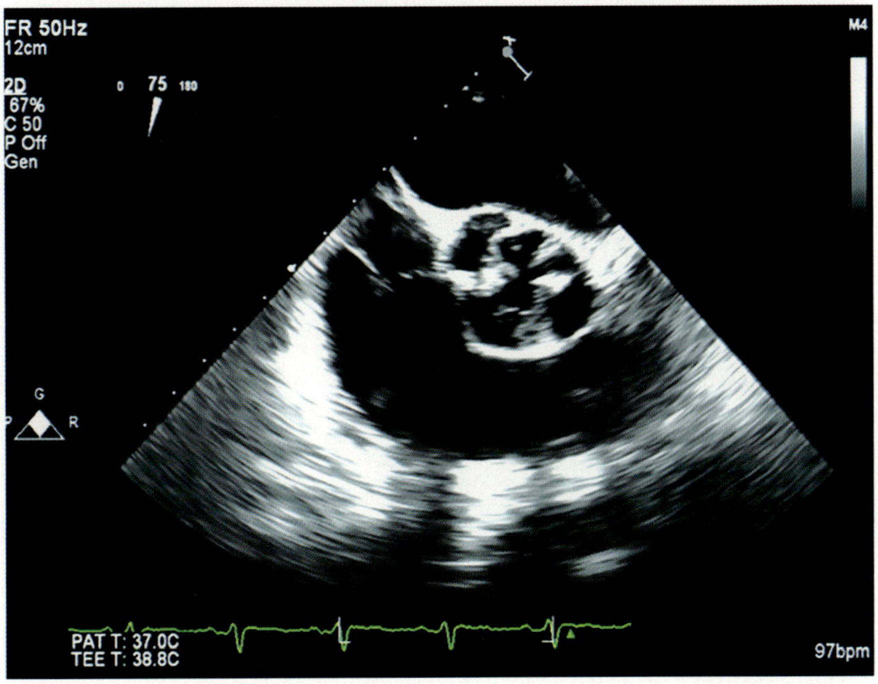

Fig. 22: Transesophageal short-axis view demonstrating bicuspid aortic valve in left-right configuration. Thickening and calcification of valve leaflets is visualized.

- Incidence of bicuspid aortic valve (BAV) is 1–2% of general population.
- It may be associated with aortopathy, leading to dilatation of ascending aorta.
- Risk of dissection is 5–9 times higher than in general population.
- Twenty percent of patients develop severe aortic regurgitation between 10 and 40 years of age.

SEVERE MITRAL REGURGITATION (FIG. 23)

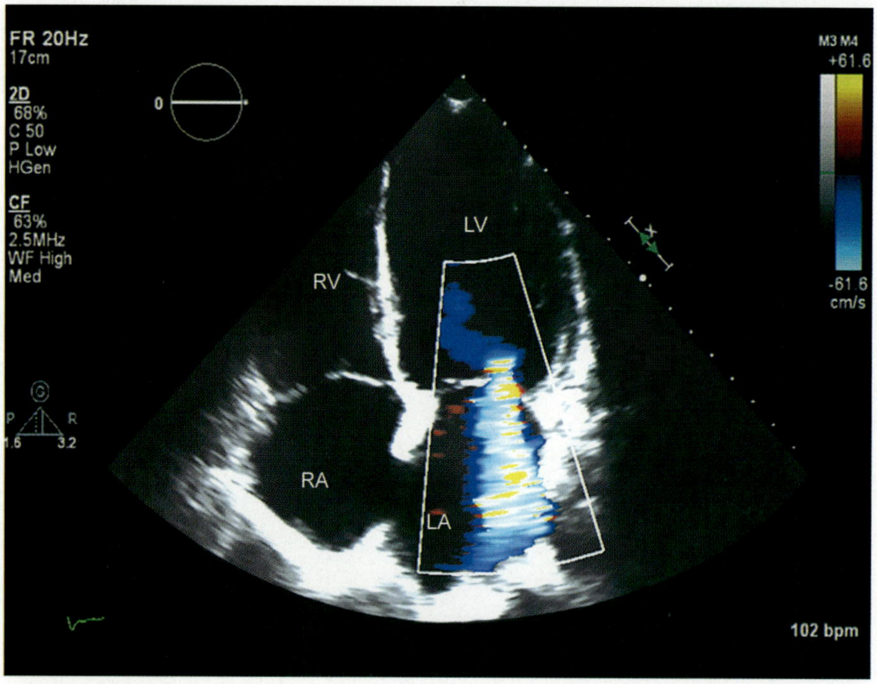

Fig. 23: Transthoracic apical four-chamber view showing dilated left ventricle and severe central mitral regurgitation.

- Main causes of mitral regurgitation (MR) are—mitral valve prolapse, rheumatic heart disease, infective endocarditis, mitral annular calcification, cardiomyopathy, ischemic heart disease.
- MR can be classified as—
  - Primary (degenerative)—due to disease of mitral leaflets.
  - Secondary (functional)—due to diseases of left ventricle or mitral annulus.

CORE VALVE (FIGS. 24A AND B)

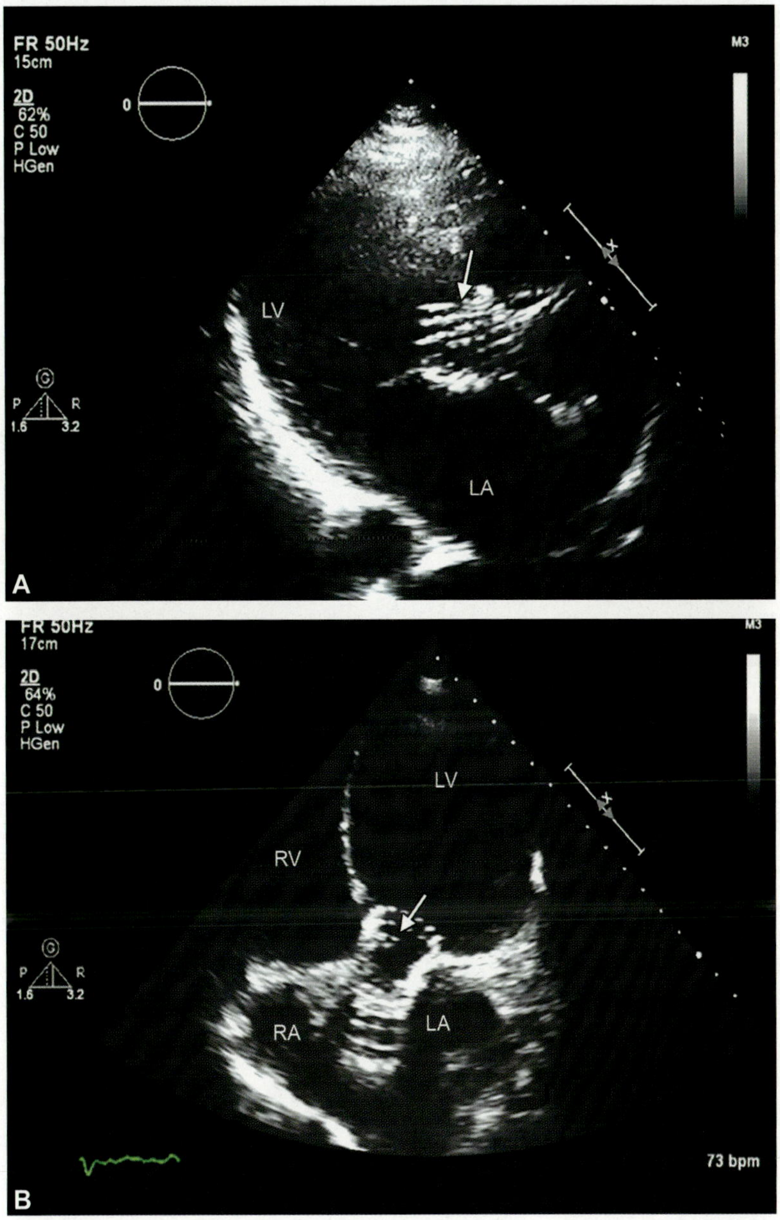

Figs. 24A and B: (A) Post-transcatheter aortic valve replacement (TAVR) patient: core valve seen *in situ*. Parasternal long-axis view; and (B) Post-TAVR patient: core valve seen *in situ*. Apical five-chamber view.

- Transcatheter aortic valve replacement (TAVR) is an alternative to surgical AVR in patients of symptomatic severe aortic stenosis with high surgical risk.
- Two types of valve are in use—self-expanding and balloon expanding.
  - Self-expanding—Core Valve, Core Valve Evolute R, Core Valve Evolute Pro, etc.
  - Balloon expanding—Edwards SAPIEN THV system, Edwards SAPIEN XT, Edwards SAPIEN S3, etc.

TRICUSPID REGURGITATION (FIGS. 25A AND B)

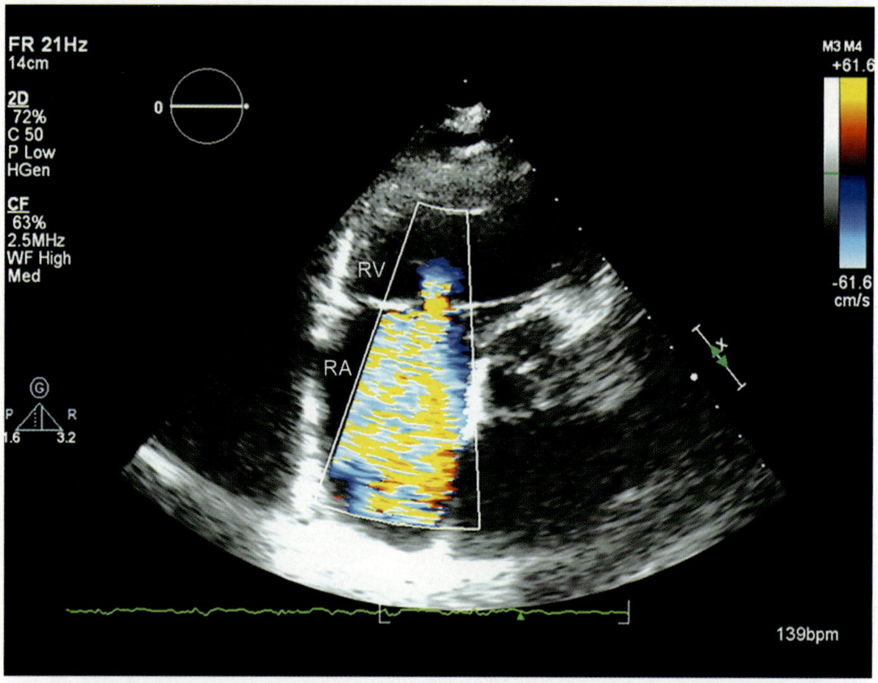

Fig. 25A: Transthoracic right ventricle focused view demonstrating severe tricuspid regurgitation.

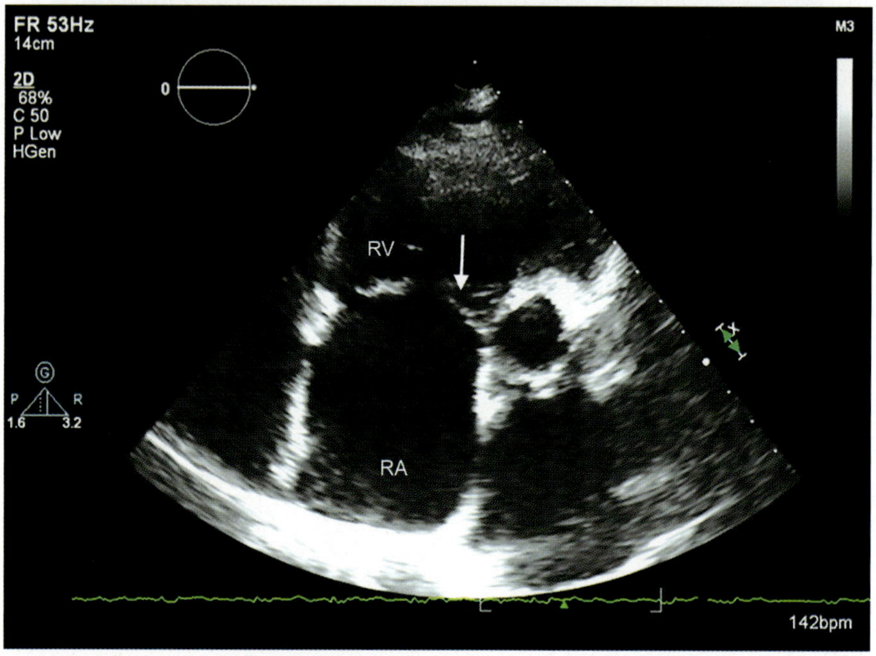

Fig. 25B: Transthoracic right ventricle focused view. Dilated tricuspid annulus resulting in non-coaptation of leaflets, dilated right atrium and right ventricle.

- Most common cause of tricuspid regurgitation (TR) is dilatation of right ventricle and tricuspid annulus (secondary TR).
- Other causes of TR are—RV infarction, pulmonary stenosis and pulmonary hypertension.
- Organic TR can occur in Ebstein's anomaly, rheumatic heart disease (RHD), AV canal defect.

RHEUMATIC DISEASE OF TRICUSPID VALVE (FIG. 26)

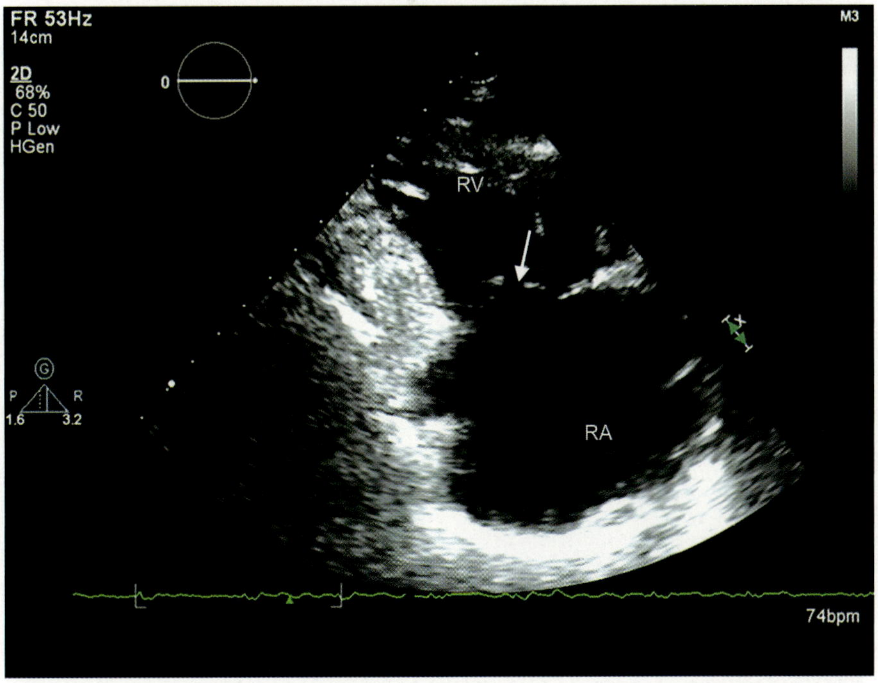

Fig. 26: Right ventricle inflow view in a patient of rheumatic heart disease. Thickening and non-coaptation of leaflets are visualized.

- It is associated with rheumatic disease of mitral and tricuspid valve.
- May result in tricuspid regurgitation alone due to malcoaptation of leaflets or in association with tricuspid stenosis.

INFECTIVE ENDOCARDITIS (FIGS. 27A TO D)

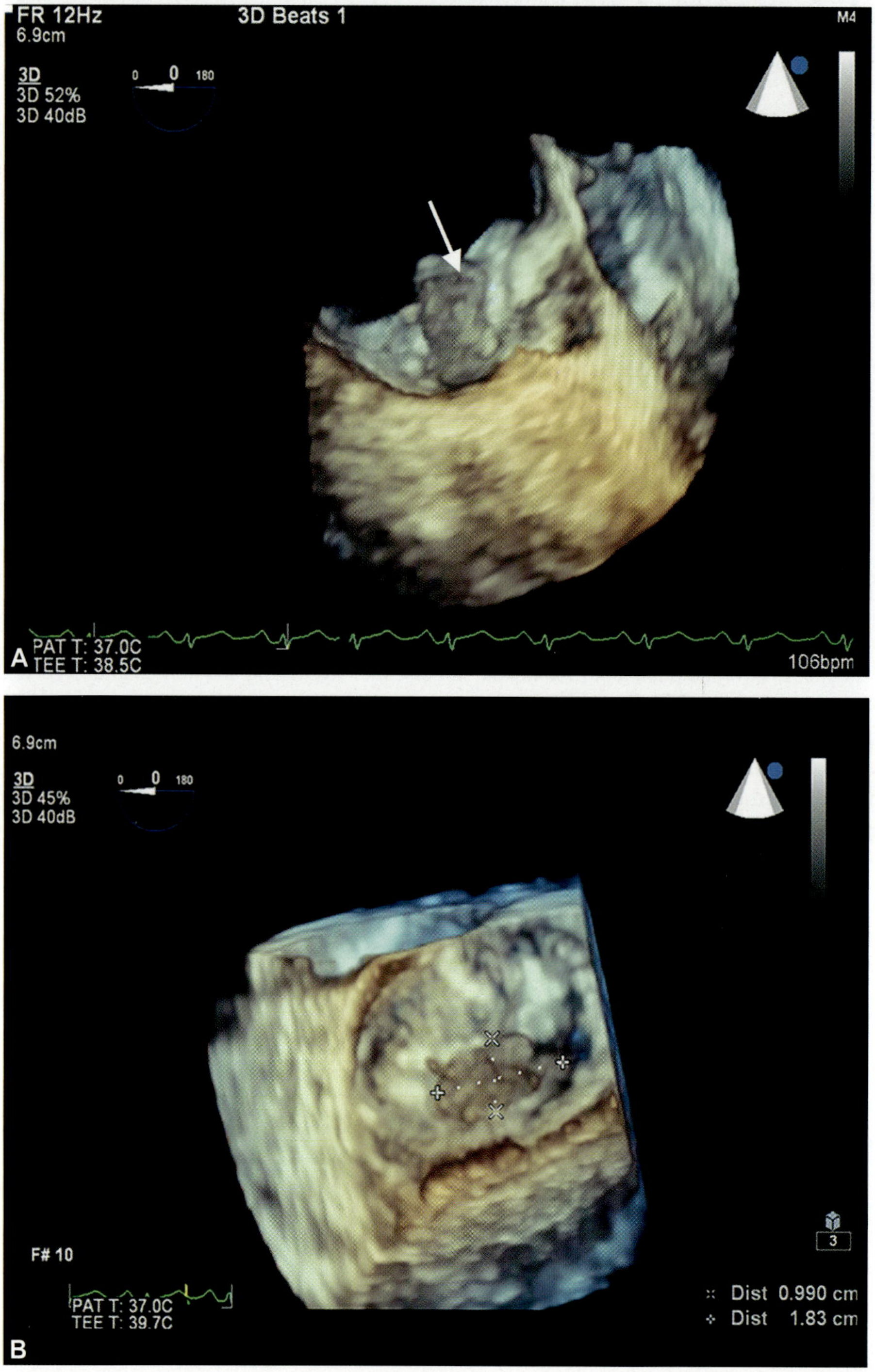

Figs. 27A and B: Transesophageal 3D image showing large vegetation on posterior mitral leaflet (PML).

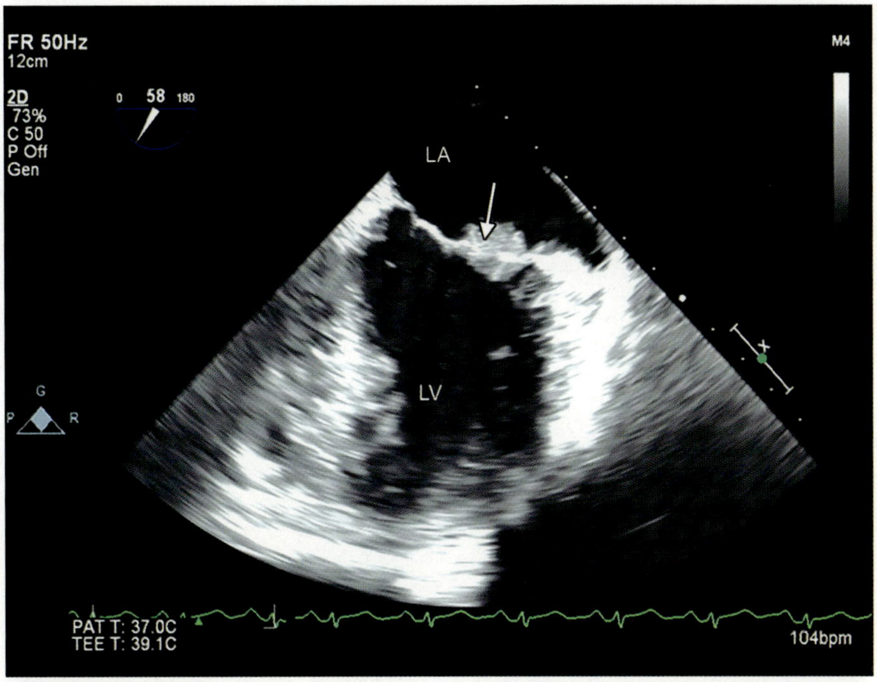

Fig. 27C: Transesophageal bicommissural view in a patient of recurrent stroke. Large vegetation involving the base and midportion of posterior mitral leaflet (PML) with multiple small oscillating fronds like extensions.

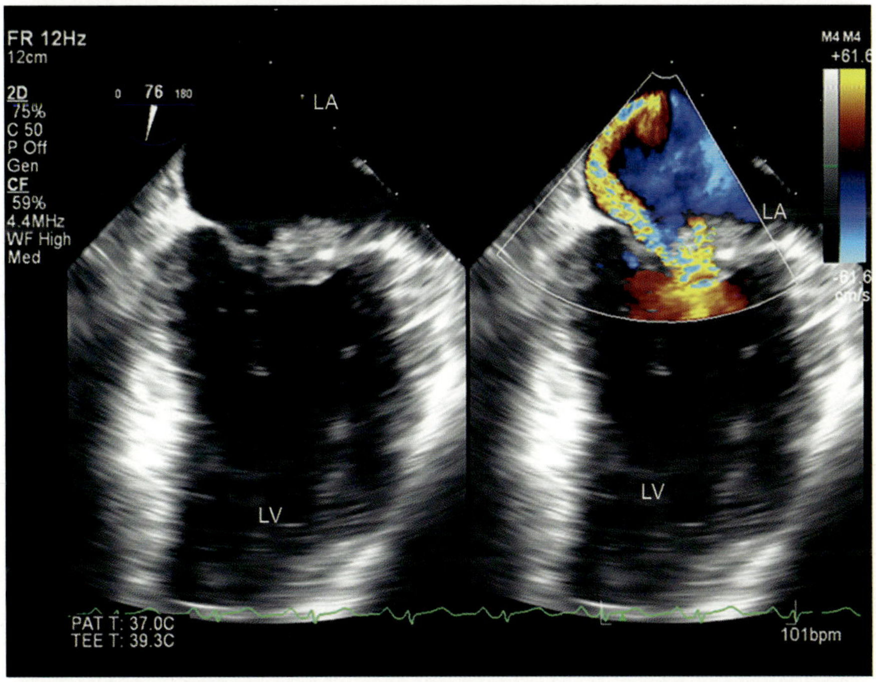

Fig. 27D: Transesophageal bicommissural color compare view showing eccentric anteriorly directed jet of severe mitral regurgitation. Another jet through the perforation in a patient of infective endocarditis.

- Clinical diagnosis is based on modified Duke's criteria.
- Acute cardiovascular complications of infective endocarditis (IE) include perforation of leaflets, rupture of papillary muscle, chordae tendinae leading to severe regurgitation; embolization to systemic and/or coronary circulation.

RIGHT VENTRICLE MYXOMA (FIG. 28)

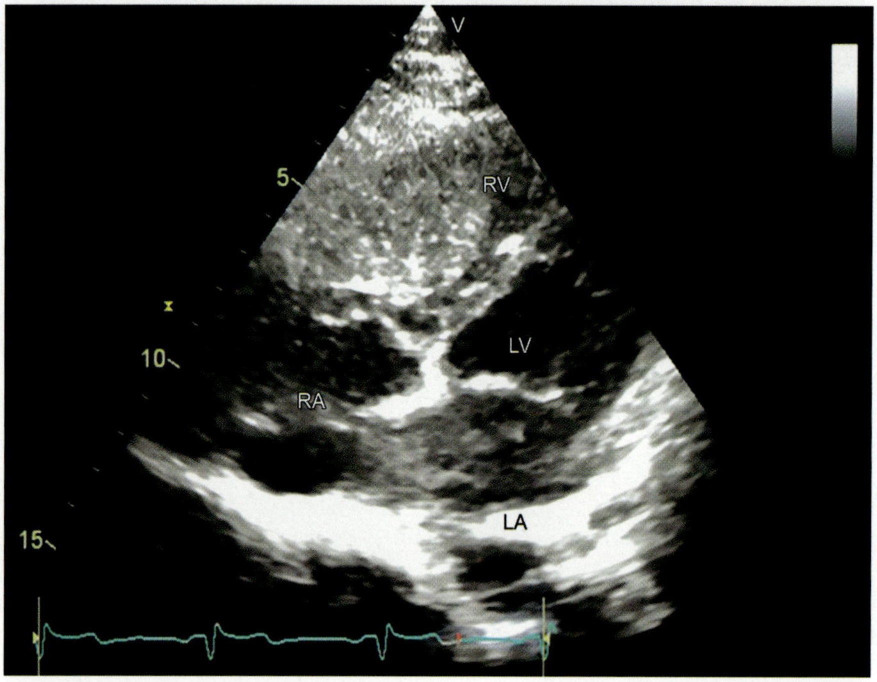

Fig. 28: Transthoracic right ventricle (RV) focused view in a patient of RV myxoma. Myxoma is filling the RV apex, midcavity, and to some extent basal cavity with sparing of tricuspid valve.

- Myxomas are the most common benign tumors of heart in adults.
- Mostly found in left atrium, but are also found in right atrium, right ventricle and left ventricle.
- More common in females (3:1).
- Definitive treatment is surgical removal.
- Recurrence rate varies from 5% to 14%.

AORTIC VALVE ANEURYSM (FIGS. 29A AND B)

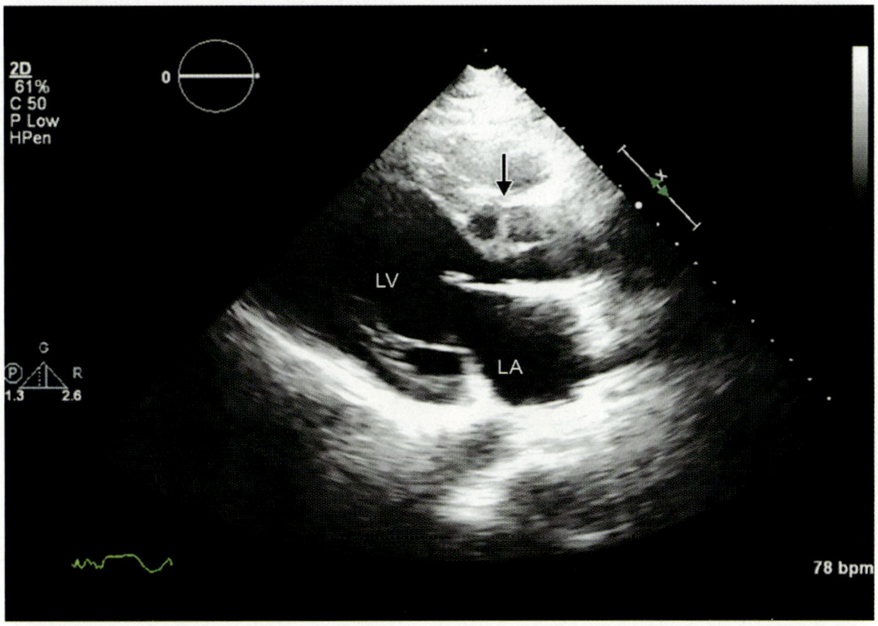

Fig. 29A: Transthoracic parasternal long-axis view in a patient of severe aortic regurgitation. Aneurysmal dilatation of right coronary cusp (RCC) is visualized.

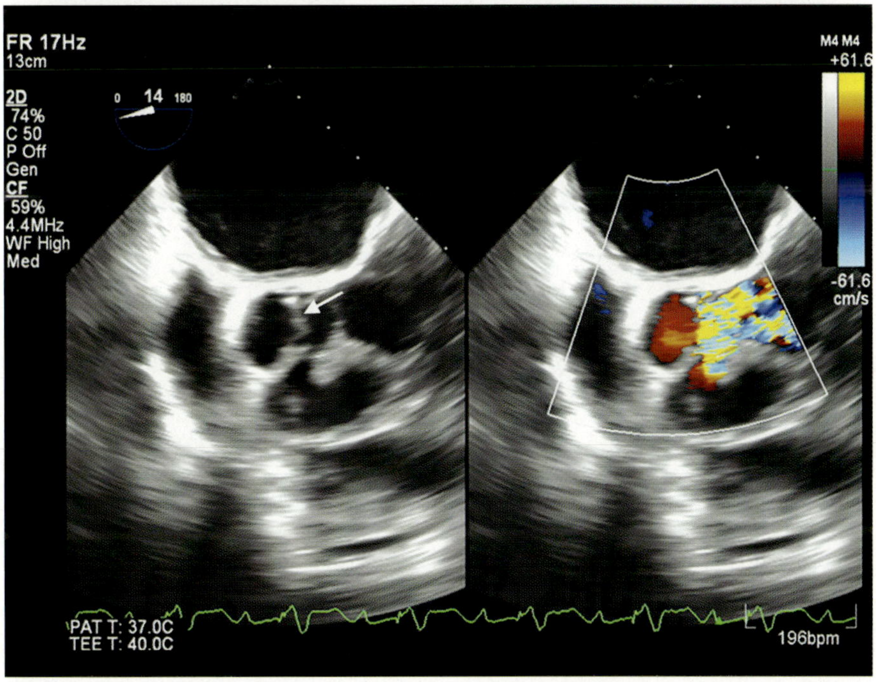

Fig. 29B: Transesophageal color compare view of aortic valve. Aneurysmal dilatation of right coronary cusps with resultant non-coaptation leading to severe aortic regurgitation.

- Aortic valve aneurysm is less frequent than mitral valve aneurysm.
- Most possible causes of aortic valve aneurysm are endocarditis and/or aortitis.
- Most frequent complication is severe aortic regurgitation.
- Management—aortic valve replacement.

QUADRICUSPID AORTIC VALVE (FIGS. 30A AND B)

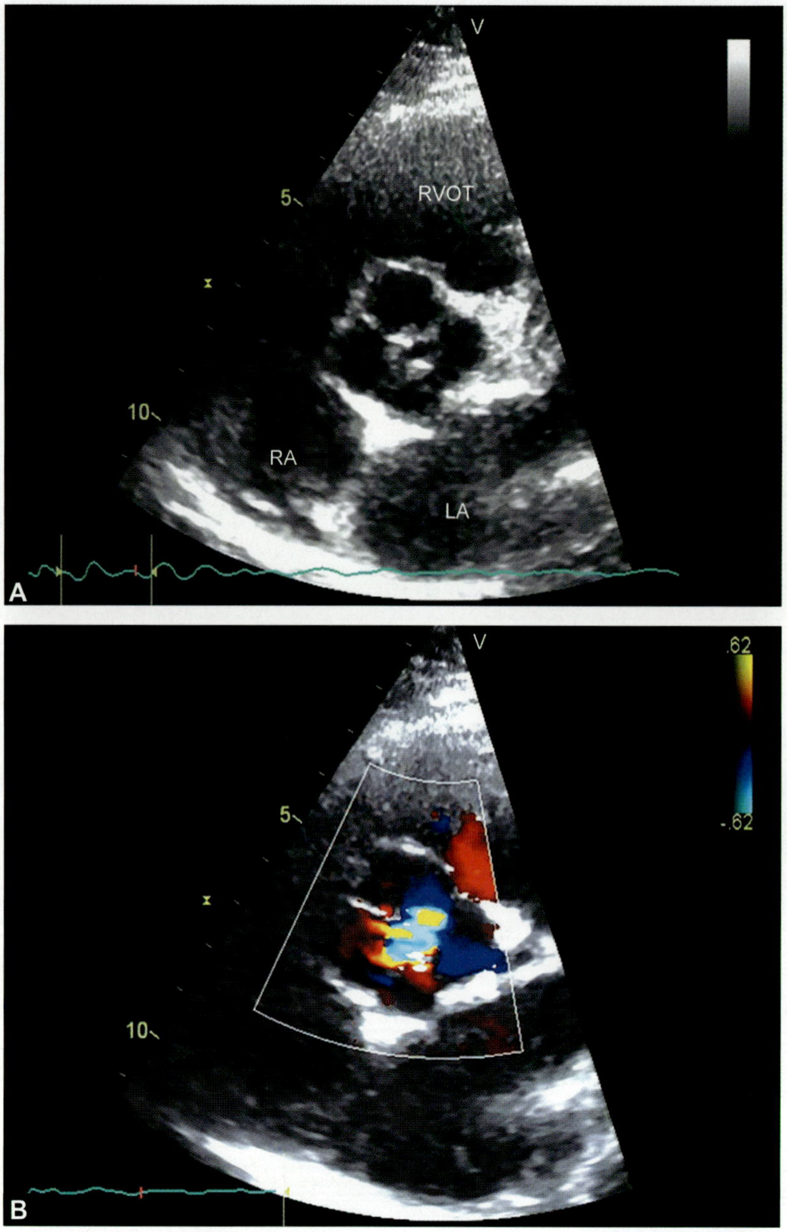

Figs. 30A and B: (A) Transthoracic short-axis view of quadricuspid aortic valve. Image obtained in diastole, note the incomplete valve closure; and (B) Color Doppler image of quadricuspid aortic valve with significant aortic regurgitation (AR).

- Rare congenital anomaly with incidence of 0.01–0.04%.
- Diagnosed in fifth to sixth decade of life.
- Hurwitz Robert classified quadricuspid aortic valve into seven types.
- Most common type is B, often associated with aortic regurgitation.
- Management includes regular follow-up and aortic valve replacement before left ventricular decompensation.

PROSTHETIC VALVE ENDOCARDITIS (FIGS. 31A AND B)

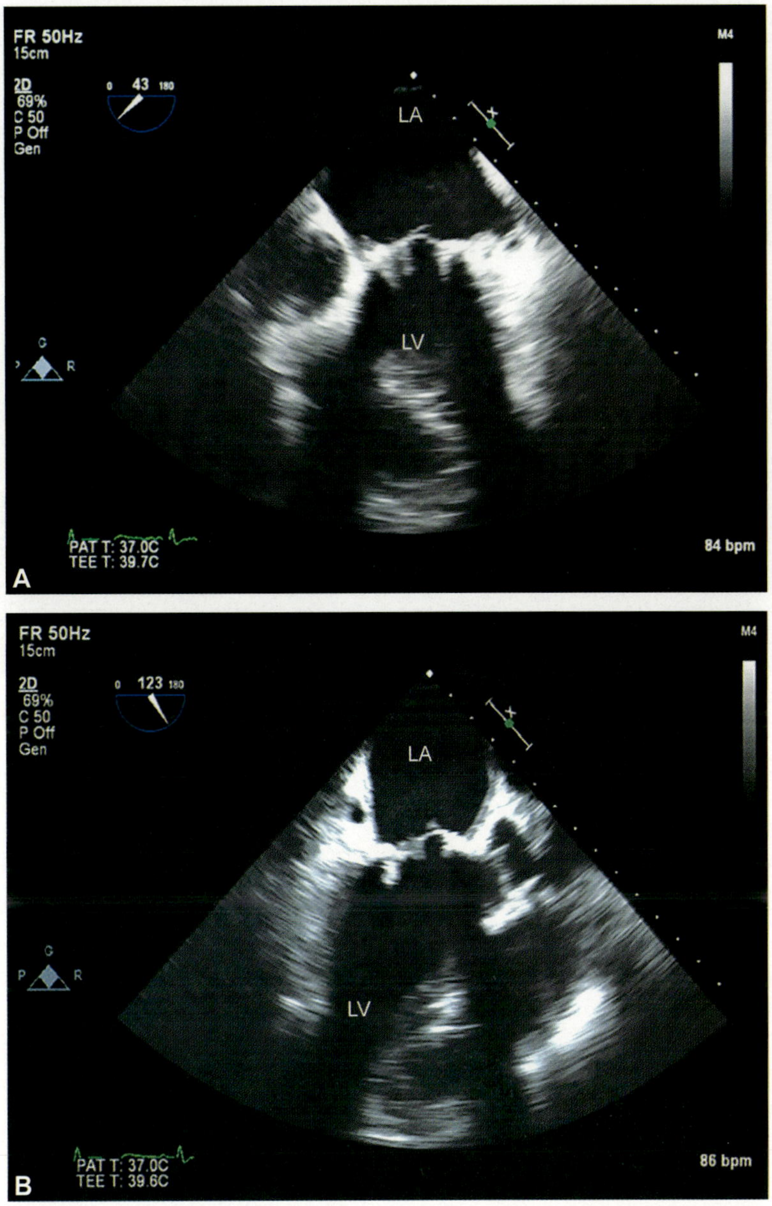

Figs. 31A and B: Multiple vegetations on mitral prosthesis visualized in transesophageal four-chamber view; and (B) Multiple vegetations on mitral prosthesis visualized in transesophageal long-axis view.

- Most severe form of infective endocarditis (IE).
- It accounts for 20% of all cases of IE.
- Bioprosthetic heart valves are at higher risk endocarditis compared to mechanical prosthesis.
- Management—medical management with appropriate antibiotics and surgical intervention in cases of large, mobile vegetation (>10 mm), embolic events, persistent sepsis and prosthesis dehiscence, etc.

LAMBL'S EXCRESCENCE (FIG. 32)

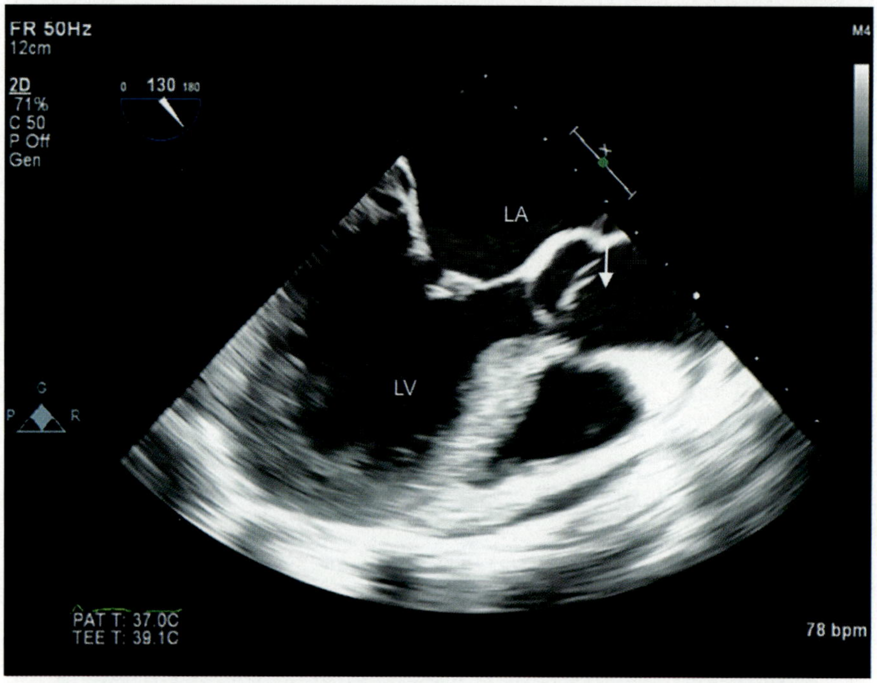

Fig. 32: Transesophageal long-axis view demonstrating Lambl's excrescences.

- These are filamentous extensions of cardiac valves.
- Mostly asymptomatic, but can be associated with thromboembolic events like ischemic stroke and acute coronary syndrome.
- Treatment modalities include dual antiplatelet therapy/anticoagulation and surgical intervention recurrent ischemic events.

LEFT ANTERIOR DESCENDING STENT ABSCESS (FIG. 33)

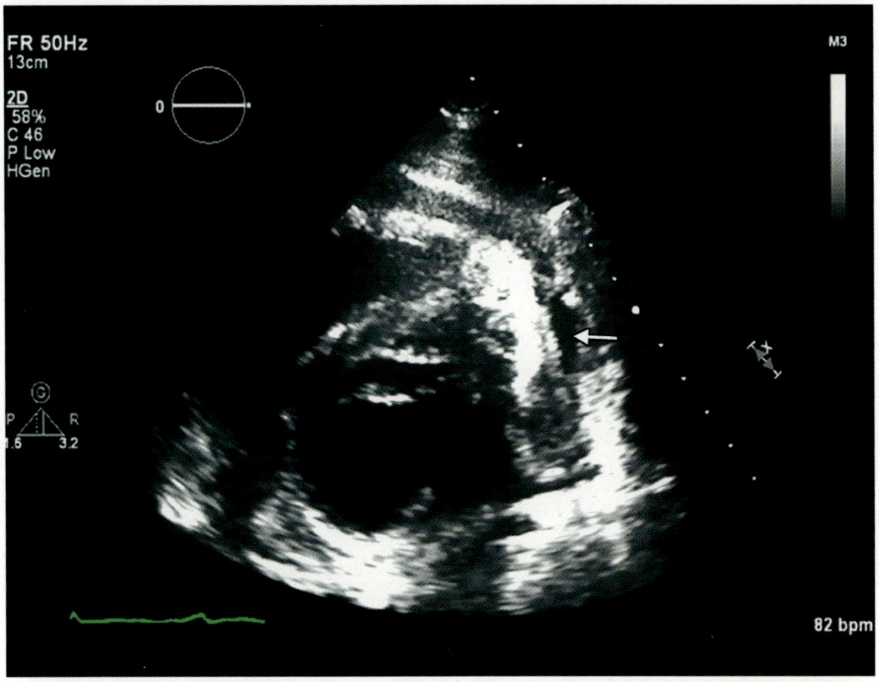

Fig. 33: Transthoracic short-axis view showing abscess around left anterior descending (LAD) stent.

- Coronary stent infection is rare but hard to treat and associated with high mortality rate.
- Early onset infection occurs in less than 10 days of stent placement and late infections after 10 days.
- Treatment of early infection includes medical management with antibiotics while late onset infection with abscess formation requires medical therapy along with surgical stent removal and abscess drainage.

LEFT VENTRICULAR CLOT (FIGS. 34A AND B)

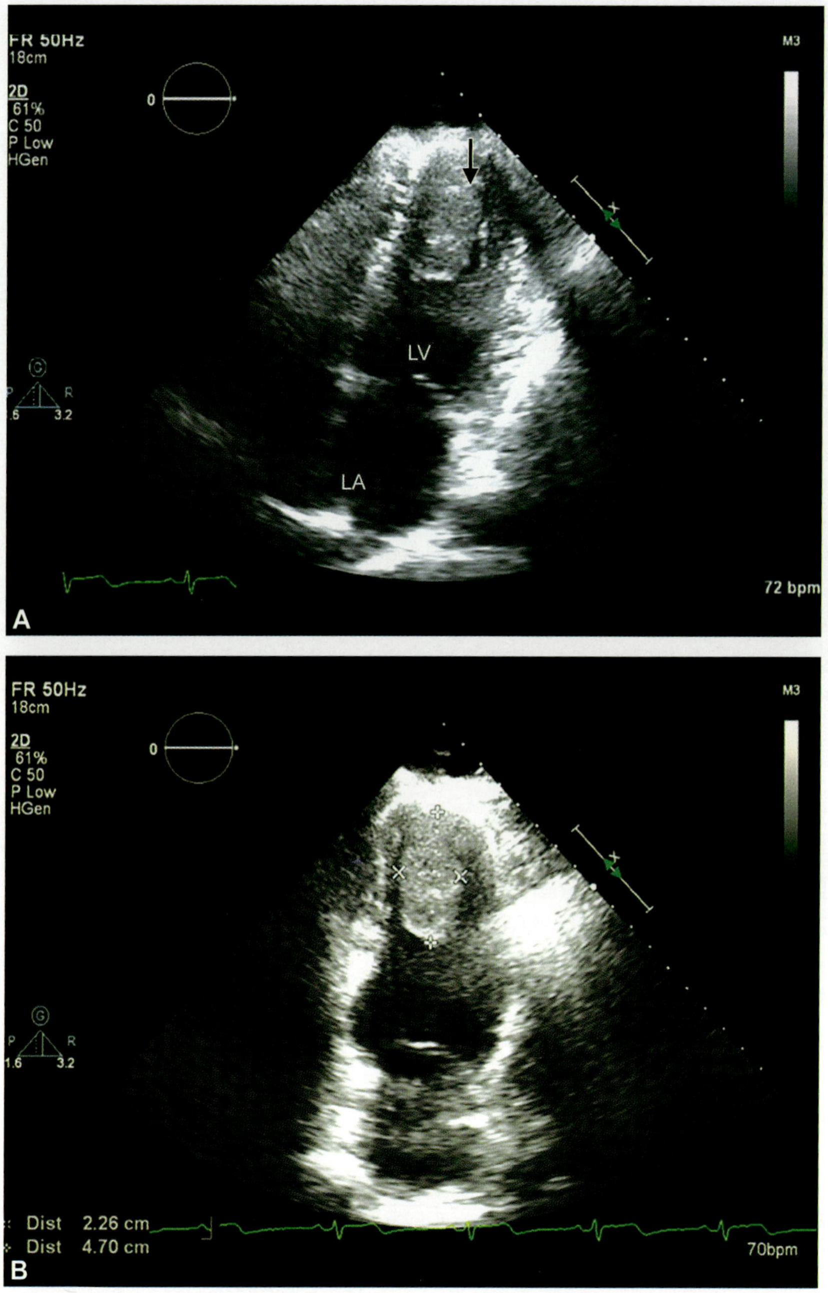

Figs. 34A and B: (A) Transthoracic four-chamber view in a patient of severe left ventricular dysfunction. Large apical clot is visualized; and (B) Transthoracic echocardiography in a patient of severe left ventricular dysfunction. Large apical clot in two-chamber view.

- Left ventricular (LV) clot is seen in patients with recent myocardial infarction, LV aneurysm or dilated cardiomyopathy.
- Most common site is apical region of left ventricle.
- It is associated with high risk of systemic embolization.
- Management—therapeutic anticoagulation.

PSEUDOANEURYSM OF LEFT VENTRICLE (FIG. 35)

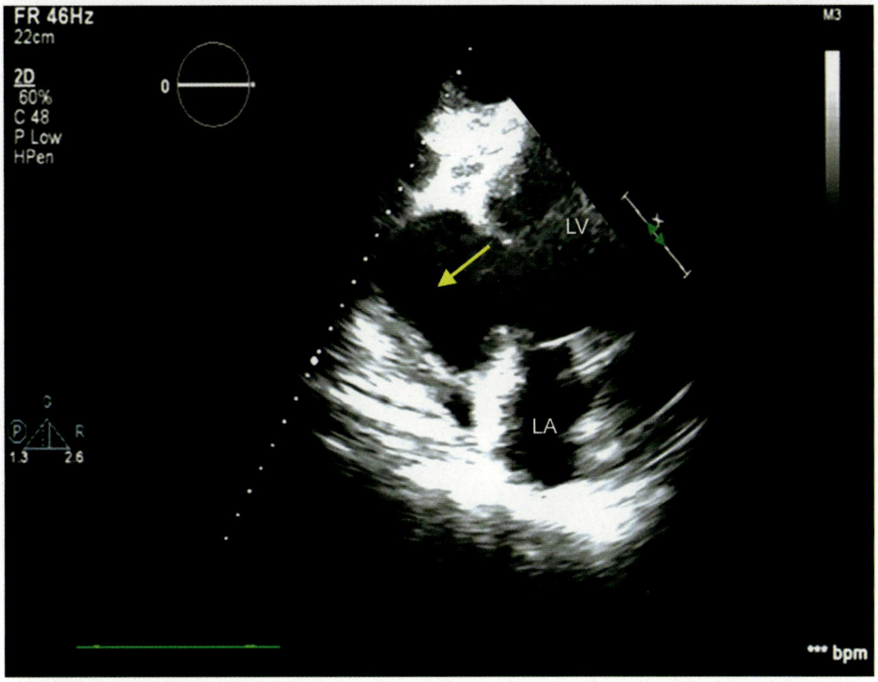

Fig. 35: Transthoracic two-chamber view showing pseudoaneurysm of inferior wall.

- Pseudoaneurysm is the contained rupture of LV free wall.
- It is a complication of acute myocardial infarction.
- Majority are seen in inferoposterior or inferolateral region.
- There is high risk of spontaneous rupture.
- Management—surgical repair.

ARRHYTHMOGENIC RIGHT VENTRICULAR DYSPLASIA/CARDIOMYOPATHY (FIG. 36)

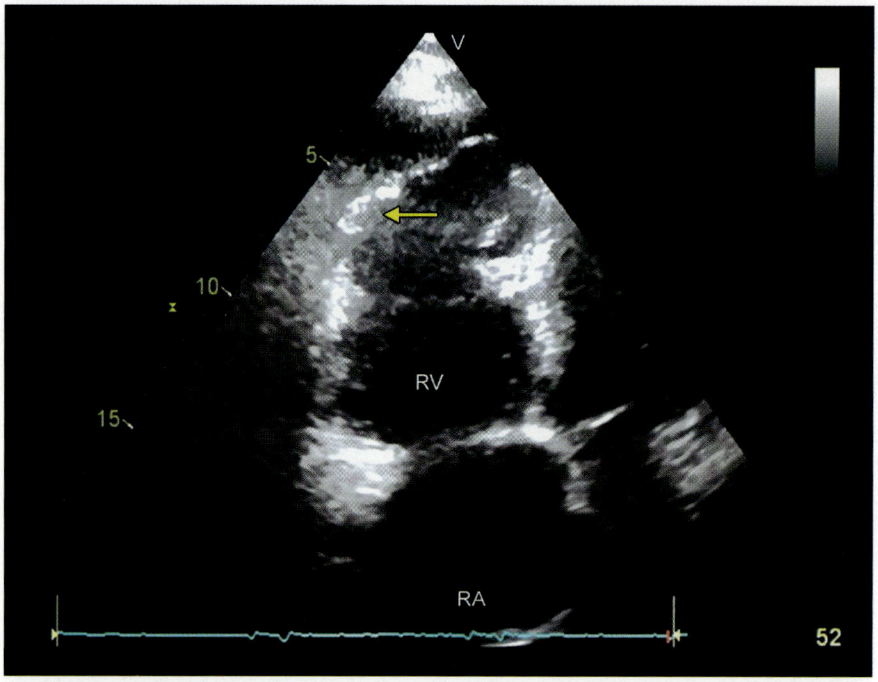

Fig. 36: Transthoracic right ventricle focused view in a patient of arrhythmogenic right ventricular dysplasia. Aneurysm of mid-right ventricular free wall.

- Genetically determined cardiomyopathy.
- Mainly involves right ventricle, but in up to 50% of cases biventricular involvement and in a small percentage predominantly left ventricular involvement can be seen.
- Most common pathological finding is RV thinning and aneurysm formation in areas of right ventricular outflow tract (RVOT) and below tricuspid annulus.
- Typical ECG findings are monomorphic ventricular tachycardia with left bundle branch block (LBBB) and superior axis.
- Usually affects teens and young adults.
- Arrhythmogenic right ventricular dysplasia (ARVD) can cause sudden cardiac arrest in young athletes.

CHAPTER

6

Cardiovascular Intervention: Equipment and Procedures

Ashok Seth, Manish Vinayak

CATHETERIZATION LABORATORY AND EQUIPMENT USED FOR CARDIAC INTERVENTIONS (FIGS. 1 TO 16)

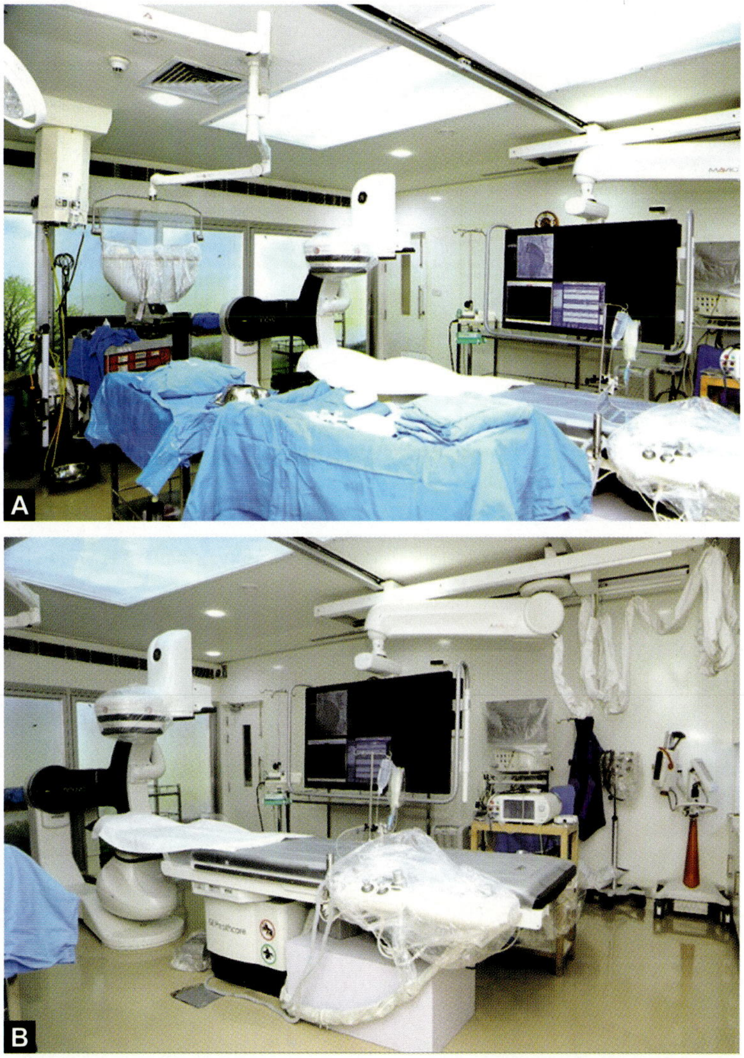

Figs. 1A and B: Catheterization laboratory. A catheterization laboratory or cath lab is an examination room in a hospital with diagnostic imaging equipment, i.e. C-ARM with radiation source, image intensifier and monitors used for angiography, angioplasty, pacemaker, implantable cardioverter defibrillator (ICD), cardiac resynchronization therapy defibrillator (CRT-D) insertion and for electrophysiological procedures.

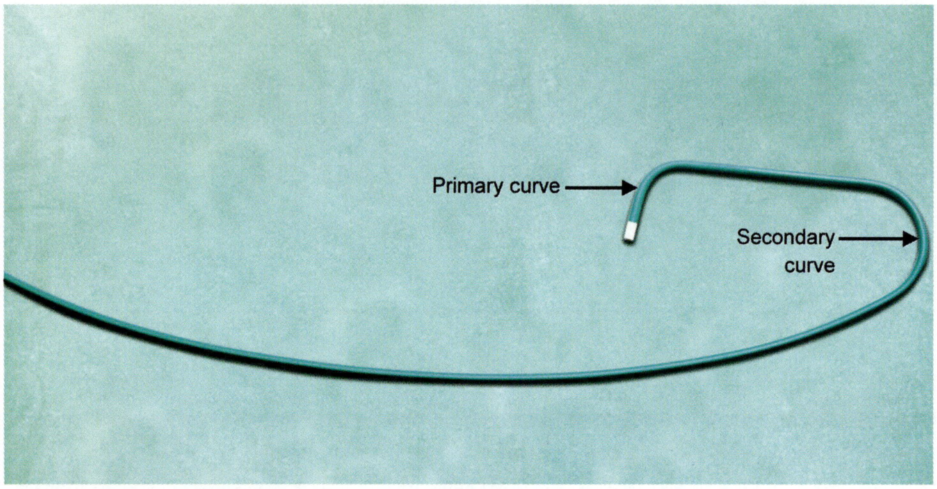

Fig. 2: Judkins left (JL) diagnostic catheter for left coronary artery angiography which has primary curve which engages coronary ostium and secondary curve which stabilizes the catheter on opposite aortic wall.

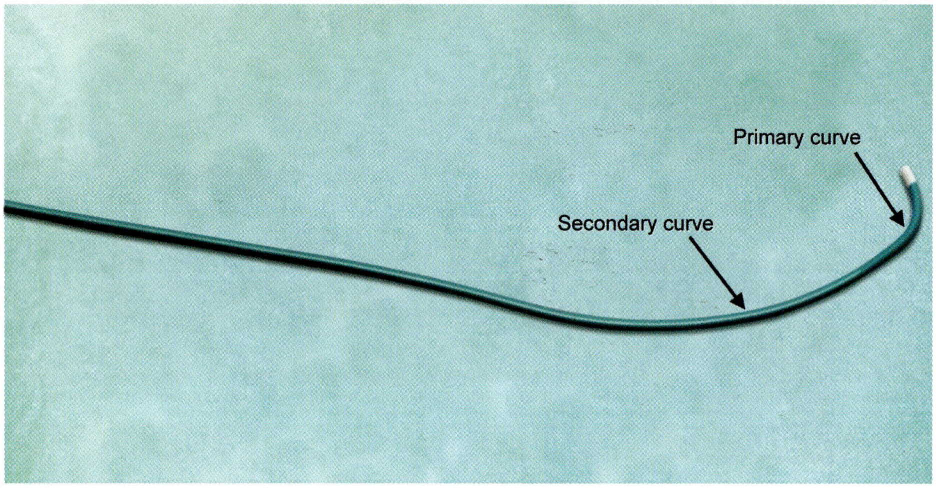

Fig. 3: Judkins right (JR) diagnostic catheter for right coronary artery angiography. JR catheter has sharp primary curve and shallow secondary curve.

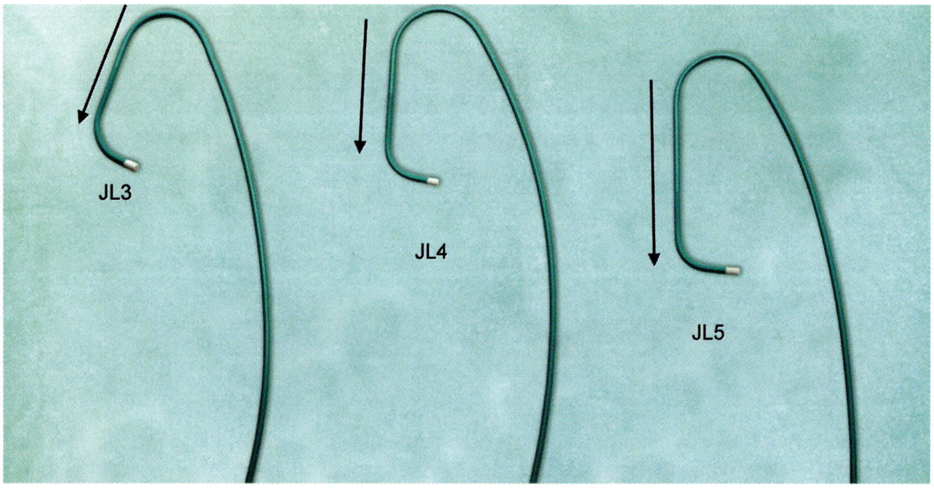

Fig. 4: Distance between primary and secondary curve determines size of catheter. Larger secondary curves are needed to engage dilated aorta.

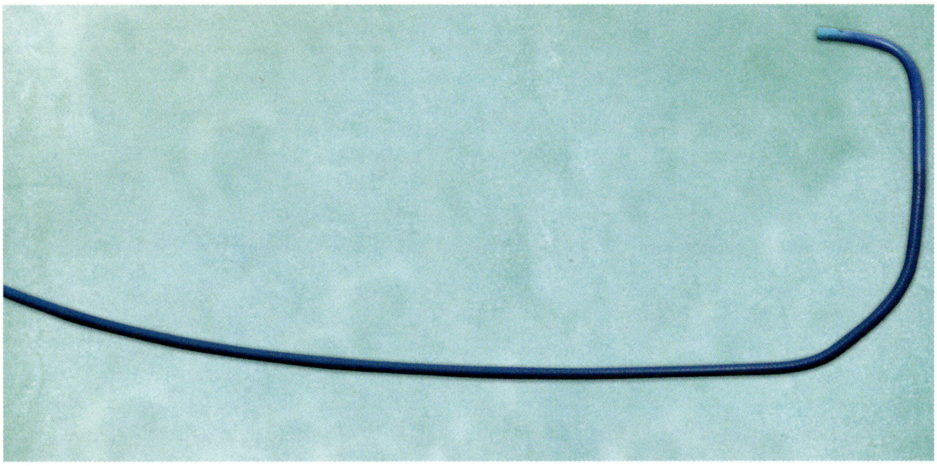

Fig. 5: Tiger diagnostic catheter for angiography through transradial route and can be used for both left as well as right coronary artery angiography.

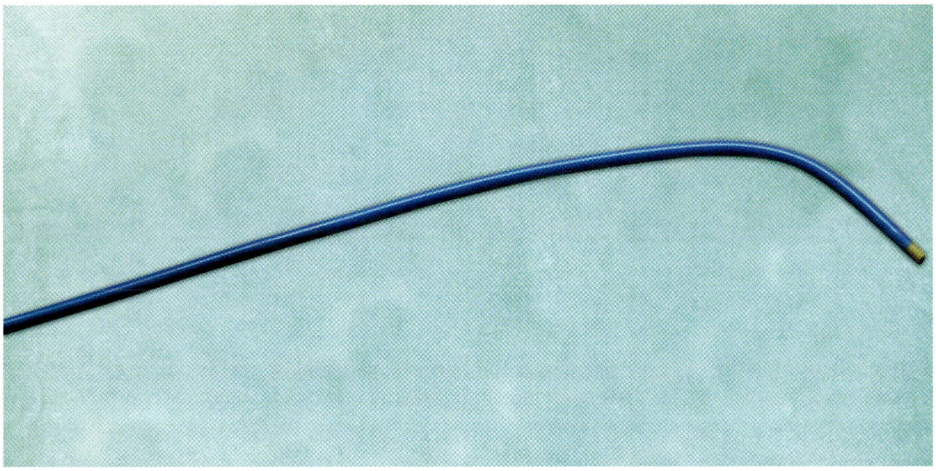

Fig. 6: MPA 1 (Multipurpose A1) diagnostic catheter with end hole only. It is used for inferior origin right coronary artery (RCA) and for saphenous vein graft (SVG)-RCA graft angiography. It can also be used to assess pulmonary artery pressures and for crossing of ductus arteriosus from pulmonary artery to aorta.

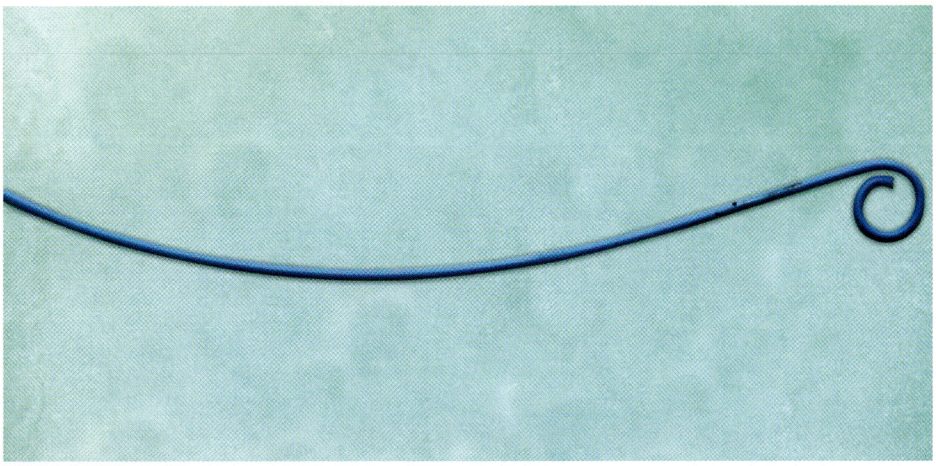

Fig. 7: Pigtail catheter. Curved diagnostic catheter with pigtail-shaped tip and with multiple side holes and end hole.

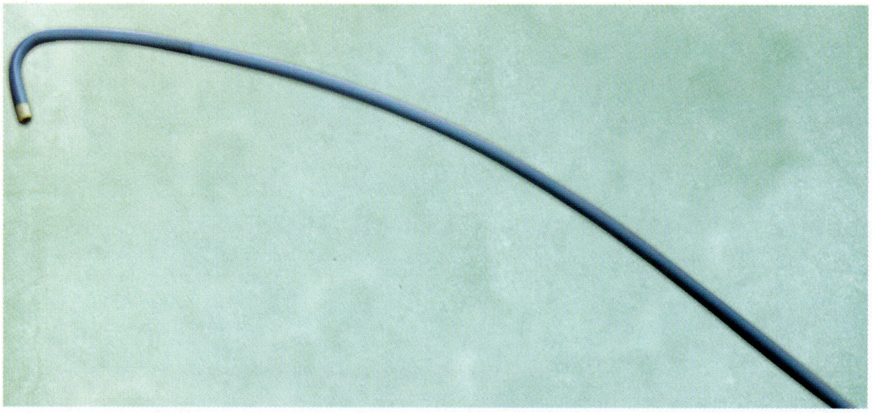

Fig. 8: Internal mammary (IM) diagnostic catheter for selective cannulation of left IM bypass graft.

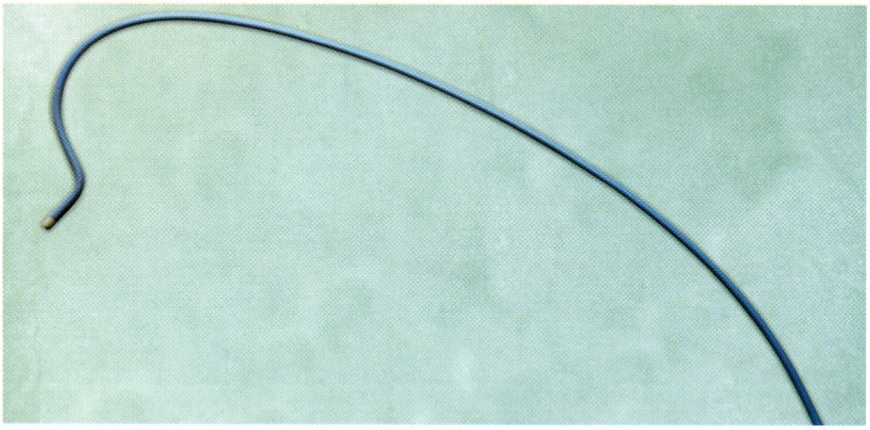

Fig. 9: Amplatz left (AL) coronary catheter used for difficult left coronary cannulation like anomalous and separate origin of left anterior descending and left circumflex arteries. It is also used to engage high anterior origin of right coronary artery.

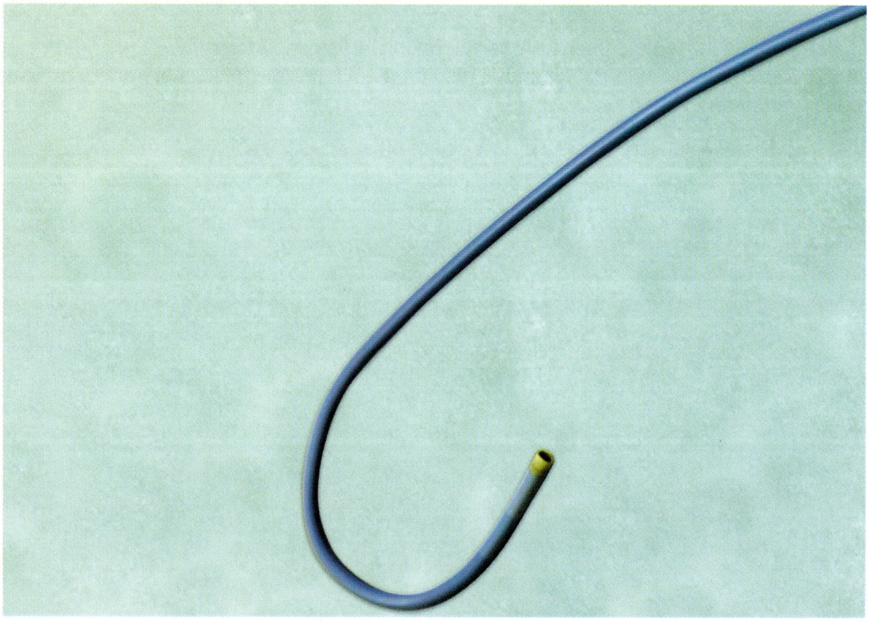

Fig. 10: XBU/EBU (extra backup). Guide catheter used for angioplasty of left system through both transfemoral and transradial route. It provides better contralateral wall support and coaxial alignment in coronary ostia.

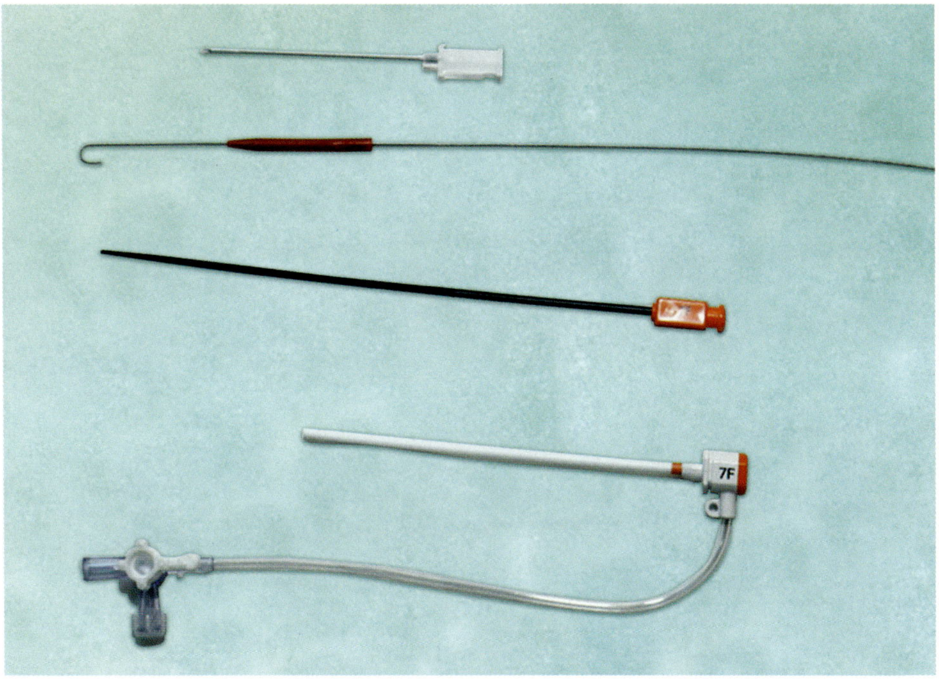

Fig. 11: Femoral sheath components.

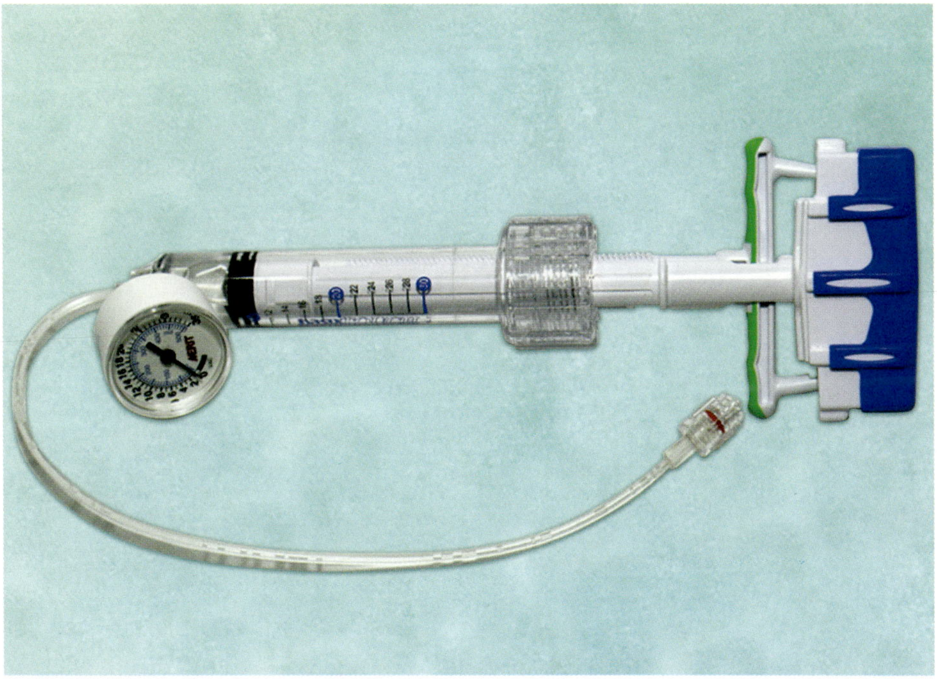

Fig. 12: Inflation device used for inflation of balloon catheter and for deployment of stent inside the coronary artery.

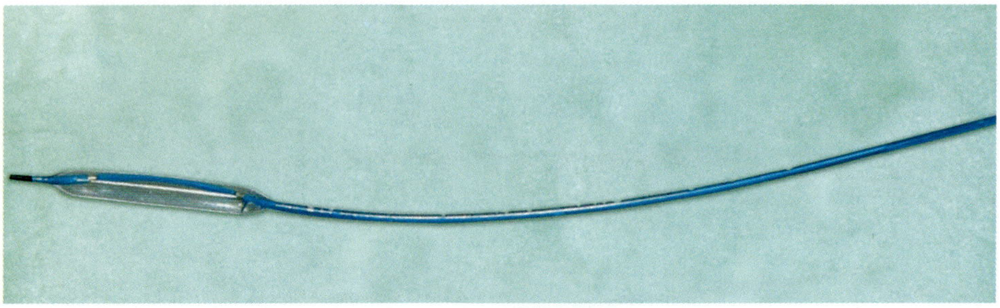

Fig. 13: Coronary predilation balloon catheter.

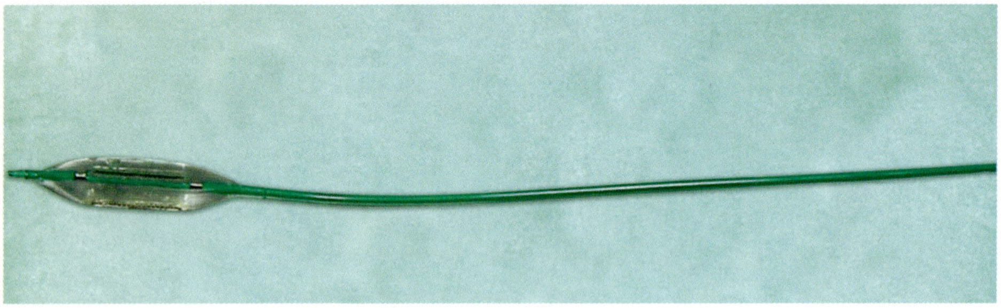

Fig. 14: Cutting balloon used for predilation in fibrotic lesions. It has blades on it which longitudinally scores the lesion rather than stretching and disrupting the plaque.

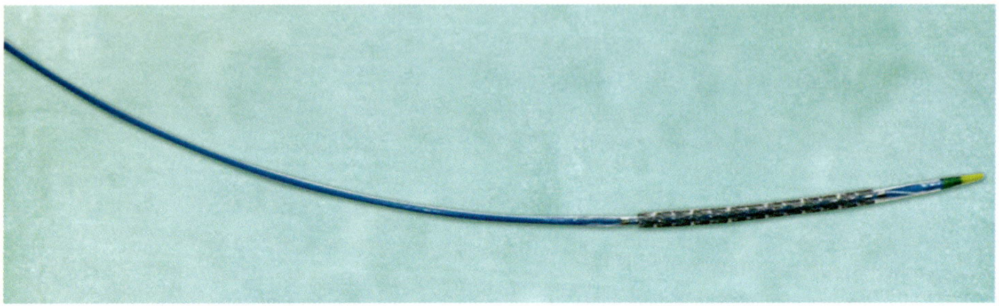

Fig. 15: Coronary stent in unexpanded position.

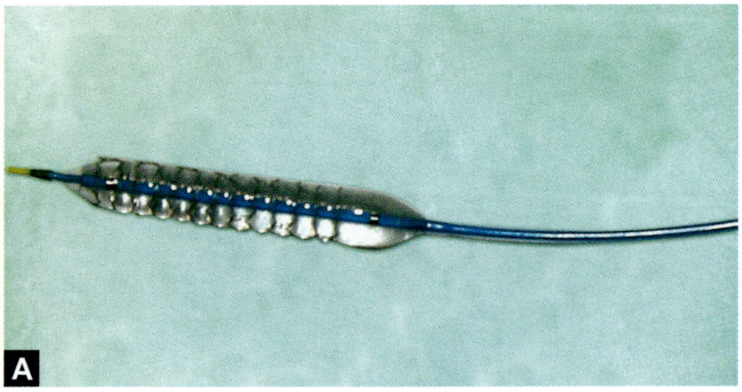

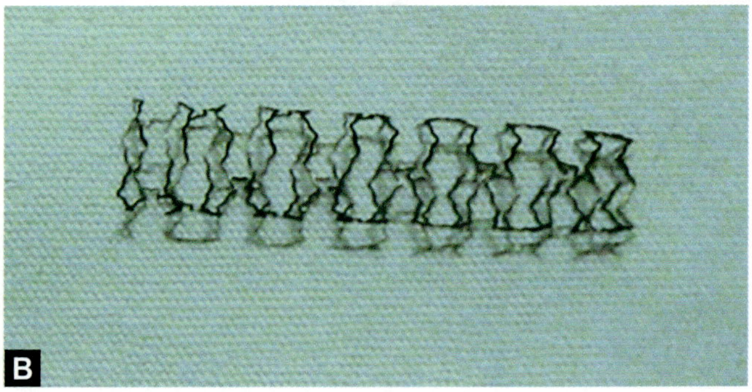

Figs. 16A and B: (A) Stent with inflated balloon; and (B) Expanded coronary stent.

FLUOROSCOPIC IMAGES (FIGS. 17 TO 23)

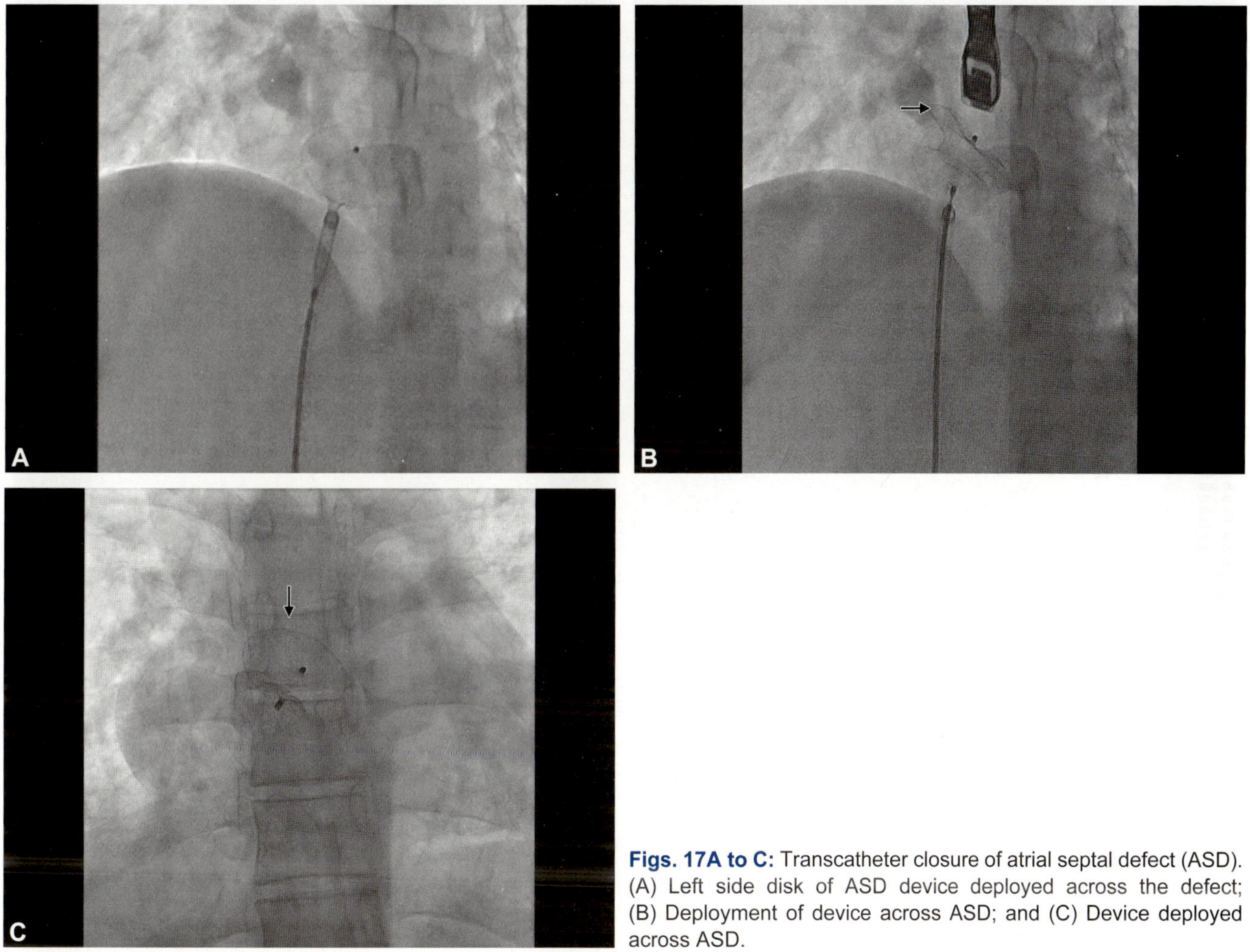

Figs. 17A to C: Transcatheter closure of atrial septal defect (ASD). (A) Left side disk of ASD device deployed across the defect; (B) Deployment of device across ASD; and (C) Device deployed across ASD.

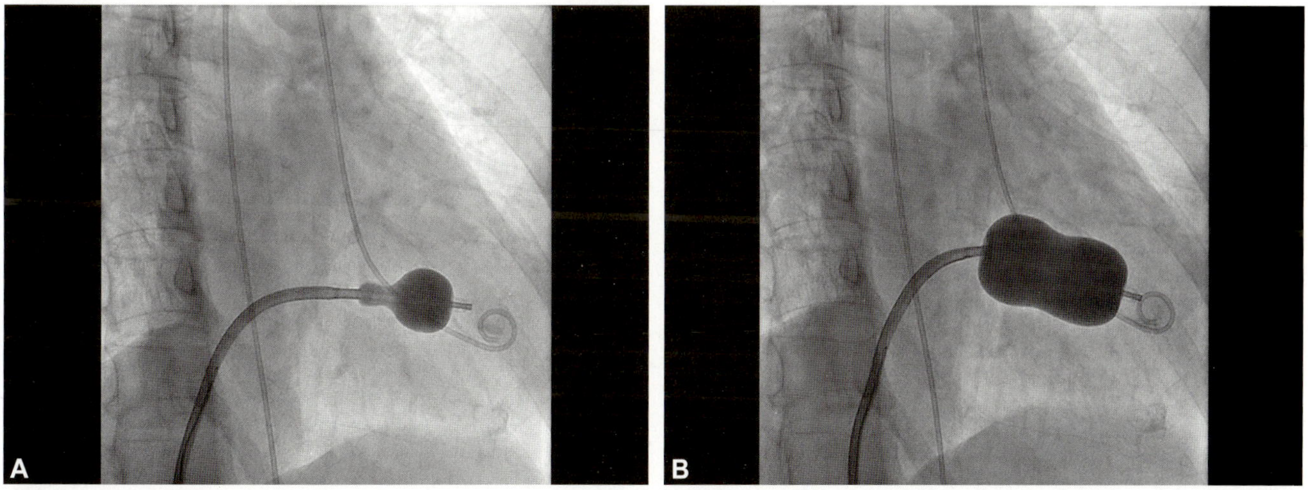

Figs. 18A and B: Balloon mitral valvotomy. (A) Inoue-balloon across mitral valve through trans-septal access and pigtail catheter in left ventricle retrogradely through aorta; and (B) Inoue-balloon inflated across mitral valve through trans-septal access in right anterior oblique view.

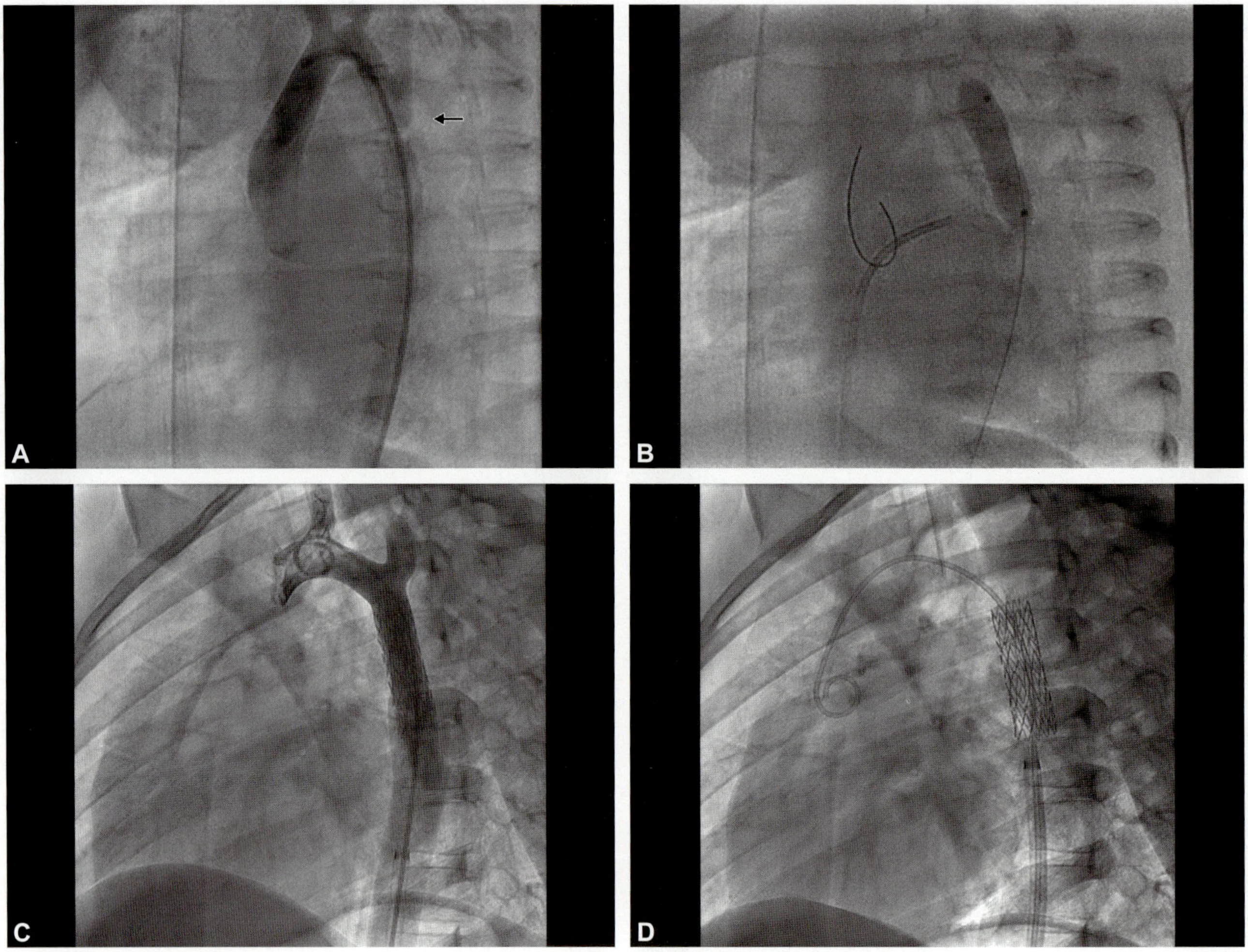

Figs. 19A to D: Coarctation of aorta. (A) Coarct segment in descending aorta; (B) Predilation of coarct segment; (C) Deployment of stent across coarct segment; and (D) Stent deployed across the coarct segment.

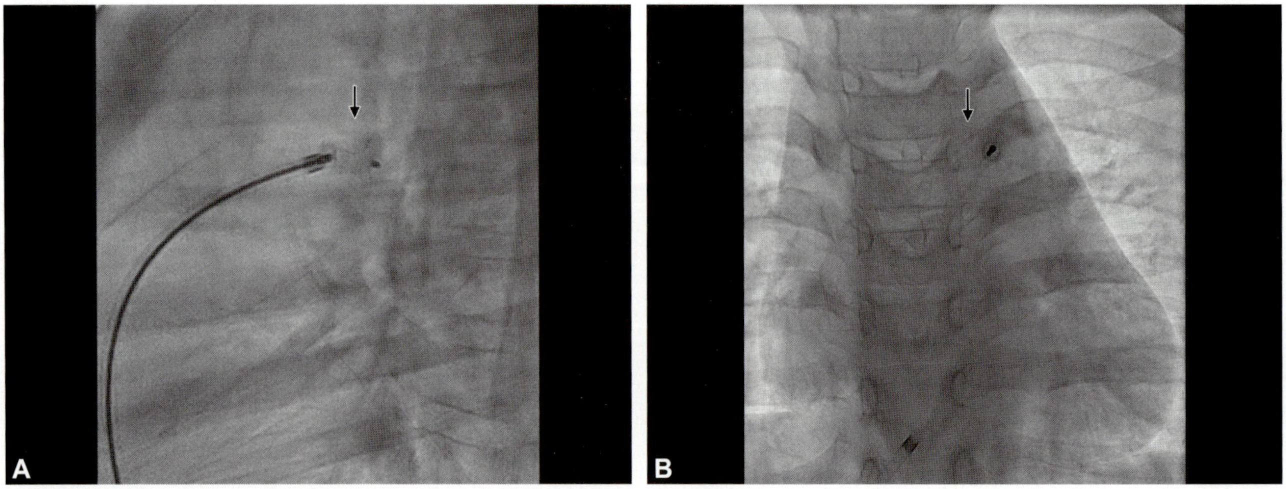

Figs. 20A and B: Patent ductus arteriosus (PDA). (A) Transcatheter closure of PDA, crossed from pulmonary artery to aorta through the ductus; and (B) Device deployed across ductus arteriosus.

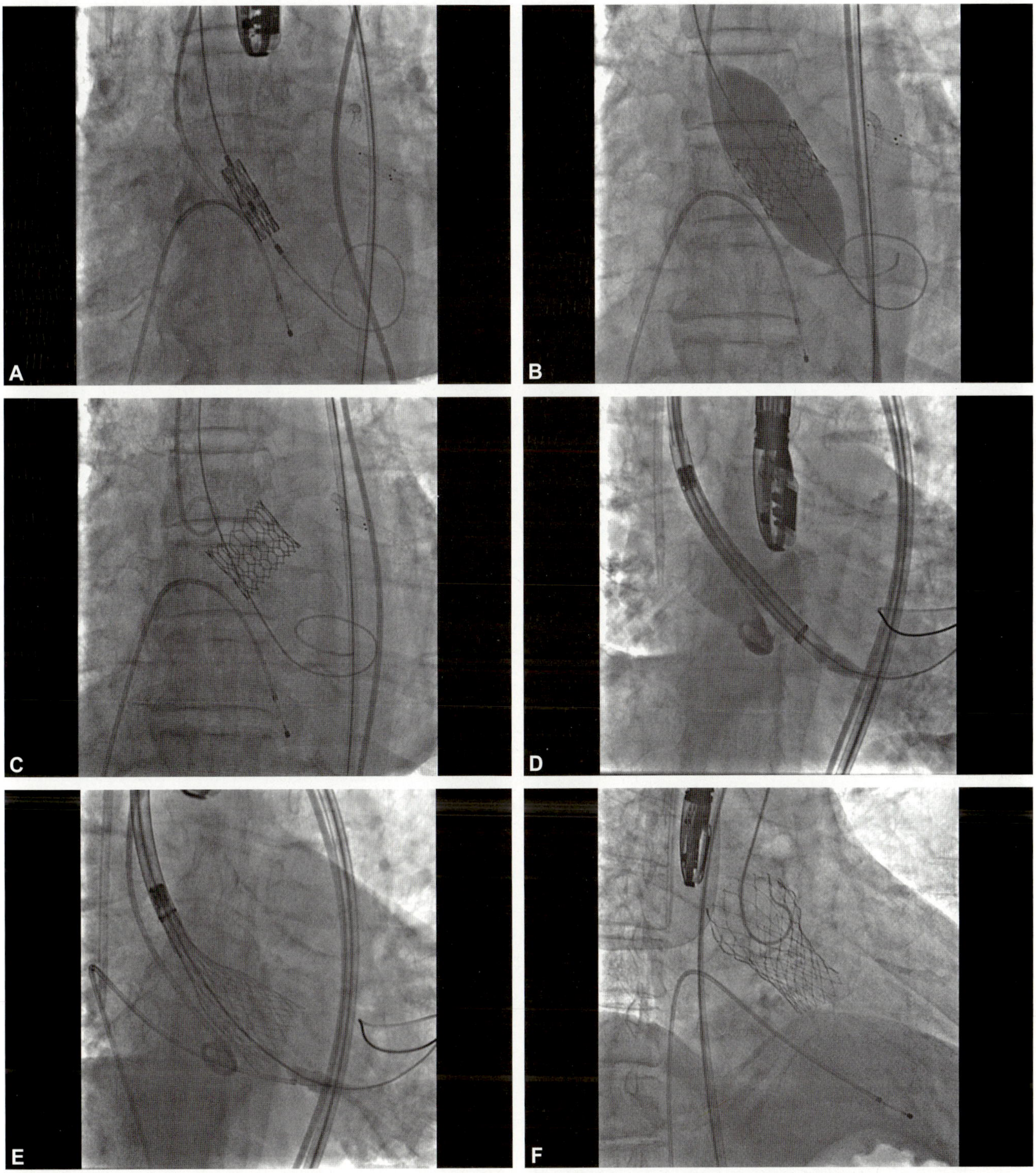

Figs. 21A to F: Transcatheter aortic valve replacement. (A) Balloon expandable Edwards valve positioned across aortic valve; (B) Inflation of balloon to deploy Edwards valve across aortic valve; (C) Edwards Sapien valve deployed across aortic valve; (D) Self-expandable Evolut-R positioned across aortic valve; (E) Deployment of Evolut-R; and (F) Evolut-R deployed across aortic valve.

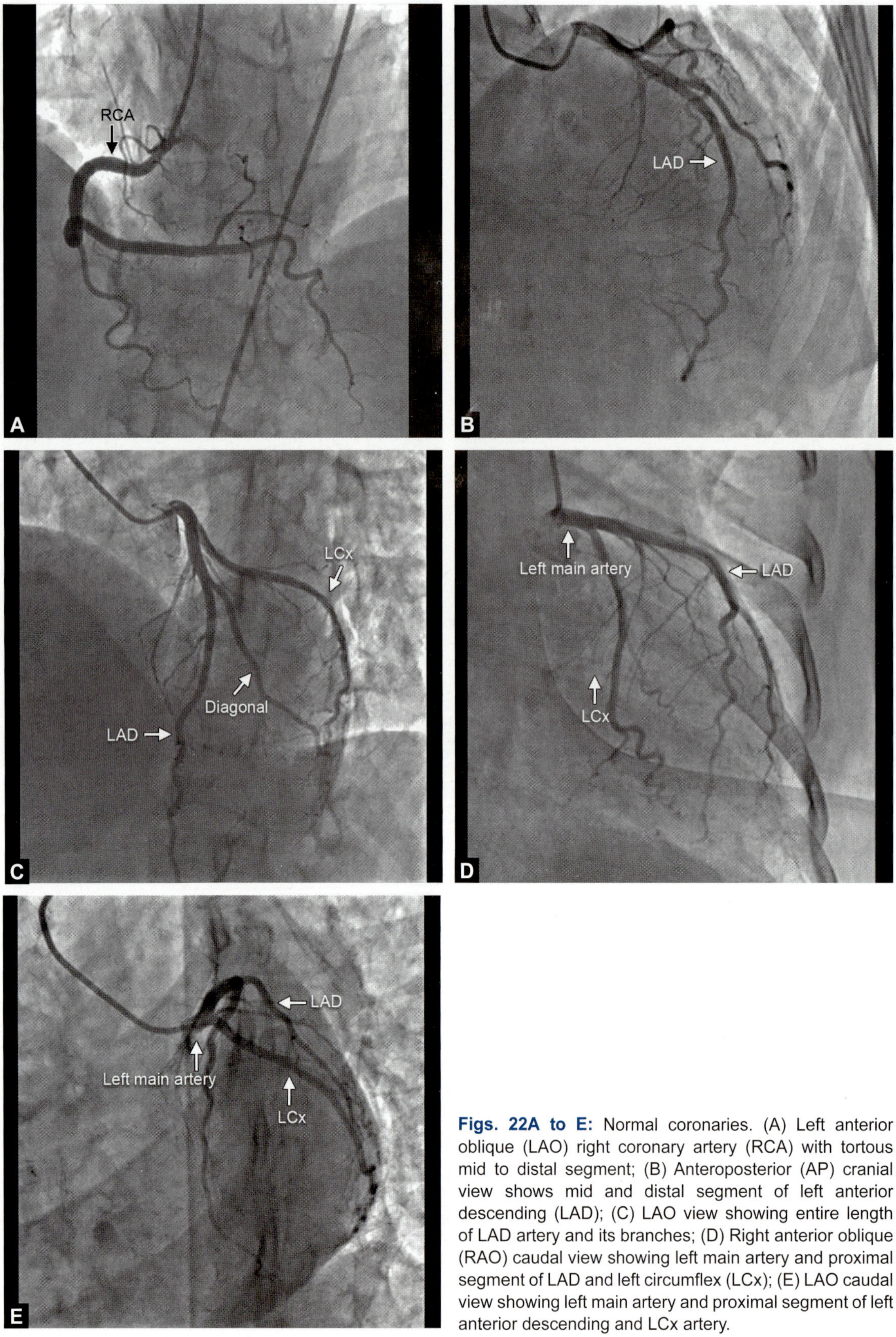

Figs. 22A to E: Normal coronaries. (A) Left anterior oblique (LAO) right coronary artery (RCA) with tortous mid to distal segment; (B) Anteroposterior (AP) cranial view shows mid and distal segment of left anterior descending (LAD); (C) LAO view showing entire length of LAD artery and its branches; (D) Right anterior oblique (RAO) caudal view showing left main artery and proximal segment of LAD and left circumflex (LCx); (E) LAO caudal view showing left main artery and proximal segment of left anterior descending and LCx artery.

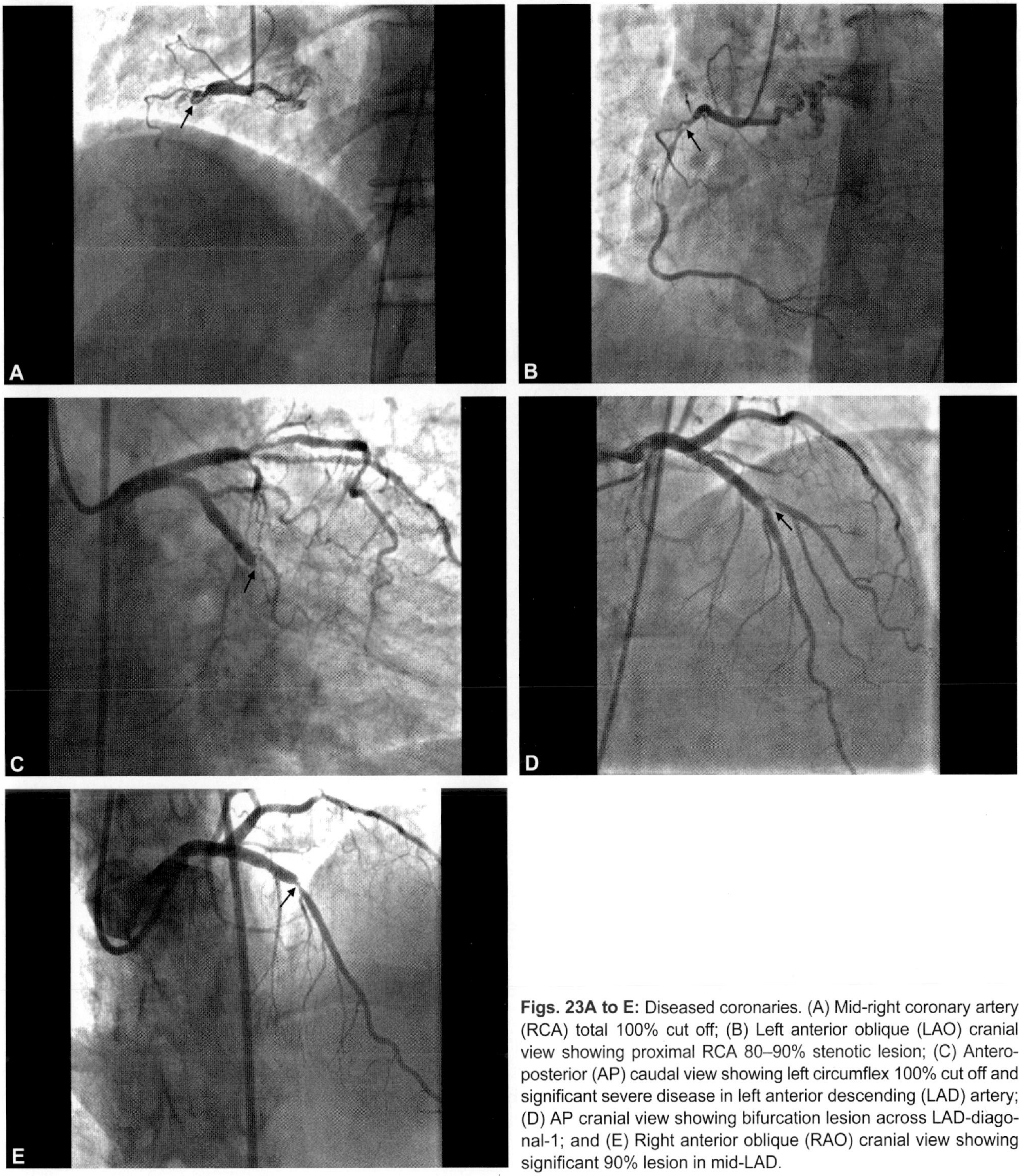

Figs. 23A to E: Diseased coronaries. (A) Mid-right coronary artery (RCA) total 100% cut off; (B) Left anterior oblique (LAO) cranial view showing proximal RCA 80–90% stenotic lesion; (C) Antero-posterior (AP) caudal view showing left circumflex 100% cut off and significant severe disease in left anterior descending (LAD) artery; (D) AP cranial view showing bifurcation lesion across LAD-diagonal-1; and (E) Right anterior oblique (RAO) cranial view showing significant 90% lesion in mid-LAD.

CHAPTER 7

Electrocardiography: Heart Blocks

Balbir Singh, Lakshme Kottu

FIRST-DEGREE ATRIOVENTRICULAR BLOCK (FIG. 1)

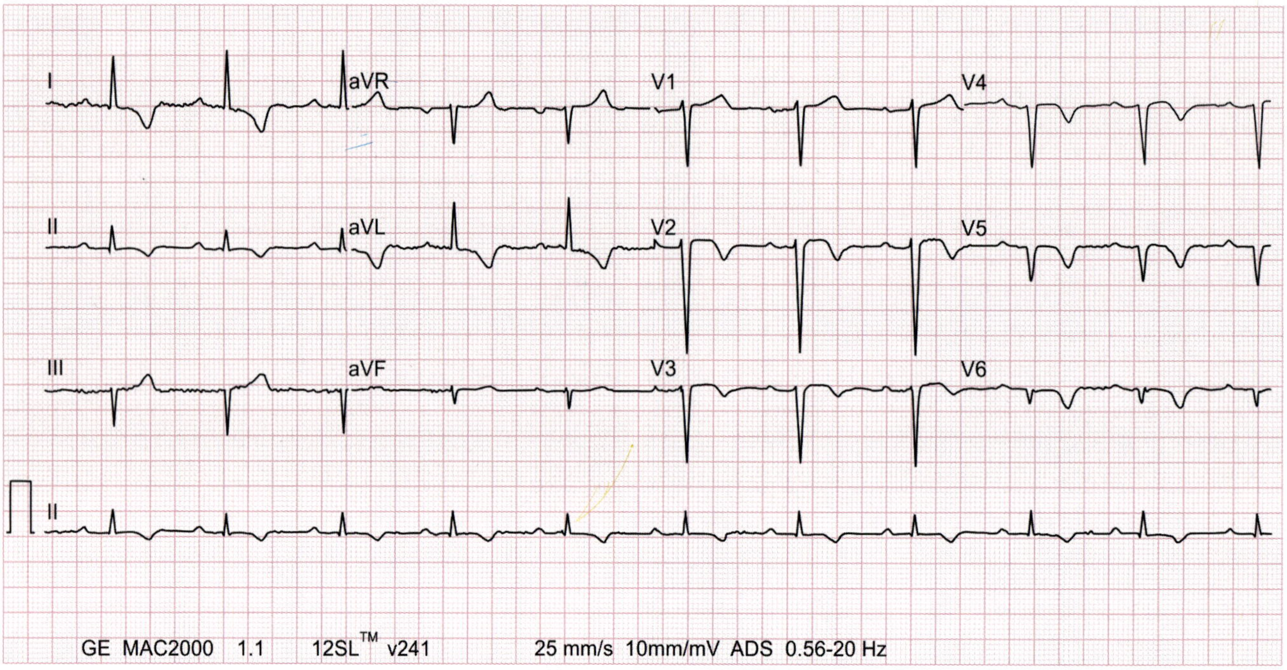

Fig. 1: First-degree atrioventricular (AV) block: Electrocardiography (ECG) showing sinus rhythm with first-degree AV block (prolonged PR interval measuring 230 ms requires monitoring).

- Atrioventricular (AV) conduction is slightly prolonged usually at AV node.
- There is 1:1 P/QRS relationship.
- It may require OPD follow-ups (identify and correct electrolyte imbalances, withhold any offending medications which causes this).

RIGHT BUNDLE BRANCH BLOCK (FIG. 2)

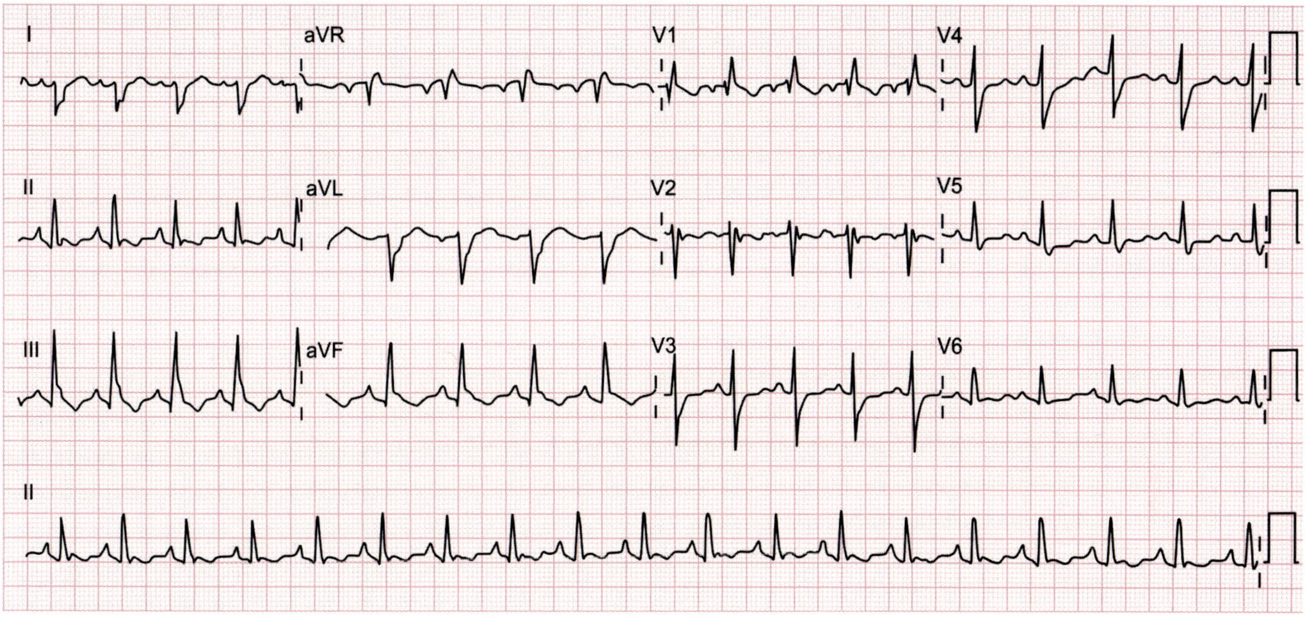

Fig. 2: Right bundle branch block (RBBB): Electrocardiography (ECG) of RBBB with right axis deviation (RAD) (*Note*: rsR' pattern in V1, V2).

- Electrocardiography (ECG) criteria for right bundle branch block (RBBB).
- QRS duration> 100 ms for incomplete RBBB and equal to or more than 120.
- Lead V1 and V2 - Rsr', rsR' or rSR' (QRS complex appears as letter "M").
- Lead V5, V6, I, aVL - S wave broad, its duration is greater than R wave duration and more than 40 ms in V6 and I.
- Common causes of RBBB in ICU—coronary artery disease, pulmonary embolism, acute cor pulmonale, postcardiac surgery, post-percutaneous coronary intervention (PCI), cardiomyopathy and chronic obstructive pulmonary disease (COPD).

COMPLETE HEART BLOCK (FIG. 3)

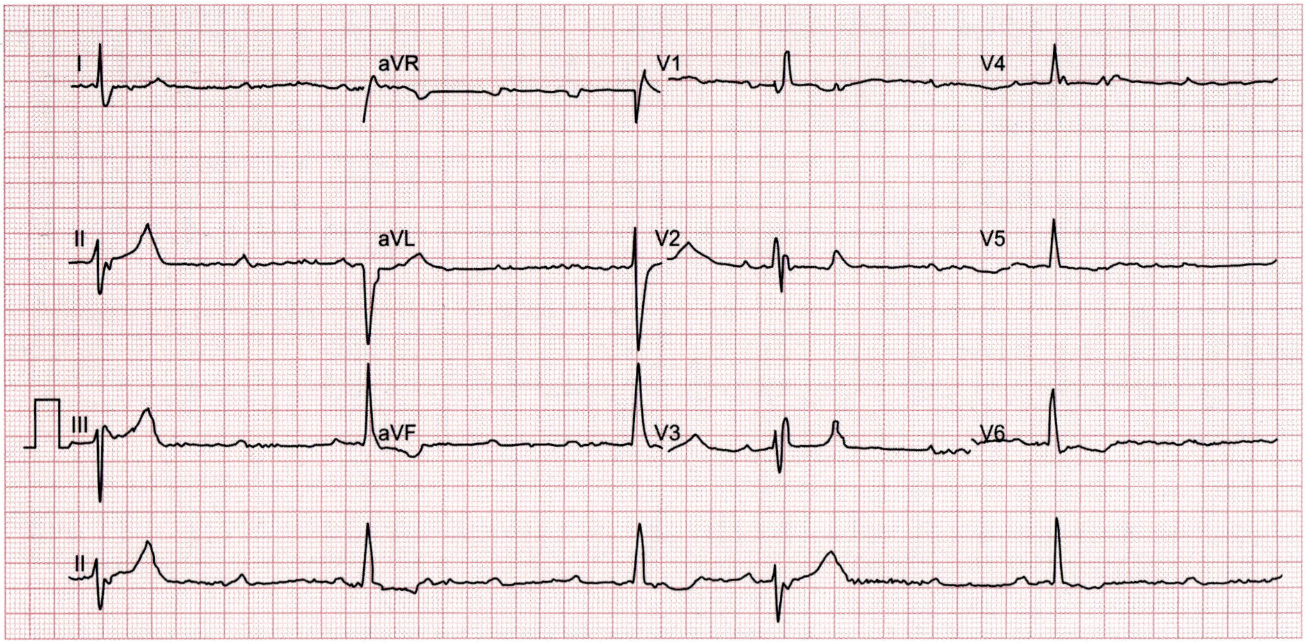

Fig. 3: Complete heart block (CHB): Electrocardiography (ECG) of a 75-year-old female patient symptomatic with CHB showing regular P-P; regular R-R intervals. PP interval is shorter than RR interval with complete AV dissociation.

- Requires temporary pacemaker implantation (TPI) urgently.
- TPI was placed in her immediately.
- Complete hear block (CHB) is also known as third degree heart block.
- ECG criteria for CHB—regular P-P interval; regular R-R interval; lack of an apparent relationship between the P waves and QRS complexes; and more P waves are present than QRS complexes.
- This is potential life-threatening rhythm requires urgent temporary pacing either intravenous or transcutaneous.
- Common causes of CHB in ICU—acute coronary syndrome, coronary artery disease, drugs (antiarrhythmics including beta and calcium channel blocker), myocarditis, certain infiltrative processes (amyloidosis, sarcoidosis, tumors, Hodgkin disease, multiple myeloma), metabolic causes (hypoxia, hyperkalemia, hypothyroidism) and toxins.

DUAL CHAMBER PACEMAKER (FIG. 4)

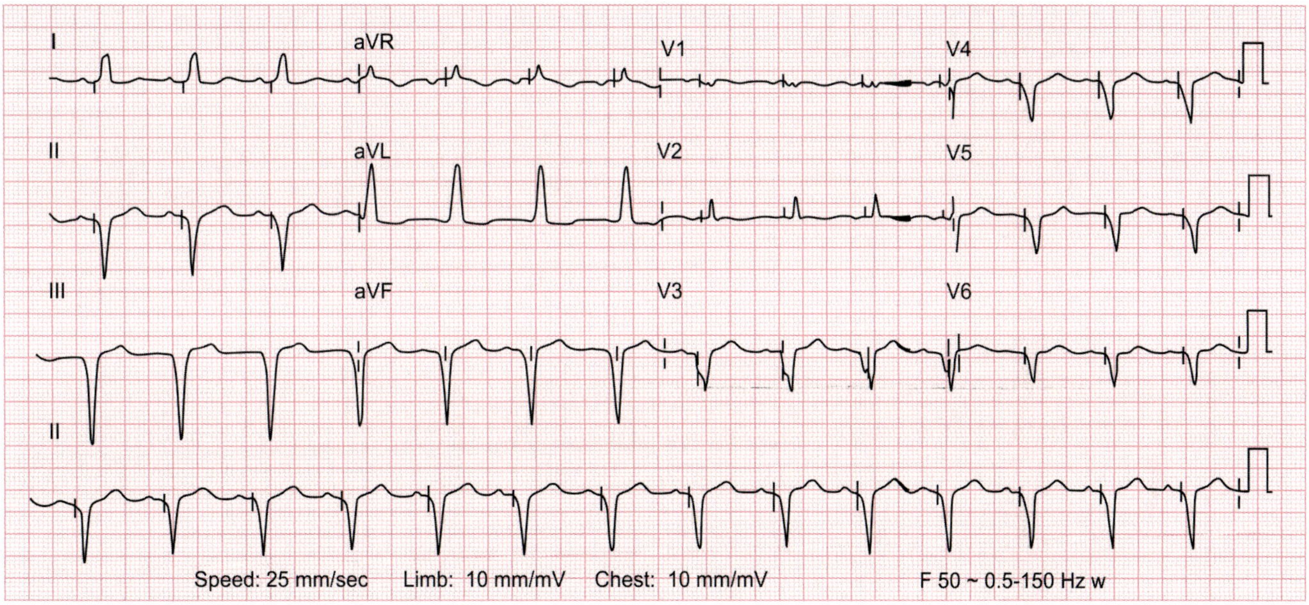

Fig. 4: Dual-chamber pacemaker: Dual-chamber (DDD) mode, note pacing spike before each QRS complex (bipolar lead used, thus small pacing spike).

- Dual-chamber (DDD) is the most common pacing mode used.
- Note vertical pacing spikes of short duration less than 2 ms.
- Bipolar leads result in much smaller pacing spike than unipolar lead.
- The absence of paced complex does not always mean pacemaker failure, as it might be due to satisfactory native conduction.

SINGLE CHAMBER TEMPORARY PACING (FIG. 5)

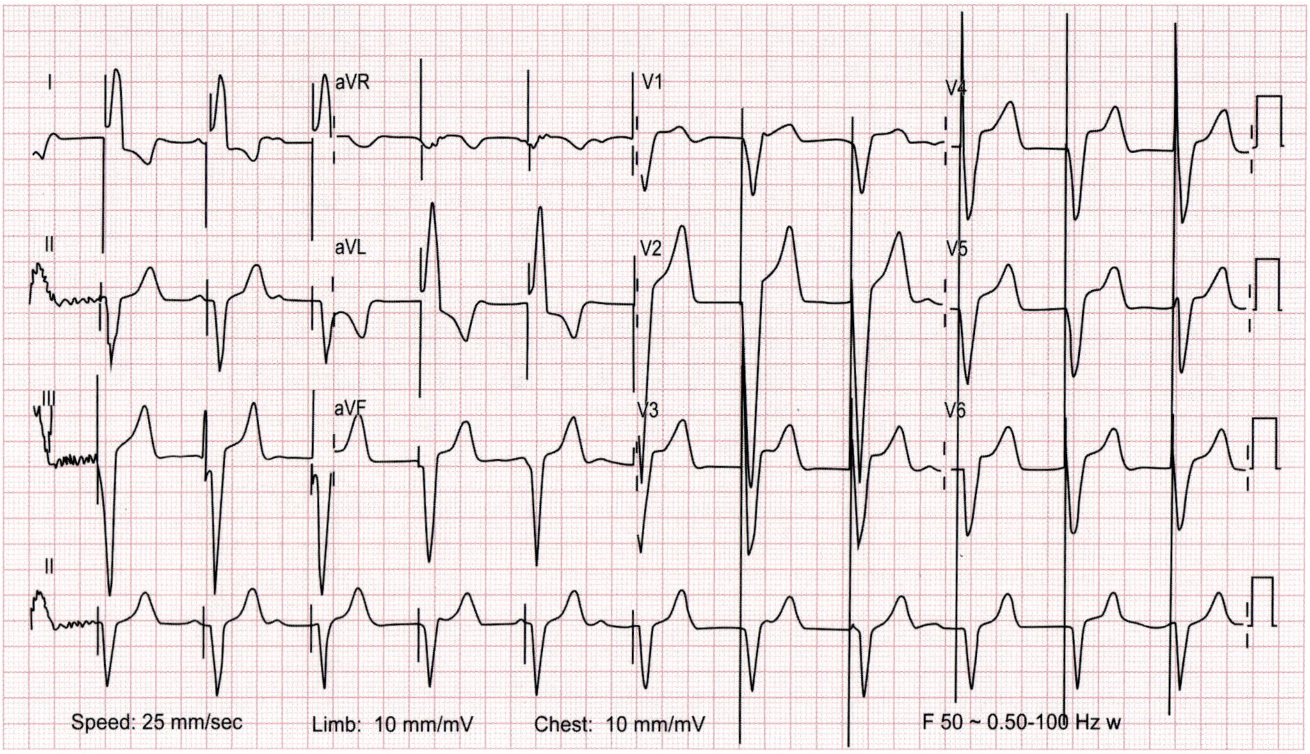

Fig. 5: Single chamber temporary pacing: ECG of a 44-year-old patient with temporary pacing.

- Used in emergency treatment of CHB/life threating or unstable bradyarrhythmias.
- Note larger pacing spike before each QRS due to use of unipolar lead.

VENTRICULAR TACHYCARDIA (FIG. 6)

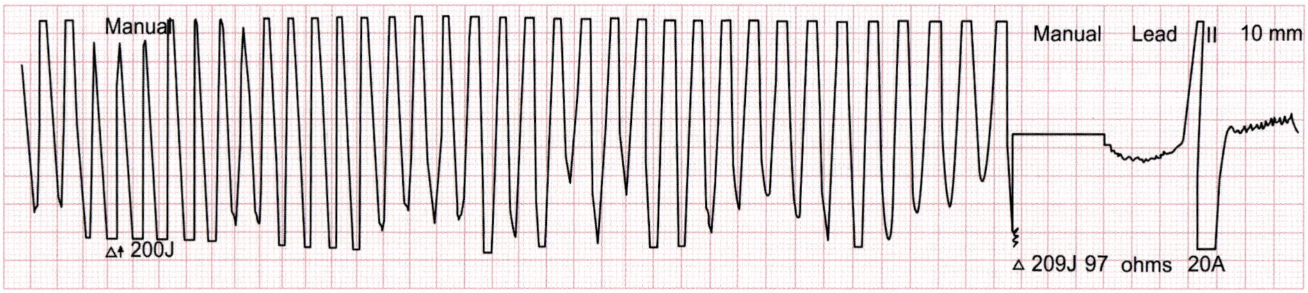

Fig. 6: Ventricular tachycardia (VT): Rhythm strip of a patient in sustained monomorphic VT, reverted to sinus rhythm by applying 200 J shock twice.

- Defibrillator delivers a therapeutic dose of electrical current at a particular moment in cardiac cycle and is the most effective resuscitation measure for cardiac arrest associated with VF/pulseless VT.
- Pharmacological cardioversion is done with antiarrhythmic drugs like Ibutilide, Flecarite.

FLUORO-RAO CAUDAL VIEW OF A SINGLE CHAMBER IMPLANTABLE CARDIOVERTER DEFIBRILLATOR (FIGS. 7A TO C)

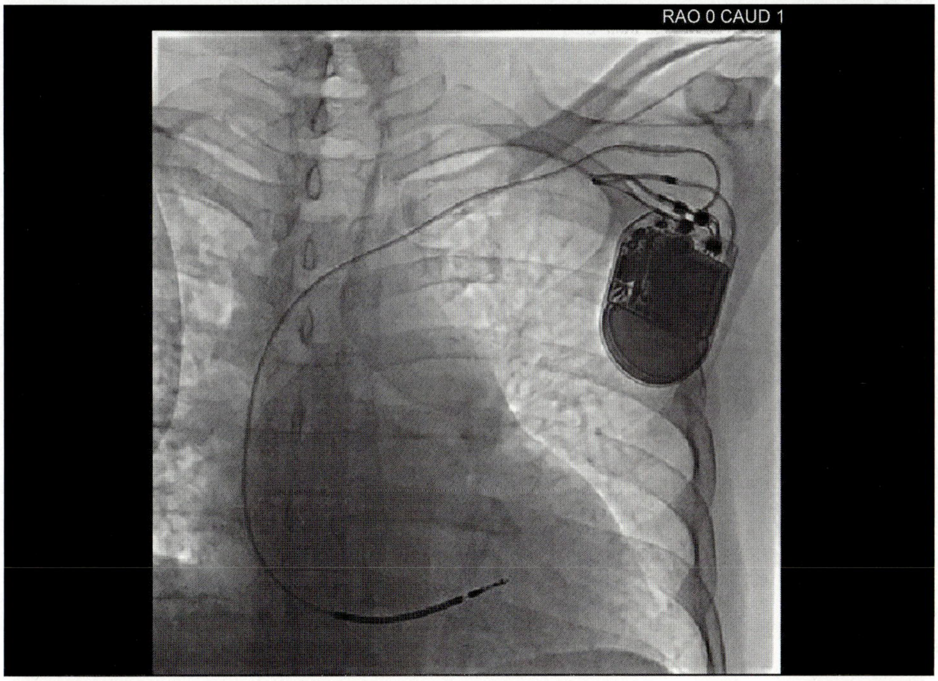

Fig. 7A: Fluoro-right anterior oblique (RAO) caudal view of a single chamber implantable cardioverter defibrillator (ICD): The ventricular lead tip in the region of the right ventricular (RV) apex. The single chamber ICD (ICD CAN) is seen in the left infraclavicular region. The lead is seen traversing the left subclavian into the left brachiocephalic vein to the superior vena cava and then to the right atrium and right ventricle. This is a single coil lead (RV COIL).

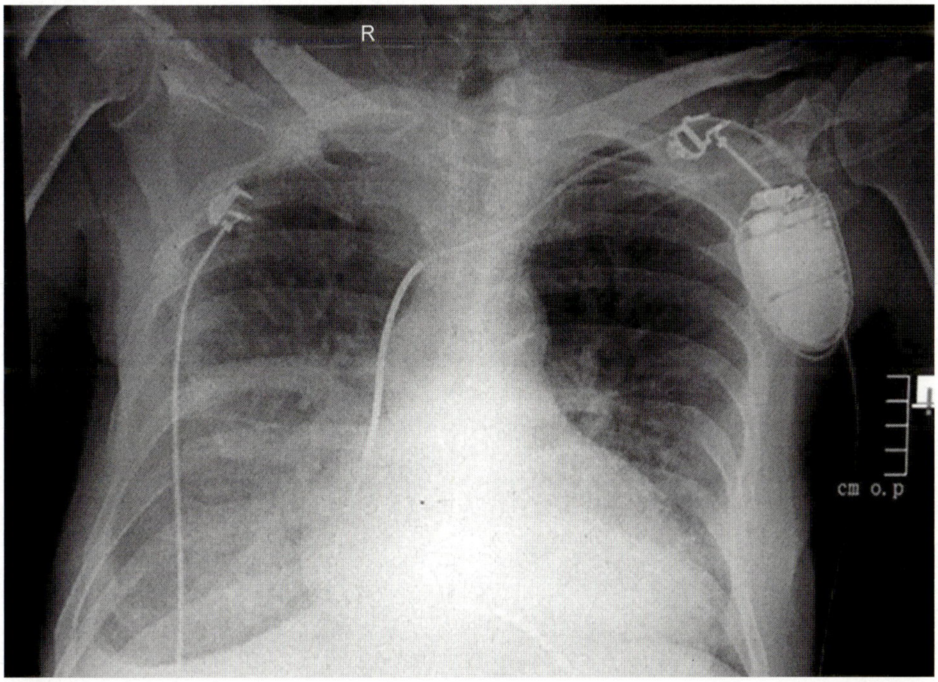

Fig. 7B: Chest X-ray anteroposterior (AP) view of a patient with single chamber implantable cardioverter defibrillator (ICD).

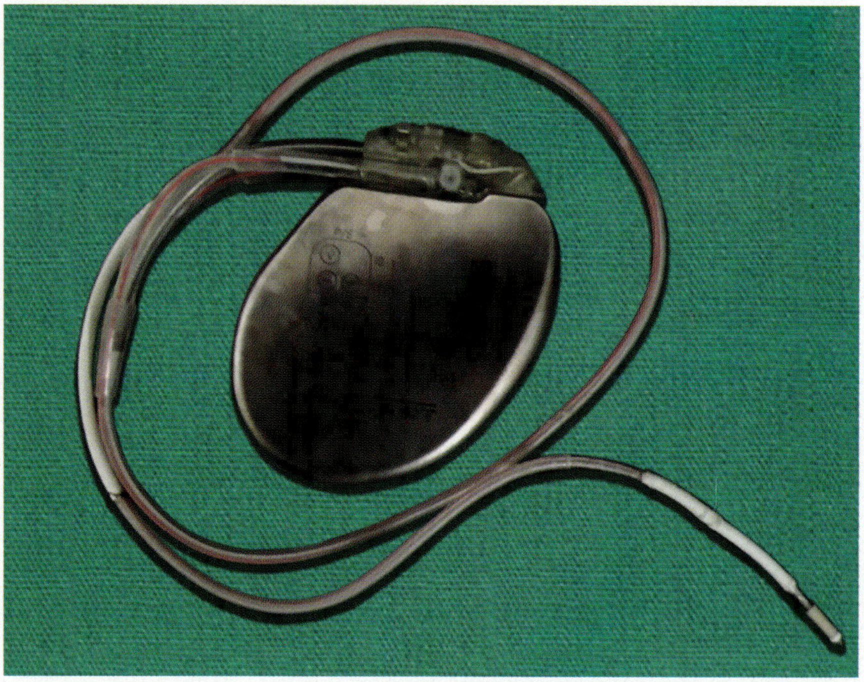

Fig. 7C: Automated implantable cardioverter defibrillator (AICD).

- Automated implantable cardioverter defibrillator (AICD) is a device implantable inside the body, able to perform cardioversion, defibrillation, and (in modern versions) pacing of the heart.
- The device is capable of correcting most life-threatening cardiac arrhythmias. Therefore, it is the first-line treatment and prophylactic therapy for patients at risk for sudden cardiac death due to ventricular fibrillation and ventricular tachycardia.
- Some of the Class I indications are:
  a. Structural heart disease and spontaneous sustained ventricular tachycardia (VT), whether hemodynamically stable or unstable.
  b. Syncope of undetermined origin with clinically relevant, hemodynamically significant sustained VT or ventricular fibrillation (VF) induced at electrophysiological study.
  c. Left ventricular (LV) dysfunction due to prior myocardial infarction (MI) who are at least 40 days post-MI, have a left ventricular ejection fraction (LVEF) ≤ 30%, and are in New York Heart Association (NYHA) Functional Class I.
  d. LVEF ≤ 35% due to prior MI who are at least 40 days post-MI and are in NYHA Functional Class II or III.
  e. Nonischemic dilated cardiomyopathy (DCMP) who have an LVEF ≤ 35% and who are in NYHA Functional Class II or III.
  f. Nonsustained VT due to prior MI, LVEF < 40%, and inducible VF or sustained VT at electrophysiological study.

FLUORO IMAGE OF LEADLESS PACEMAKER (FIG. 8)

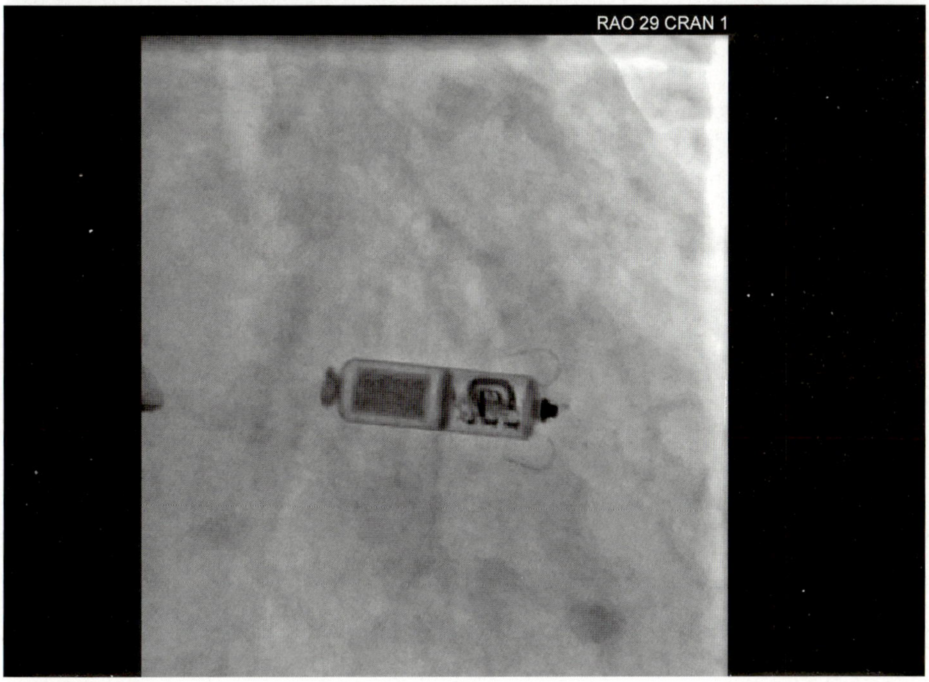

Fig. 8: Fluoro image of leadless pacemaker: Image showing the final position of leadless pacemaker (Micra device; Medtronic), its active fixation mechanism is made by tines used in patients with normal EF.

- Leadless pacemaker is small self-contained device that is inserted in the right ventricle of the heart via a transfemoral catheter approach.
- Leadless cardiac pacemaker system is a pulse generator with built-in battery and electrode. There is no requirement of pacing leads and generator. There is no need for creation of pocket by surgery. That eliminating potential transvenous lead- and pacemaker pocket-related complications.

FLUORO IMAGE—TPI LEAD (FIG. 9)

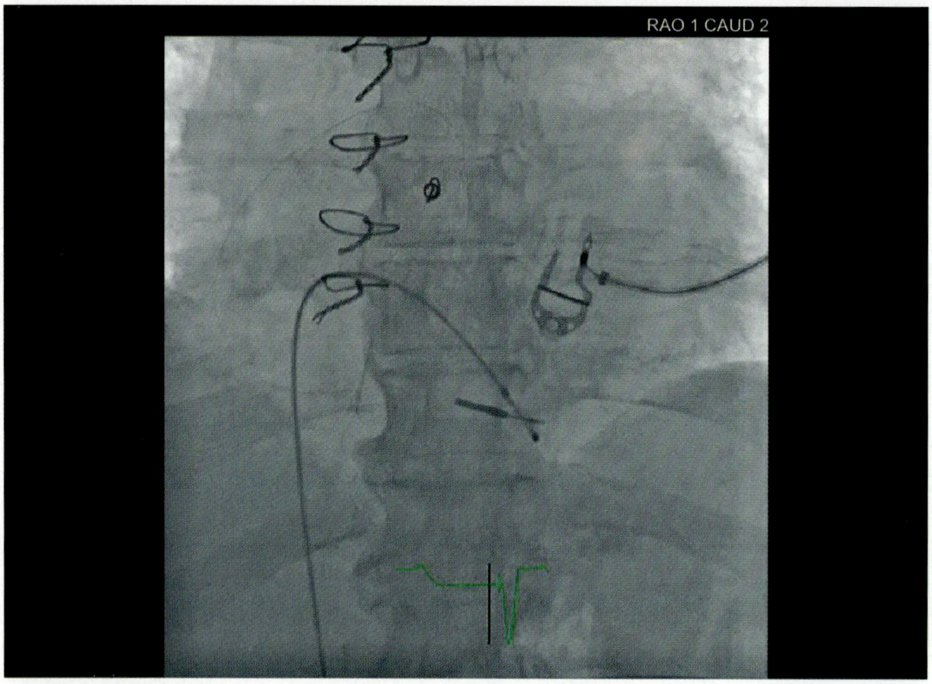

Fig. 9: Fluoro image—TPI lead.

- Done for CHB in ER/ICU.
- Femoral or right internal jugular vein (RIJV) route—transvenous.
- Also have balloon tipped wires for easy placement, once pacing is captured deflate balloon and decrease mA to find threshold.
- Confirmed by Fluoro/ECHO.

FLUORO RIGHT ANTERIOR OBLIQUE (RAO) CAUDAL VIEW OF CRT-D (FIG. 10)

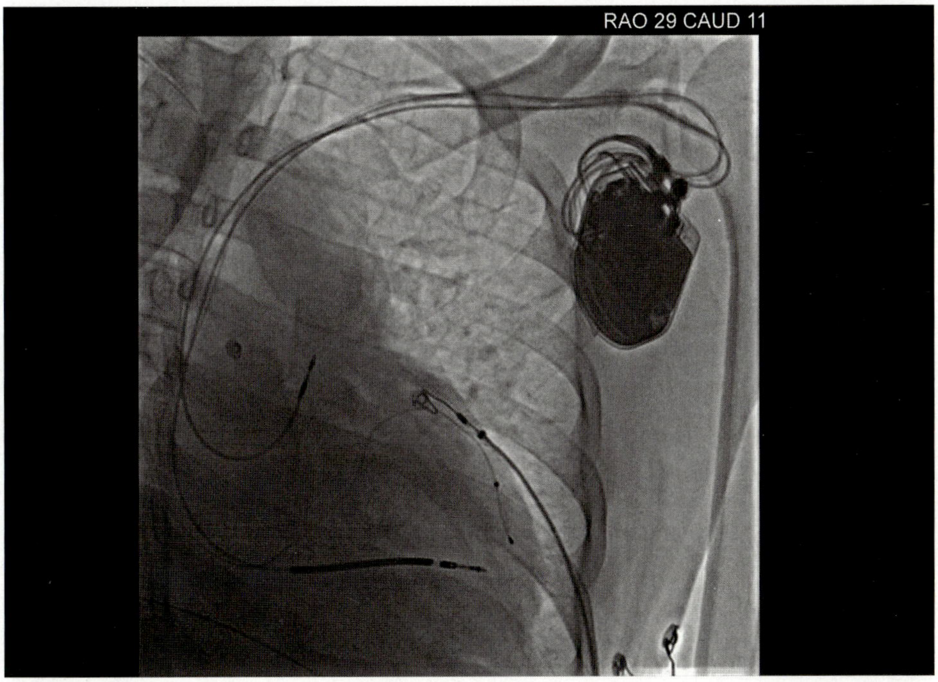

Fig. 10: Fluoroscopy image of an 81-year-old patient with CRDT in right anterior oblique (RAO) 29 degree projection.

- Cardiac resynchronization therapy (CRT) is achieved by simultaneously pacing RV and LV in a synchronized manner.
- Numerous studies demonstrated that in selected patients with ventricular dyssynchrony, CRT provided acute hemodynamic benefits while reducing myocardial energy consumption.
- Note the pulse generator along with RA; RV lead placed over the septum and LV lead placed in anterolateral cardiac vein.
- Used for patient with reduced EF.

LEFT ANTERIOR OBLIQUE CRANIAL VIEW FLUOROSCOPY OF A PATIENT WITH INTRA-AORTIC BALLOON PUMP (FIG. 11)

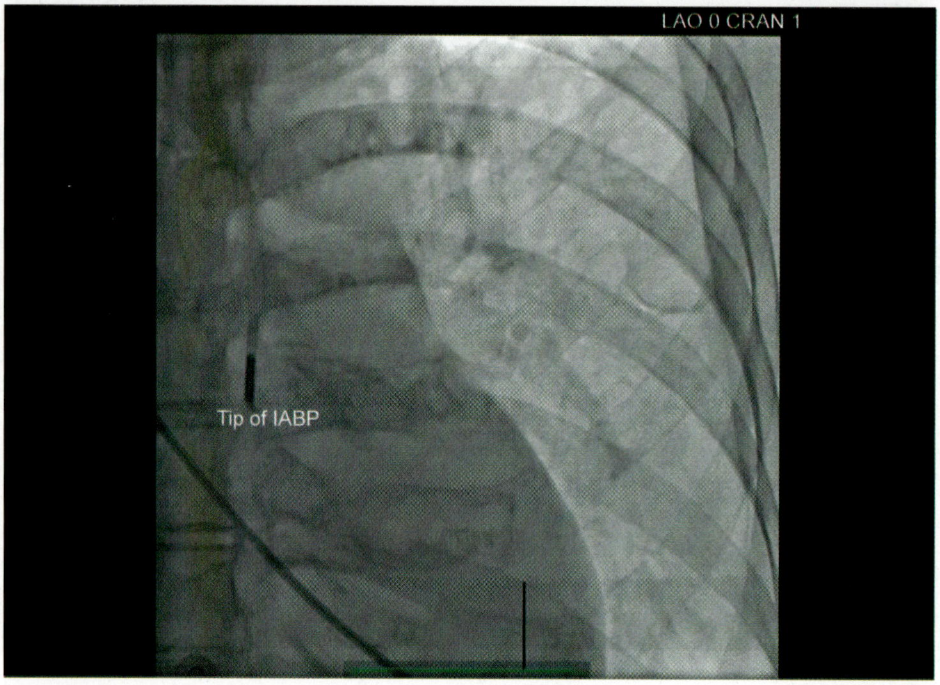

Fig. 11: Left anterior oblique (LAO) cranial view fluoroscopy of a patient with intra-aortic balloon pump (IABP): This is a fluoro image of a patient in cardiogenic shock with IABP. The balloon itself is not radiopaque, but the marker is used to assess balloon position—it should be in the proximal descending aorta (as in this case), so that it is located beyond the origin of the left subclavian artery.

- Intra-aortic balloon pump (IABP) improves coronary perfusion while reducing the afterload (MVO_2).
- Buys time for further intervention in acute decompensated heart failure (ADHF), cardiogenic shock.
- Inserted via femoral vein.
- *Complications*: Vascular injury, aortic dissection, sepsis, limb ischemia, thrombocytopenia.

Electrocardiography: Arrhythmias

CHAPTER 8

KK Talwar

ELECTROCARDIOGRAPHY: ARRHYTHMIAS (FIGS. 1 TO 33)

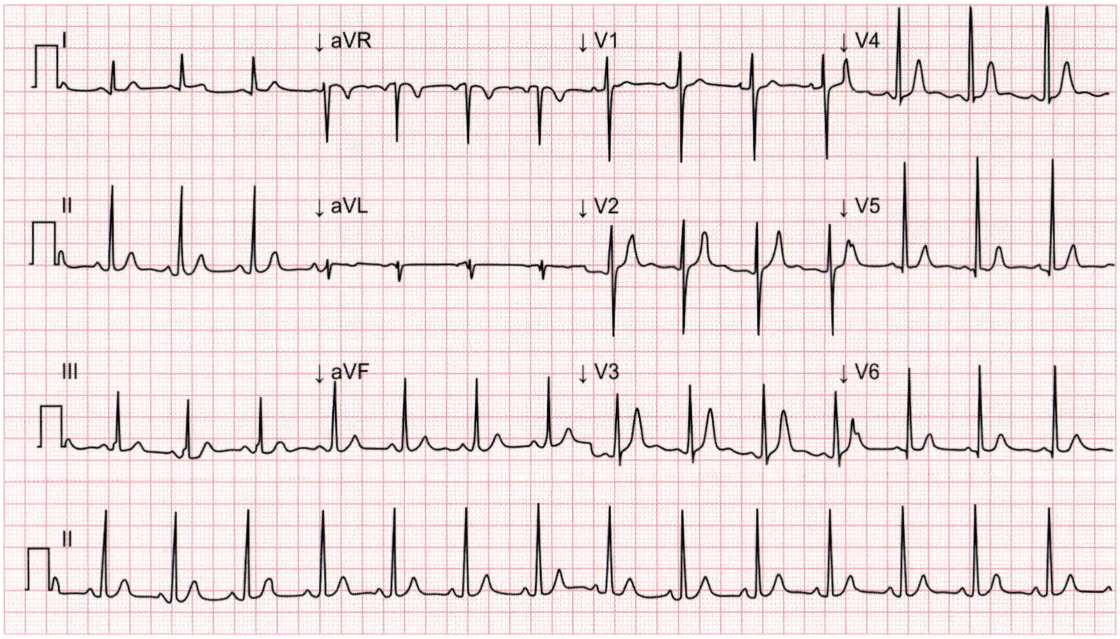

Fig. 1: Normal sinus rhythm.

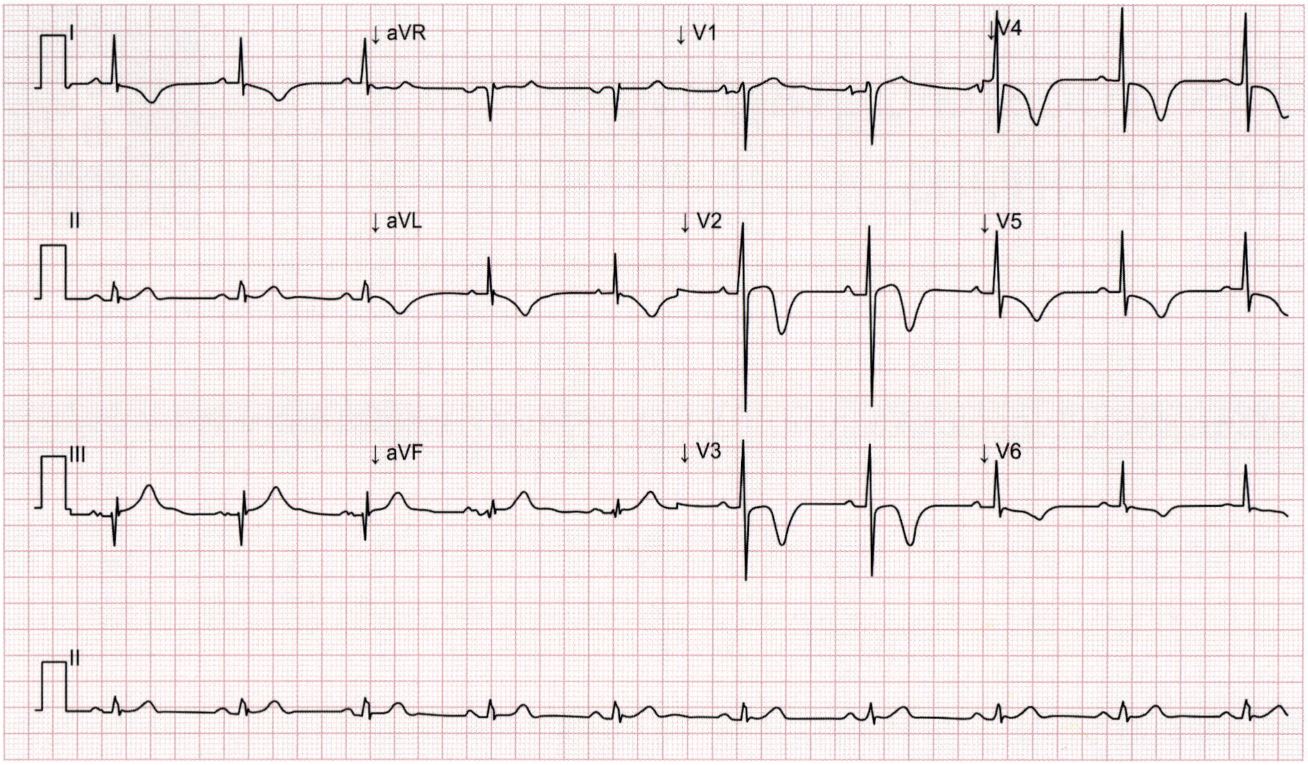

Fig. 2: Non-ST elevation myocardial infarction; deep symmetrical T wave inversion in I, aVL, V2 to V6 and preserved R wave in same leads.

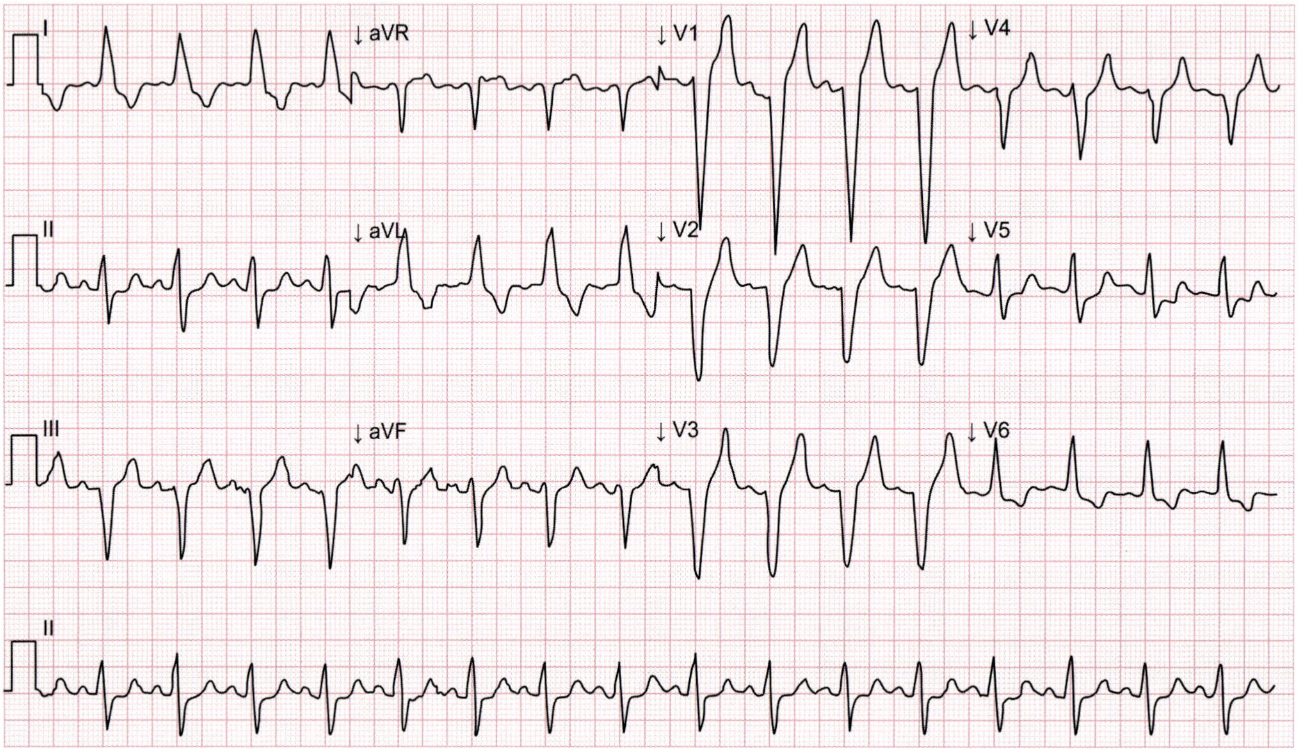

Fig. 3: Sinus rhythm with complete left bundle branch block (LBBB) with QRS duration 150 ms; etiology is idiopathic-dilated cardiomyopathy.

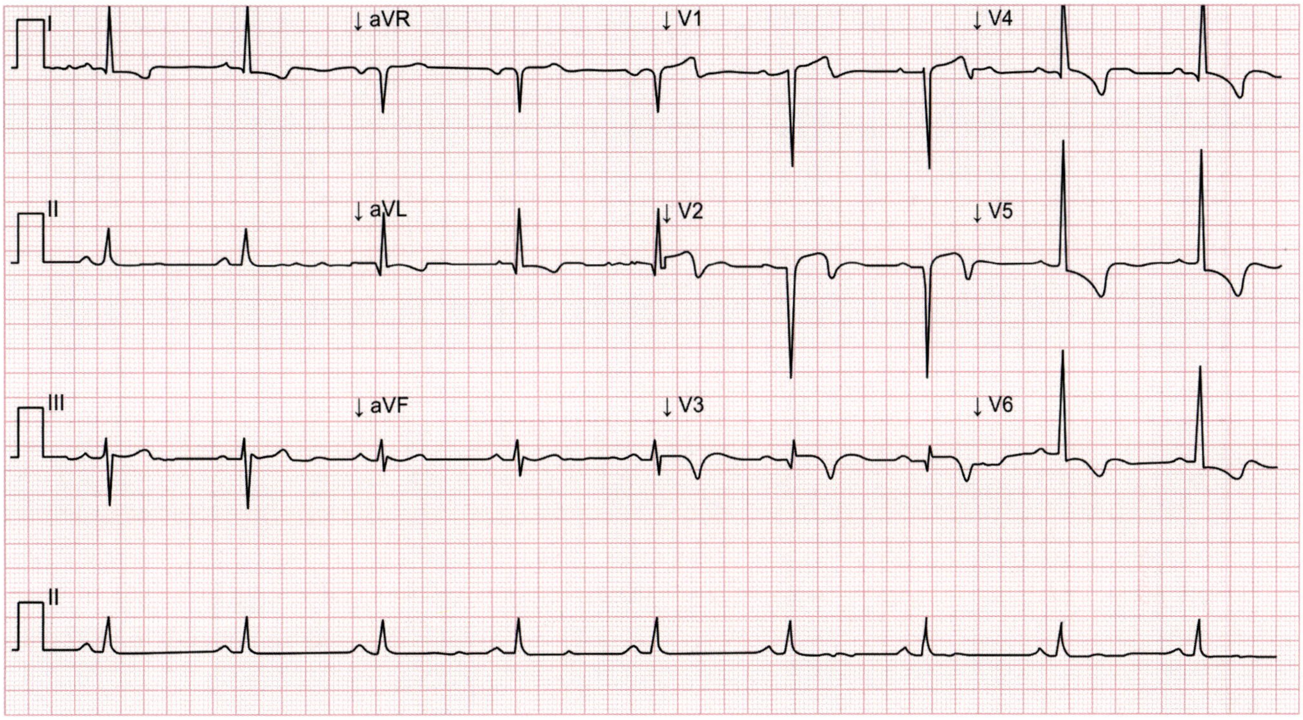

Fig. 4: Evolved anterior wall myocardial infarction (MI). Loss of R wave and presence of Q wave in V2 and V3 with T inversion I, aVL, V2 to V6.

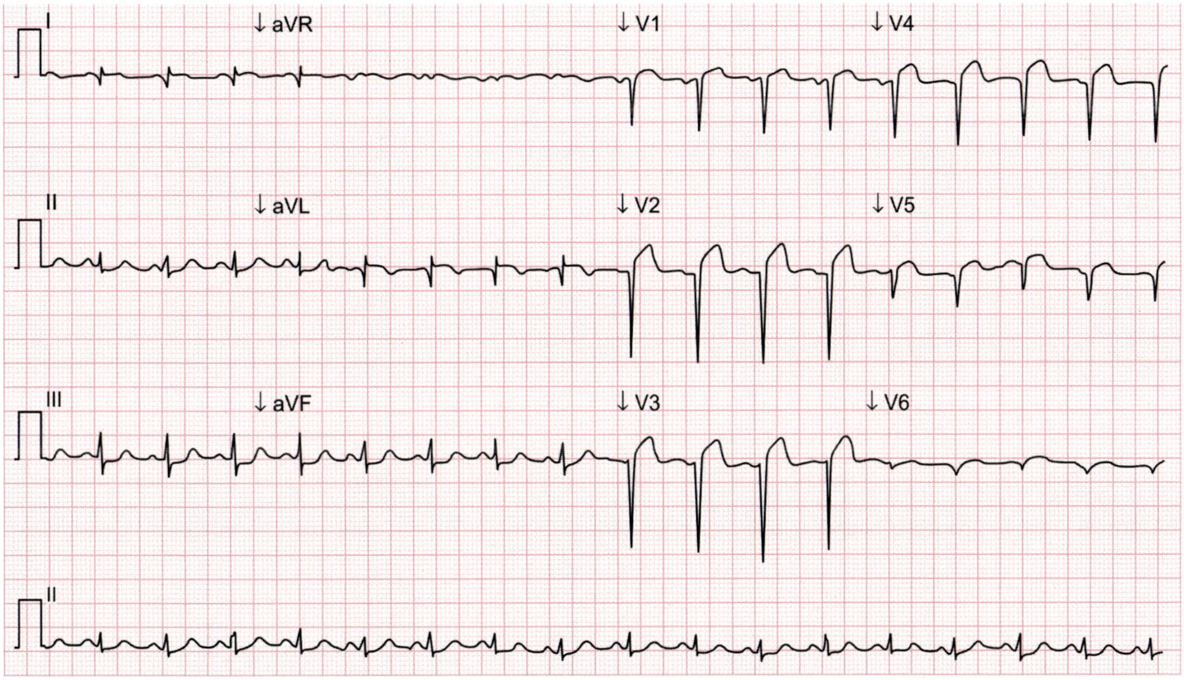

Fig. 5: Completely evolved extensive anterior wall myocardial infarction (MI); presence of Q wave and loss of R wave I, aVL, V2 to V6.

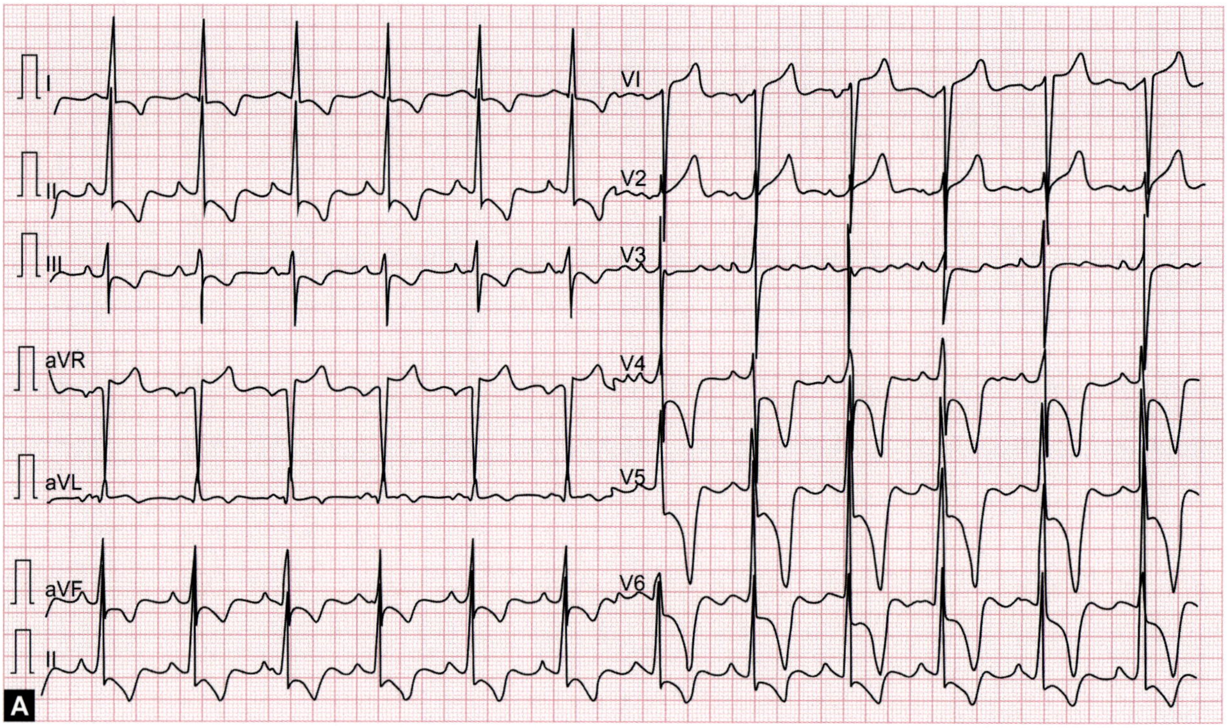

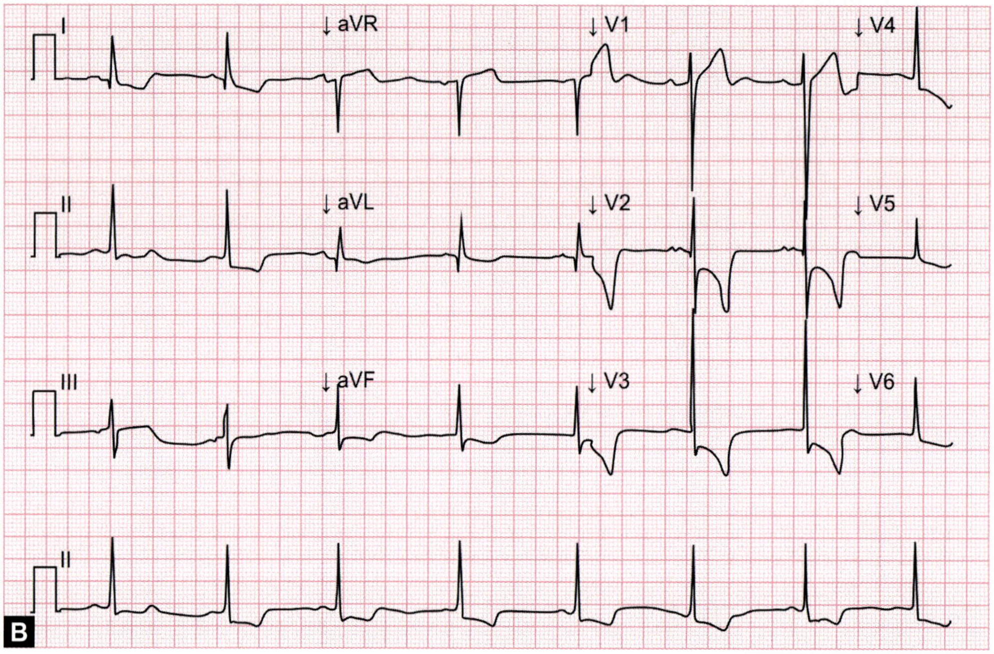

Figs. 6A and B: Sinus rhythm with significant left ventricular hypertrophy (LVH) with strain pattern; etiology—hypertrophic cardiomyopathy.

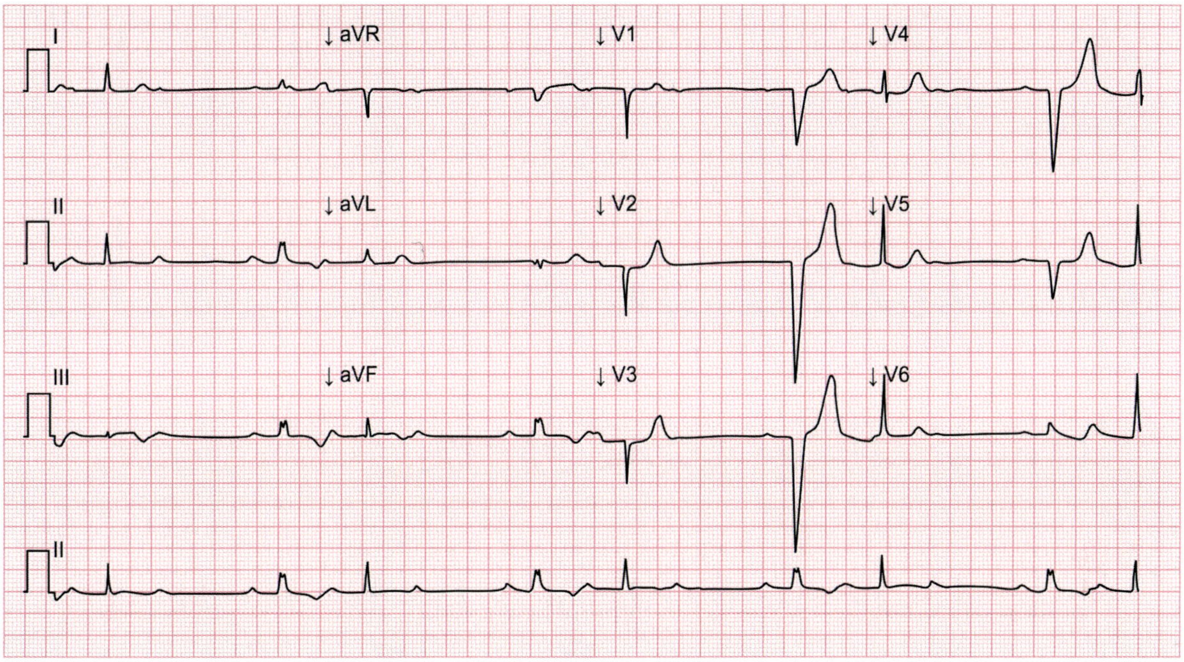

Fig. 7: Sinus rhythm with prolonger PR interval; AV Wenckebach with 3:2 AV block; subtle ST elevation and T inversion in II, III, aVF and T; etiology—inferior wall myocardial infarction (MI).

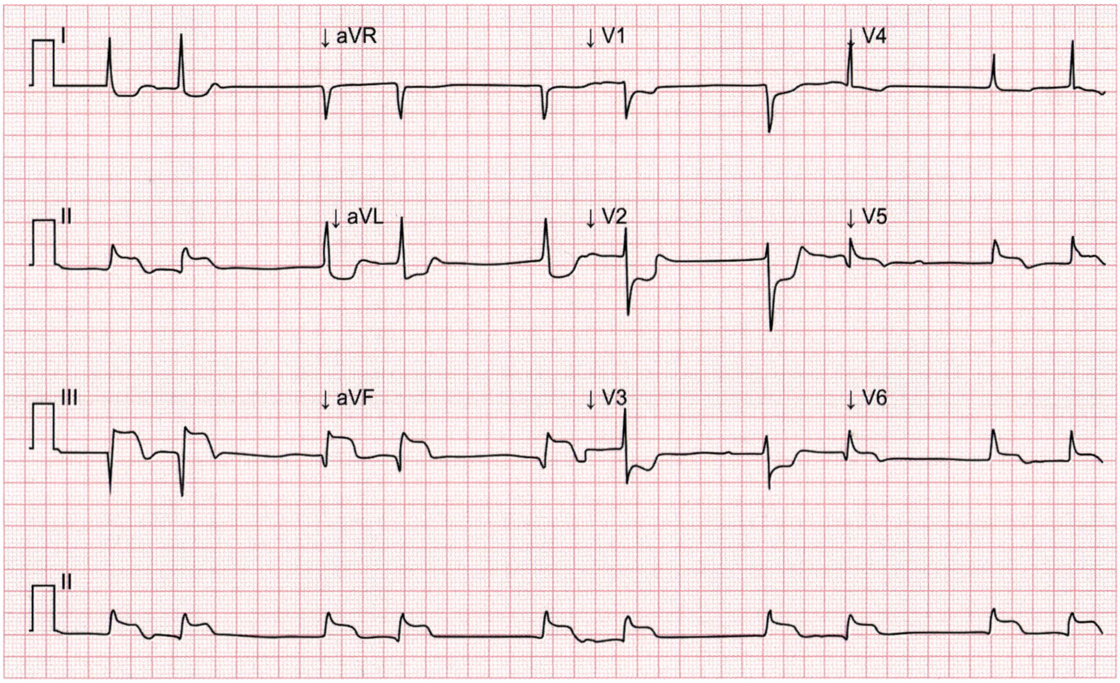

Fig. 8: Inferior wall ST elevation myocardial infarction (MI); ST elevation III more than II with junctional couplet as escape rhythm. Inferior MI associated with conduction disturbances.

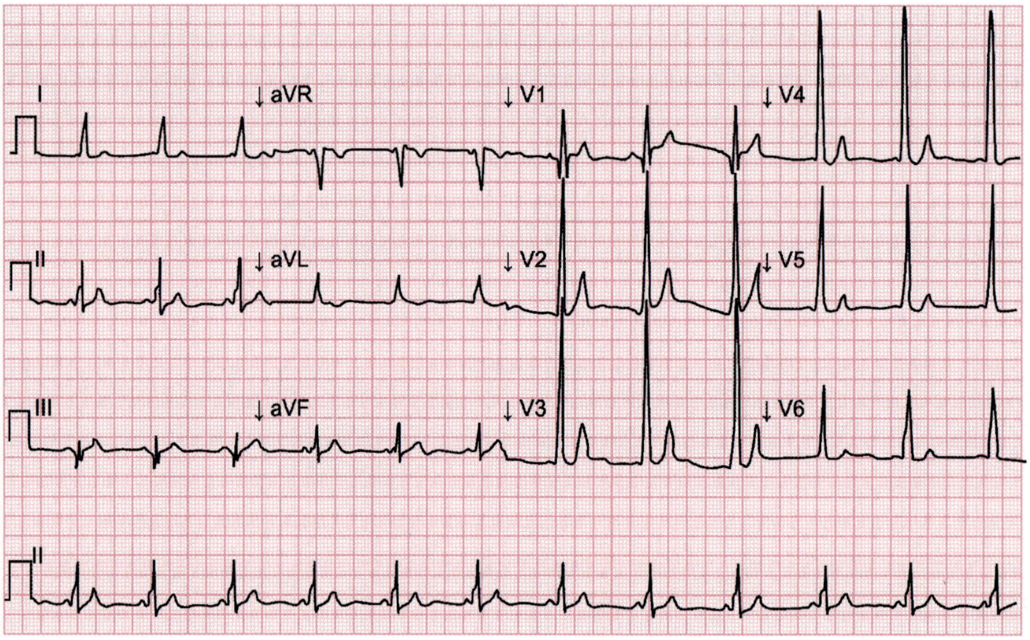

Fig. 9: Sinus rhythm with positive delta wave in lead I, II, aVL, V2 and V3; delta transition between V1 and V2 suggesting left anterior pathway.

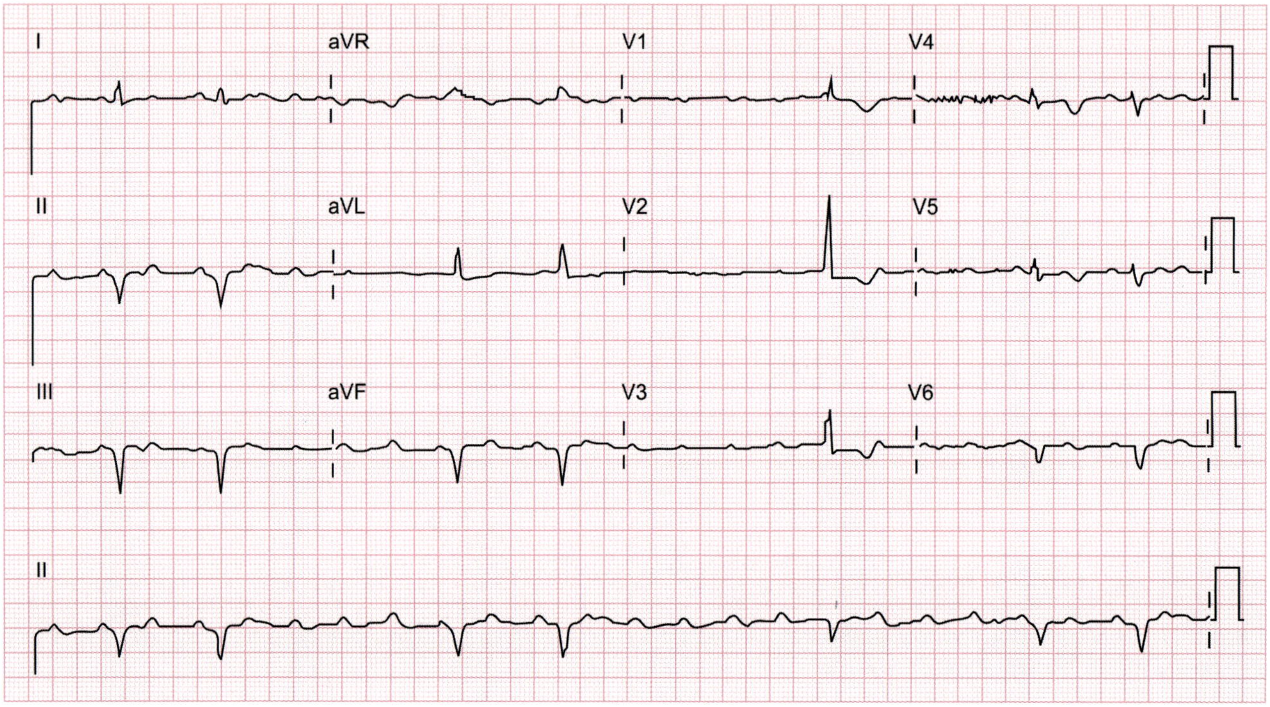

Fig. 10: Multiple P waves best seen in long lead II with variable PR interval with variable RR interval suggesting atrial tachycardia and variable AV nodal conduction.

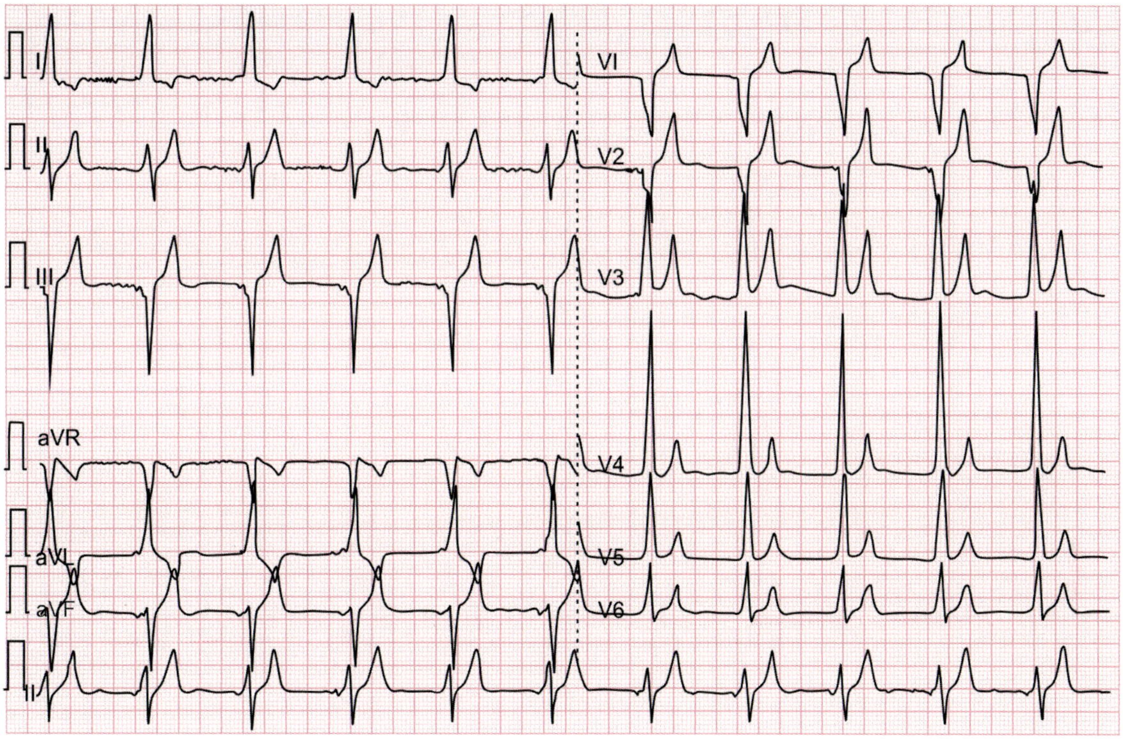

Fig. 11: Sinus rhythm with positive delta in I, aVL, and negative delta in III and aVF and V1; etiology—posteroseptal pathway.

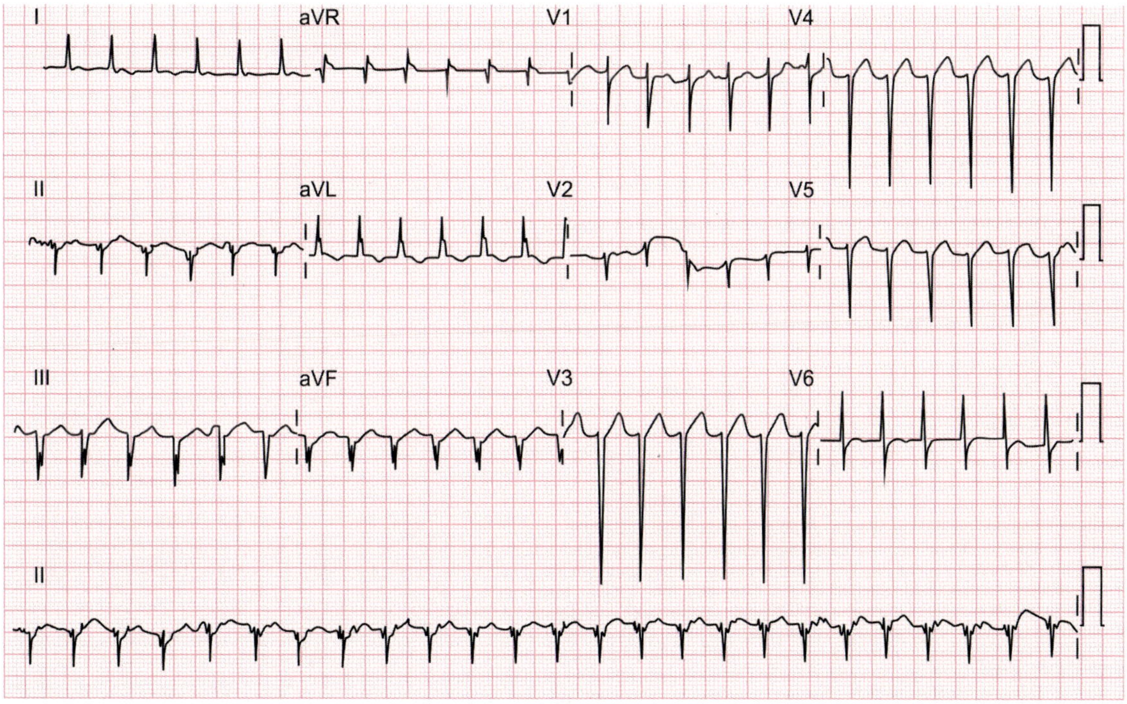

Fig. 12: Narrow complex tachycardia with pseudo S wave best seen in lead I; etiology—AV nodal re-entrant tachycardia (AVNRT).

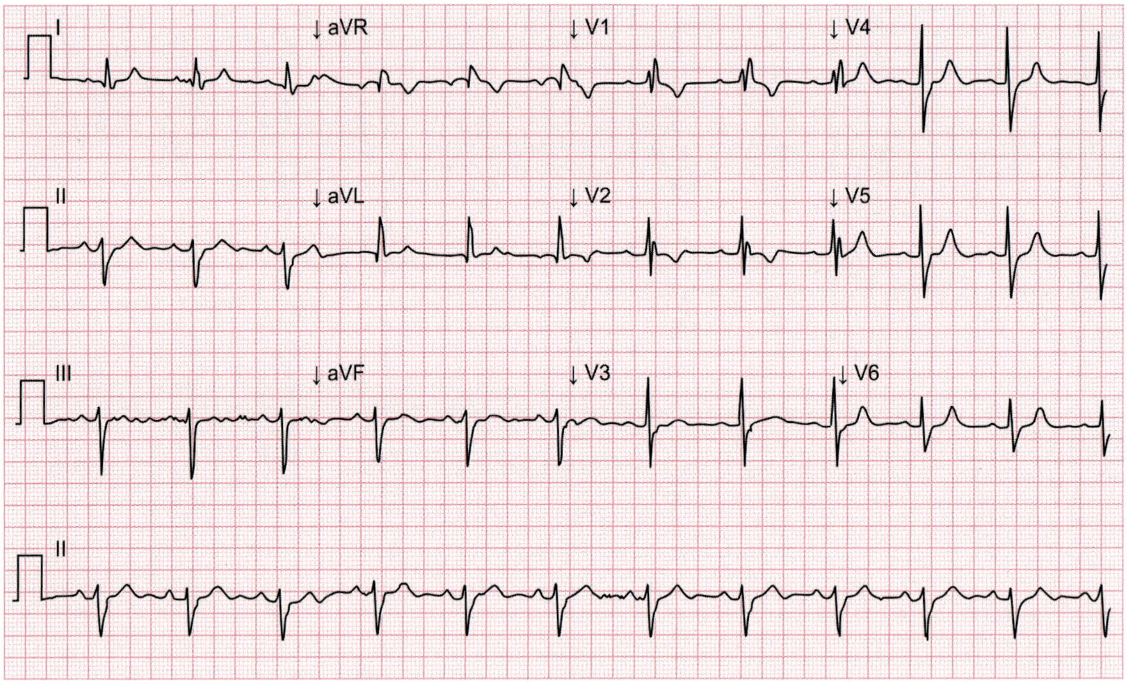

Fig. 13: Trifascicular block; right bundle branch block (RBBB) with left axis with PR interval 220 ms. *Note:* 'M' pattern in V1 - V5.

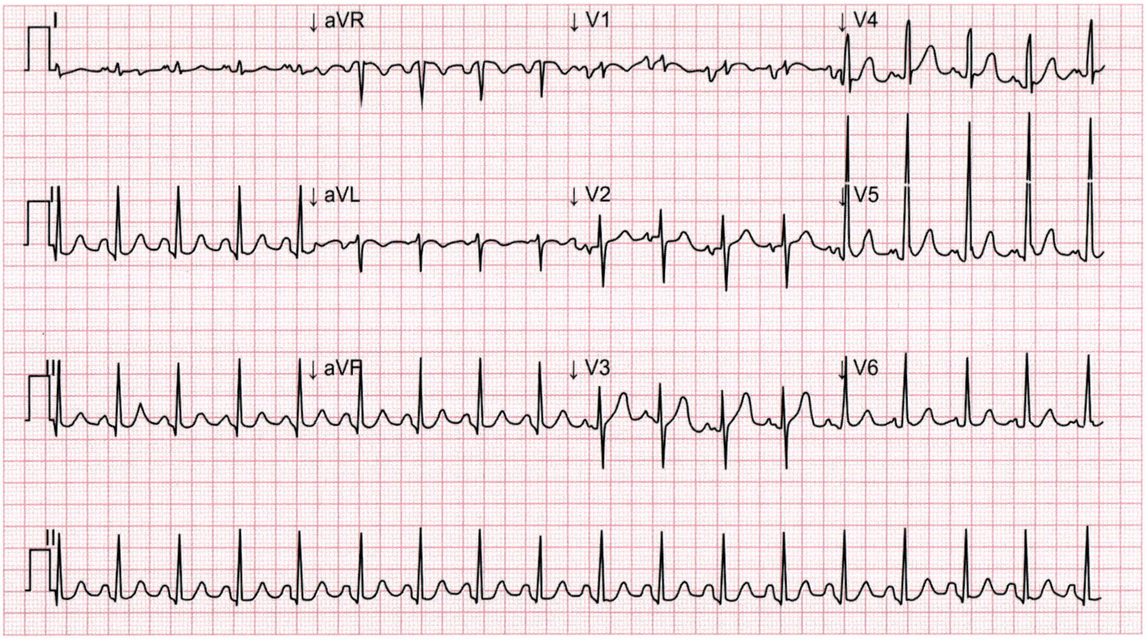

Fig. 14: Sinus rhythm with P pulmonale and P mitrale; etiology—rheumatic heart disease with mitral stenosis with severe pulmonary artery hypertension (PAH).

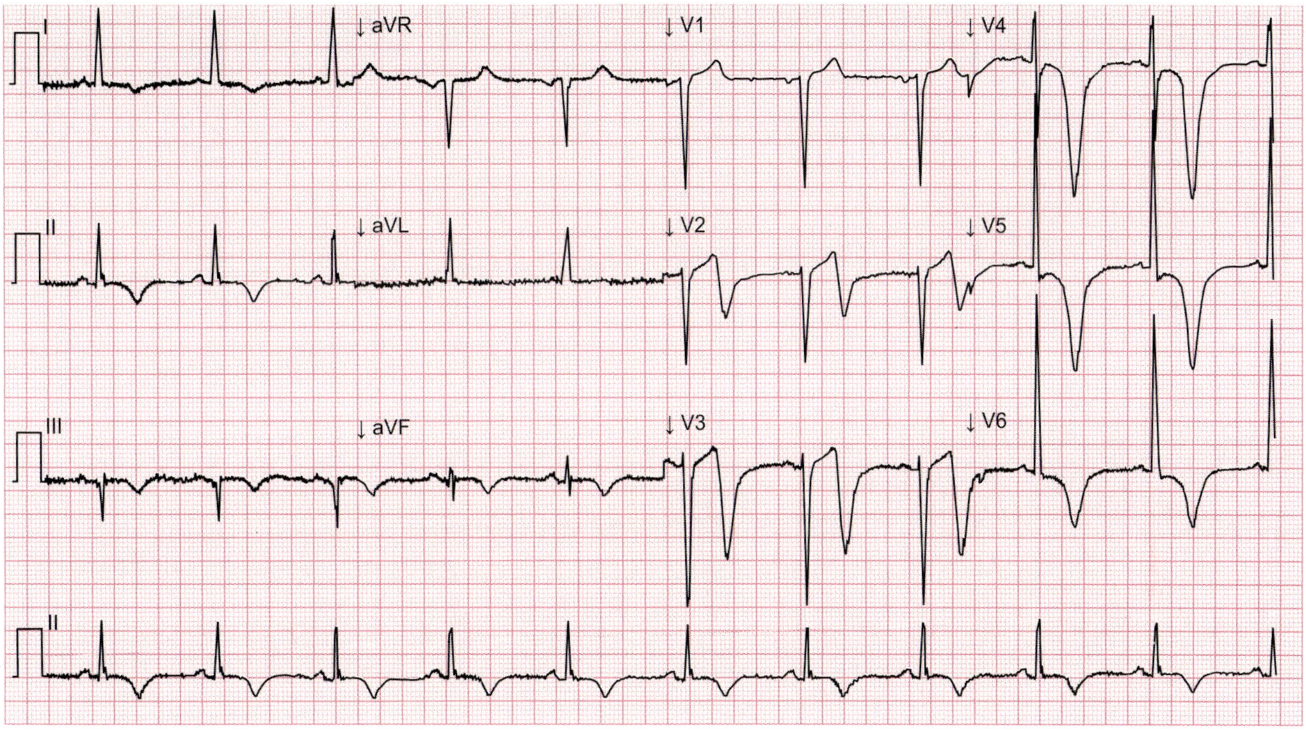

Fig. 15: Anterior wall myocardial infarction with deep symmetrical T wave inversion and loss of R wave.

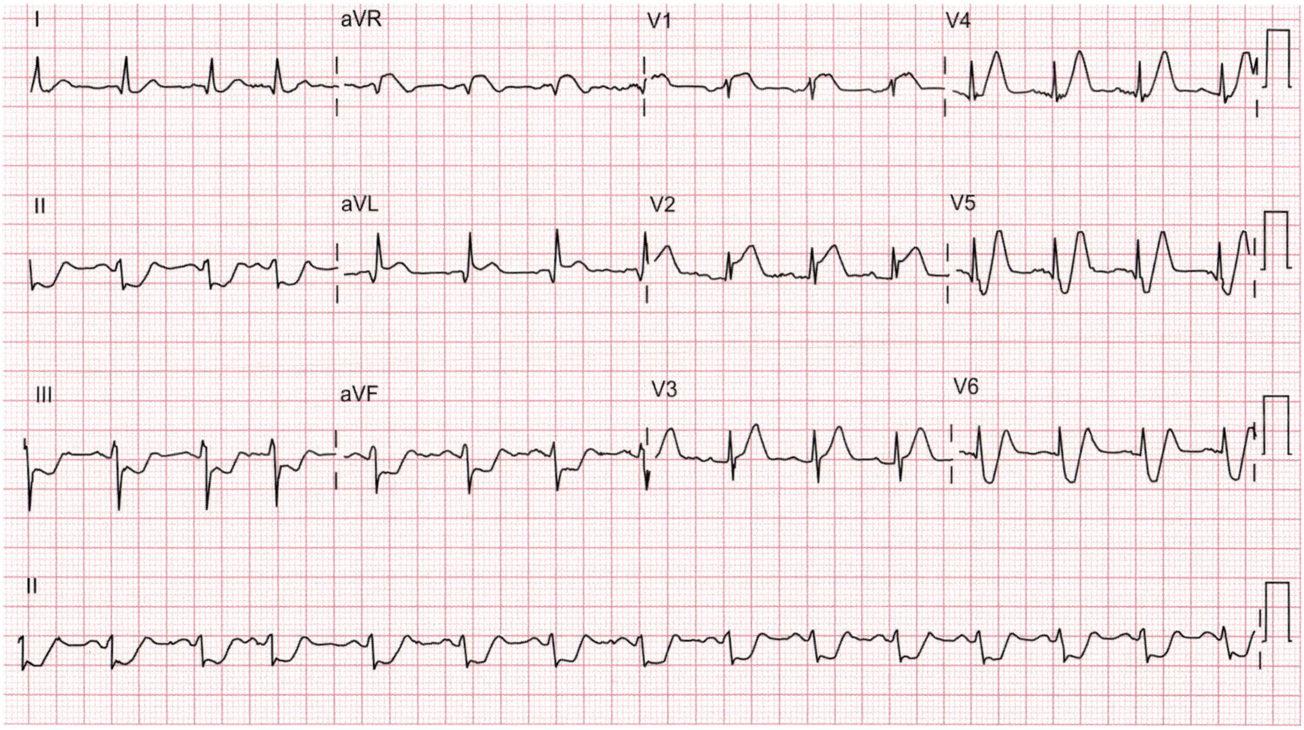

Fig. 16: Anteroseptal myocardial infarction (MI); ST elevation in V1 and V2 with ST depression in II, III, and aVF.

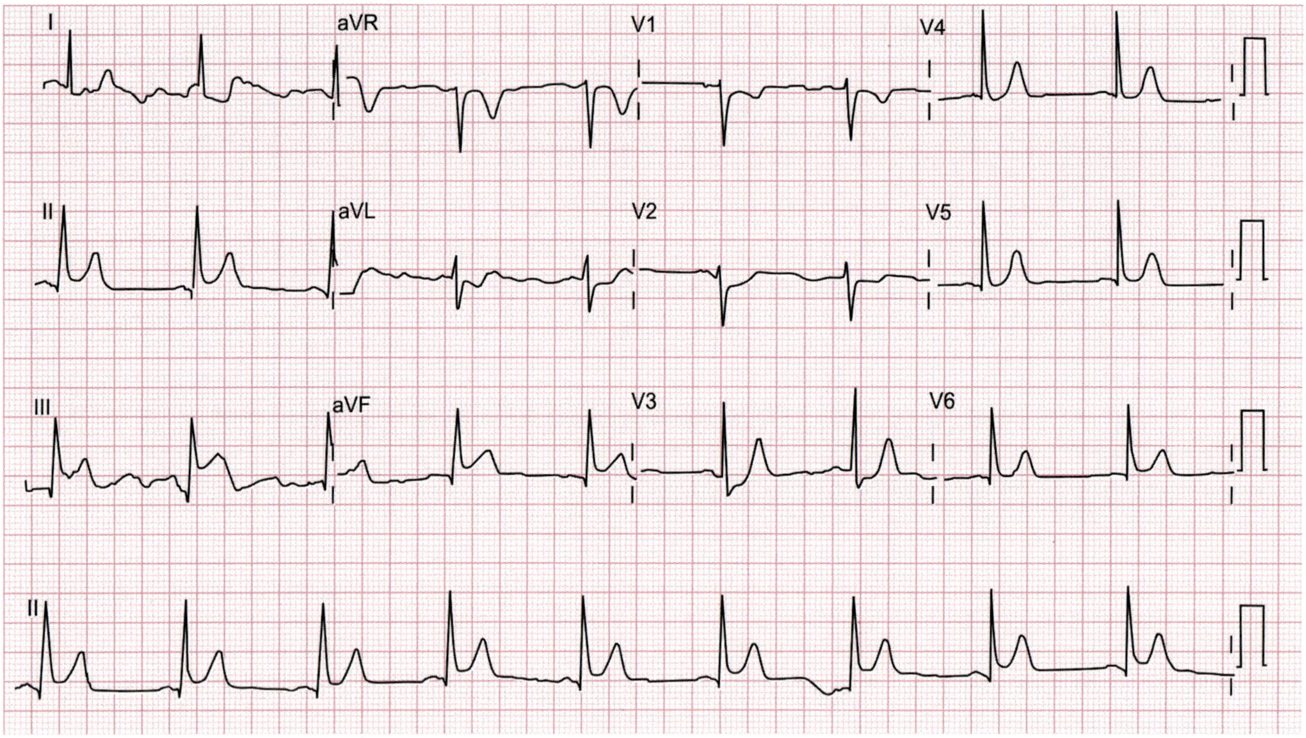

Fig. 17: Inferior wall myocardial infarction with ST elevation in III more than II and reciprocal ST depression in I and aVL.

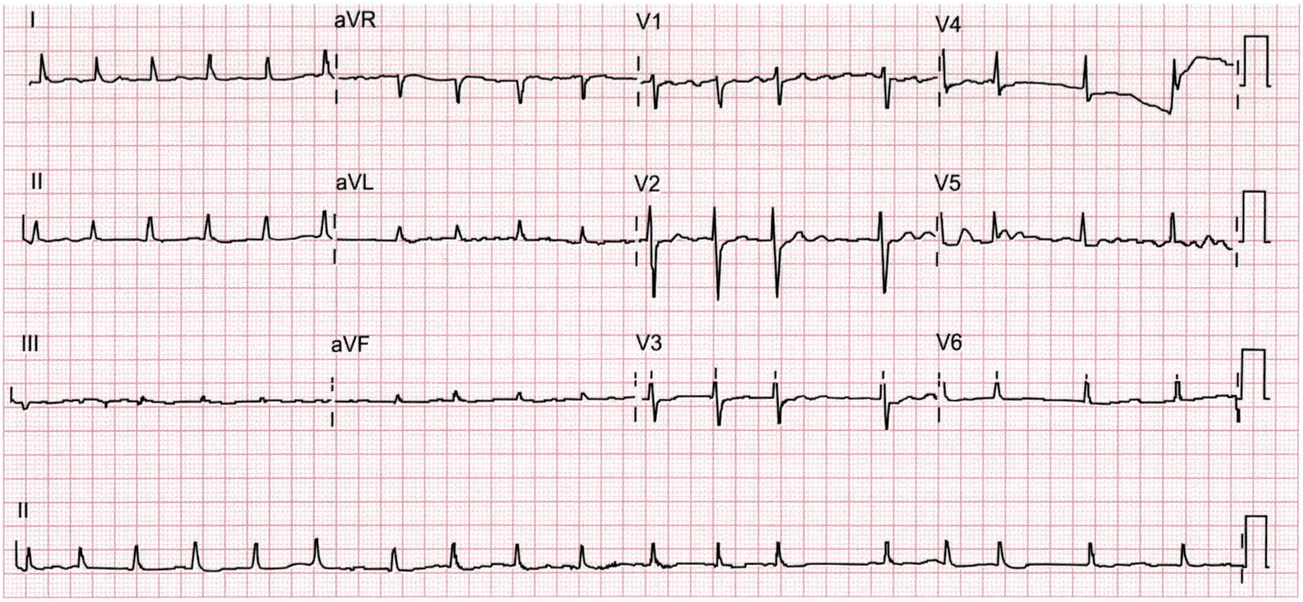

Fig. 18: Atrial fibrillation and fast ventricular rate.

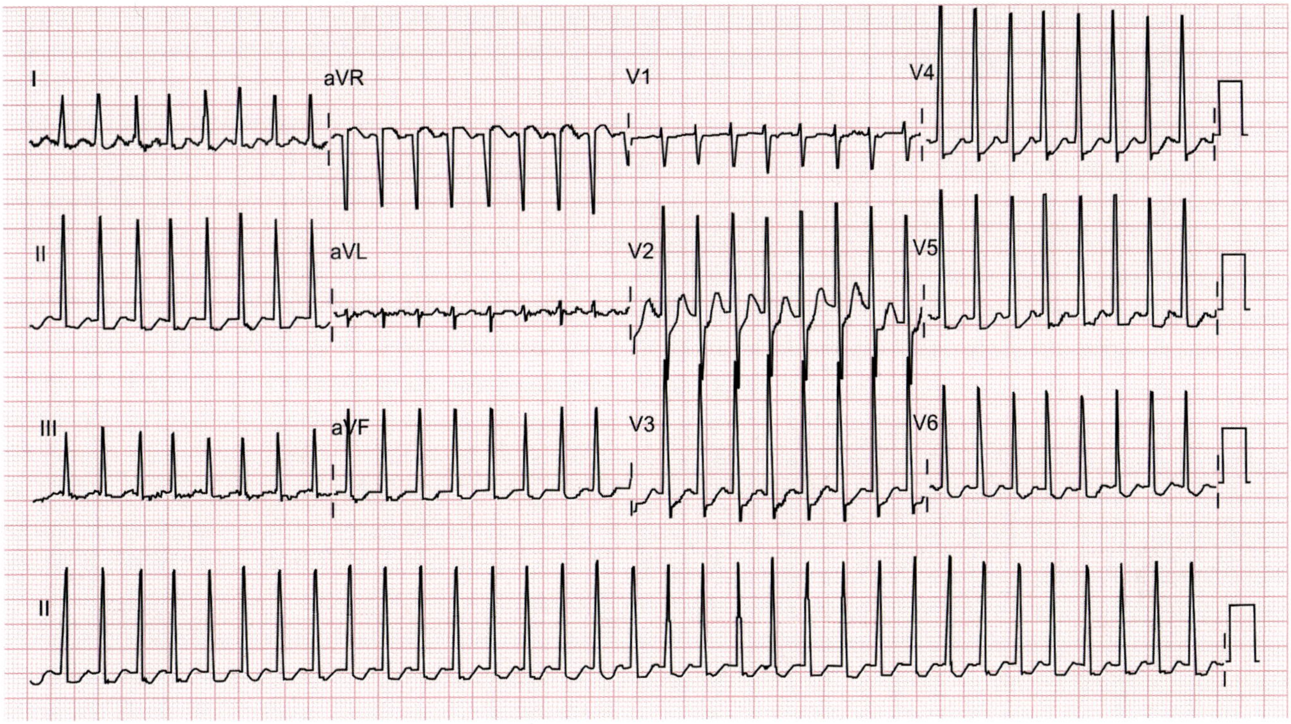

Fig. 19: Narrow complex tachycardia with 1.5 mm ST depression; etiology—possibly AV nodal re-entrant tachycardia (AVNRT).

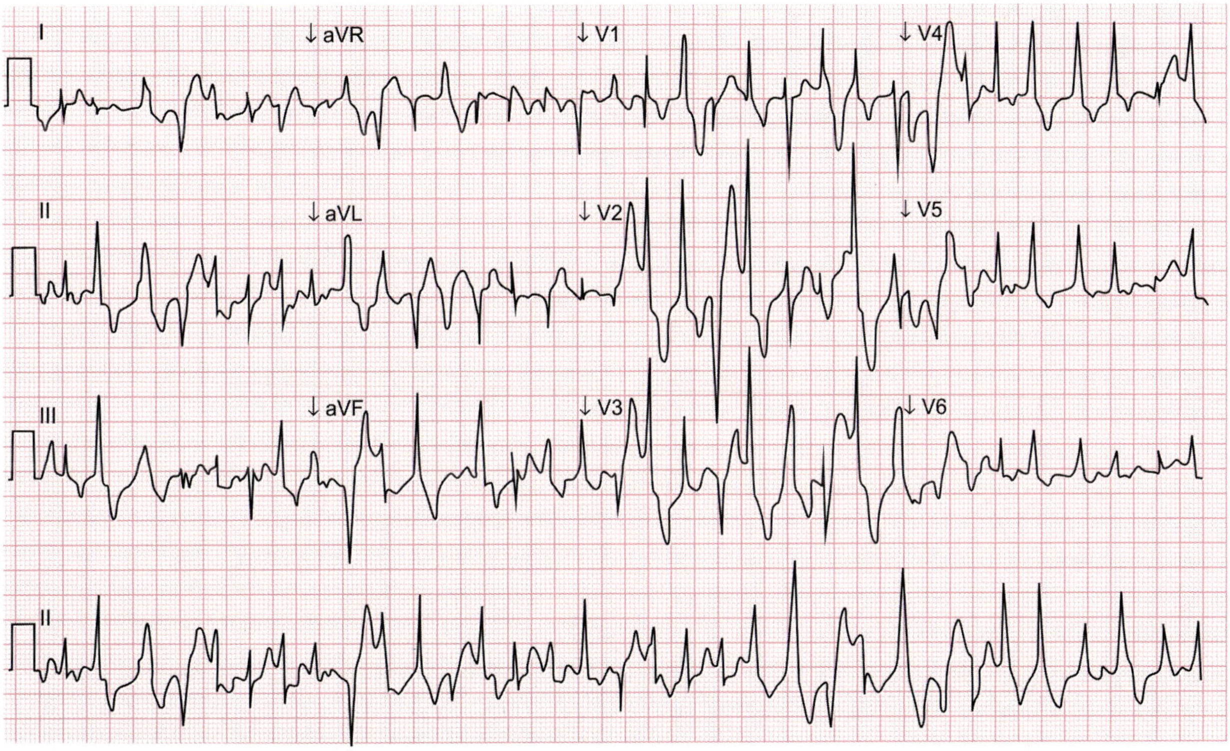

Fig. 20: Polymorphic ventricular premature contraction (VPC) with alternating axis of QRS confirming a diagnosis of bidirectional VPC/VT; etiology—catecholaminergic polymorphic ventricular tachycardia (VT).

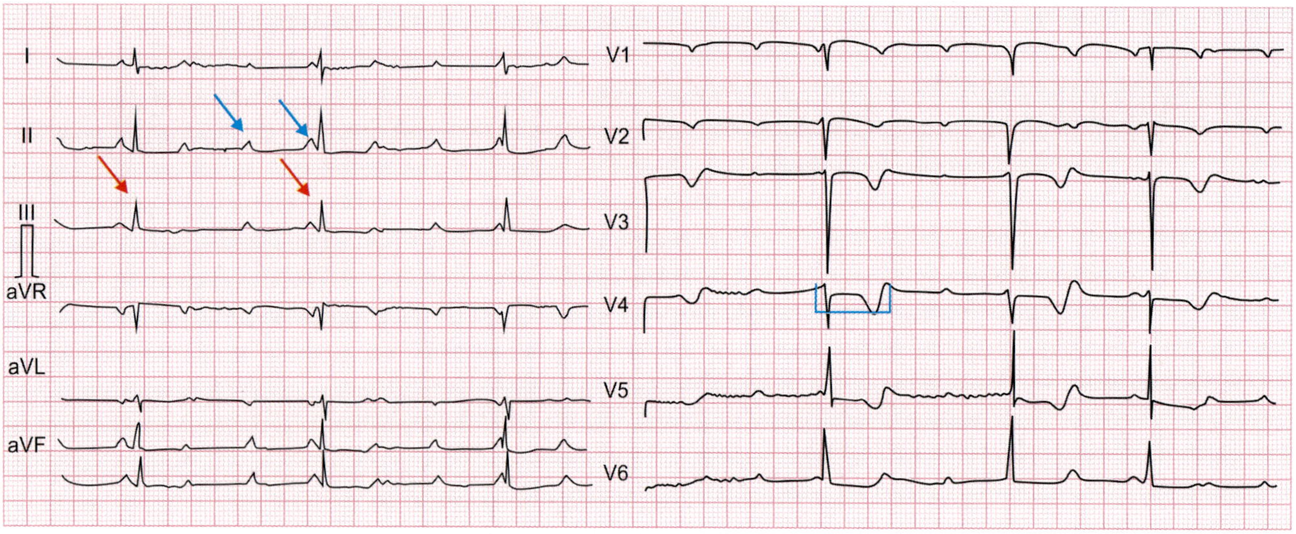

Fig. 21: Complete heart block with AV dissociation; atrial rate 90 beats/min and ventricular rate of around 30 beats/min with prolonged QT interval. Needs urgent temporary pacemaker implantation (TPI).

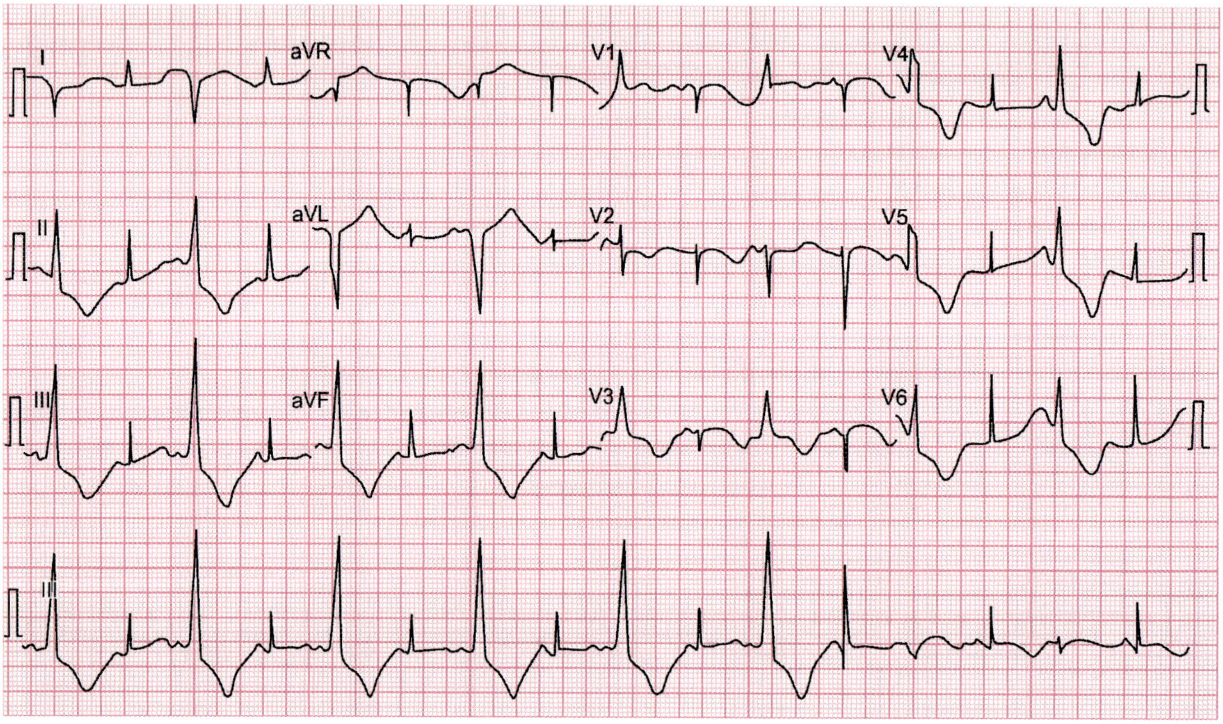

Fig. 22: Congenital long QT syndrome with QT interval measured to be 550 ms; alternating QRS having deep T wave inversion with long QT interval.

Drug-induced prolonged 'QT' in ICU, common drugs amiodarone, haloperidol, fluconazole, erythromycin can lead to torsade de pointes (polymorphic VT) t/t: Magnesium.

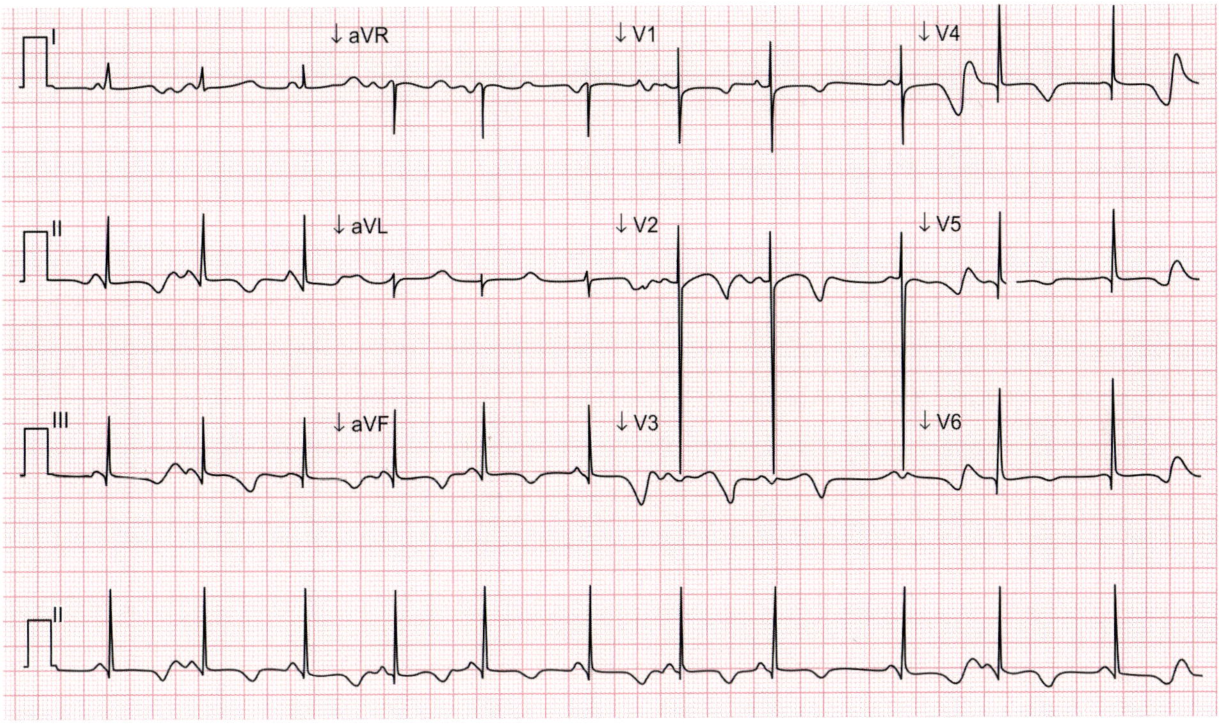

Fig. 23: Long QT interval type III with corrected QT interval of 600 ms.

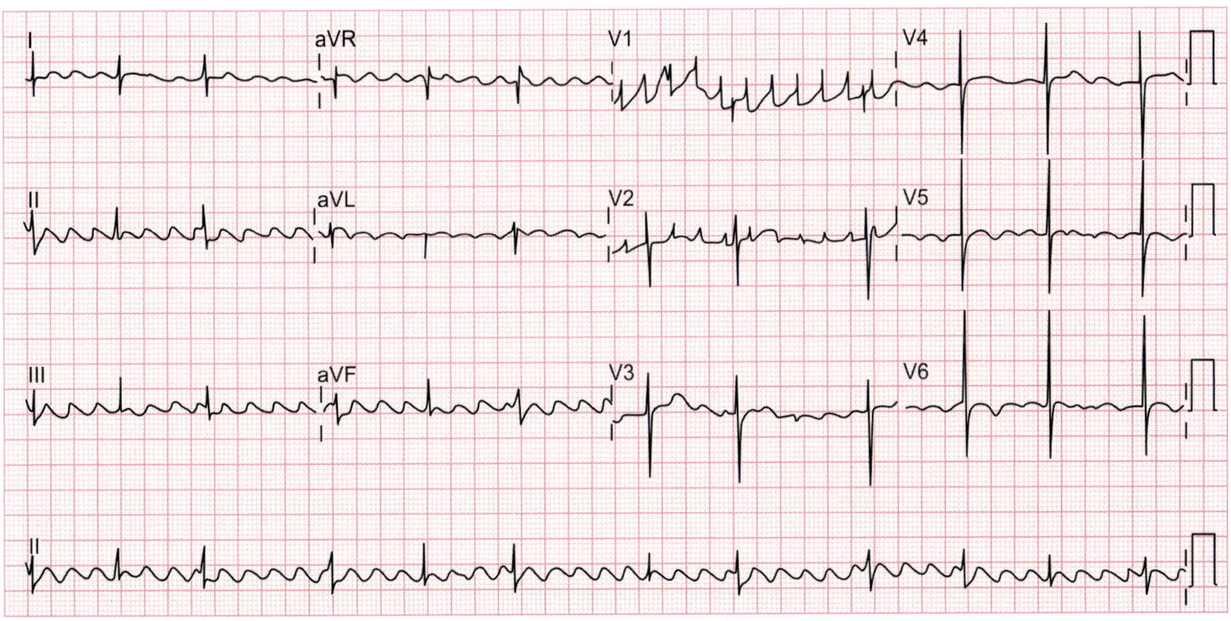

Fig. 24: Atrial flutter with typical inverted saw tooth appearance in lead II, III, and aVF; large P wave in lead V1; left ventricular hypertrophy; etiology—hypertrophic cardiomyopathy with atrial flutter.

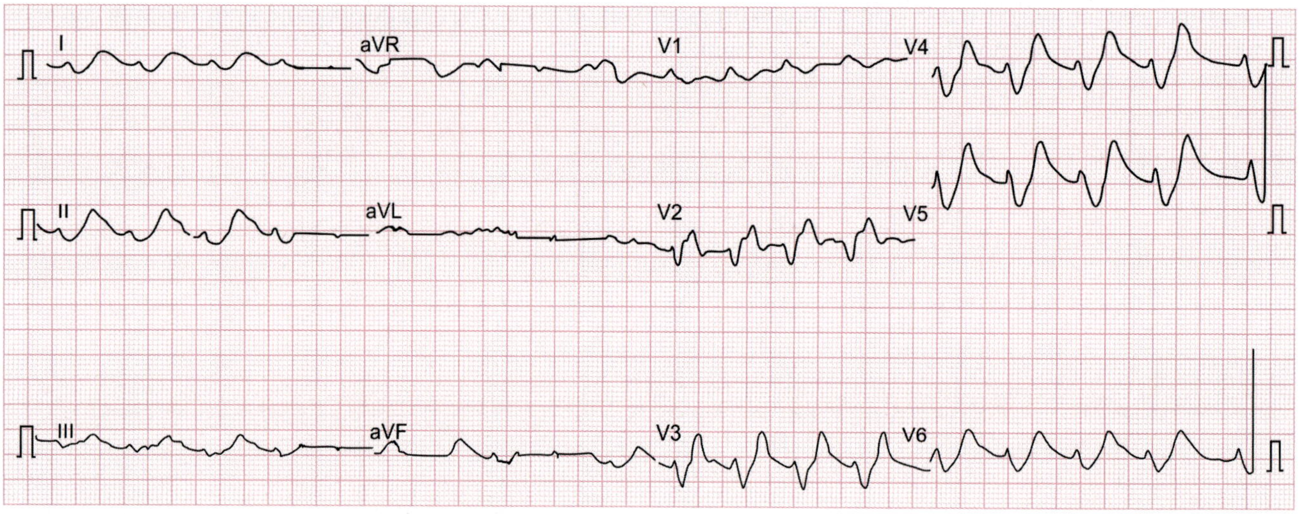

Fig. 25: Sinus rhythm with blunted P wave with prolonged PR interval with tall T waves with short QT segment; etiology—hyperkalemia.

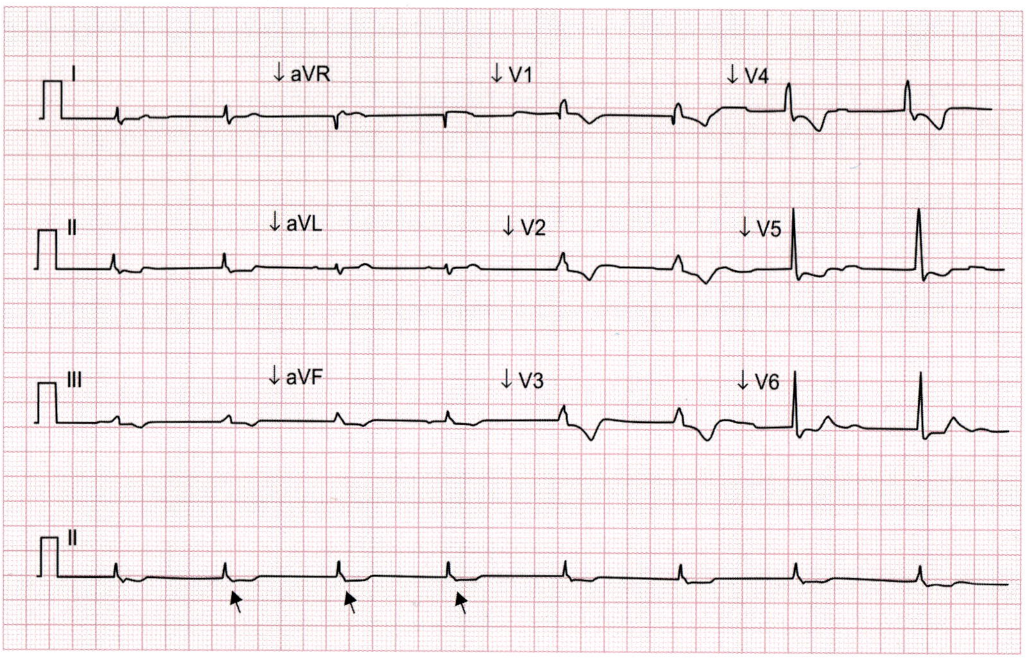

Fig. 26: Junctional rhythm with right bundle branch block escape; etiology—sclerodegenerative sinus and AV nodal disease.

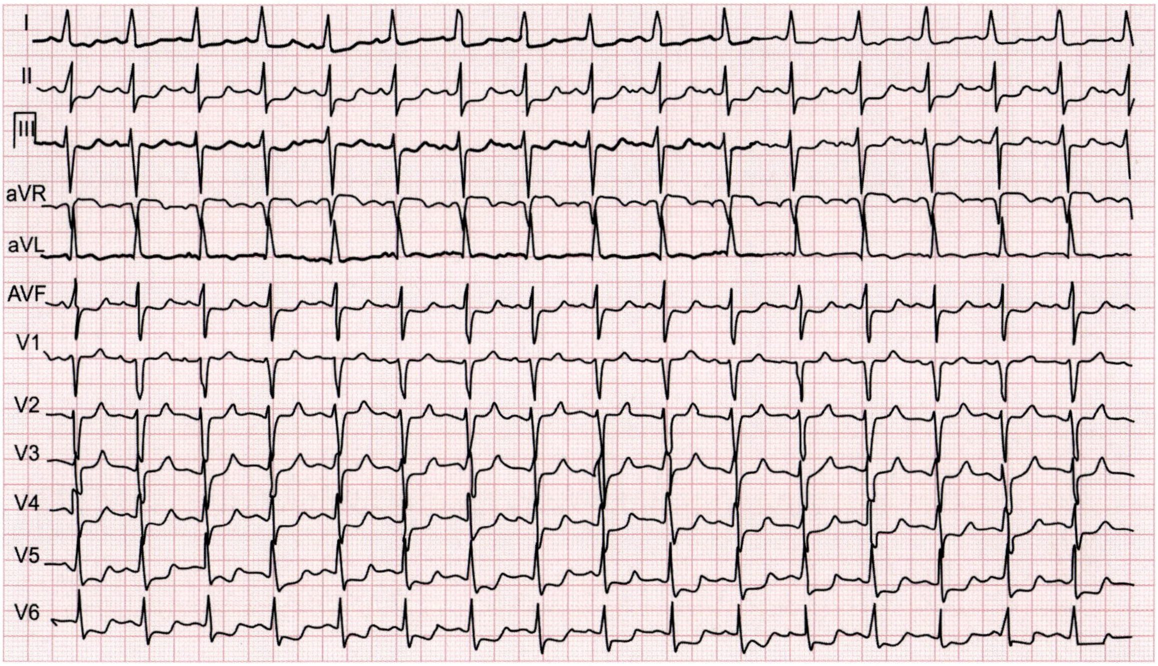

Fig. 27: Sinus rhythm with global ST depression with aVR ST elevation; etiology—left main significant coronary artery disease.

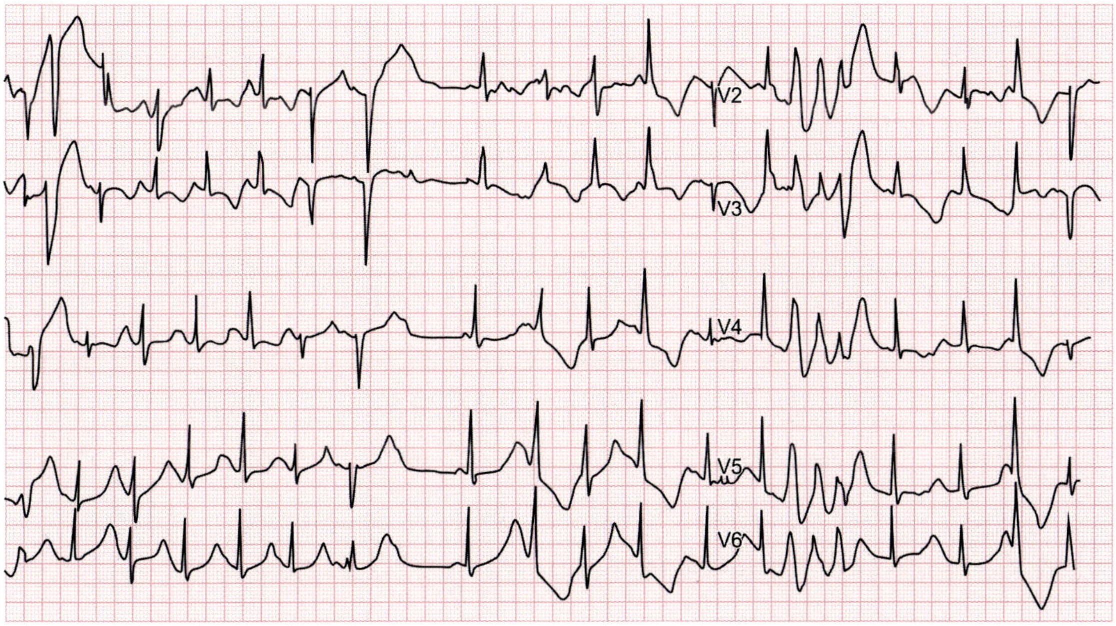

Fig. 28: Congenital long QT syndrome with degeneration into polymorphic VPC's.

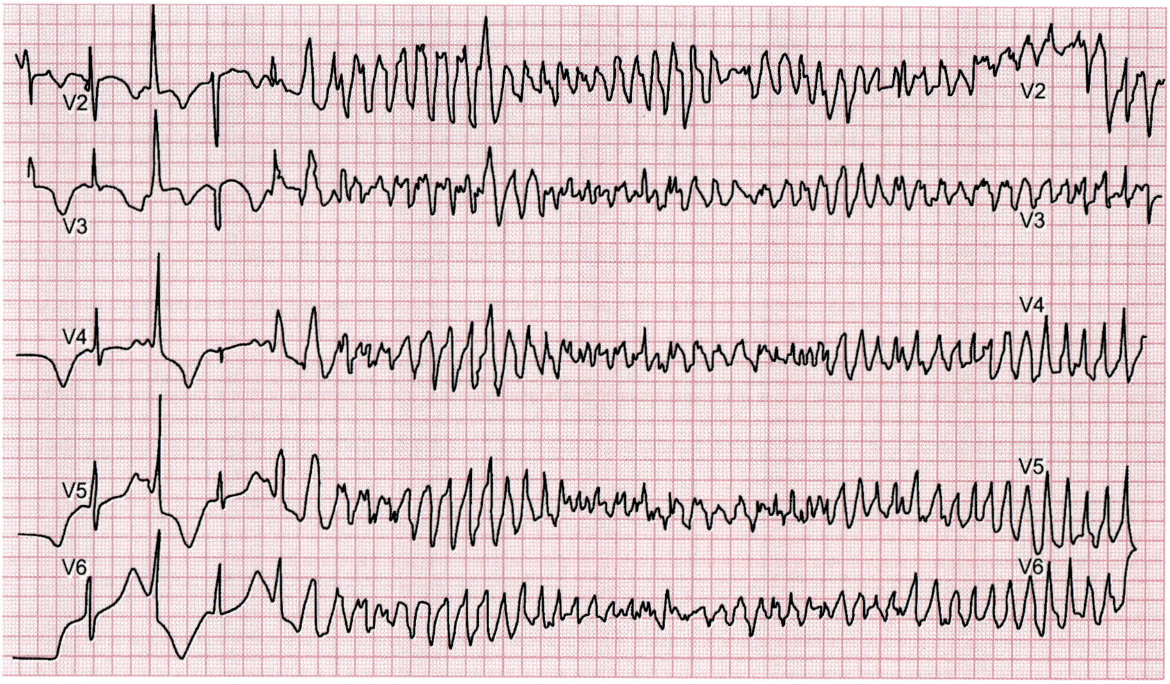

Fig. 29: Congenital long QT syndrome degenerating into torsades de pointes.

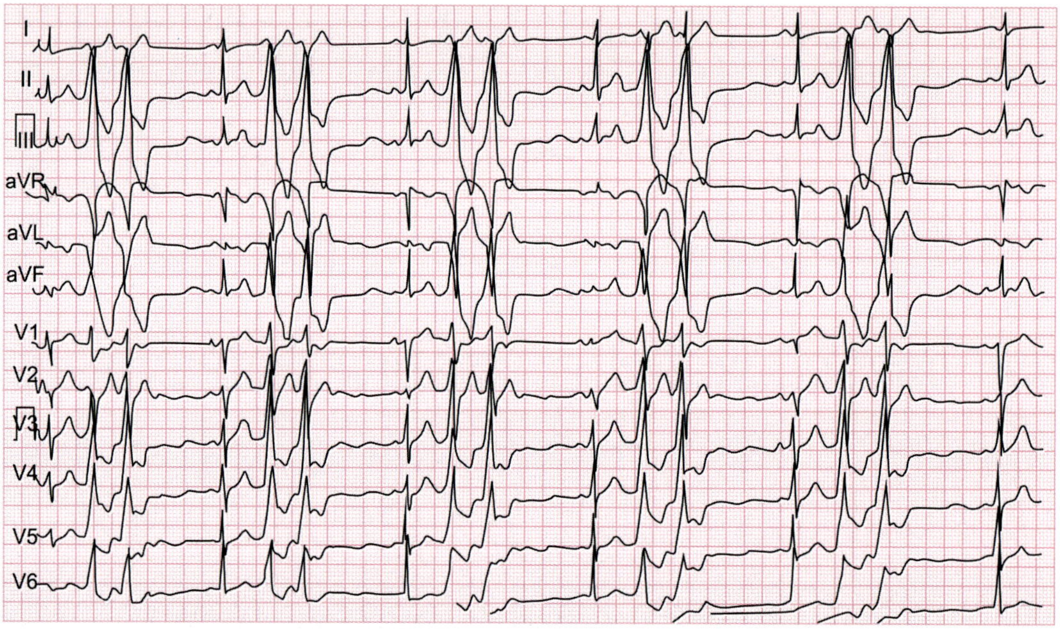

Fig. 30: Sinus rhythm with ventricular couplets; couplet morphology shows positive R in V1 to V6 with inferior axis; etiology—ventricular premature contraction (VPC) arising from LV summit.

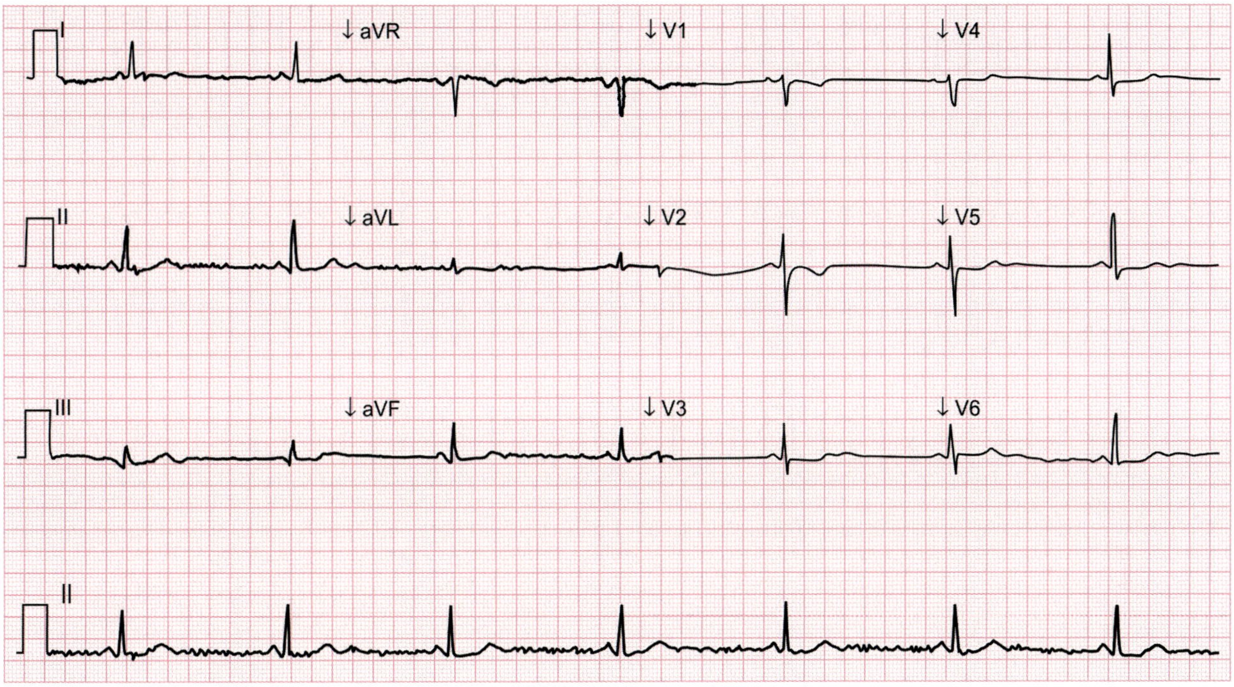

Fig. 31: Sinus bradycardia.

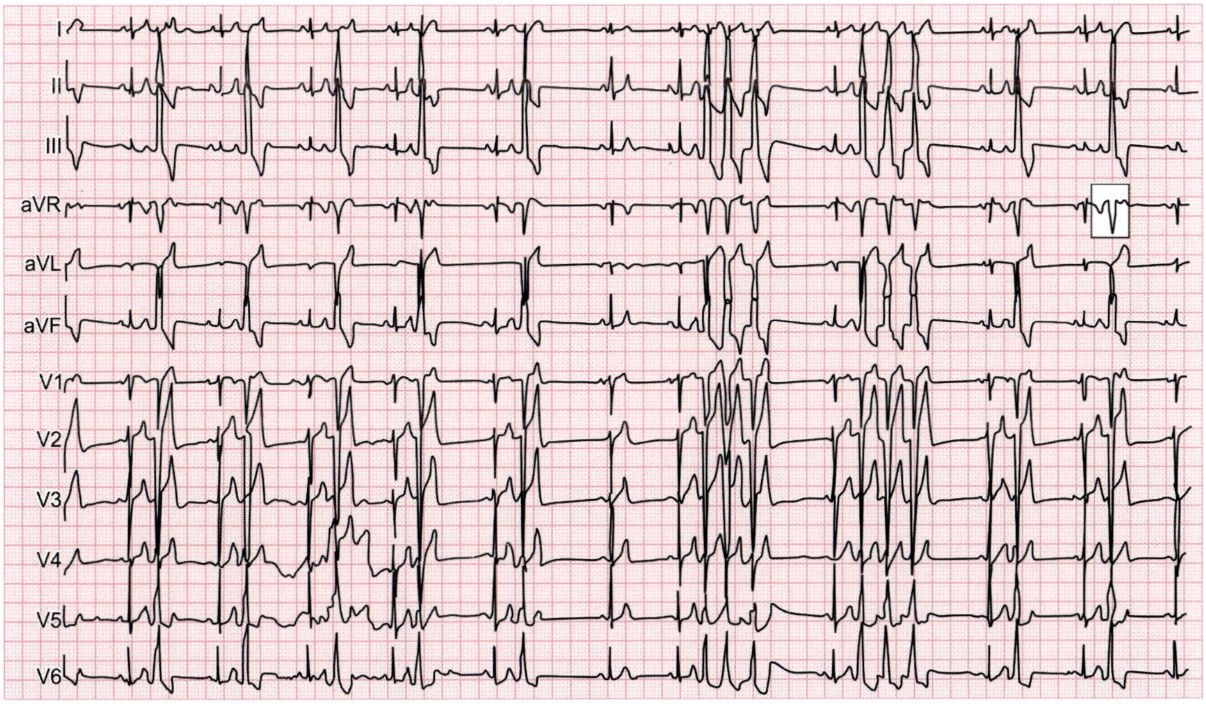

Fig. 32: Sinus rhythm with initial part of ECG showing ventricular bigeminy; later part shows nonsustained ventricular tachycardia (VT); morphology of VPC suggests left bundle branch block (LBBB) and inferior axis suggesting right ventricular outflow tract VT.

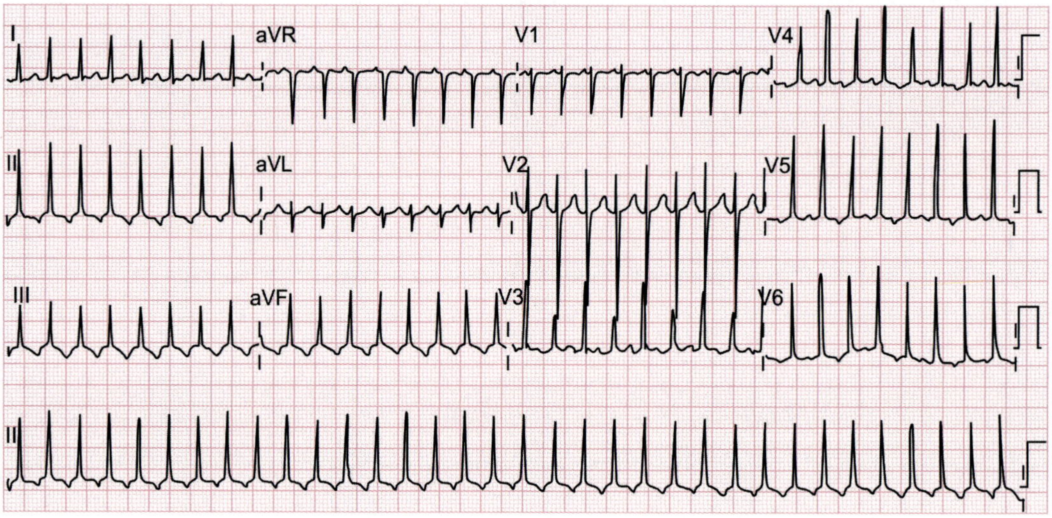

Fig. 33: Narrow complex tachycardia with long RP interval; etiology in this case was permanent junctional re-entrant tachycardia (PJRT).

CHAPTER 9

Interesting Pictures in Cardiac ICU

Raja Babu Panwar, Dinesh Choudhary

CLINICAL APPEARANCE (FIGS. 1 AND 2)

Phlegmasia Cerulea Dolens (Fig. 1)

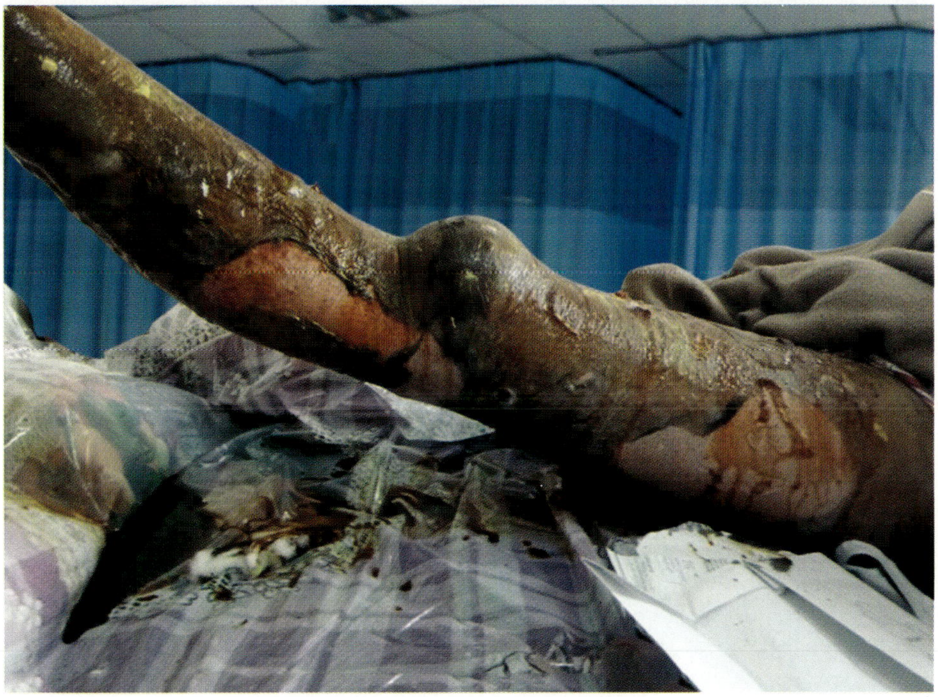

Fig. 1: Phlegmasia cerulea dolens.

- It is used in reference to extreme case of lower extremity deep venous thrombosis (DVT) that cause critical limb ischemia and limb loss.
- It is characterized by severe swelling and cyanosis and is a life-threatening condition. Usually needs thrombolytic therapy and limb salvage.

Postpuncture Site—after Coronary Interventions via Radial Route (Fig. 2)

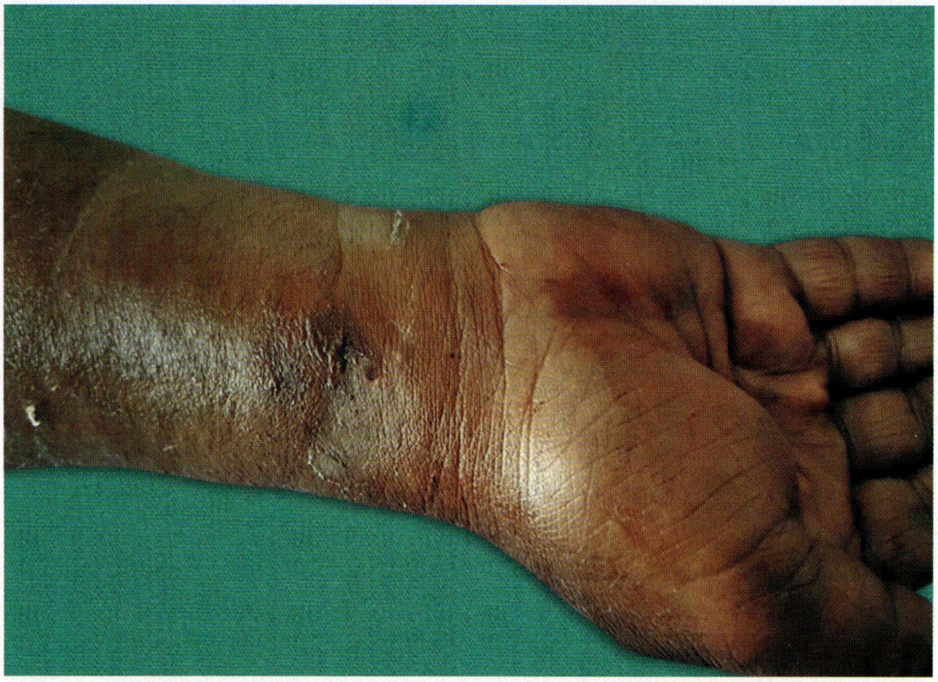

Fig. 2: Postpuncture site—after coronary interventions via radial route.

- Radial route is preferred over femoral route now-a-days because of early mobilization of patients and less vascular complications.
- Before opting for radial route, vascular integrity of palmar arch should be confirmed by Allen test or Doppler to avoid ischemic complications of the hand.

CHEST X-RAY WITH CARDIAC PATHOLOGY (FIGS. 3 TO 7)

Atrial Septal Defect Eisenmenger (Fig. 3)

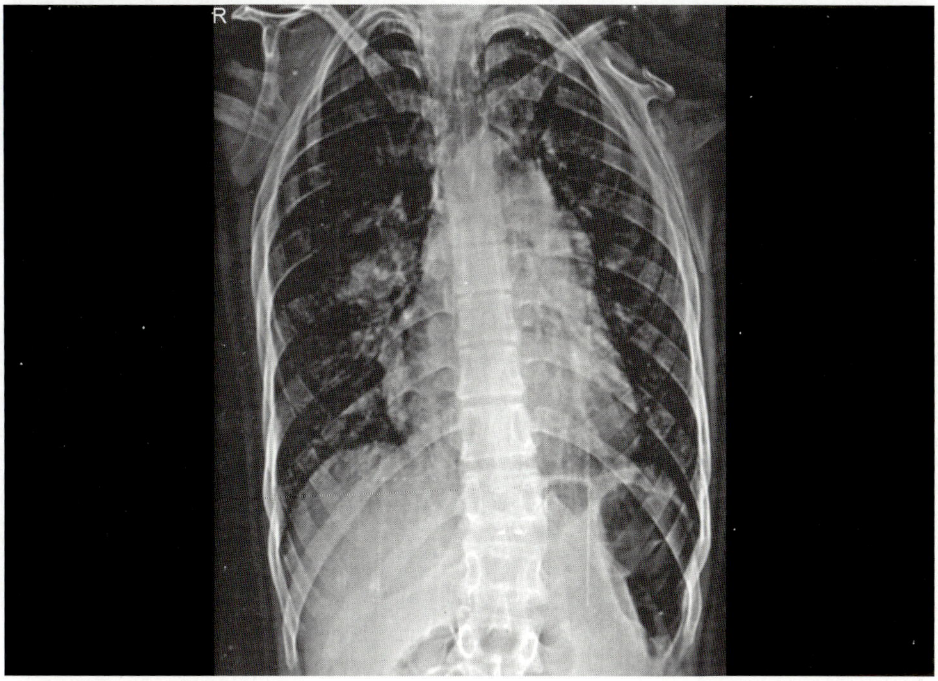

Fig. 3: Atrial septal defect (ASD) Eisenmenger—note dilated main pulmonary artery (MPA) and prominent vascular markings.

- Chest X-ray PA view showing cardiomegaly with RV type of apex and features suggestive of associated pulmonary hypertension with prominent central vascular markings and peripheral pruning and dilated MPA.
- If such situation occurs there is no benefit of surgical closure of ASD.

Large Pericardial Effusion (Fig. 4)

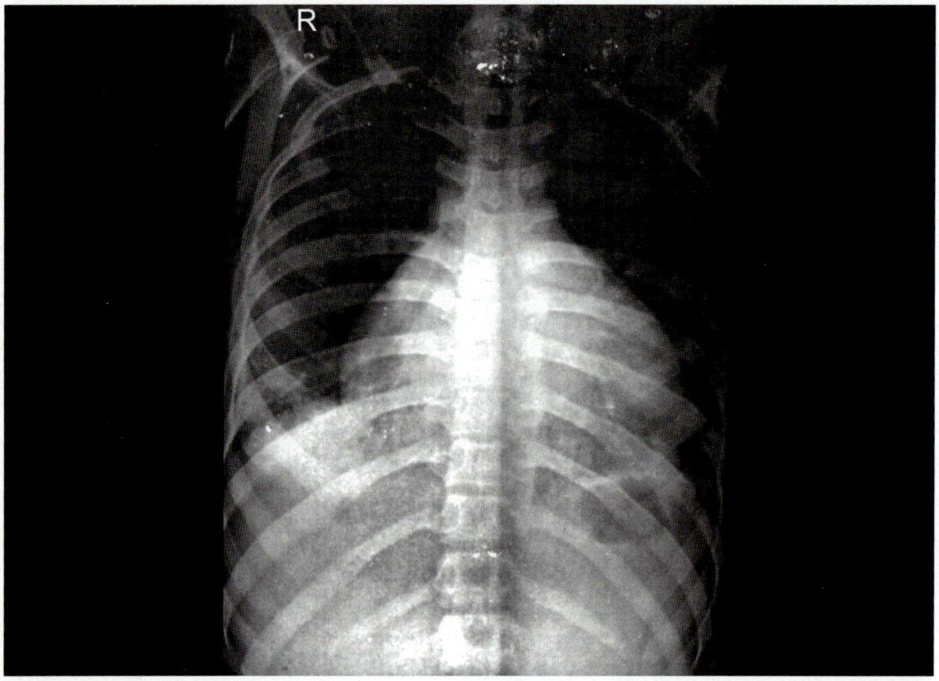

Fig. 4: Chest X-ray showing large pericardial effusion.

- Chest X-ray PA view showing massive cardiomegaly without any specific chamber enlargement, with narrow pedicle and pulmonary oligemia and obscuring hilar prominence.
- This is an acute cardiac emergency which may lead to rapid hemodynamic decompensation.
- Needs urgent pericardiocentesis after echo confirmation.

Chest X-ray of Primary Pulmonary Hypertension (Fig. 5)

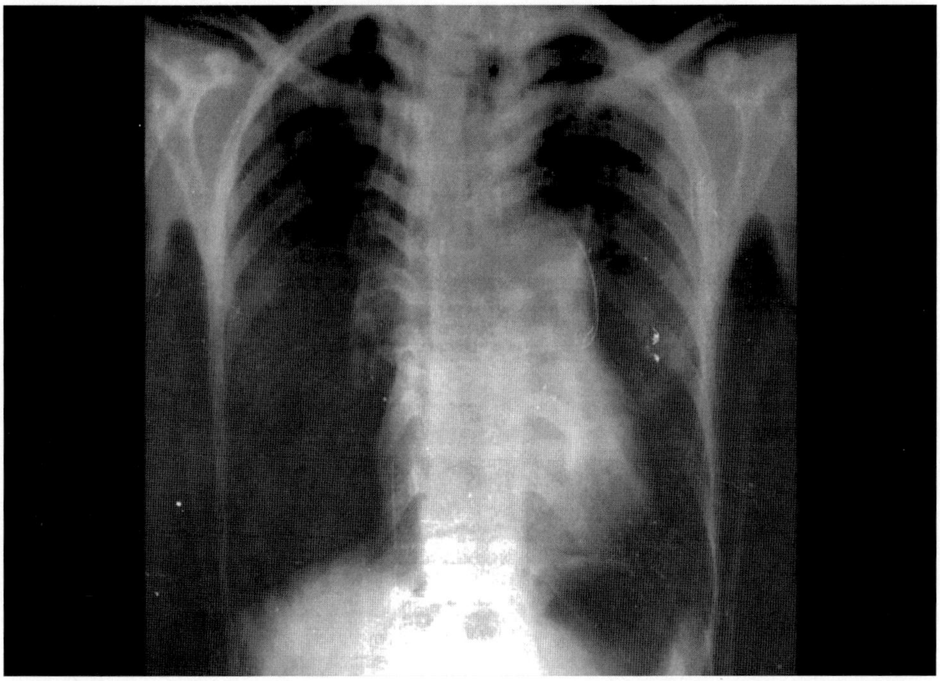

Fig. 5: Chest X-ray in pulmonary hypertension (HTN)—note the dilated pulmonary artery.

- Chest X-ray PA view showing cardiomegaly with RV type apex, dilated main PA and pulmonary oligemia suggestive of severe pulmonary hypertension (HTN).
- It may be of primary or secondary forms.
- Primary pulmonary HTN is of unknown etiology whereas secondary pulmonary HTN is due to lung disease or extrinsic to lung.

Chest X-ray of Severe Mitral Stenosis (Fig. 6)

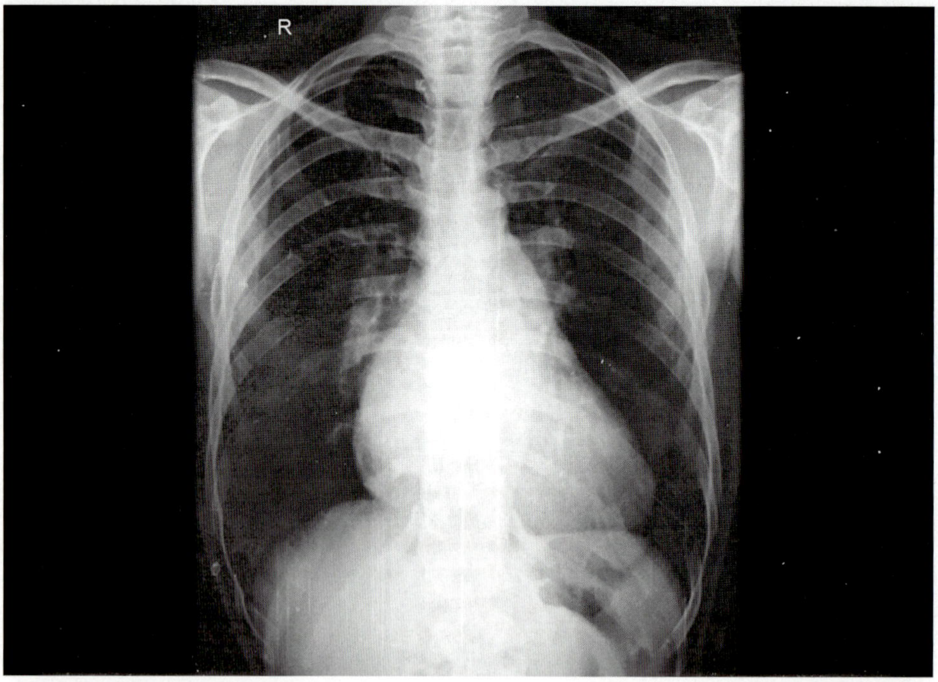

Fig. 6: Chest X-ray of severe mitral stenosis (MS)—note dilated pulmonary artery, straightening of left heart border, and double atrial shadow and right ventricular (RV) type apex.

- Chest X-ray showing cardiomegaly with right ventricular (RV) type of apex dilated, straightening of left heart border because of dilated left atrial (LA) appendage and dilated main pulmonary artery and double atrial shadow.
- Other chest X-ray findings can be associated, i.e. mitral annular calcification and pulmonary edema.
- Rheumatic heart disease (RHD) is the most common etiology in developing nations leading to mitral stenosis.

Chest X-ray TOF (Fig. 7)

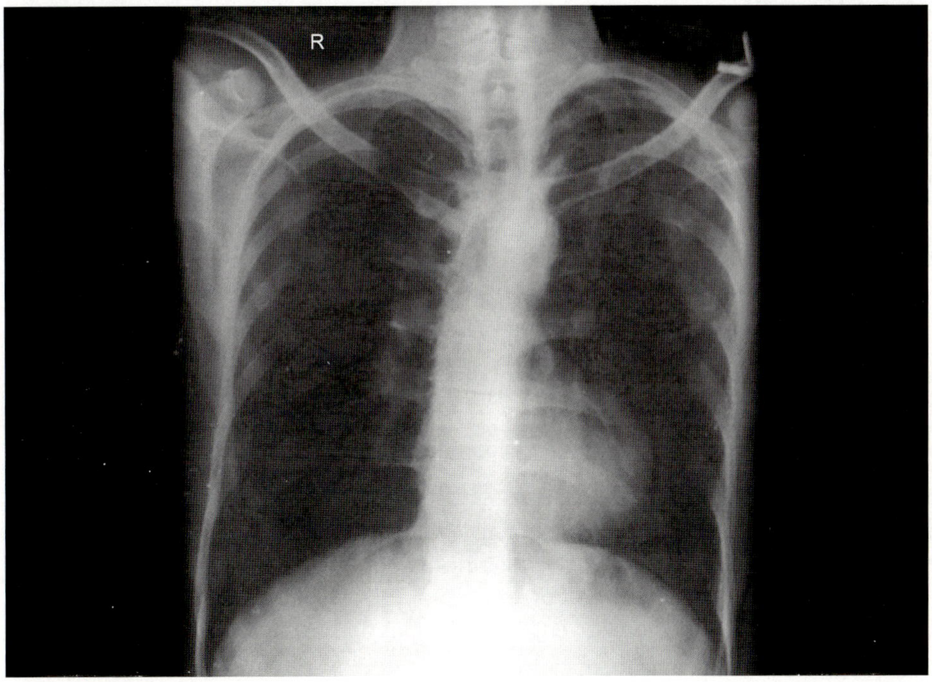

Fig. 7: Chest X-ray tetralogy of Fallot (TOF)—note the pulmonary bay and boot-shaped heart.

- Chest X-ray PA view showing characteristic boot-shaped heart classically known as coeur-en-sabot.
- It may also be seen in tricuspid atresia.
- It is produced due to underfilled LV positioned upon horizontal septum with underlying hypertrophied RV.

ELECTROCARDIOGRAPHY (FIGS. 8 TO 17)

Atrial Fibrillation (Fig. 8)

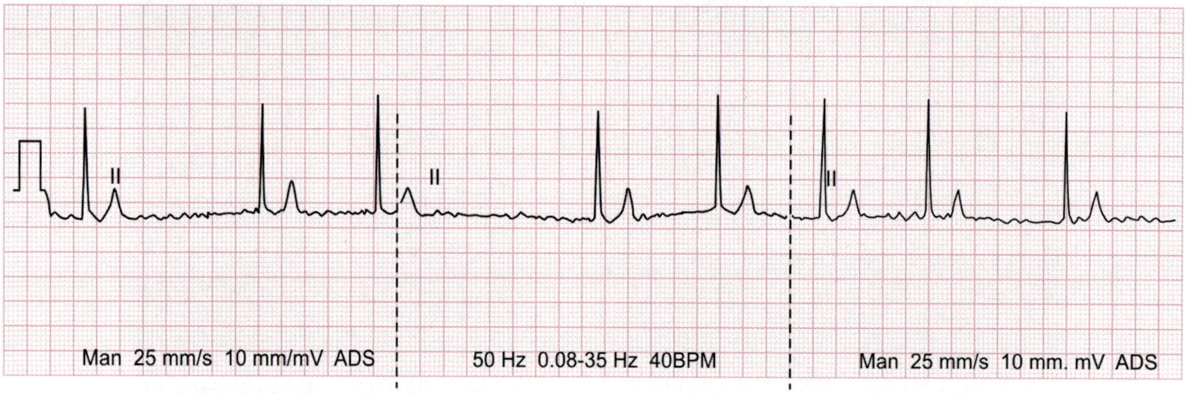

Fig. 8: Atrial fibrillation-irregularly irregular occurring R-waves with loss of definite P-waves.

- Long lead 2 suggestive of irregularly irregular occurring R waves with loss of definite P waves diagnostic of AF.
- It can cause thromboembolic events, i.e. stroke, worsening of heart failure and other complications. Symptoms often include palpitations, dizziness and shortness of breath.
- It has to be managed by controlling the fast ventricular rate and anticoagulation to prevent the thromboembolic complications.

Situs Inversus with Dextrocardia (Fig. 9)

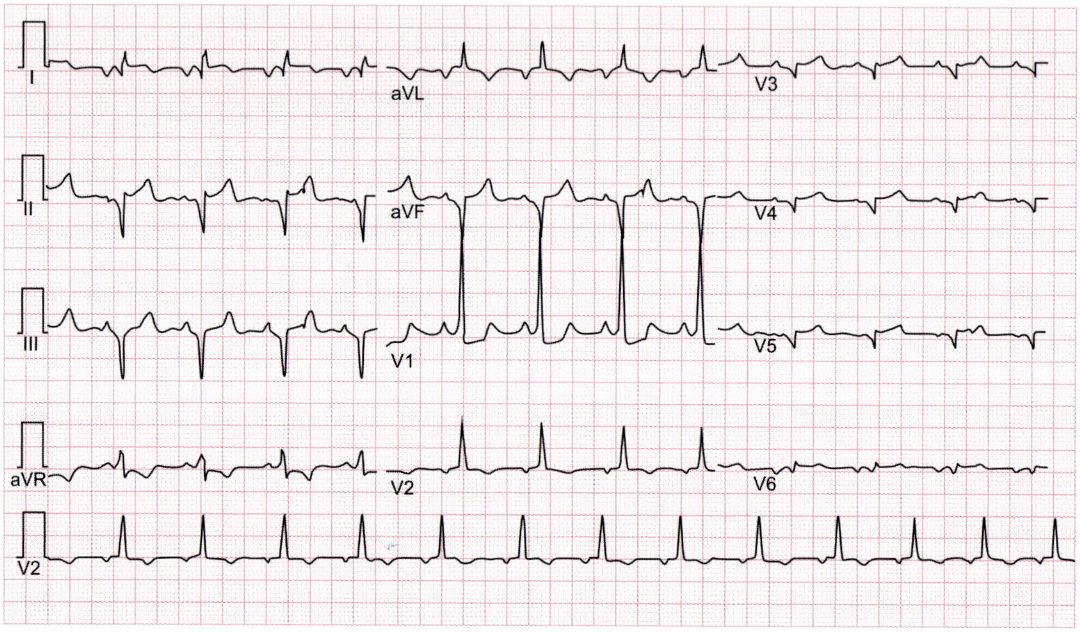

Fig. 9: Situs inversus with dextrocardia—note inverted P waves in leads 1 and augmented vector left (aVL) and upright P waves in augmented vector right (aVR), with opposite progression of R wave in anterior leads.

- 12 lead ECG showing inverted P waves in leads 1 and aVL and upright P waves in aVR, with reverse progression of R wave in anterior leads.
- In this condition heart is in the right side of thorax and visceral organs' position is reversed to their normal anatomical location.
- Incidence of associated congenital heart disease is less as compared to other cardiac malpositions.

ECG of Pulmonary Hypertension (Fig. 10)

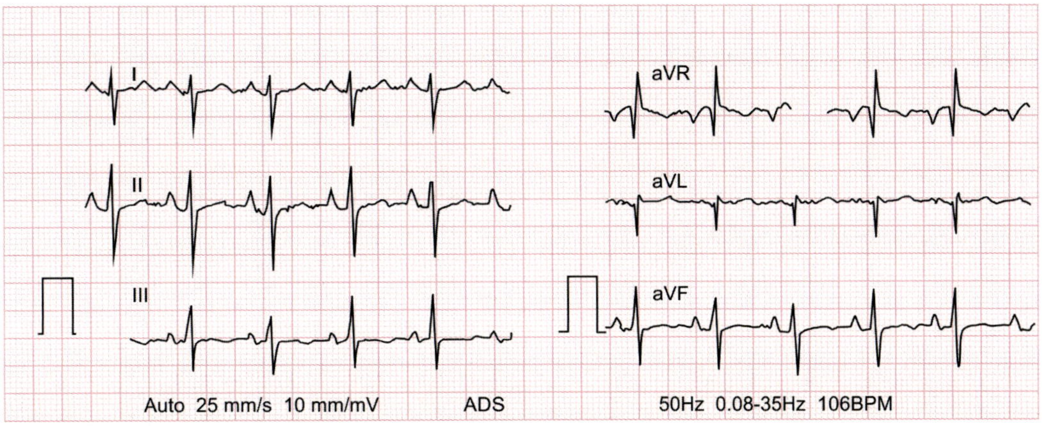

Fig. 10: Electrocardiography in pulmonary hypertension—note right ventricular hypertrophy (R > S in V1) and right axis deviation.

- Electrocardiography (ECG) showing tall P waves with amplitude exceeding 2.5 mV, with extreme right axis deviation (RAD) and R>S in V1.
- Right bundle branch block (RBBB) may also be seen in pulmonary hypertension (HTN). Higher the pulmonary artery pressure, more sensitive is the ECG.
- Chest X-ray is inferior to ECG in detecting pulmonary HTN.

Ventricular Premature Complexes (Fig. 11)

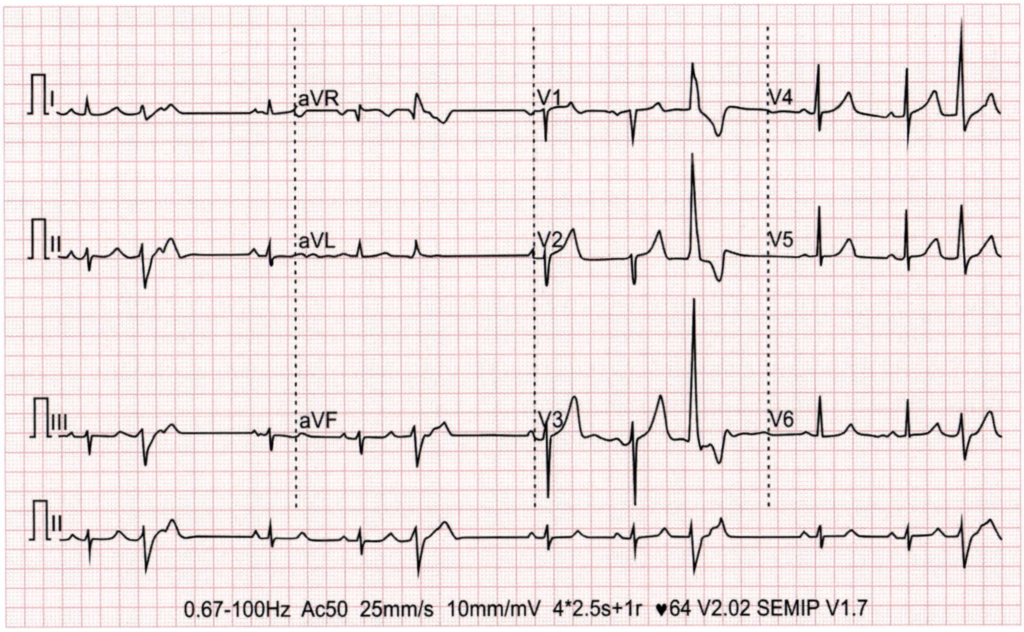

Fig. 11: Ventricular premature complexes.

- 12 lead ECG showing right bundle branch block (RBBB) morphology with superior axis ventricular premature complexes (VPCs), likely of LV exit.
- These are extra beats that originates from ventricles and may cause disruption of regular heart rhythm causing symptoms of fluttering or skipped beat in chest, it may be of left bundle branch block (LBBB) or RBBB morphology depending on the origin and associated with compensatory pause, mostly are benign but may lead to malignant arrhythmia like VT, VF.

Electrocardiography of Tetralogy of Fallot (Fig. 12)

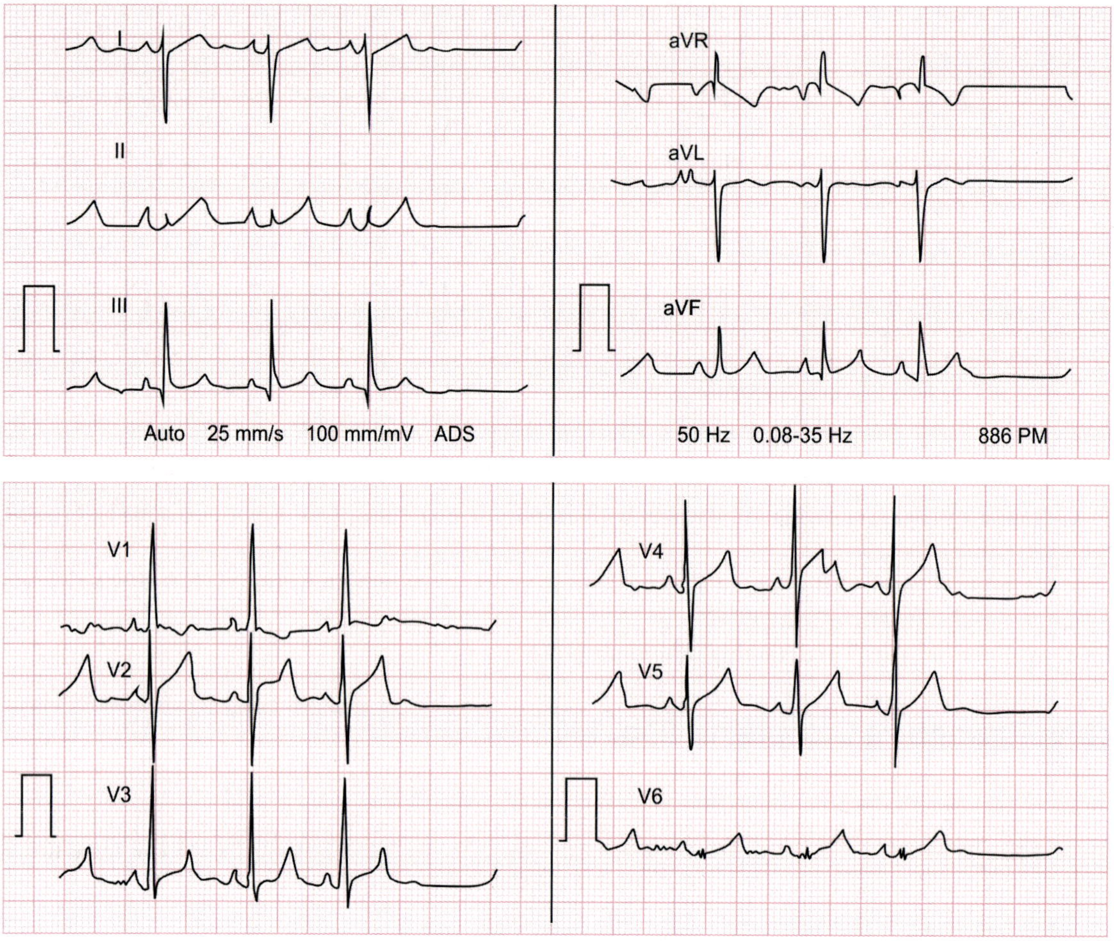

Fig. 12: Electrocardiography (ECG) in tetralogy of Fallot (TOF)—right axis deviation and right ventricular hypertrophy.

- ECG suggestive of RAD, with RVH and sudden transition of R wave in V2, with clockwise loop.
- It is the most common cyanotic heart disease characterised by large ventricular septal defect (VSD), with aortic override and RVH and right ventricular outflow tract (RVOT) obstruction most commonly infundibular.
- Definitive management is complete intracardiac repair.

Evolving Anterior Wall Motion Index (Fig. 13)

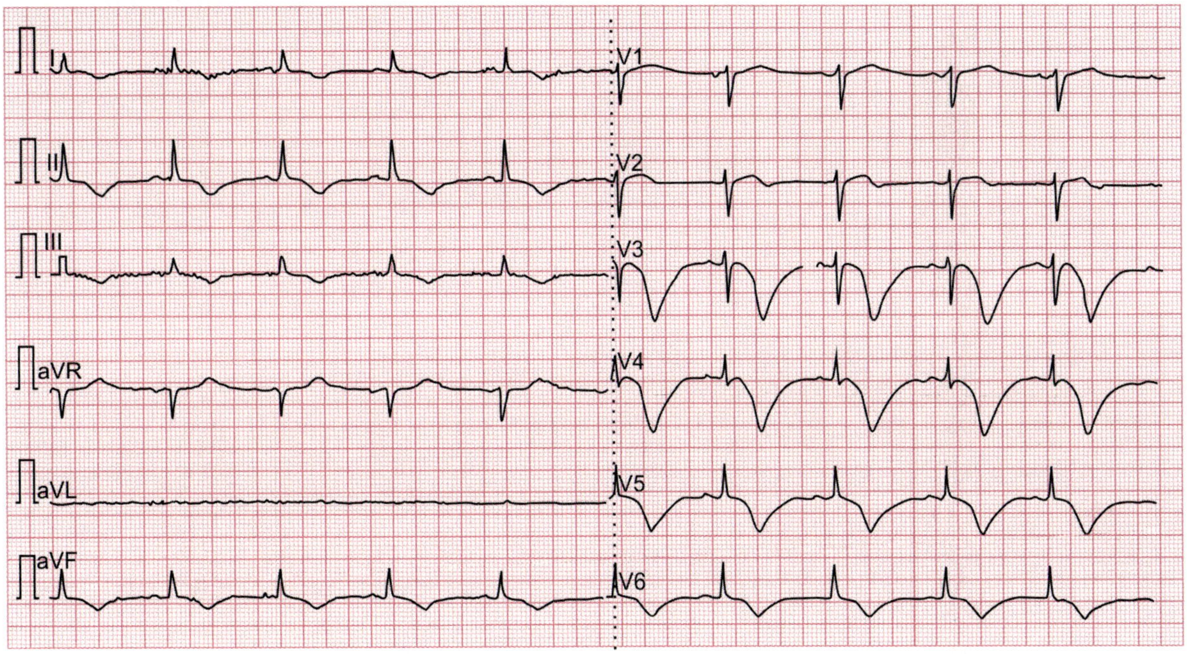

Fig. 13: Anterior wall motion index (AWMI).

- ECG showing deeply symmetrical T wave inversion in precordial leads with associated convex upwards ST elevation in V2 to V6 suggestive of acute anterior wall motion index (AWMI).
- Treatment consist of urgent reperfusion therapy in the form of thrombolysis or percutaneous coronary intervention (PCI).

Complete Heart Block (Fig. 14)

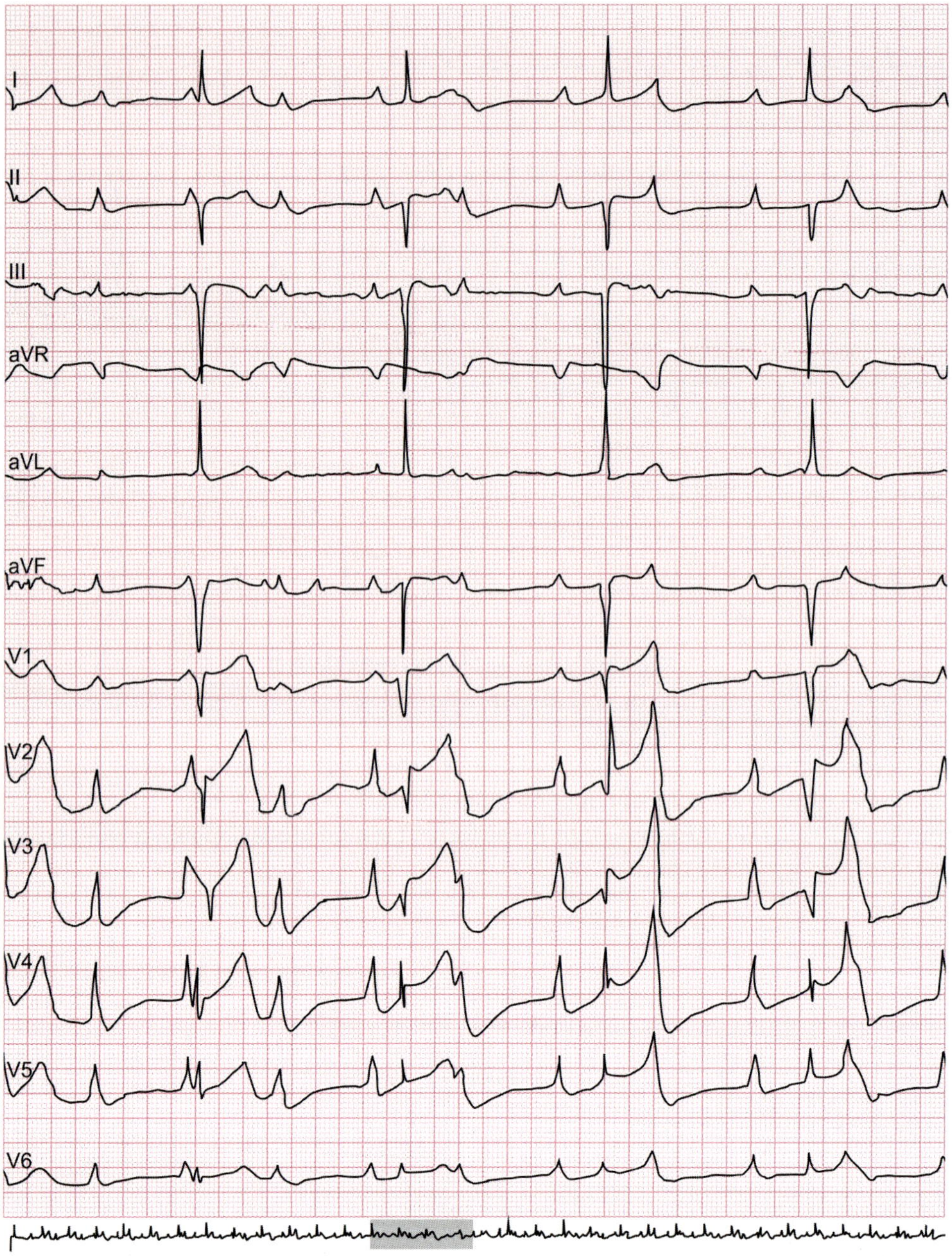

Fig. 14: Complete heart block (CHB)—complete dissociation between P and QRS complexes.

- ECG complete dissociation between P and QRS complexes.
- Features suggestive of complete heart block (CHB) are fixed P-P interval, fixed R-R interval and no relation between P and QRS complexes and ventricular rate is usually half of atrial rate.
- It may be of varied etiologies like congenital, ischemic heart disease, degenerative conduction system defect or infectious.

  Treatment is pacemaker implantation where no reversible cause is found.

Atrial Fibrillation (Fig. 15)

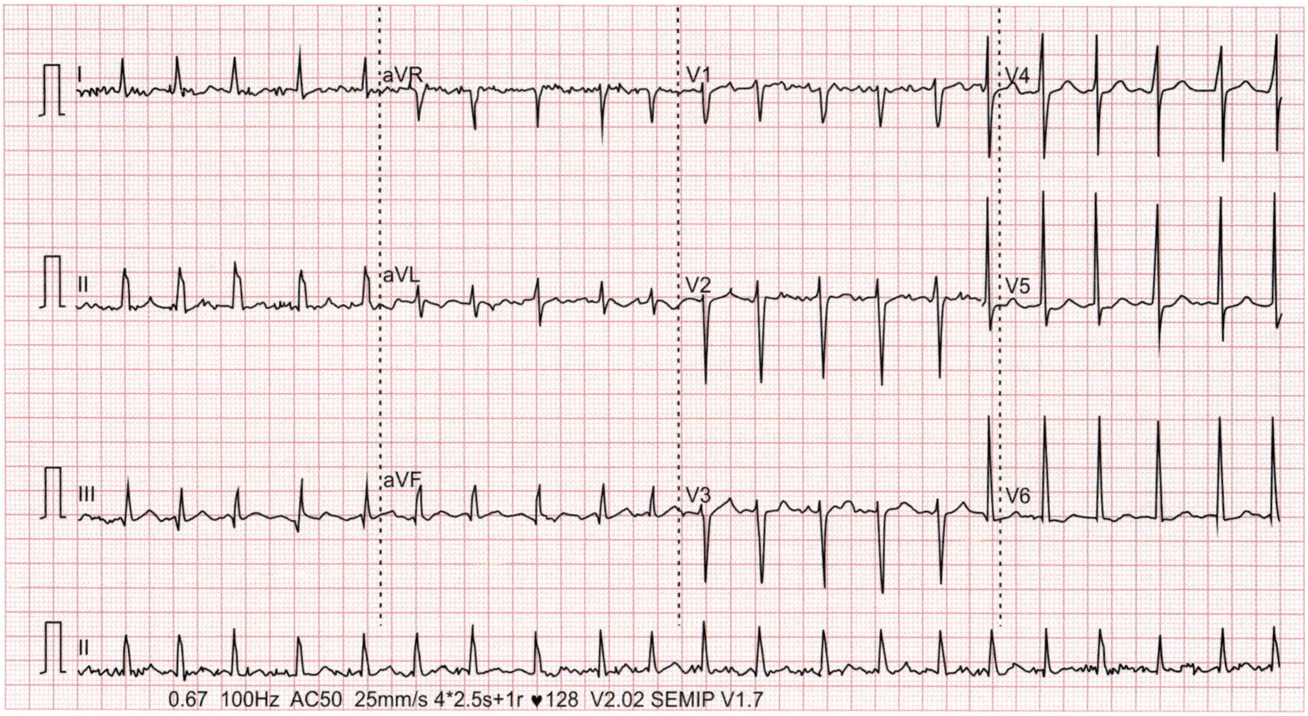

Fig. 15: Atrial fibrillation (AF) with fast ventricular response (FVR).

Low Voltage Complexes in ECG (Fig. 16)

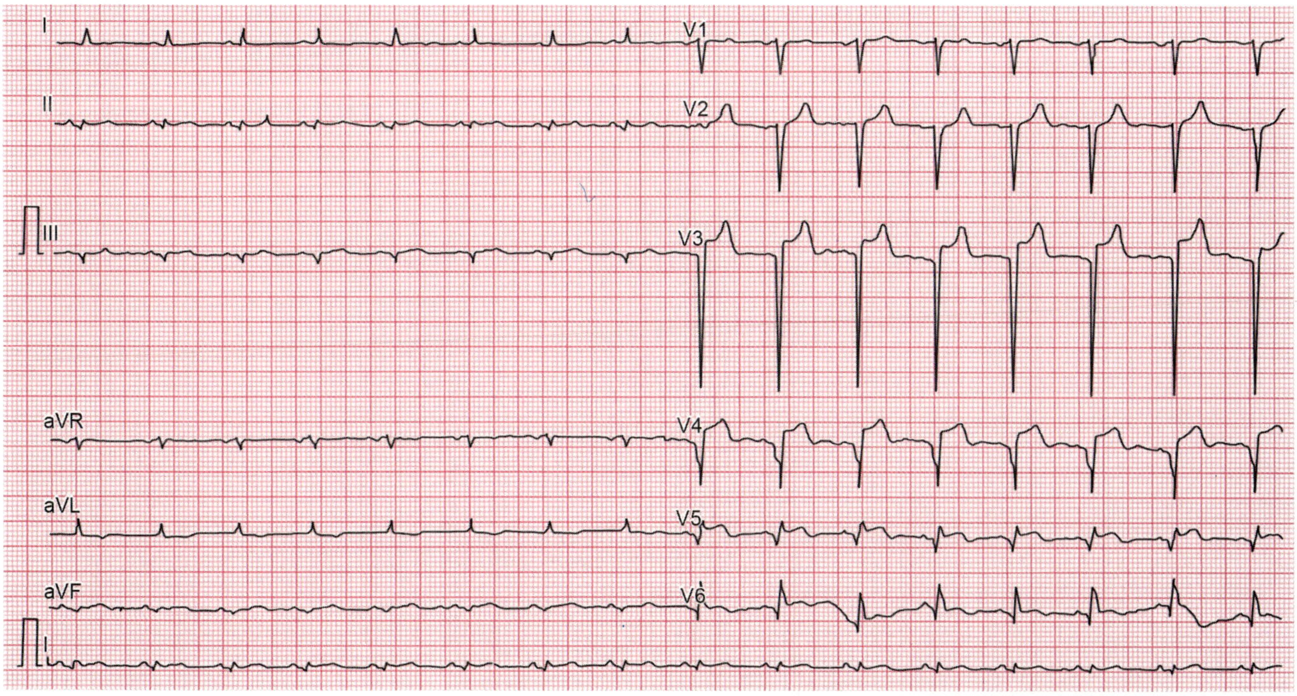

Fig. 16: ST-elevation V3 to V6 with Q waves in V3 to V6 and inferior leads; low voltage complexes in limb leads.

Electrocardiography (ECG) of Ventricular Paced (Fig. 17)

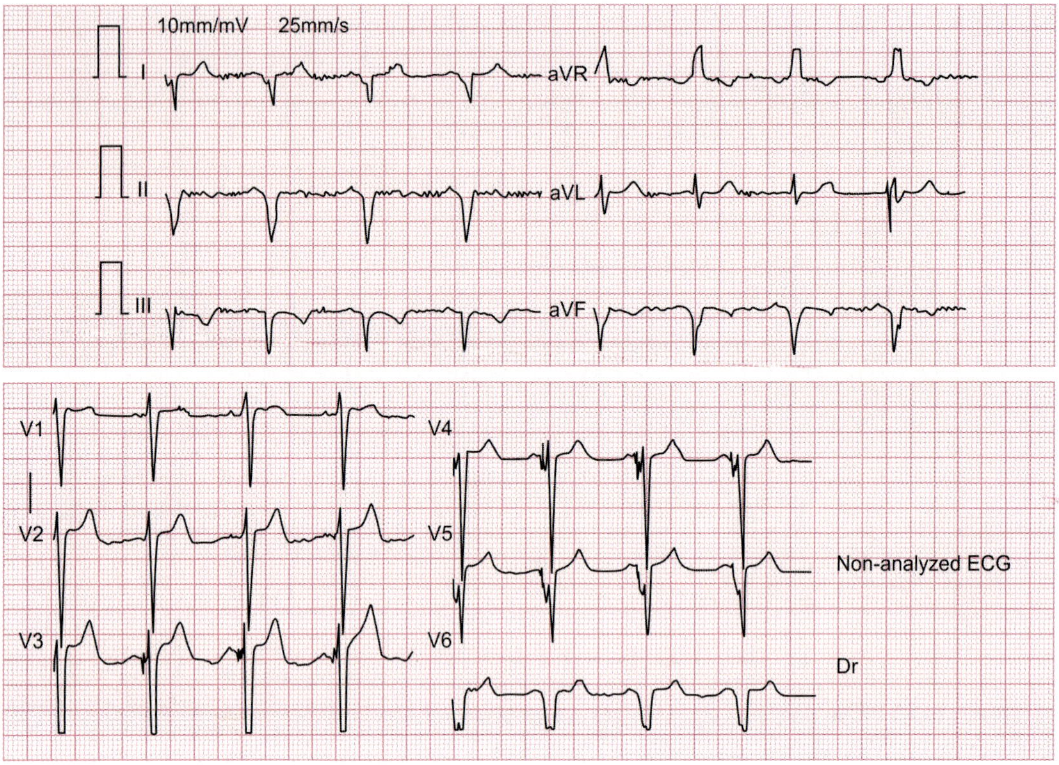

Fig. 17: Sinus P wave followed by paced QRS complex; ventricular paced, atrial sensed rhythm, maintaining AV synchrony.

ECHOCARDIOGRAPHY (FIGS. 18 TO 37)

Ostium Secundum ASD (Fig. 18)

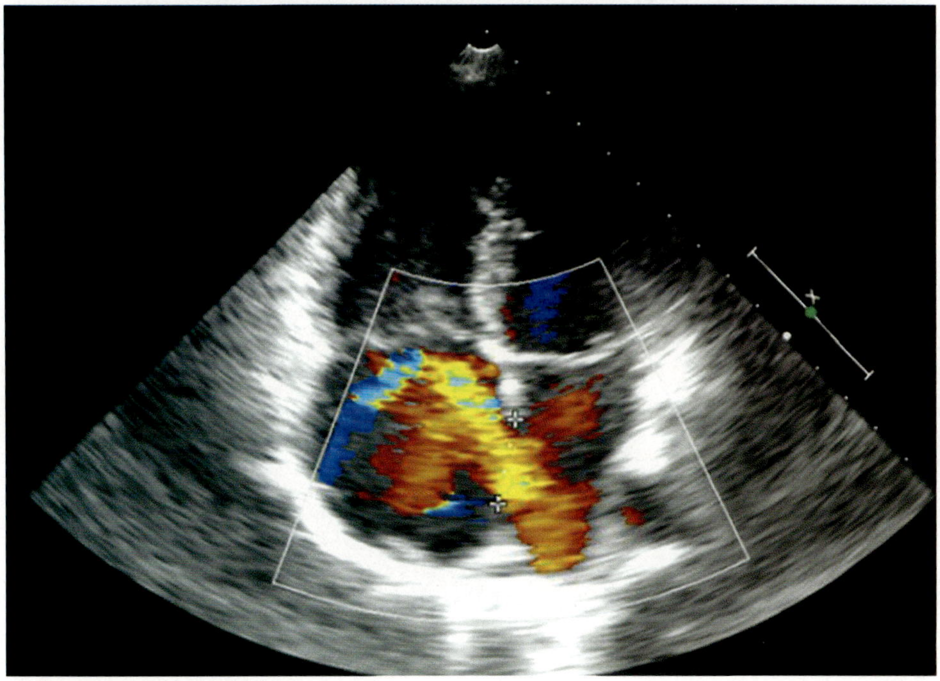

Fig. 18: Ostium secundum ASD—apical four-chamber view on transthoracic echocardiography (TTE) showing gap in interatrial septum (IAS) with red flows indicating L-to-R shunt.

- Apical four-chamber view showing gap in interatrial septum (IAS) with red flows indicating L to R shunt.
- Among all types of ASD, OS-ASD is most commonly encountered. 3–8 mm of ASD closes spontaneously in 80% cases, and size more than 8 mm rarely closes spontaneously.
- Such type of ASD can be easily closed through percutaneous device closure in most cases.

Contrast Echo in ASD (Fig. 19)

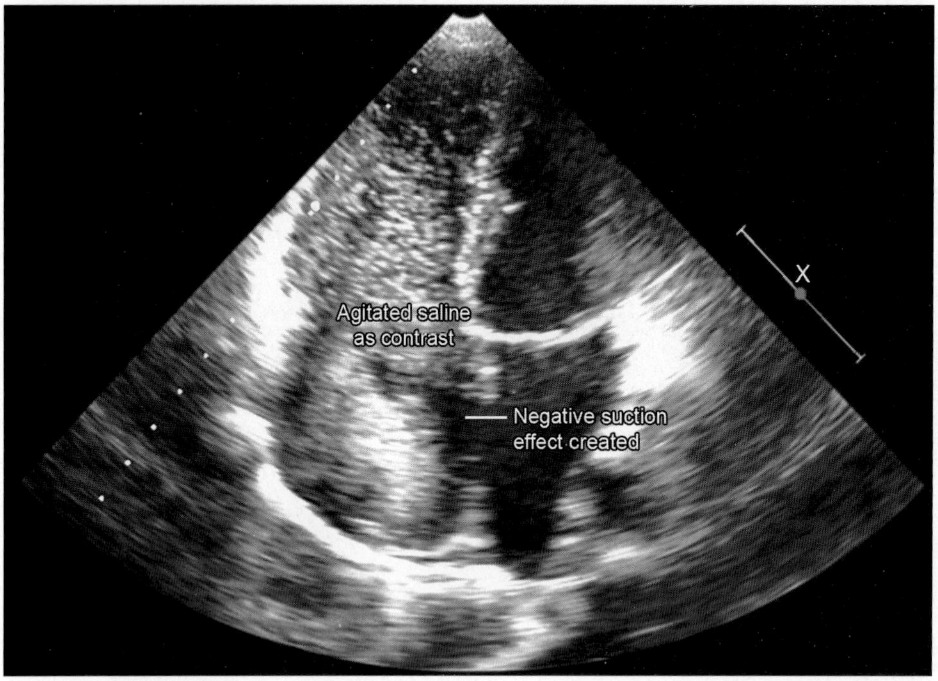

Fig. 19: Contrast echo in ASD.

- Four-chamber view of 2 D echo showing defect in IAS. No flow was seen across the defect.
- In such cases bubble contrast echocardiography is very helpful in delineating the defect and as shown negative bubble contrast is seen due to the L-R flow across the IAS defect.
- Further confirmation can be done through TEE.

Left Ventricular Clot (Fig. 20)

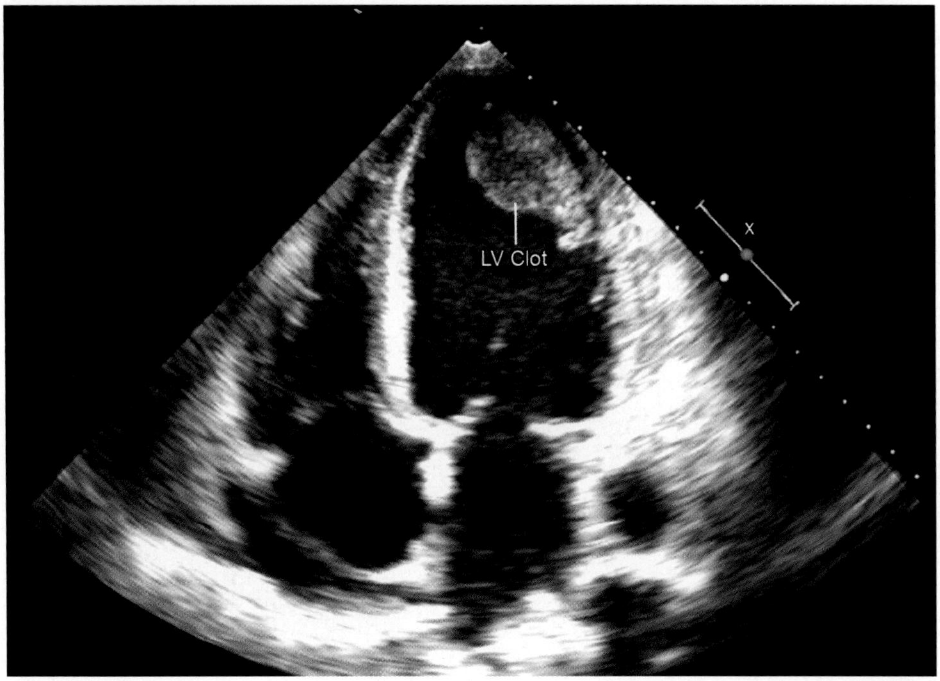

Fig. 20: Left ventricular (LV) clot—apical four-chamber view on TTE showing globular LV with clot attached to LV apex.

- Apical four-chamber view showing globular echogenic shadow, attached to the LV apex suggestive of clot in LV.
- It is frequently associated with underlying motion abnormality of LV.
- It may embolise to various organ system most commonly to central nervous system (CNS) leading to stroke.
- Management includes anticoagulation therapy and associated treatment of ischemic heart disease (IHD).

Infective Endocarditis (Fig. 21)

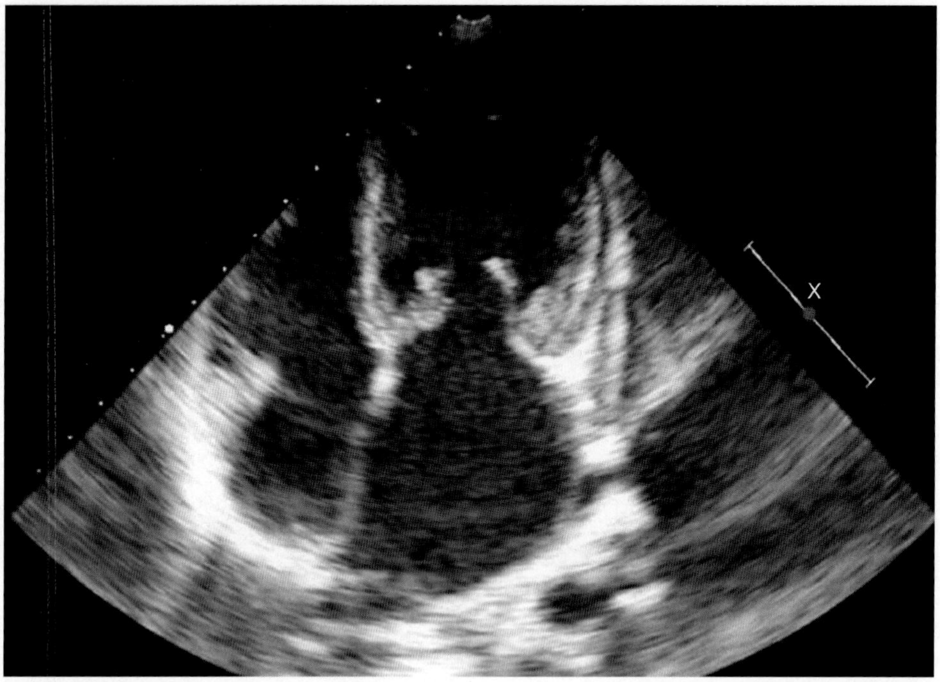

Fig. 21: Infective endocarditis—apical four-chamber view on TTE showing thickened mitral valve.

- Apical four-chamber view in diastole showing opened mitral valve leaflet with an echogenic shadow attached to undersurface of both the leaflets of mitral valve suggestive of vegetation.
- It may produce symptoms like fever, heart failure and may lead to embolic manifestations.
- Management consist of immediate blood culture and prolonged antibiotic therapy as per guidelines and the organism isolated.

Mitral Regurgitation (Fig. 22)

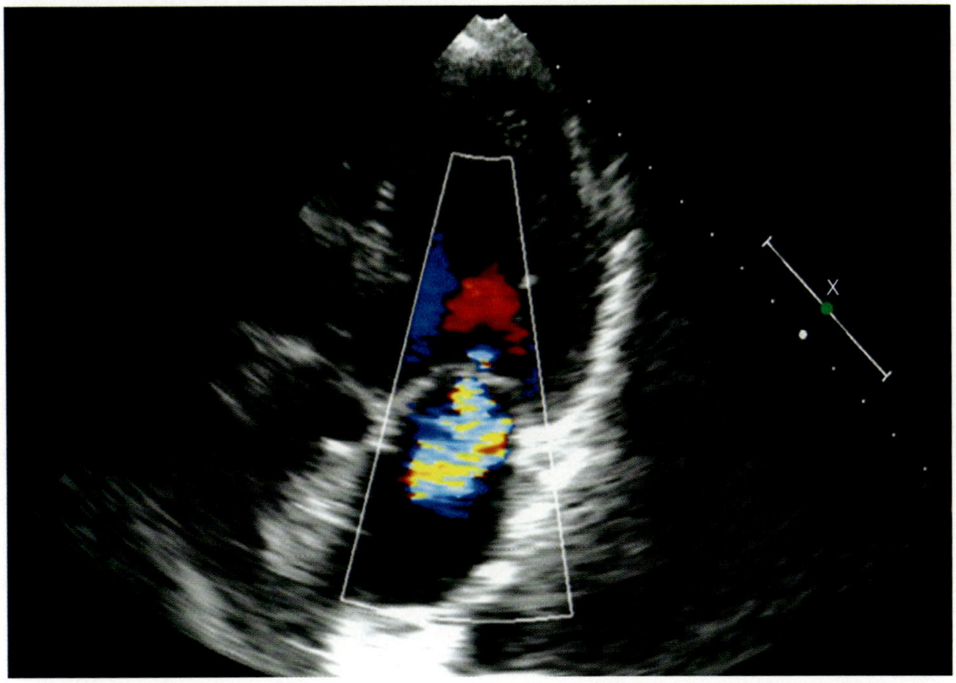

Fig. 22: Mitral regurgitation (MR)—apical four-chamber view on TTE showing MR.

- Apical four-chamber view showing regurgitation of mitral valve can also be seen in parasternal long-axis view.
- It may be of varied etiologies like rheumatic heart disease (RHD), mitral valve prolapse (MVP) or in ischemic and degenerative conditions.
- It can be chronic or acute in presentation acute MR is a cardiological emergency as it may lead to fulminant pulmonary edema.

Stuck Mitral Valve (Fig. 23)

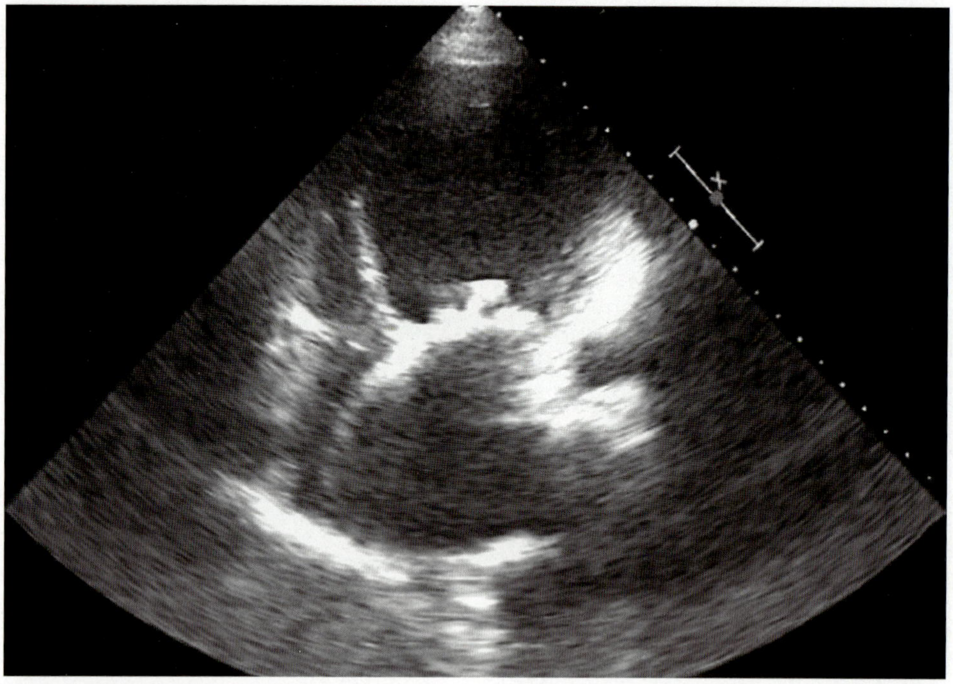

Fig. 23: Stuck mitral valve (MV)—apical four-chamber view on TTE showing dilated left atrium (LA) and stuck MV.

- Apical four-chamber view showing dilated LA and stuck MV.
- It is a dreaded complication following implantation of mechanical prosthetic valve due to thrombus formation in prosthesis leading to mitral inflow obstruction.
- Most commonly due to subtherapeutic anticoagulation.
- Management needs thrombolytic therapy or resurgery.

Pericardial Effusion (Fig. 24)

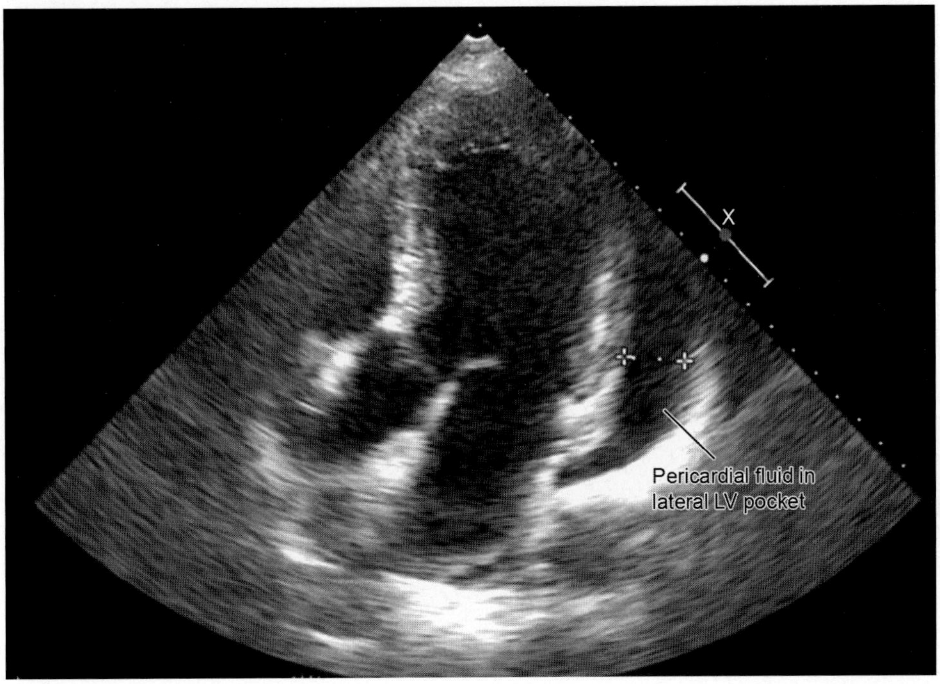

Fig. 24: Pericardial effusion on TTE.

- Apical four-chamber view showing localized pericardial effusion along the lateral wall of LV.
- Most effusions are asymptomatic but sometimes rapidly collecting effusions may lead to tamponade, commonly seen in postcardiac surgery patients.

SAM in HOCM (Fig. 25)

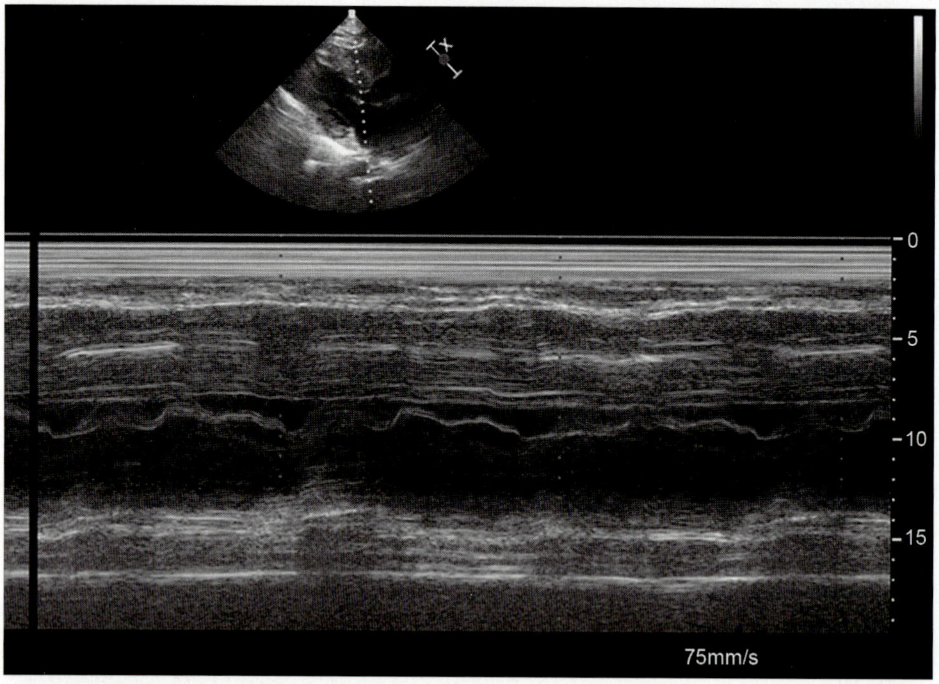

Fig. 25: Systolic anterior motion (SAM) in hypertrophic obstructive cardiomyopathy (HOCM). Upper image TTE, lower image 'M' mode ECHO.

- It is systolic anterior motion of anterior mitral leaflet (AML) leading to LV outflow obstruction during LV systole.
- It can be graded as follows:
  - Grade 1—AML buckling towards LVOT 10 mm away from septum.
  - Grade 2—AML buckling towards LVOT within 10 mm from septum.
  - Grade 3—AML buckling and touching septum but less than 30% of systole.
  - Grade 4—AML buckling and touching septum but more than 30% of systole.

Asymmetric Septal Hypertrophy in HOCM (Fig. 26)

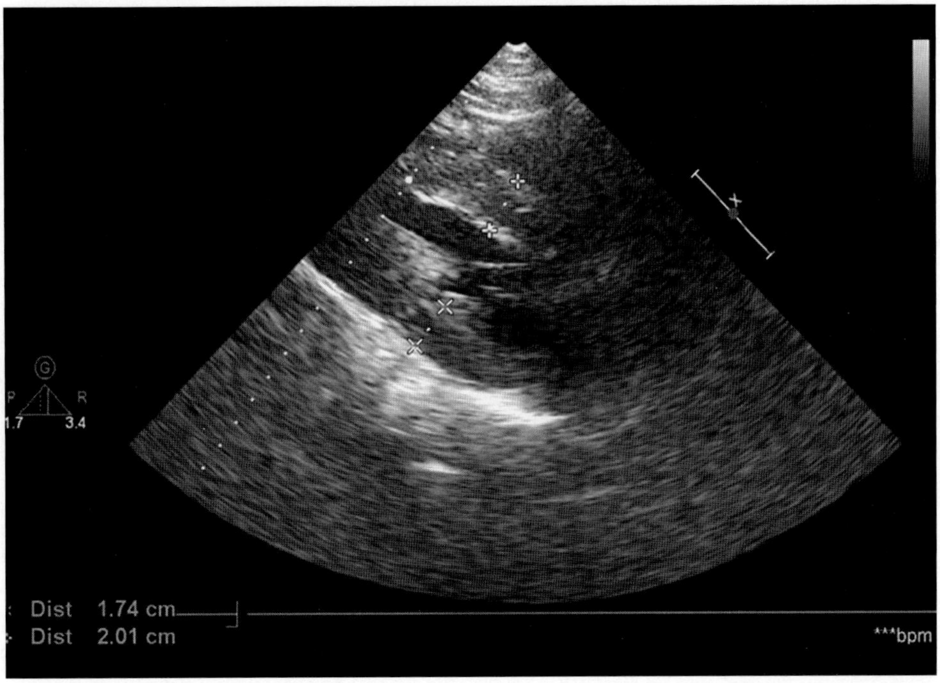

Fig. 26: On TTE asymmetric septal hypertrophy in hypertrophic obstructive cardiomyopathy (HOCM).

- Parasternal long-axis view showing interventricular septal (IVS) hypertrophy.
- It is most commonly seen in hypertrophic cardiomyopathy (HCM) but may be seen in other conditions like hypertensive heart disease.
- It may be of various types like involvement of substantial portions of both the ventricular septum and anterolateral left ventricular free wall, hypertrophy confined to the anterior portion of the ventricular septum, involving the entire ventricular septum but not the left ventricular free wall or in regions of the left ventricle other than the basal anterior ventricular septum.

LVOT Gradient in HOCM (Fig. 27)

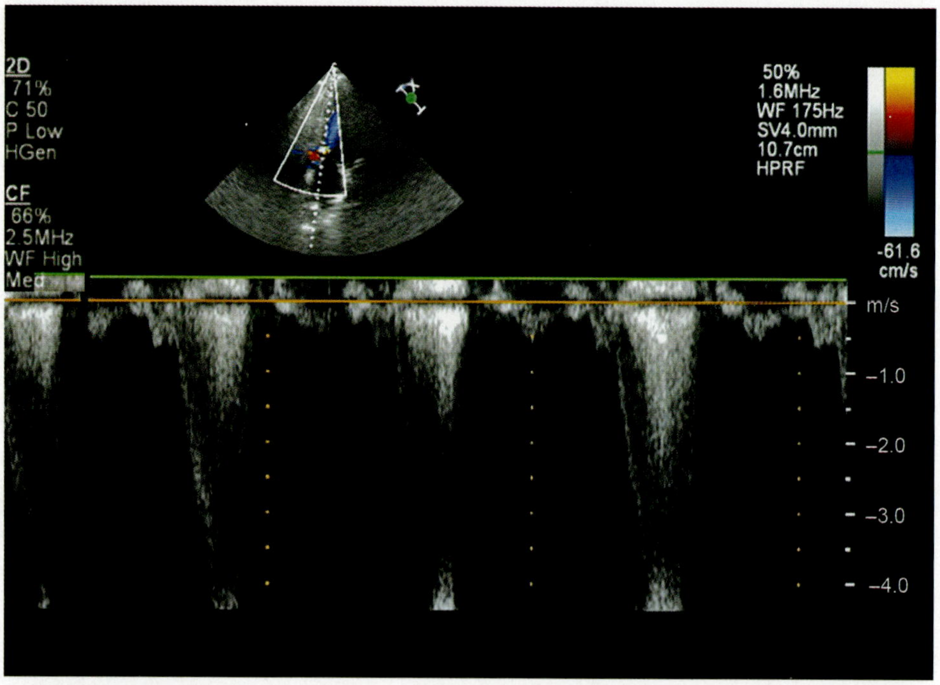

Fig. 27: Left ventricular outflow tract (LVOT) gradient in HOCM—note its typical dagger-shaped appearance.

- Note its typical dagger-shaped appearance.
- The gradient varies with dynamic maneuvers and it has to be differentiated from gradients of fixed LV outflow obstruction and mitral regurgitation.

Transmitral Variation in CCP (Fig. 28A)

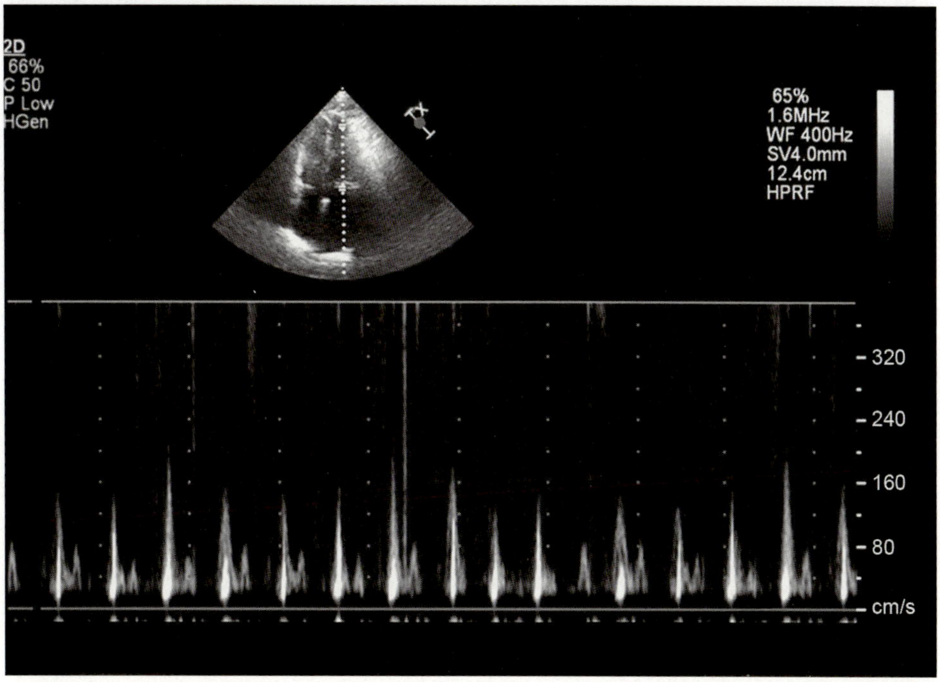

Fig. 28A: Transmitral variation in chronic constrictive pericarditis (CCP). Upper image 'TTE', lower image 'M' mode echo.

Noncollapsing Dilated IVC in CCP (Fig. 28B)

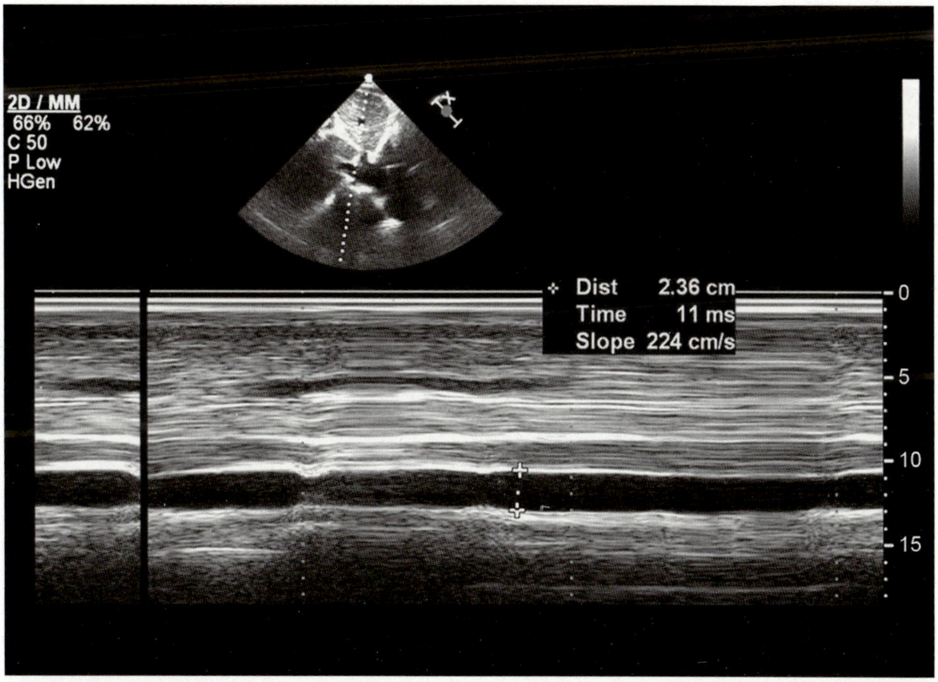

Fig. 28B: Noncollapsing dilated inferior vena cava (IVC) in chronic constrictive pericarditis (CCP). Upper image 'TTE', lower image 'M' mode echo.

Subaortic Membrane (Fig. 29)

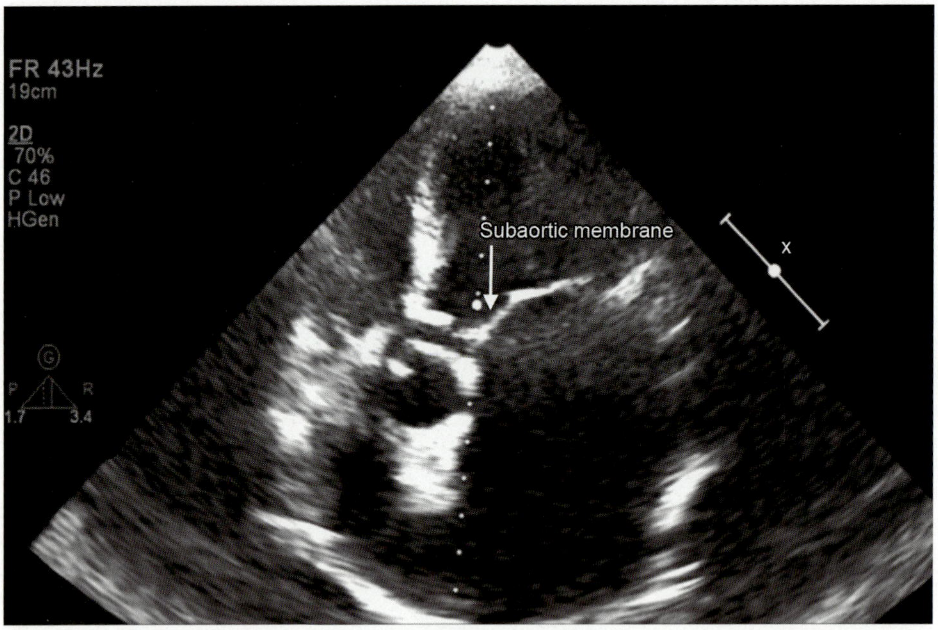

Fig. 29: Subaortic membrane.

- Apical four-chamber view showing membrane below aortic valve.
- It is a shelf like membrane that forms under the aortic valve leading to obstruction of blood flow into aorta.
- It can occur alone or associated with other congenital anomalies like Shone's complex or septal defect and may also be associated with regurgitation of aortic valve.

More Images of Echocardiography (Figs. 30 to 39)

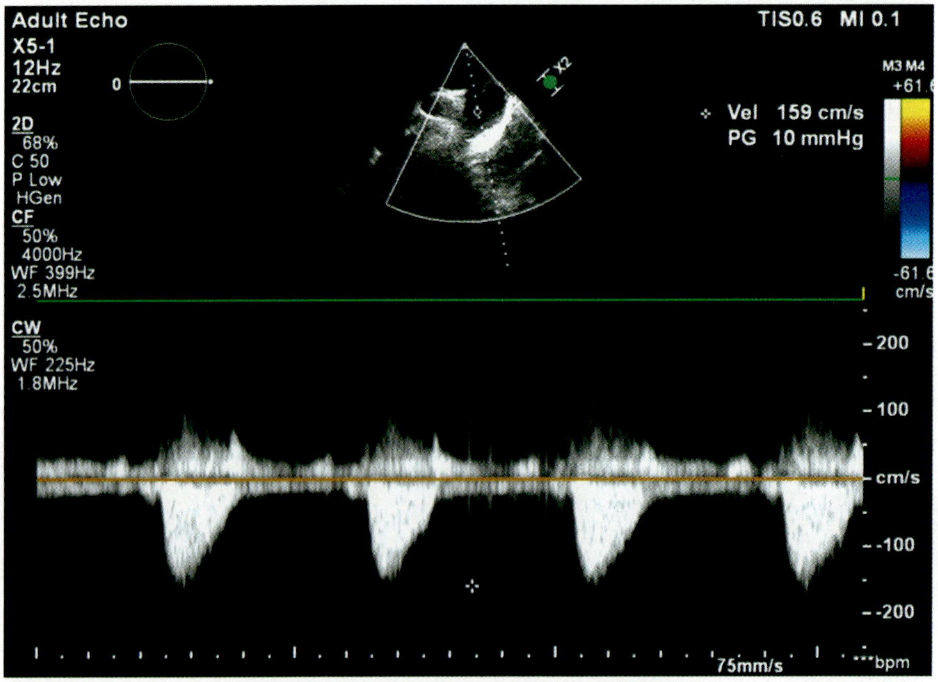

Fig. 30: Dilated main pulmonary artery (MPA).

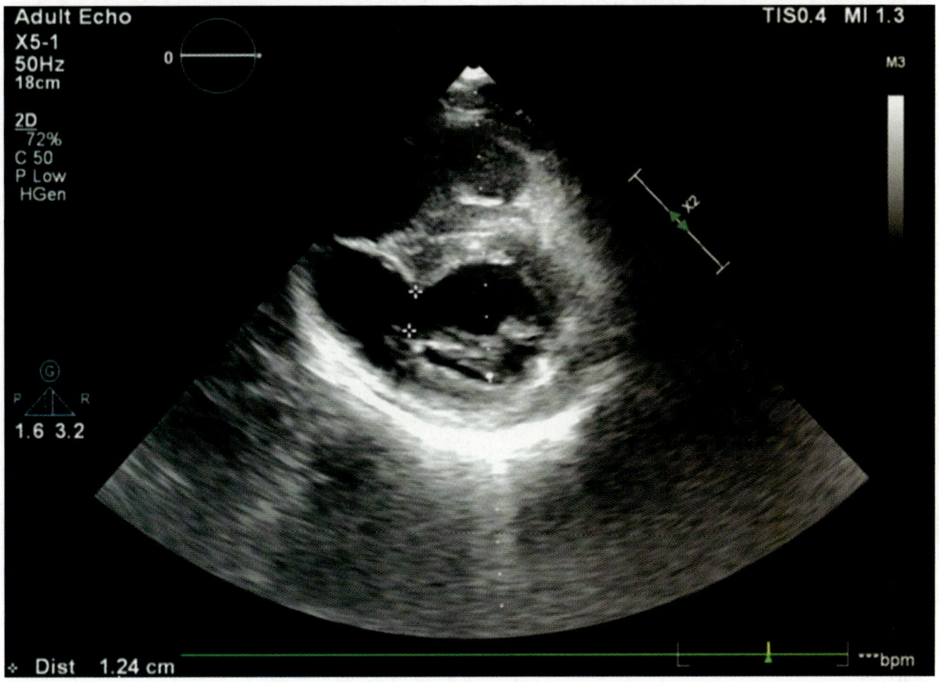

Fig. 31: Muscular VSD with inlet extension.

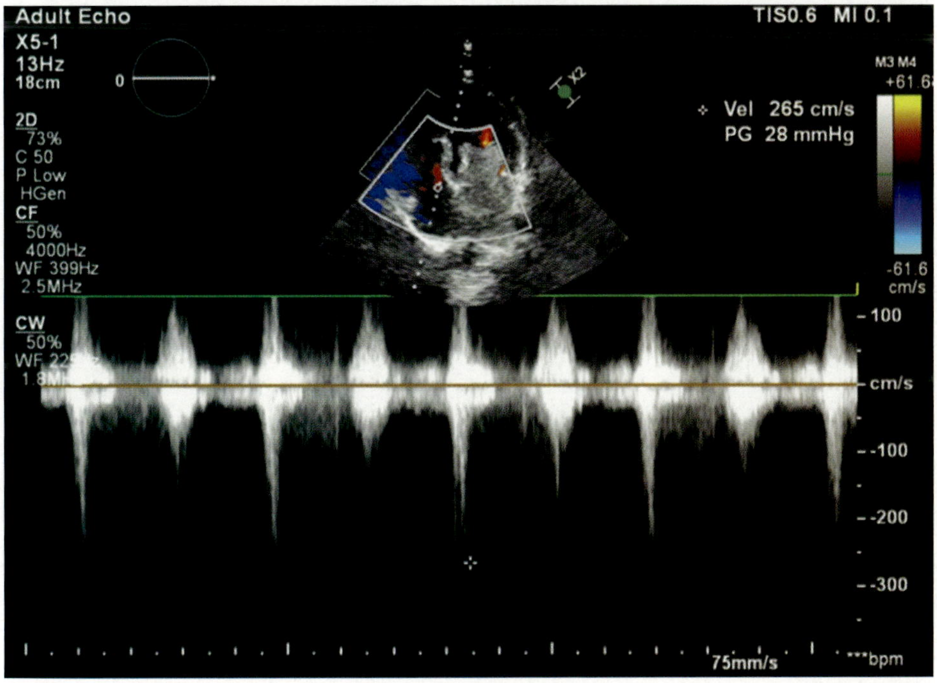

Fig. 32: Large LA clot.

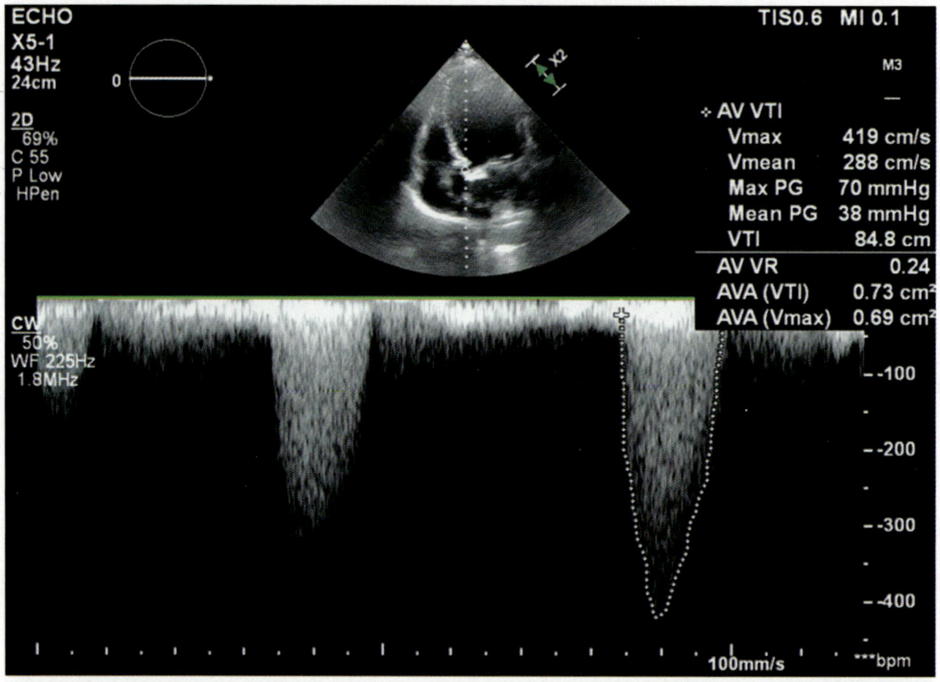

Fig. 33: Apical five-chamber view: Severe AS, CW tracing showing Vmax of 4.2 m/s.

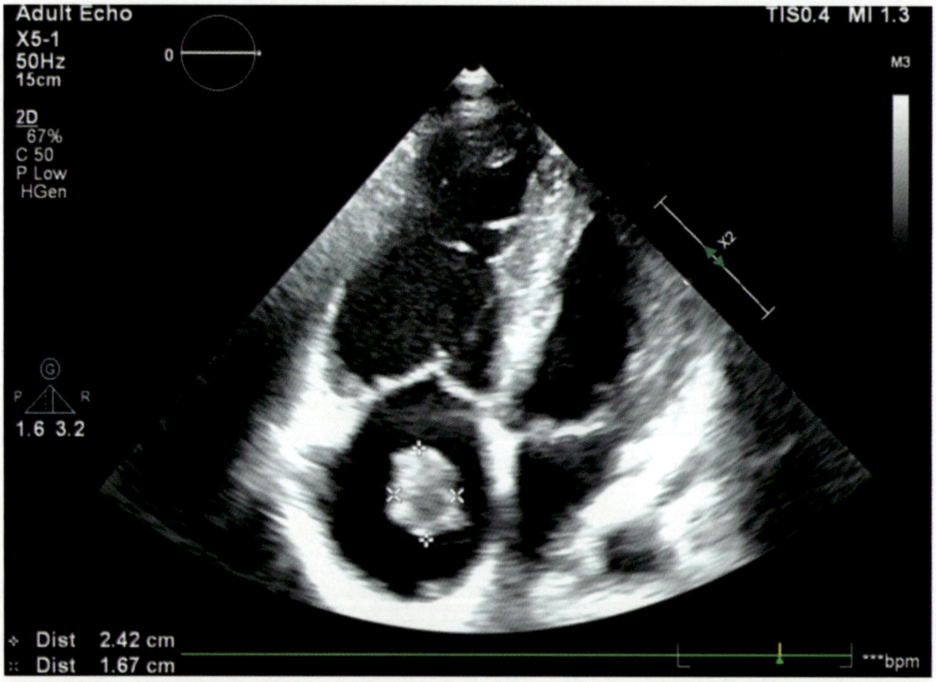

Fig. 34: Apical four-chamber view showing enlarged RA/RV with RA clot and spontaneous echo contrast in RV.

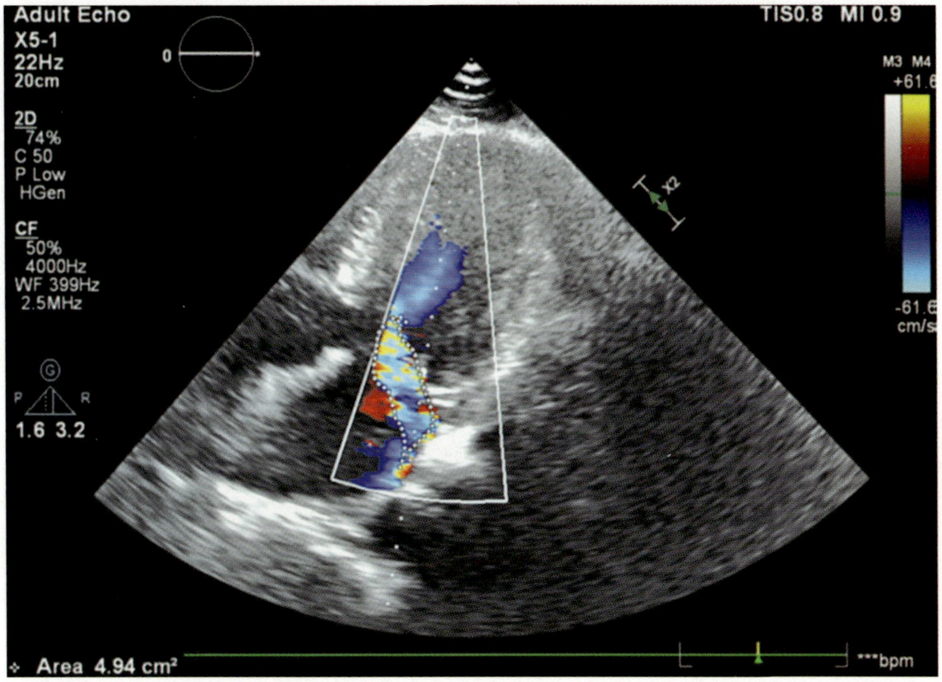

Fig. 35: Apical five-chamber view showing eccentric MR jet in LA.

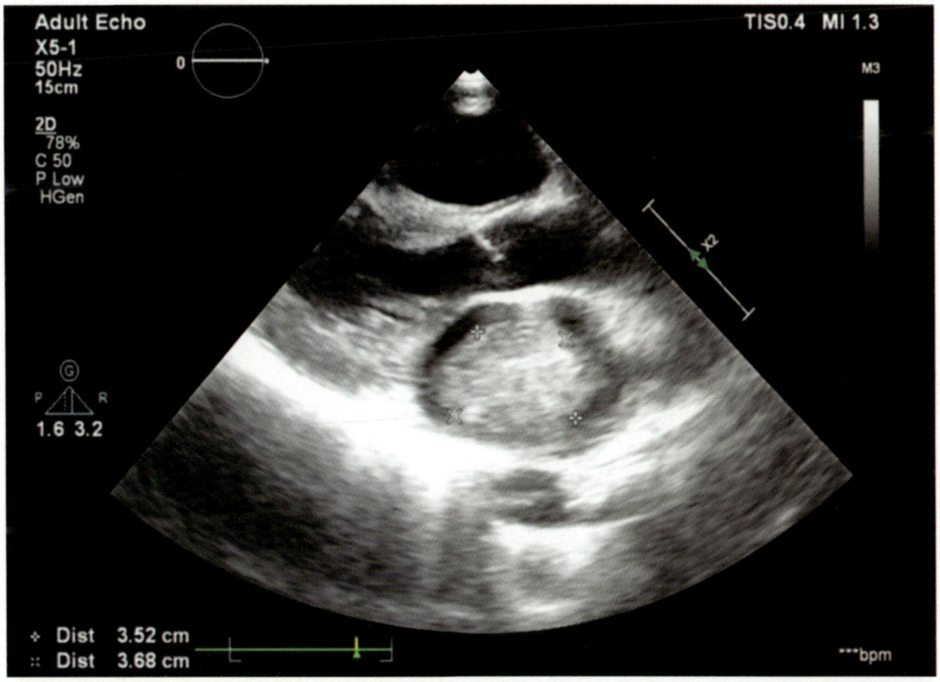

Fig. 36: Large LA clot.

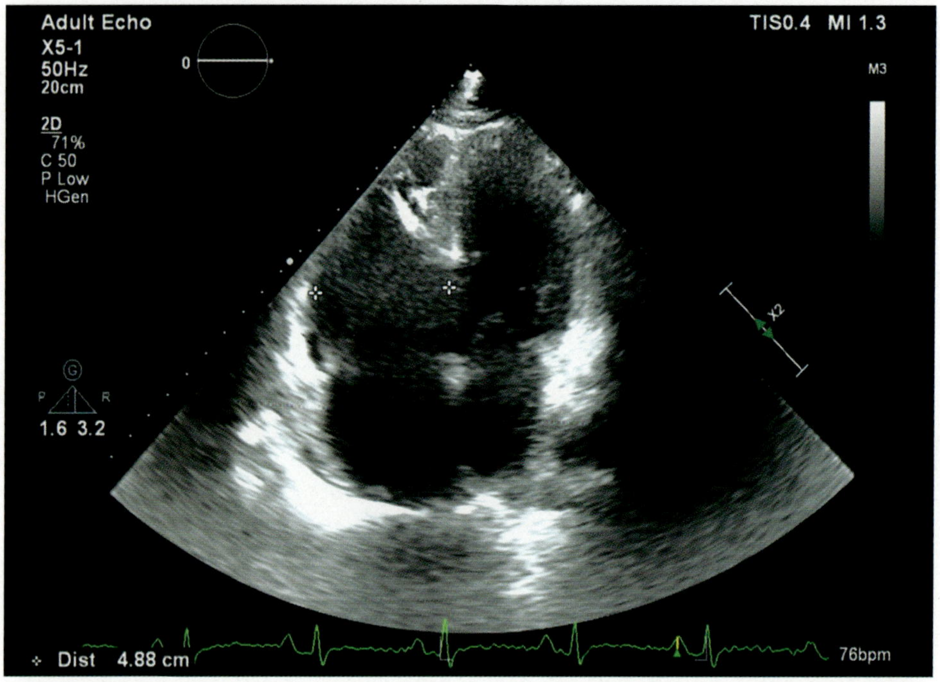

Fig. 37: Ebstein's anomaly; note the displaced septal leaflet of TV as compared to mitral valve.

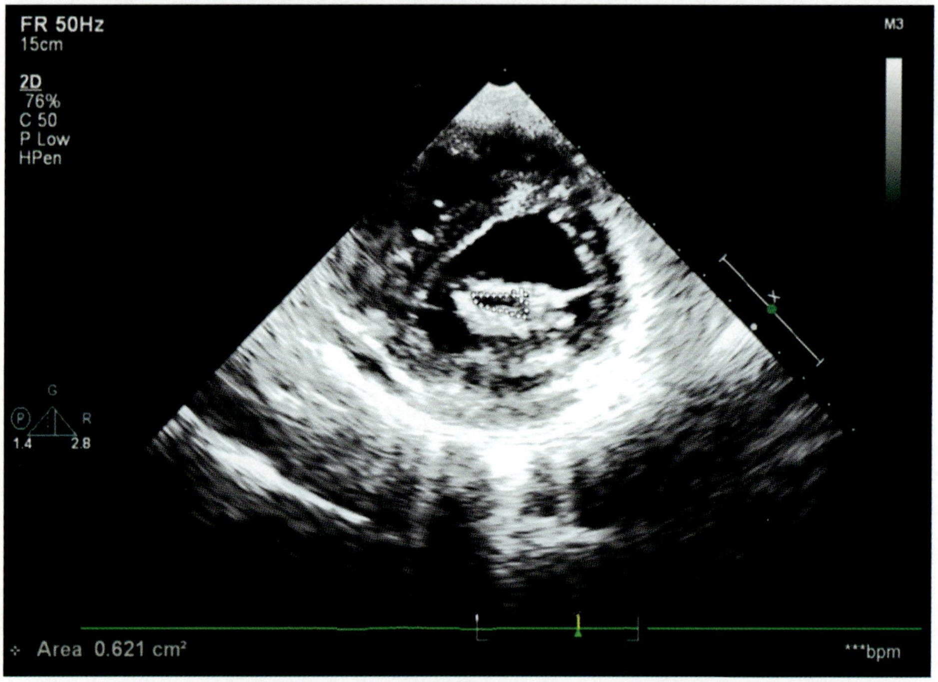

Fig. 38: Fish mouth appearance of mitral valve in severe rheumatic MS in short-axis view.

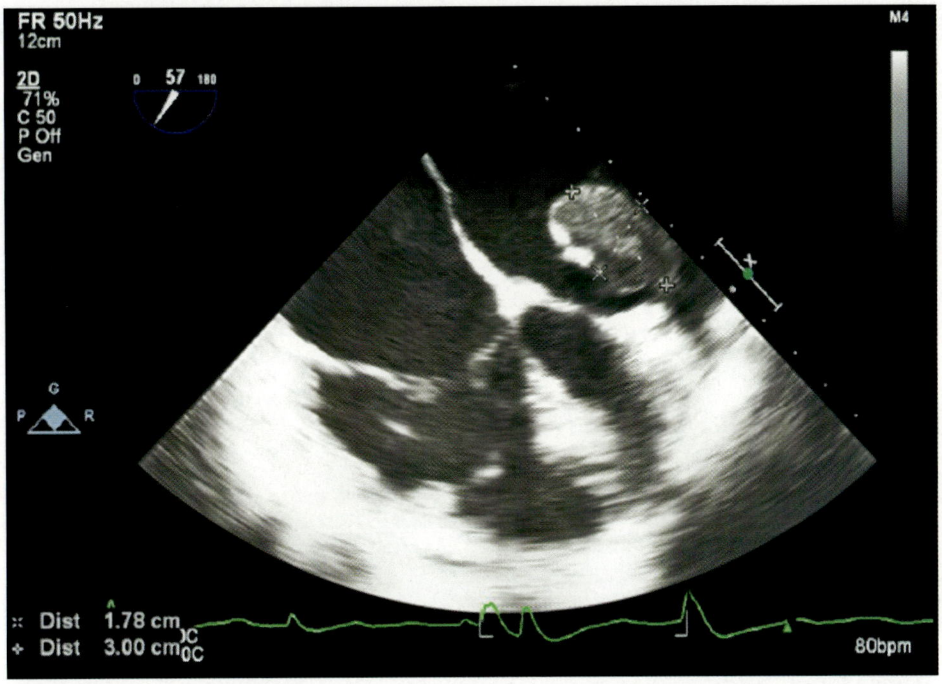

Fig. 39: TEE image showing large LA clot at the mouth of LAA.

FLUOROSCOPIC IMAGES (FIGS. 40 TO 42)

Stent Upper-edge Dissection (Fig. 40)

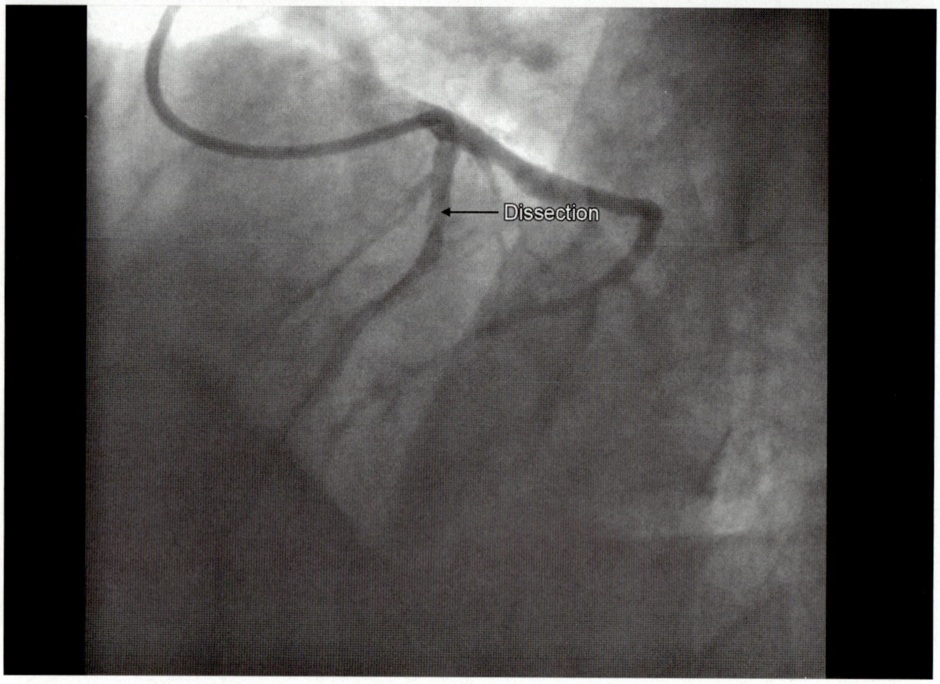

Fig. 40: Coronary angiogram showing stent upper-edge dissection.

- Stent dissection is a procedural complication of percutaneous coronary intervention (PCI).
- It may occur at proximal edge or distal edge of stent during stent dilation.
- Residual stent-edge dissection specially with smaller residual lumen area may lead to stent thrombosis or restenosis leading to repeat revascularization.

Ulcerated Lesion in RCA (Fig. 41)

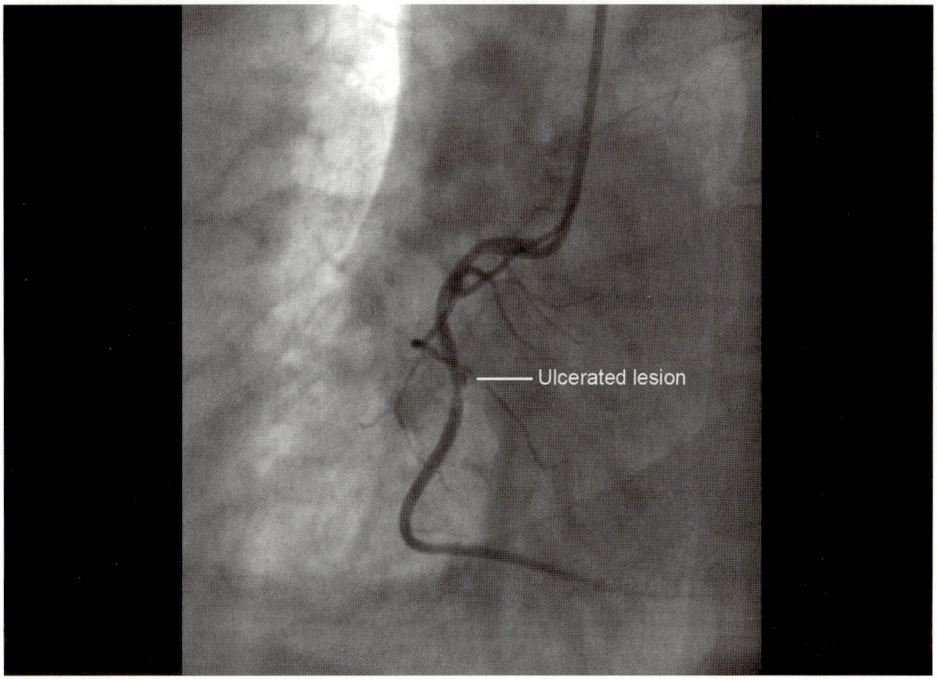

Fig. 41: Ulcerated lesion in right coronary artery (RCA).

- Coronary angiogram showing ulcerated plaque in mid-RCA.
- An ulcerated lesion is defined as a cavity in the vessel wall with disruption of the intima and flow observed within the plaque cavity.
- Coronary artery ulceration is assessed visually using a well-defined grading system.
- Grade 0 corresponds to no angiographic evidence of ulceration, grade 1 ulceration is present when the lesion contains a neck with contrast material dissecting under the plaque either proximally or distally, and grade 2 ulceration is present when there is distinct extravascular extravasation of contrast material with the appearance of a mushroom.

Fluoro Image of Massive Pericardial Calcification (Fig. 42)

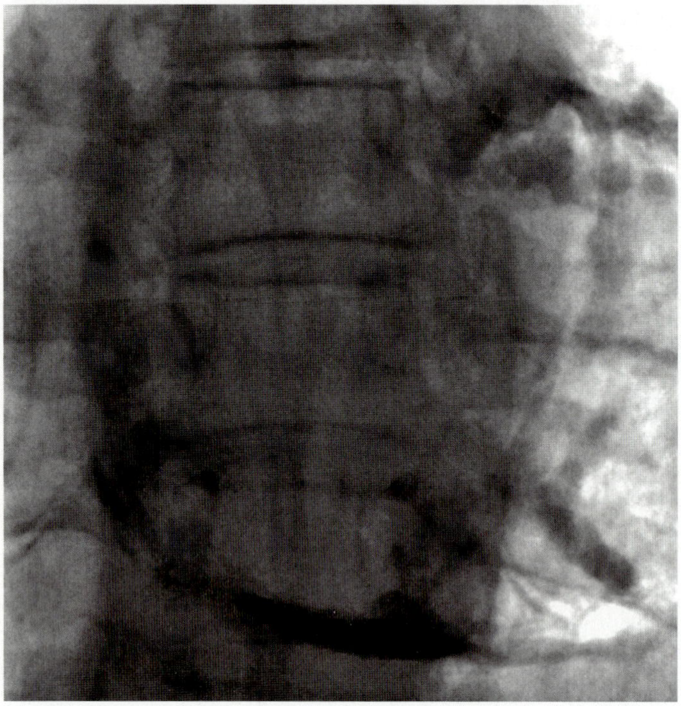

Fig. 42: Fluoroscopic image of massive pericardial calcification.

- Chronic constrictive pericarditis (CCP) is inflamed, scarred and thickened pericardium due to varied etiology.
- It has varied constellation of echo findings.
- Common findings include (1) respiration-related ventricular septal shift, (2) variation in mitral inflow E velocity, (3) medial mitral annular e' velocity $\geq$ 9 cm/s, (4) ratio of medial mitral annular e' to lateral e', and (5) hepatic vein expiratory diastolic reversal ratio.

INTRAVASCULAR ULTRASOUND (FIGS. 43A TO D)

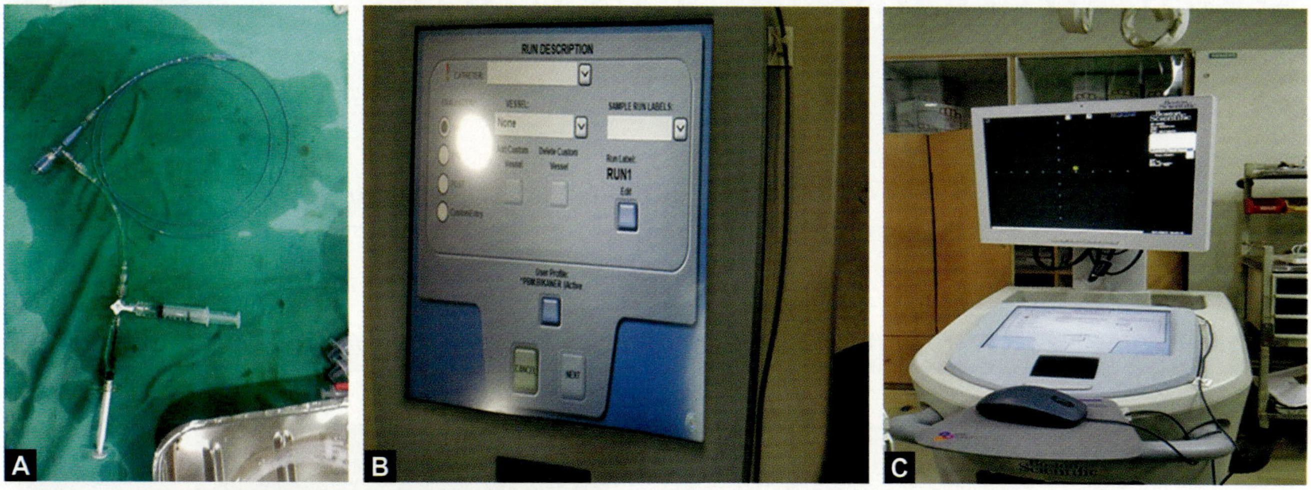

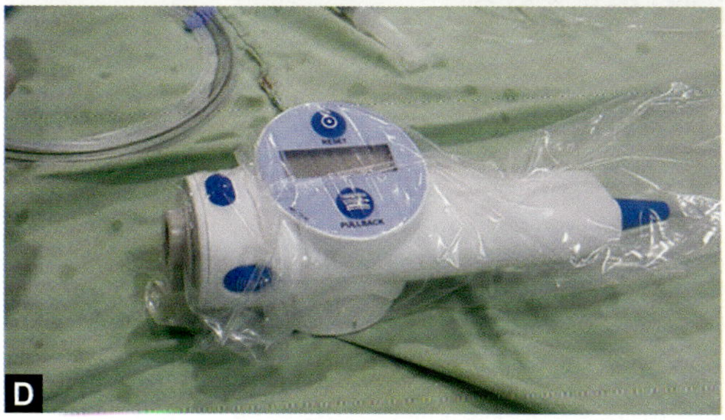

Figs. 43A to D: Intravascular ultrasound (IVUS). (A) IVUS catheter; (B) IVUS screen; (C) IVUS system; (D) IVUS.

- It is a medical imaging methodology using specially designed catheter with a miniature ultrasound probe attached to the distal end of the catheter.
- Proximal end of catheter is attached to computerized ultrasound equipment.
- It allows us to see coronary artery from inside out.
- Cross-sectional view can aid in stent sizing and appropriate positioning of the stent.
- Should be used in left main percutaneous transluminal coronary angioplasty (PTCA).

CHAPTER

10

Transesophageal Echocardiography and Aortic Aneurysm

Dheeraj Arora, Jeetendra Sharma, Mukesh K Gupta, Yatin Mehta

INTRAMURAL HEMATOMA (FIG. 1)

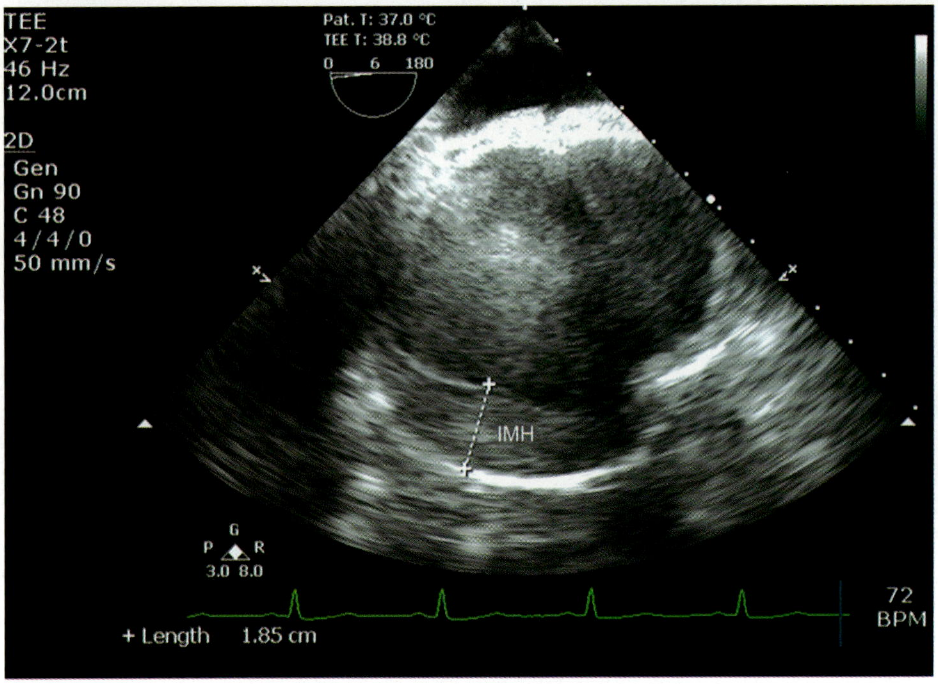

Fig. 1: Intramural hematoma (IMH) of aorta.

- Transesophageal echocardiography (TEE) midesophageal (ME) descending thoracic aorta short axis (SAX) view showing intramural hematoma (IMH).
- IMH is a life-threatening aortic disease within acute aortic syndrome along with aortic dissection and penetrating aortic ulcer.
- It is a contained aortic wall hematoma with bleeding within the media but without initial intimal flap formation, involving ascending aorta and warrants urgent surgery.

PLEURAL EFFUSION (FIG. 2)

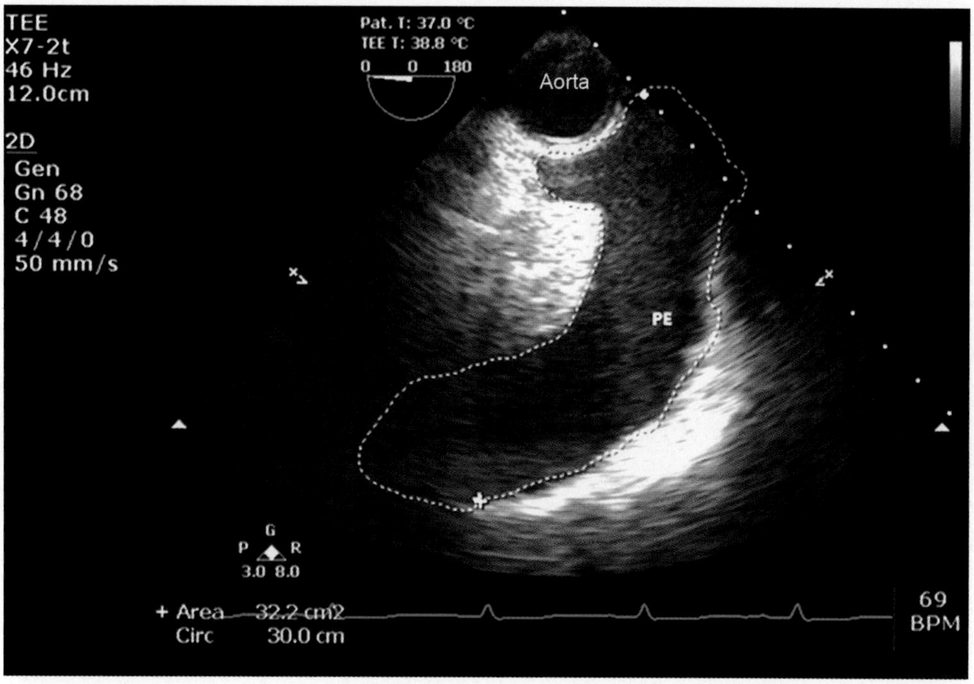

Fig. 2: Pleural effusion (PE).

- TEE image showing pleural effusion (PE) in dotted line and descending thoracic aorta at the top.
- PE is the abnormal collection of fluid in the pleural space, usually resulting from excess fluid production and/or decreased lymphatic absorption.
- TEE is one of the diagnostic modalities for PE and also helps in quantification and insertion of pigtail catheter.
- Cardiac tamponade associated with PE can also be detected.

LEFT VENTRICLE ANEURYSM (FIG. 3)

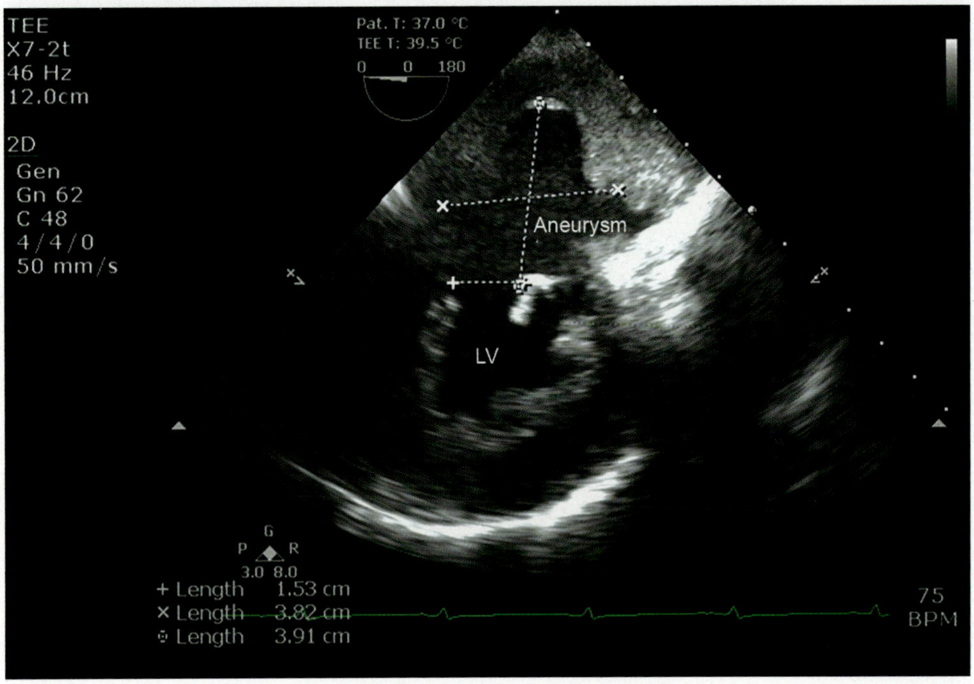

Fig. 3: Left ventricle (LV) aneurysm.

- TEE—Transgastric (TG) midpapillary short axis view of left ventricle (LV) showing aneurysm of the inferior wall (with dimensions).
- Left ventricular true aneurysms are discrete, dyskinetic areas of the LV wall with a broad neck. They develop in less than 5% of all patients with ST-elevation myocardial infarctions (STEMI) and may be associated with LV thrombus which can embolize.
- It may present with decompensated cardiac failure and echocardiography is diagnostic.
- Mortality is up to six times higher than in these patients. Major cause of sudden death is ventricular tachyarrhythmia.

MITRAL REGURGITATION (FIG. 4)

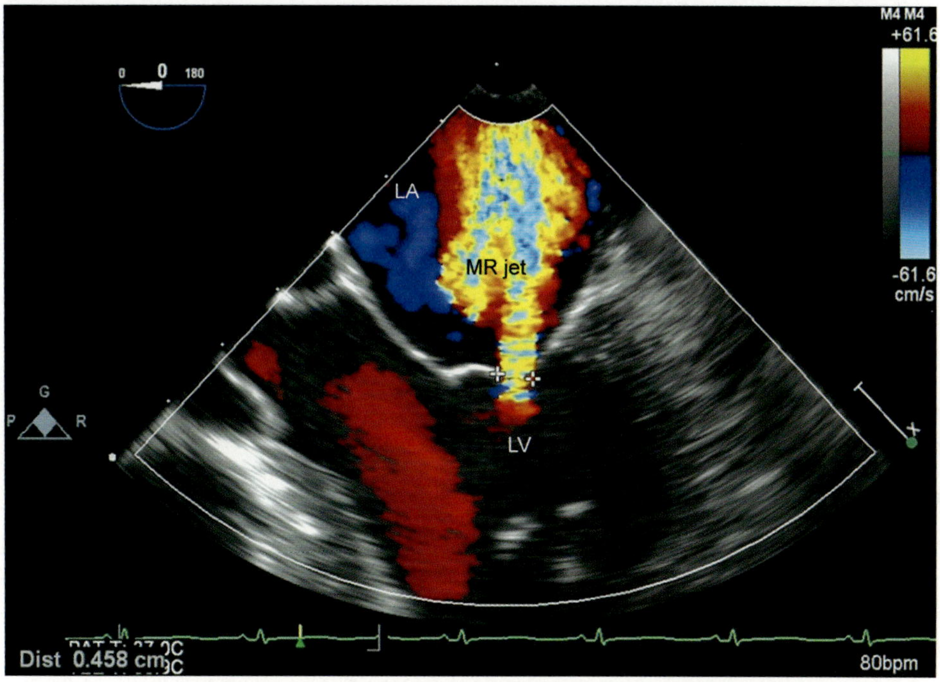

Fig. 4: Mitral regurgitation (MR). (LA: Left atrium; LV: Left ventricle)

- TEE midesophageal (ME) five-chamber view showing mitral regurgitation (MR) jet in left atrium (LA).
- During systole, contraction of the left ventricle (LV) causes abnormal backflow into the LA.
- Echocardiography is an important tool for quantification of MR and can be used in the pre-, intra- and postoperative period.
- Acute MR happens after STEMI with papillary muscle rupture.
- In chronic heart failure, MR may be associated with annular dilatation of mitral valve (MV).

MITRAL STENOSIS (FIG. 5)

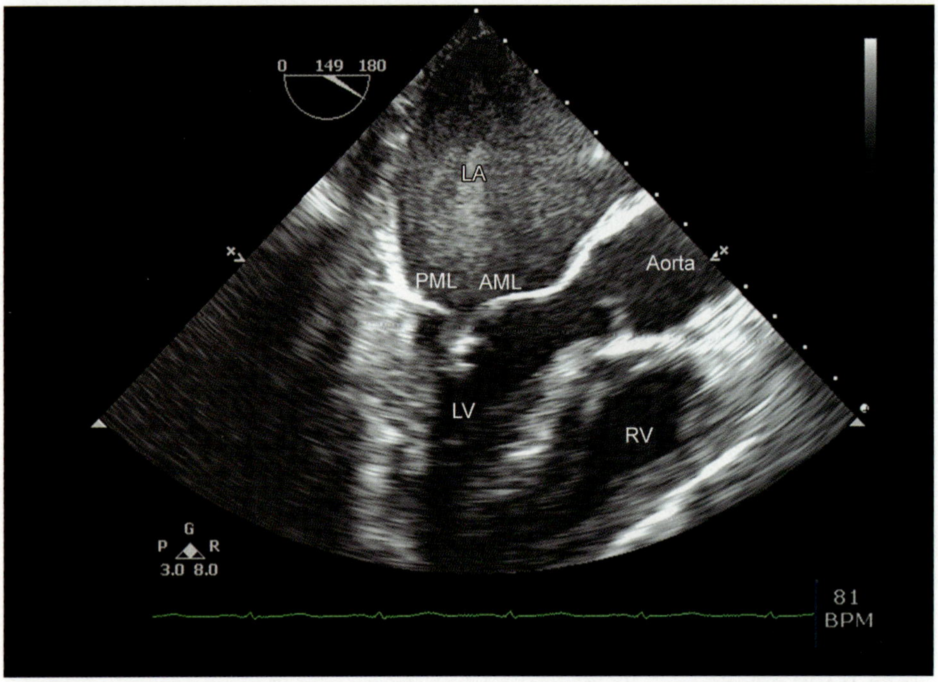

Fig. 5: Mitral stenosis (MS). (LA: Left atrium; PML: Posterior mitral leaflet; AML: Anterior mitral leaflet; LV: Left ventricle; RV: Right ventricle)

- TEE—ME long axis (LAX) view showing mitral stenosis (MS). The MV leaflets are thick and calcific. There is a "hockey stick" appearance of anterior mitral leaflet (AML) in MS.
- Left atrium (LA) is dilated and spontaneous echo contrast (SEC) is also present.
- Echocardiography is used to assess the severity and quantification of MS.
- Wilkins' score is calculated by echocardiography to have the suitability for balloon mitral valvotomy (BMV).
- MS is usually associated with atrial fibrillation (AF) and sometimes with LA thrombus which can embolize.
- Before cardioversion (CV) in patients with AF of more than 48 hours duration, it is advisable to do TEE to rule out LA thrombus.
- In presence of LA thrombus, CV is contraindicated then anticoagulation/medical management should be done.

ACUTE AORTIC DISSECTION (FIGS. 6A AND B)

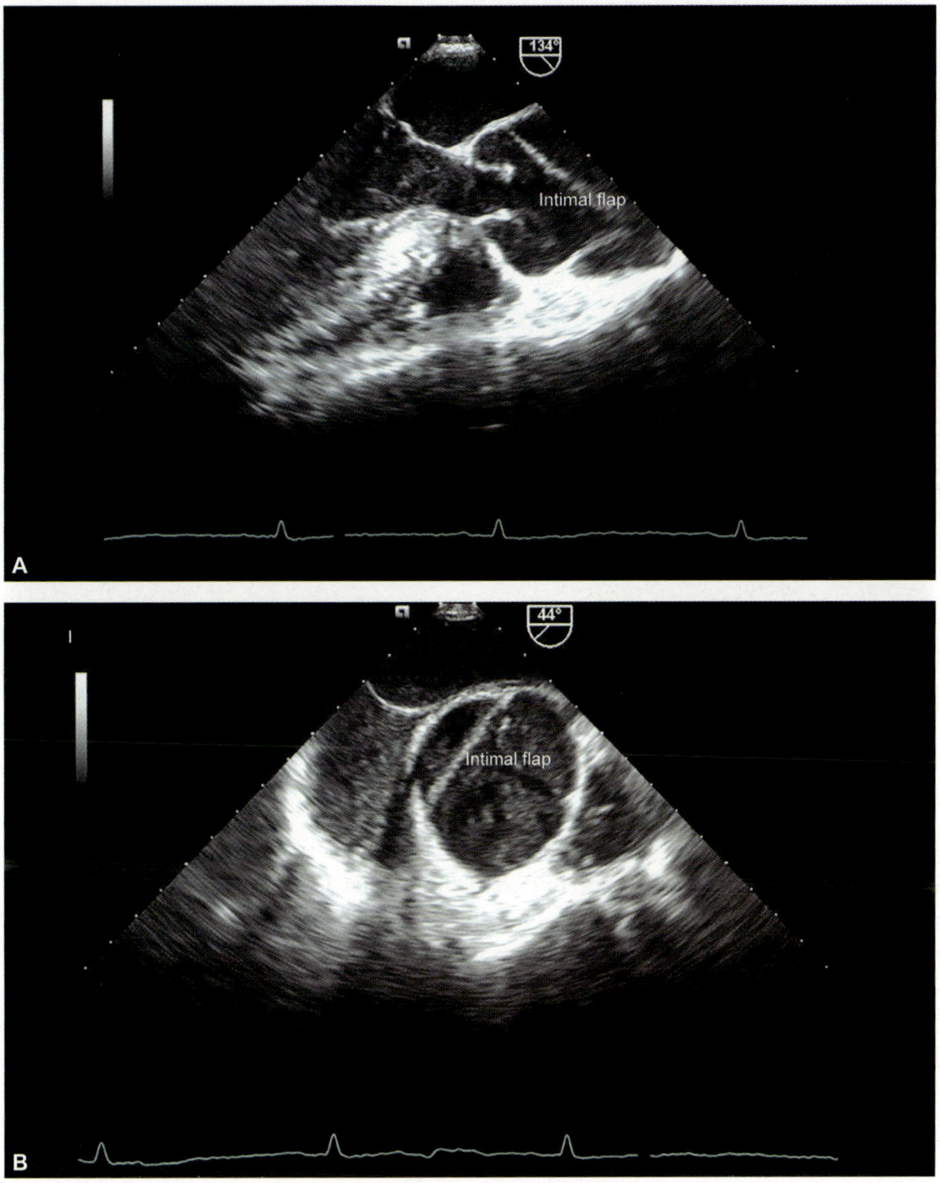

Figs. 6A and B: Acute aortic dissection.

- TEE—ME long axis (LAX) view (Fig. 6A) showing intimal flap in the ascending aorta and SAX view (Fig. 6B) showing the intimal flap in descending thoracic aorta.
- Aortic dissection (AD) is the part of acute aortic syndrome that requires urgent intervention. Common causes are trauma, hypertension and arteritis.
- TEE is helpful in diagnosing the intimal flap with sensitivity of 94% and specificity of 77–100%.
- TEE is most suitable for hemodynamically unstable patients who are not fit for radiology or cath procedures.
- It also helps in detecting the extent of the dissection, intimal tear location, aortic insufficiency, principal aortic branch involvement and signs of blood extravasation (pericardial effusion or aortic rupture).

PERICARDIAL EFFUSION (FIG. 7)

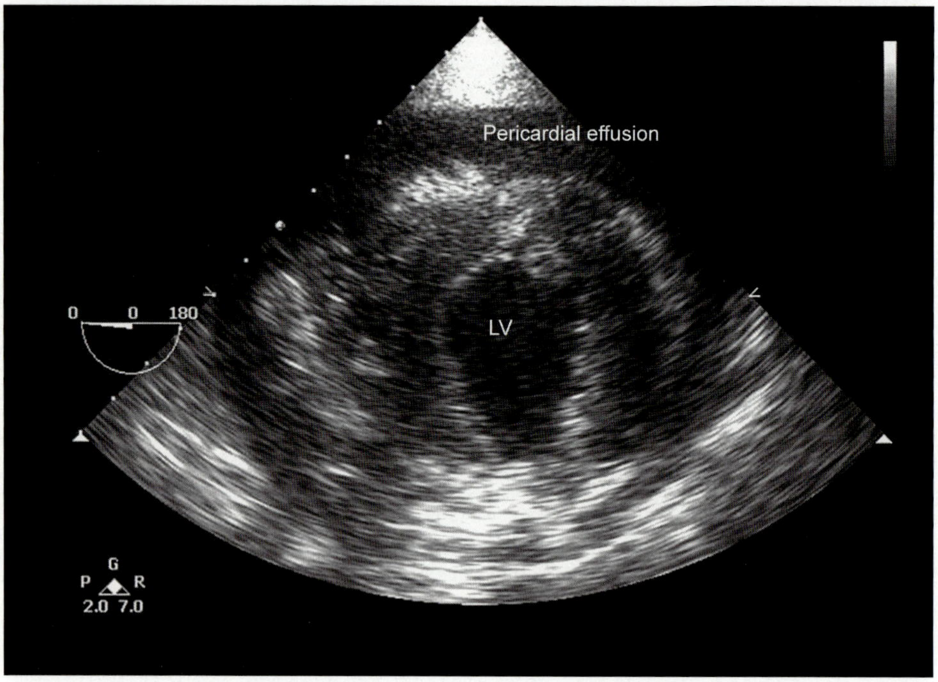

Fig. 7: Pericardial effusion. (LV: Left ventricle)

- TEE TG SAX view showing pericardial effusion encircling left ventricle (LV).
- PE is the abnormal collection of fluid in the pericardial cavity due to local or systemic cause. It may be seen in immediate postcardiac surgical patients.
- It can be life-threatening because of low cardiac output.
- Beck' triad (muffled heart sound, hypotension and jugular venous distension) is classical of pericardial tamponade.
- Echocardiography is the diagnostic modality of choice and also aids in pericardiocentesis.

PULMONARY EMBOLISM (FIG. 8)

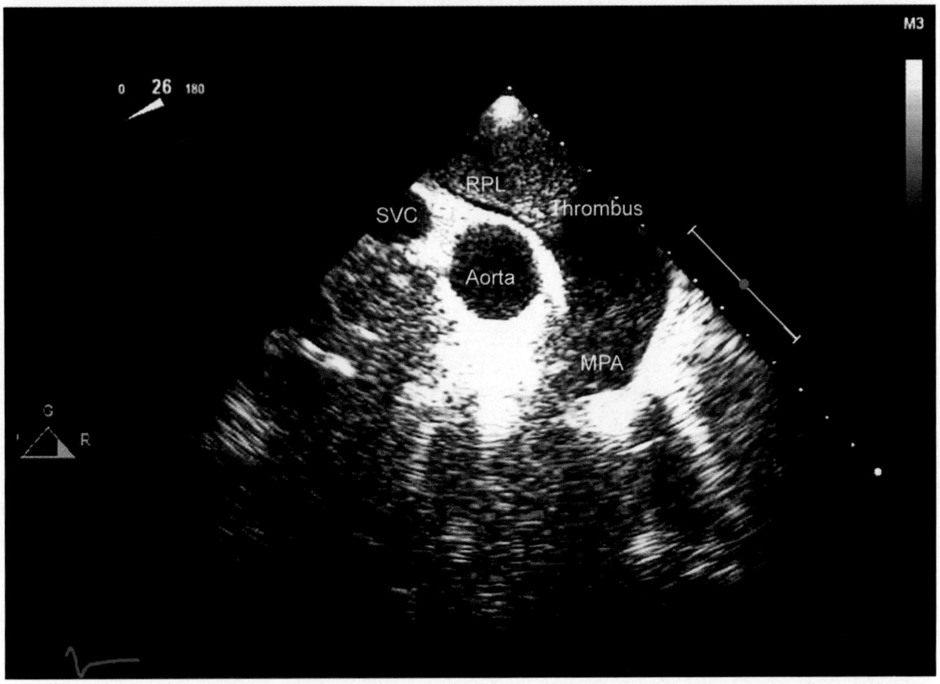

Fig. 8: Pulmonary embolism (PE). (MPA: Main pulmonary artery; RPA: Right pulmonary artery; SVC: Superior vena cava)

- TEE upper esophageal (UE) view showing the main pulmonary artery (MPA) and thrombus in the right pulmonary artery (RPA).
- Pulmonary embolism (PE) is secondary to the thrombi originating from the deep vein systems of the lower extremities and causes hemodynamic compromise.
- Classical presentation is sudden onset chest pain, shortness of breath and hypoxia.
- TEE is an important tool to detect PE although computerized tomography pulmonary angiography (CTPA) is diagnostic.
- It can be safely done in hemodynamically unstable patients who are not fit for radiology or cath procedures.
- Management includes immediate anticoagulation, thrombolytic therapy or surgical intervention.

INFECTIVE ENDOCARDITIS (FIGS. 9A AND B)

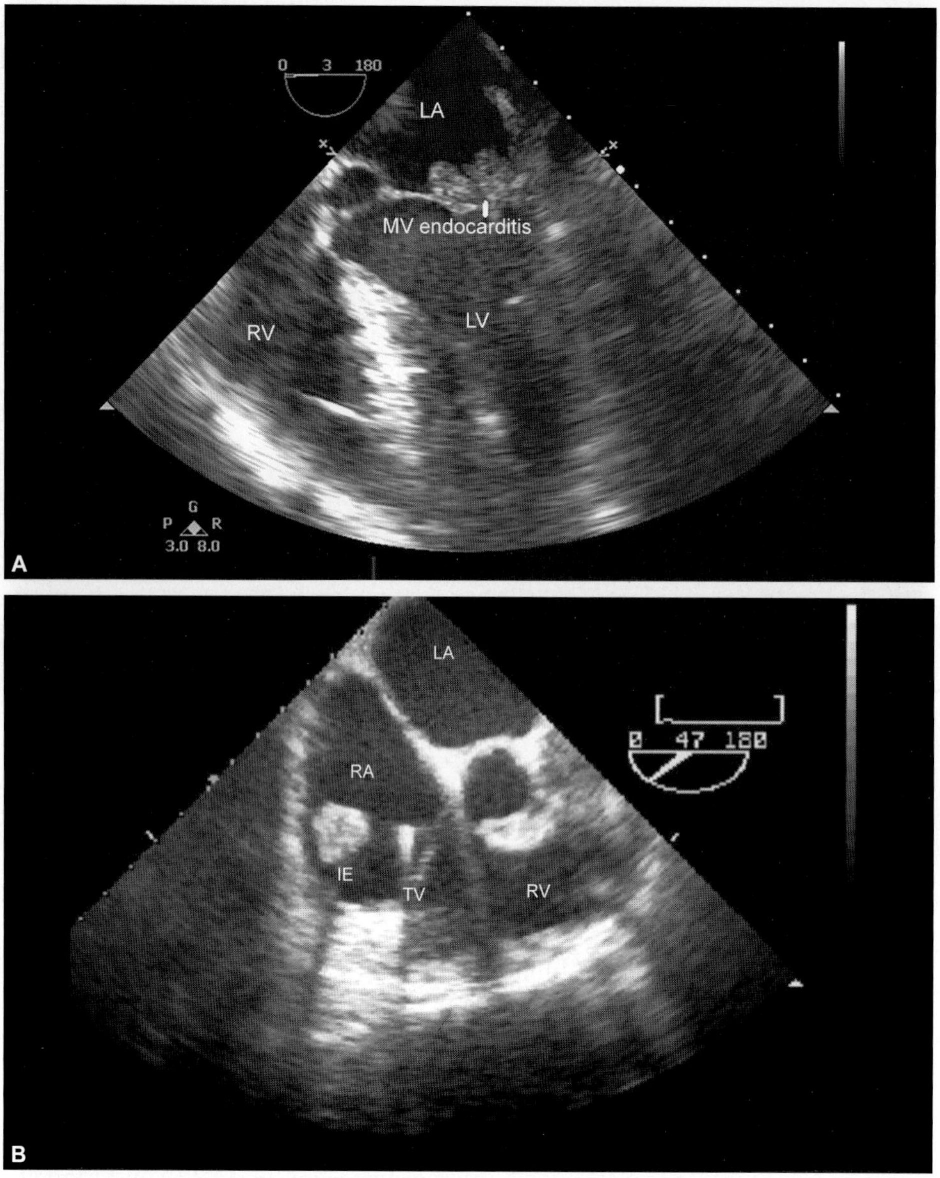

Figs. 9A and B: (A) Infective endocarditis; (B) Mass on the tricuspid valve (TV). (LA: Left atrium; LV: Left ventricle; MV: Mitral valve; RV: Right ventricle; IE: Infective endocarditis; TV: Tricuspid valve)

- TEE ME four-chamber view showing irregular mass on mitral leaflet suggestive of infective endocarditis (IE). Figure 9B shows mass on the tricuspid valve (TV).
- IE is defined as infection of endocardial surface of the heart that may involve one or more valves. It may lead to MR, abscess formation causing congestive heart failure.
- Duke diagnostic criteria (major and minor) include clinical, microbiological and echocardiographic characteristics.
- Tricuspid valve endocarditis is common in drug addicts.
- Antibiotics are the main stay of treatment after blood cultures and surgical treatment should be reserved for refractory cases.
- This should be suspected when other causes of fever or sepsis cannot be ruled out in the ICU.

LEFT ATRIAL THROMBUS (FIG. 10)

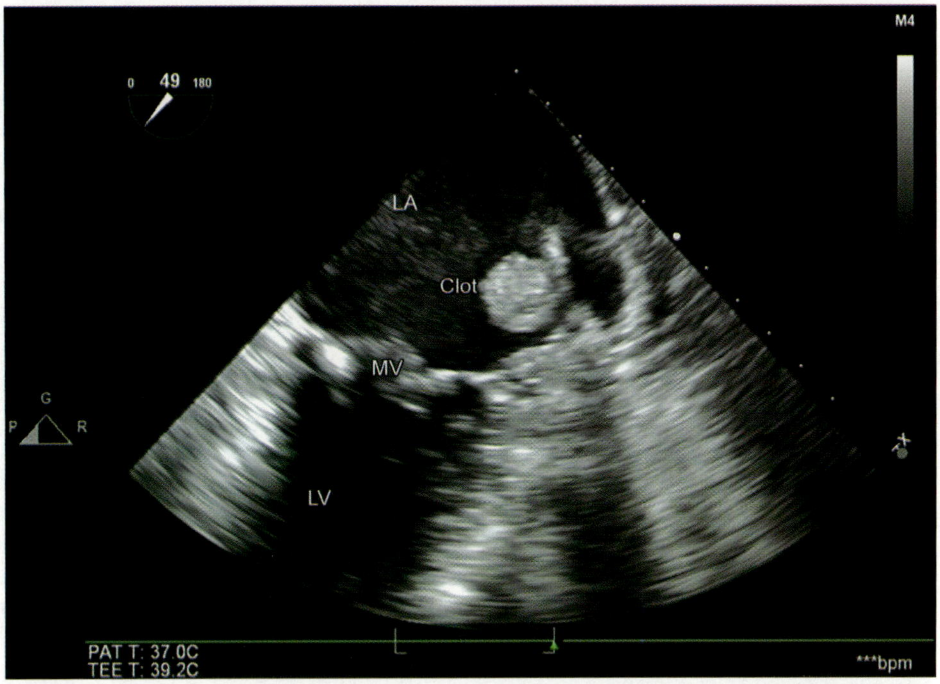

Fig. 10: Left atrial thrombus. (LA: Left atrium; MV: Mitral valve; LV: Left ventricle)

- TEE ME two-chamber view showing an echodense shadow in the LA, most likely a clot originating from LA appendage (LAA). MV is also thickened and calcified.
- LAA is the most common site of cardiac thrombus and TEE is the most appropriate modality to diagnose the same.
- It is commonly associated with atrial flutter or fibrillation as low flow velocities lead to rouleaux formation of red blood cells.
- If left untreated, it may lead to stroke and embolism in the peripheral vasculature and other organ systems.

ATRIAL SEPTAL DEFECT (FIGS. 11A AND B)

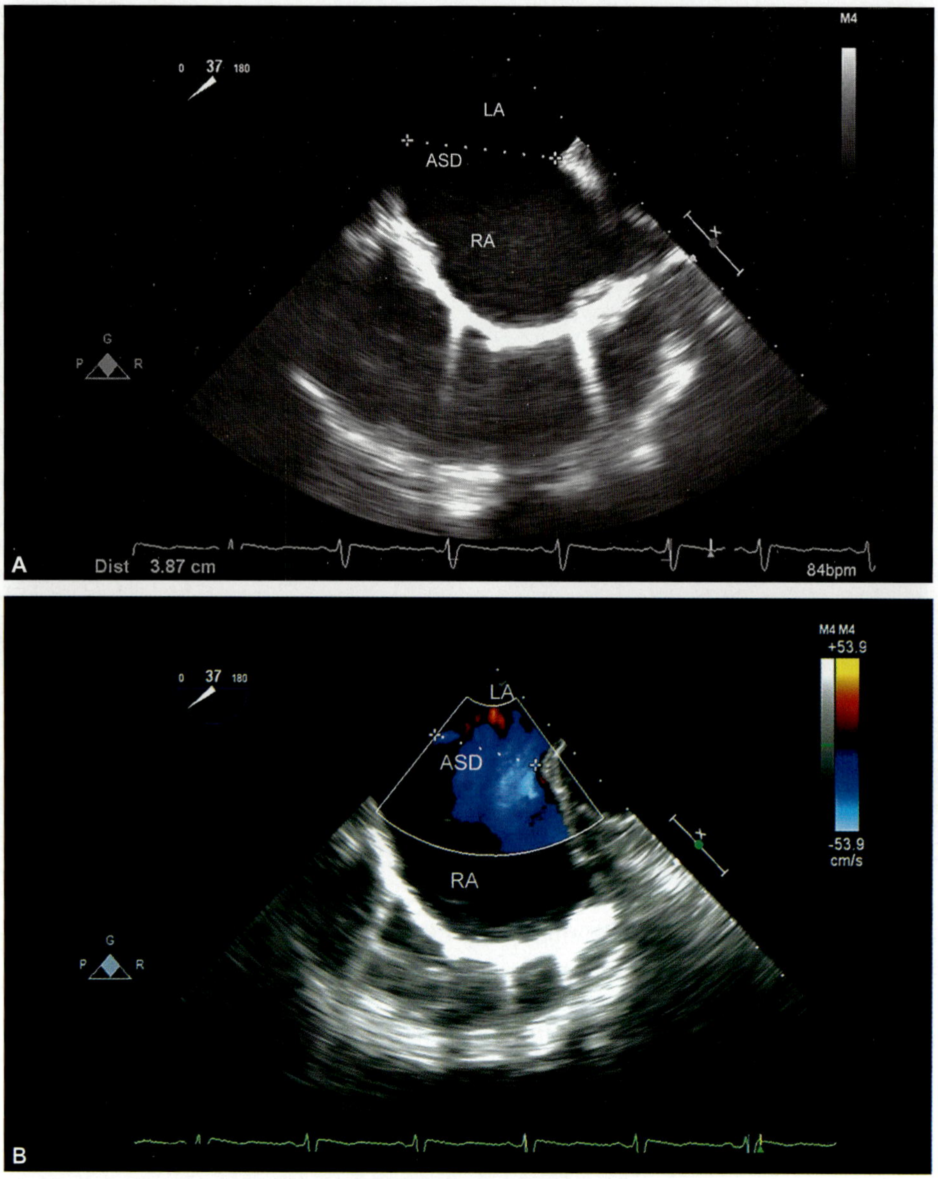

Figs. 11A and B: (A) ASD with measurement of size; (B) Color flow Doppler across the defect. (LA: Left atrium; ASD: Atrial septal defect; RA: Right atrium)

- TEE bicaval view showing ostium secundum atrial septal defect (ASD) (Fig. 11A) and color flow Doppler (Fig. 11B) showing flow from LA to RA.
- Atrial septal defect is one of the common congenital cardiac defects presenting in childhood.
- The incidence of ASD has increased with routine use of echocardiography.
- Echocardiography helps in evaluation of the RA, RV, and pulmonary arteries shunt fraction, however, TEE is required in cases of sinus venosus ASD.
- It may be a source of paradoxical embolism.

LEFT VENTRICLE HYPERTROPHY (FIG. 12)

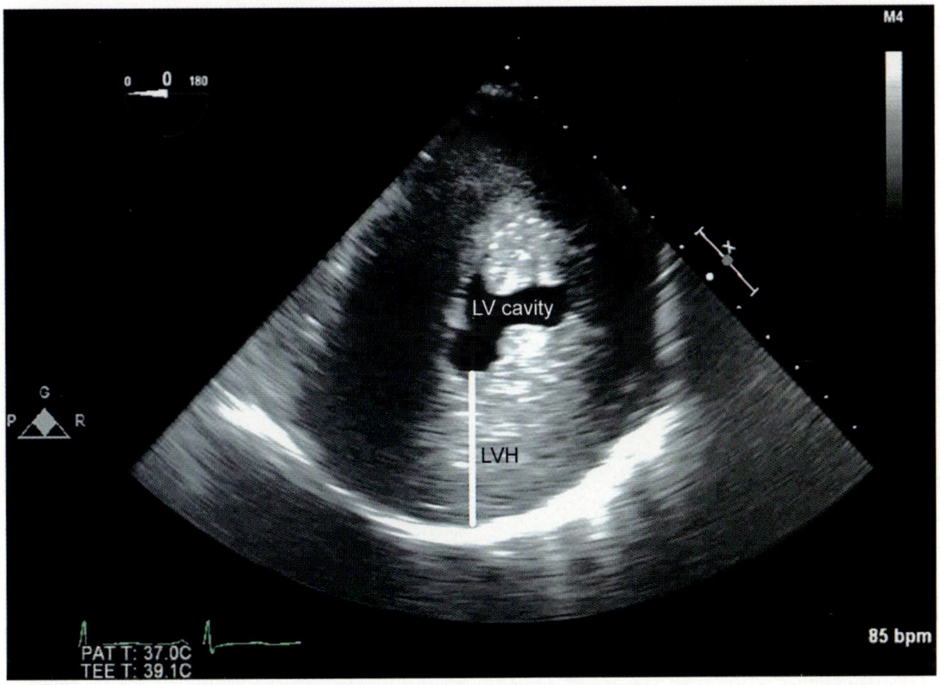

Fig. 12: Left ventricle hypertrophy (LVH).

- TEE TG midpapillary SAX view of LV showing left ventricular hypertrophy (LVH) and LV cavity.
- LVH is ventricular remodeling secondary to increase afterload usually seen in aortic stenosis or regurgitation and hypertension. It may occur due to primary disease of muscle as seen in hypertrophic obstructive cardiomyopathy (HOCM).
- Echocardiography helps in assessing thickness of myocardium, LV mass index and systolic anterior motion (SAM) of mitral leaflets leading to MR.
- LVH is a risk factor and strongly predicts cardiovascular morbidity and overall mortality.
- Pressure indices of cardiac filling may be misleading in these patients. They may need higher filling pressures and also prone to myocardial ischemia and arrhythmias.

DILATED CARDIOMYOPATHY (FIGS. 13A AND B)

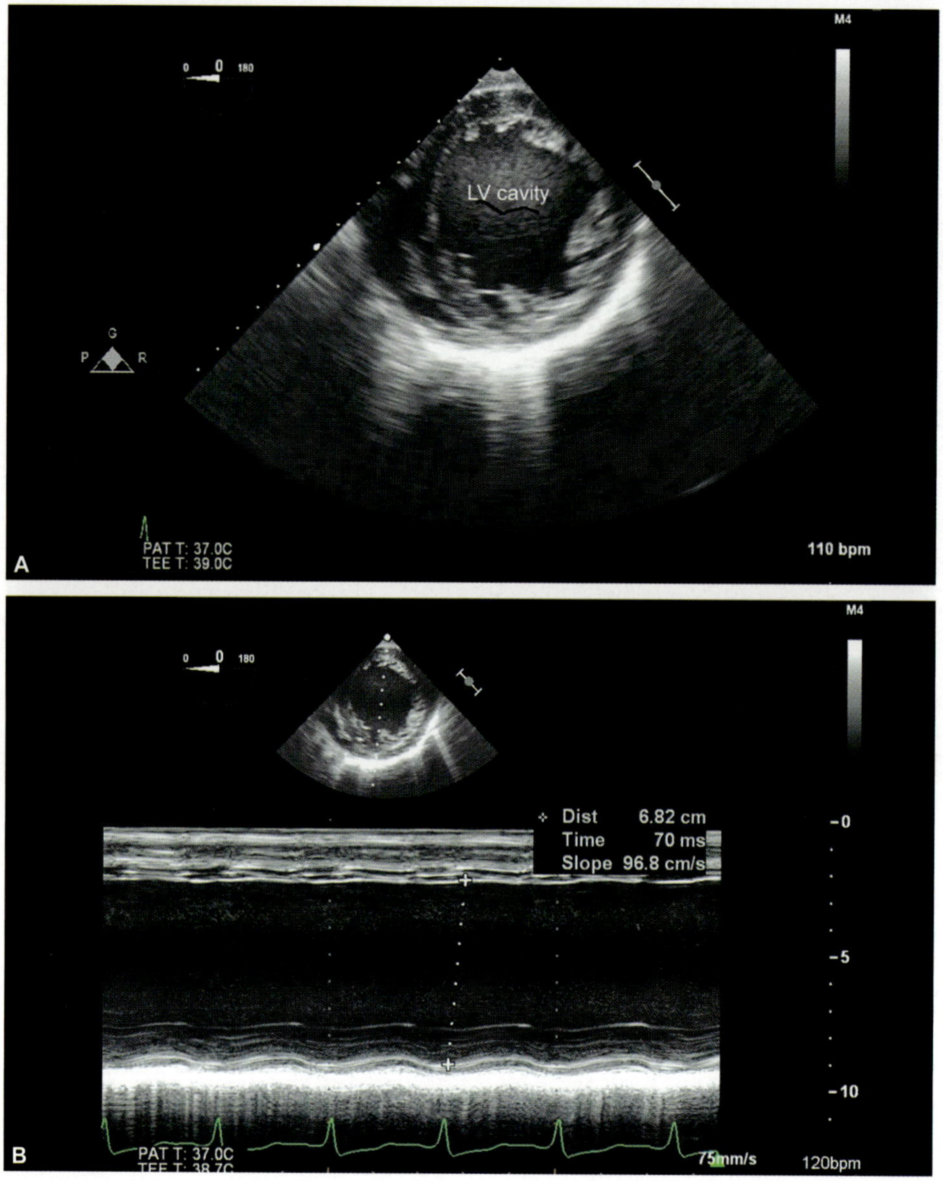

Figs. 13A and B: (A) Left ventricle (LV) dysfunction; (B) M-mode across LV showing cavity size.

- TEE TG midpapillary SAX view of LV showing dilated LV (Fig. 13A) and M-mode across LV showing cavity size (Fig. 13B).
- Dilated cardiomyopathy (DCMP) is cardiac muscle disorder usually secondary to myocardial infarction. Heart chambers are dilated and is associated with poor LV function.
- Commonly associated with valvular regurgitation, congestive heart failure, life-threatening arrhythmia and sudden death.
- Echocardiography shows thin-walled LV with dilatation, valvular dysfunction and reduced globally ejection fraction.

LEFT ATRIAL MYXOMA (FIG. 14)

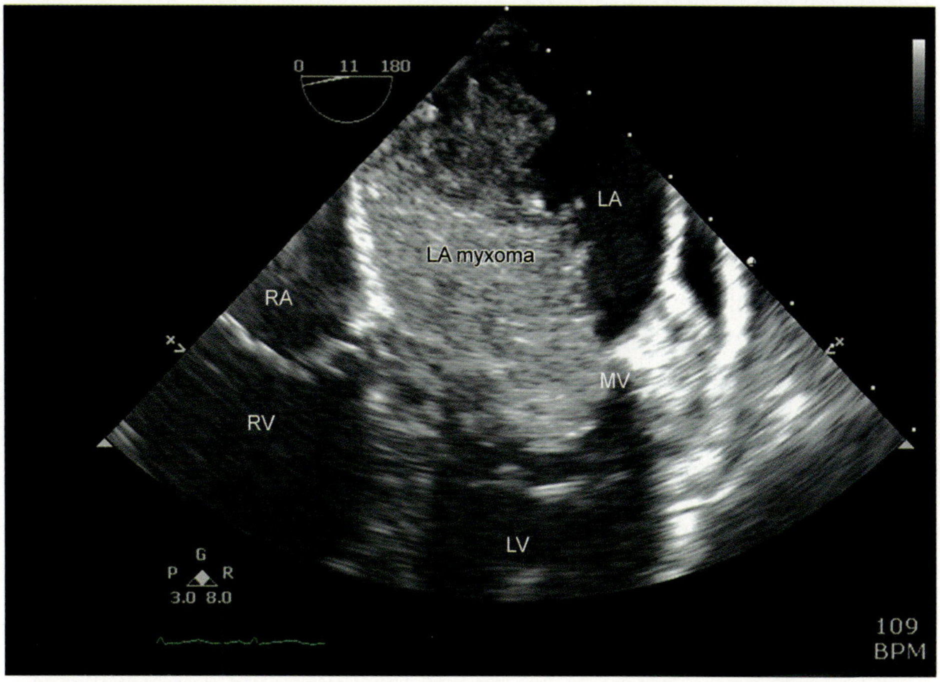

Fig. 14: Left atrial myxoma. (LA: Left atrial; RA: Right atrium; RV: Right ventricle; LV: Left ventricle; MV: Mitral valve)

- TEE ME four-chamber view showing LA myxoma originating from interatrial septum and crossing MV.
- Atrial myxoma is the most common primary heart tumor (40–50%). Myxomas are usually benign polypoid, round, or oval and most common site of attachment is at the border of the fossa ovalis in the LA.
- Echocardiography is the diagnostic modality of choice as it assesses tumor location, size, attachment, and mobility. TEE has better specificity and 100% sensitivity.
- Surgical removal of the tumor through midsternotomy or thoracotomy is the conventional treatment.

AORTIC ANEURYSM (FIGS. 15A TO F)

- An aneurysm is defined as a focal dilatation of an artery that exceeds the normal diameter by at least 50%.
- Crawford classification of thoracoabdominal aortic aneurysms.
- Type I, distal from origin of left subclavian artery to above renal arteries.
- Type II, distal from the left subclavian artery to the infrarenal aorta.
- Type III, from the sixth intercostal space to the infrarenal aorta.
- Type IV, from the thirteenth intercostal space to the aortic bifurcation.
- Type V, below the sixth intercostal space to the renal arteries.

Aneurysm classified as a True or False

- True aneurysm results from a progressive weakening of the structural elements of the arterial wall, and both radial and longitudinal lengthening involving all three mural layers (intima, media, and adventitia).
- False aneurysms, or "pseudoaneurysms," form as a result of injury to the aortic wall and the flow of extraluminal blood, which is contained by surrounding tissue.

Aneurysms are also classified According to their Shape

- Fusiform aneurysms are characterized by a symmetric dilatation of the complete circumference of the aortic wall.
- Saccular aneurysm when they exhibit an outpouching of only a portion of the circumference of the aortic wall.

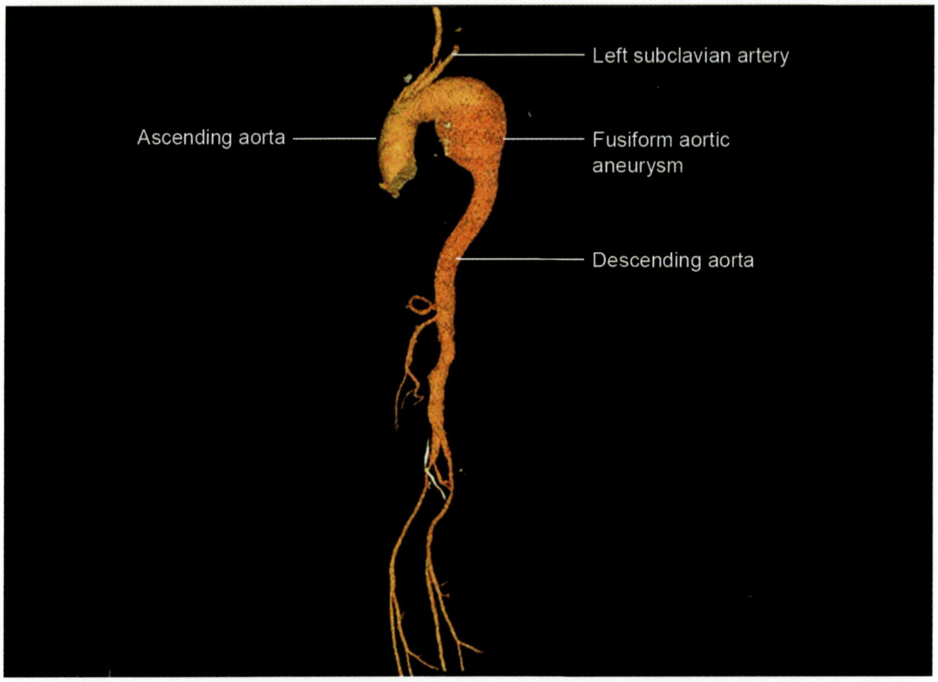

Fig. 15A: 3D reconstruction of CT aortogram.

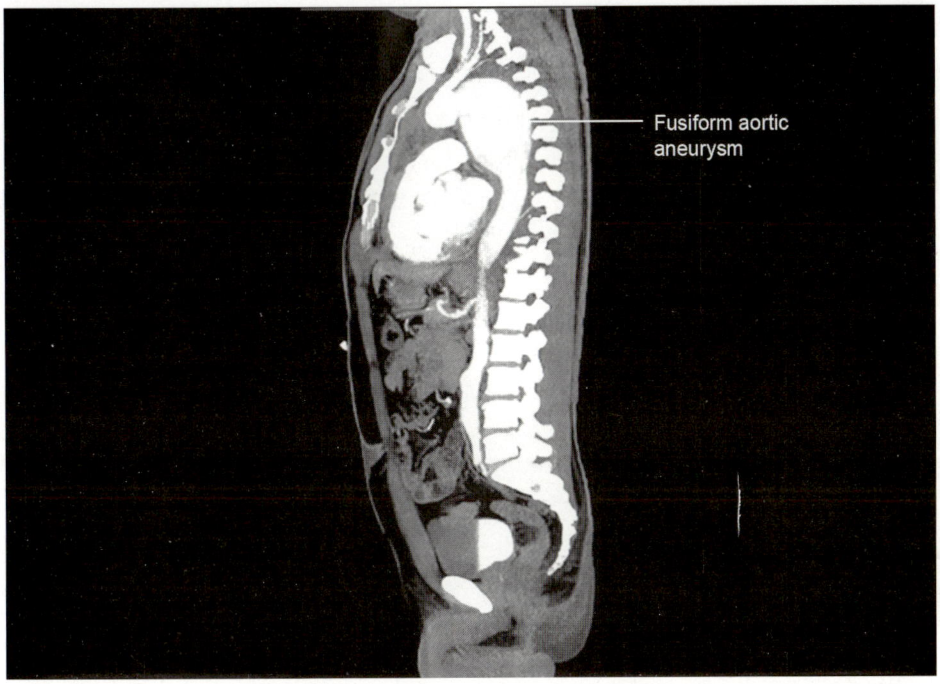

Fig. 15B: Sagittal view of CT aortogram.

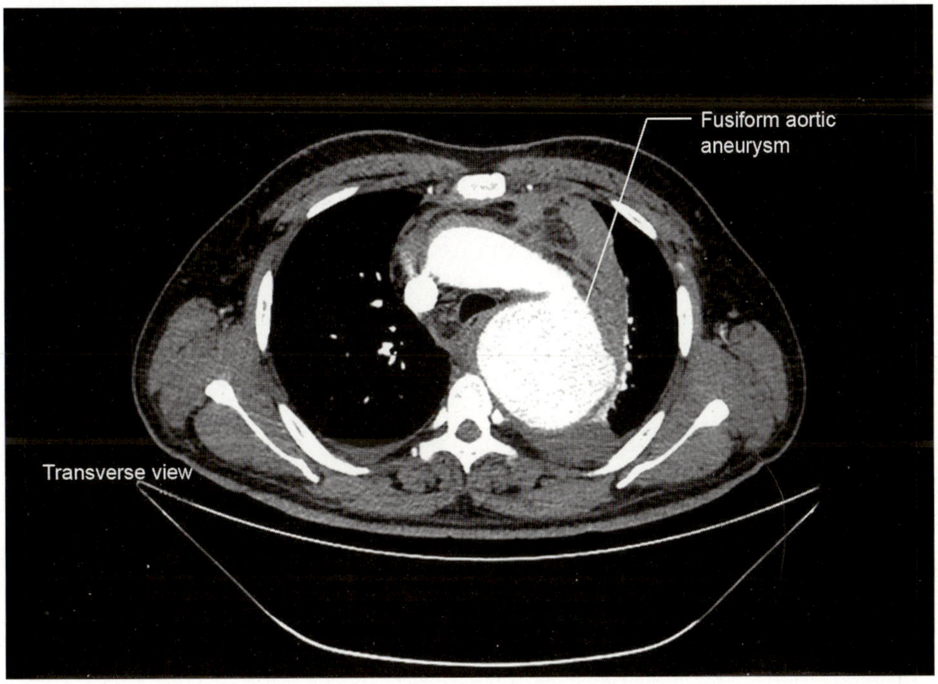

Fig. 15C: Transverse view of CT aortogram.

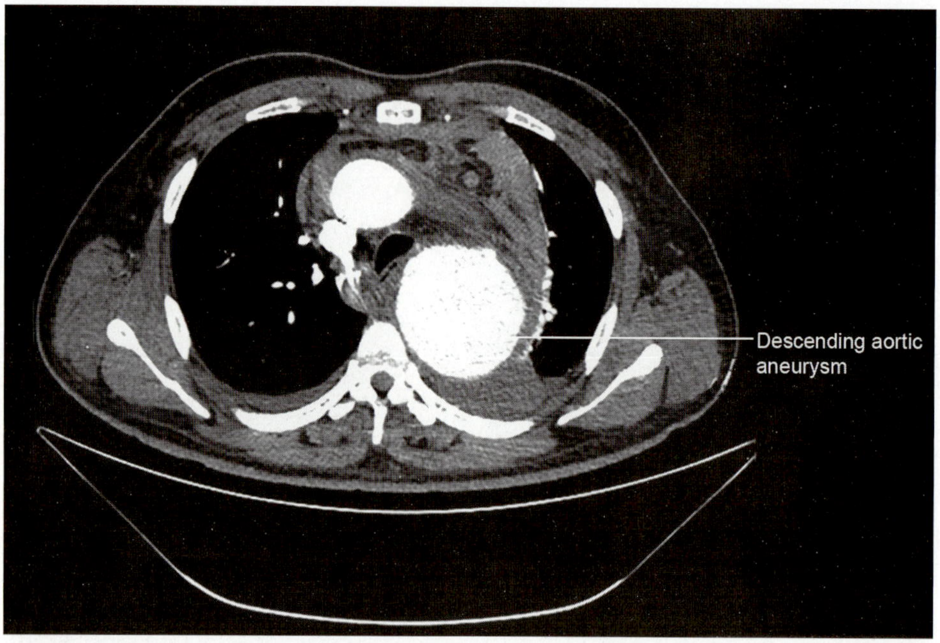

Fig. 15D: Transverse view of CT aortogram.

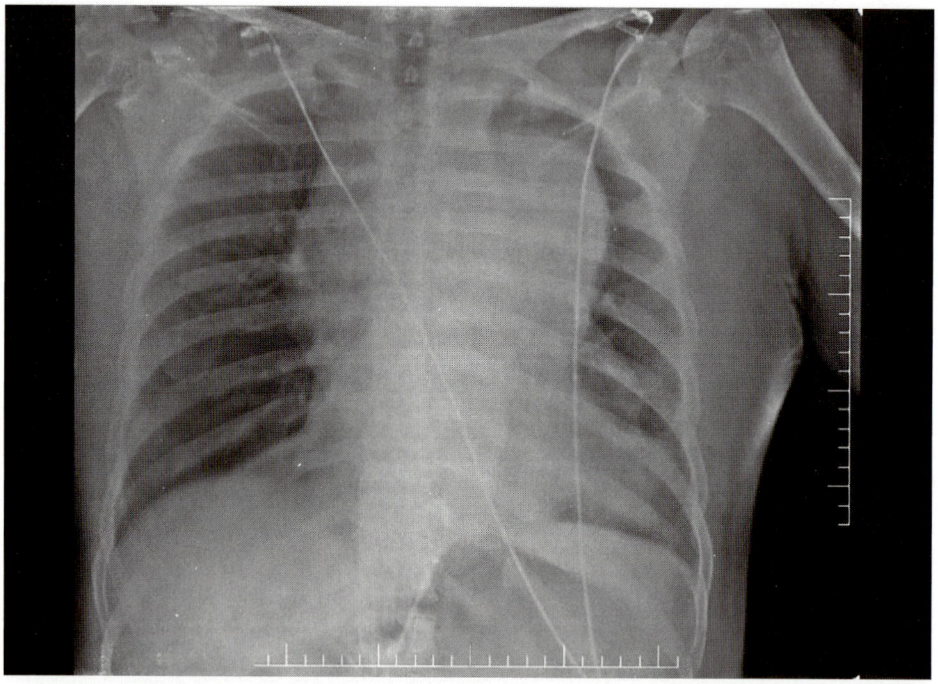

Fig. 15E: Chest X-ray of thoracic aortic aneurysm before intervention.

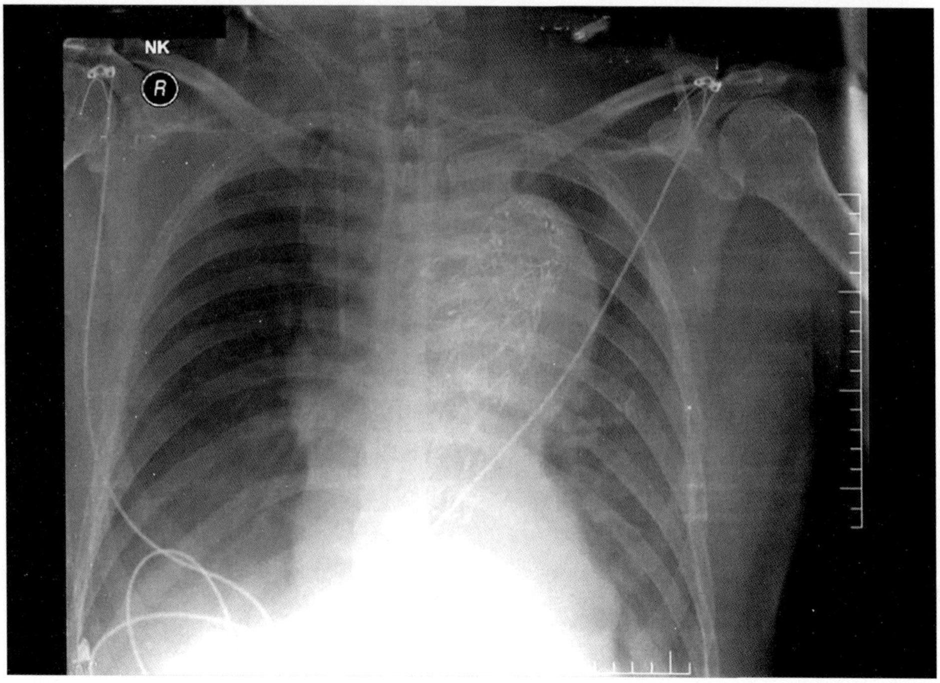

Fig. 15F: Chest X-ray of thoracic aortic aneurysm postendovascular stent.

SECTION 4

Gastroenterology

CHAPTER

11

Endoscopic Images

Randhir Sud, Deepika Parmar

COLONIC LESIONS (FIGS. 1 TO 10)

Colonic Growth (Fig. 1)

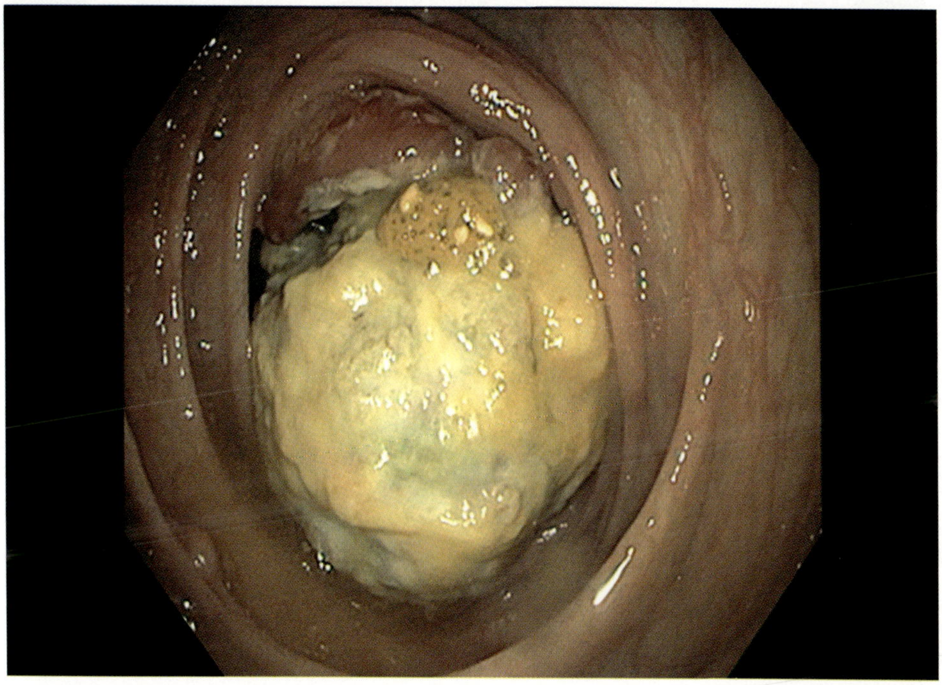

Fig. 1: Colonic growth: Ulceroproliferative growth in the ascending colon causing luminal narrowing.

- Ulceroproliferative growth in colon can present with features of obstruction or gastrointestinal (GI) bleed along with various constitutional symptoms.
- Colonoscopy can help confirm the nature of lesion with help of biopsies taken from the growth.

Colonic Stricture (Fig. 2)

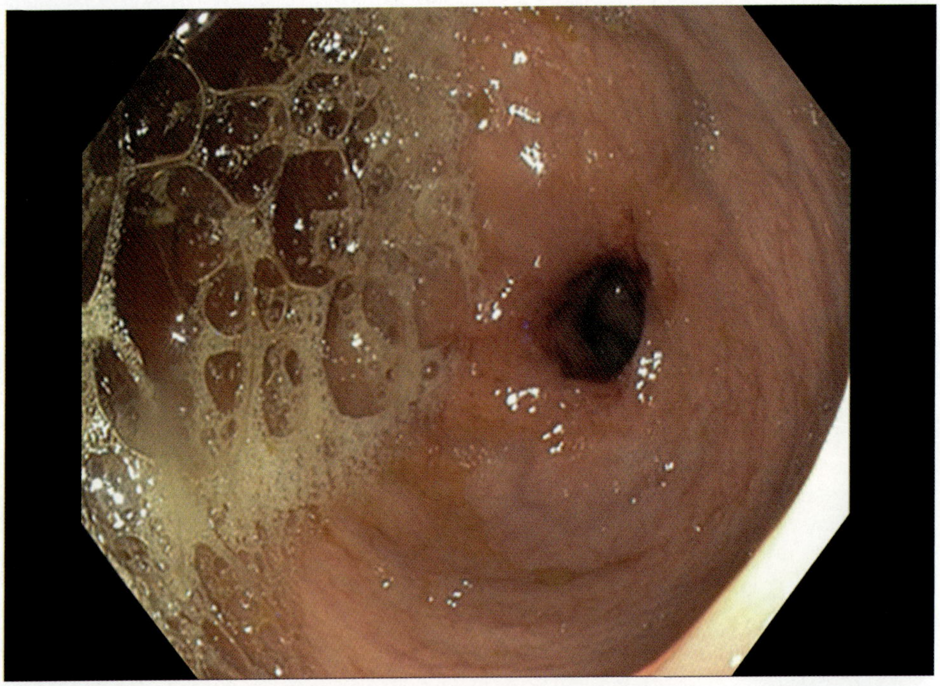

Fig. 2: Colonic stricture: Smooth narrowing of the colonic lumen indicative of benign stricture.

- The margins and length of the stricture helps us to differentiate benign from malignant stricture.
- Smooth margins and longer length of the stricture usually favors a benign etiology.

Pseudomembranous Colitis (Fig. 3)

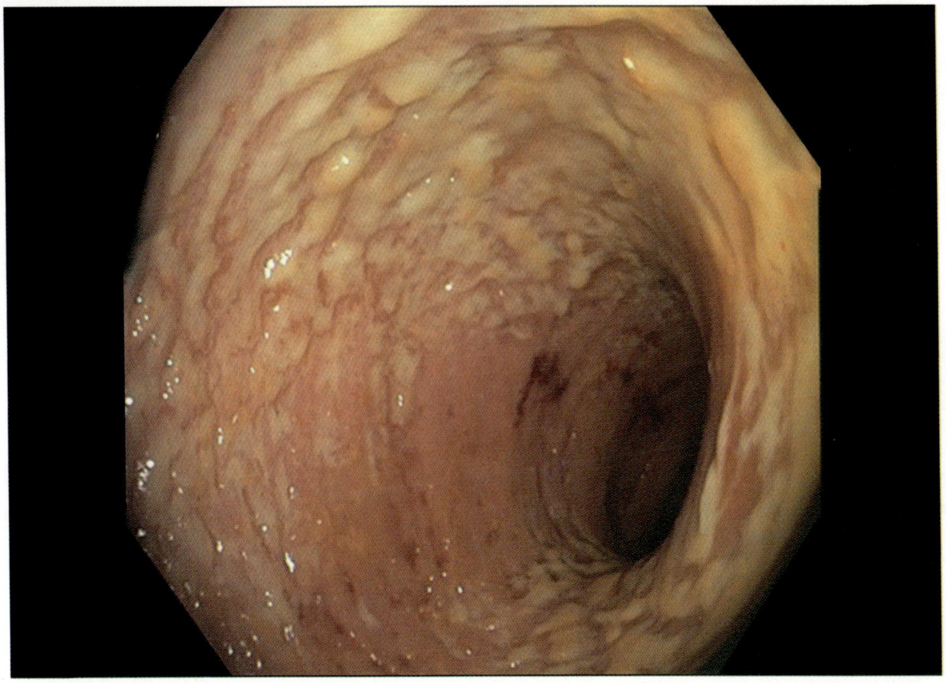

Fig. 3: Pseudomembranous colitis: Large colonic ulcers with yellowish pseudomembrane coating the surface of ulcers.

- Pseudomembranous colitis refers formation of yellowish pseudomembranes covering the surface of ulcers due to exudates and can be seen in variety of inflammatory diseases of colon, but most commonly associated with *Clostridium difficile* infection.

Colonic Ulcer (Fig. 4)

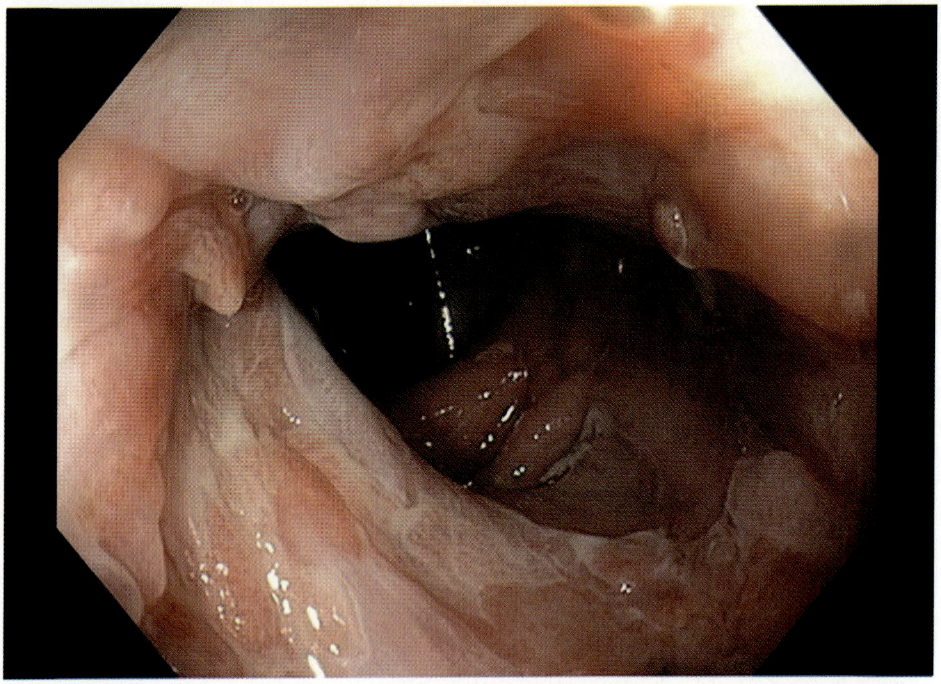

Fig. 4: Colonic ulcer: Circumferential ulcer in the colon causing partial luminal narrowing indicative of possible tubercular etiology.

- Circumferential ulcer involving colon (commonly ascending colon and cecum) with partial luminal narrowing is commonly suggestive of tubercular stricture secondary to *Mycobacterium tuberculosis* infection especially in Indian setting.
- Biopsies are required to confirm the diagnosis. Tissue culture and Gene Xpert Tb-PCR may help increasing the yield of diagnosis.

Colonic Crohn's (Fig. 5)

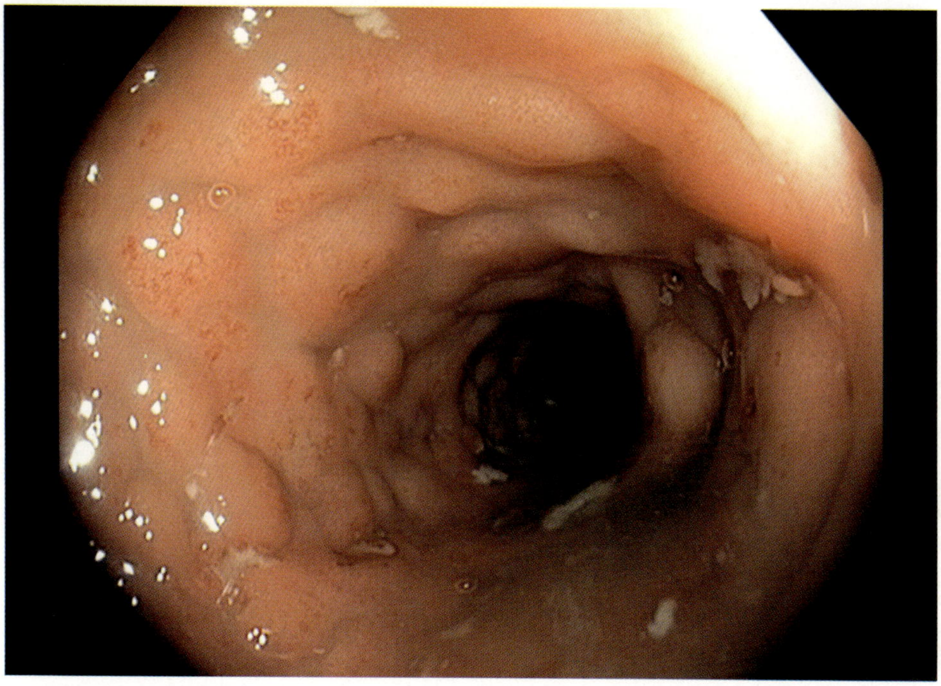

Fig. 5: Colonic Crohn's: Multiple colonic ulcers with cobblestoning of colonic mucosa suggestive of Crohn's disease.

- Multiple longitudinal or long segment ulcers with intervening normal areas (Skip areas) and cobblestoning pattern is seen in patients with Crohn's disease.
- Associated involvement of ileum and other parts of GI tract may be strong indicator of inflammatory bowel disease (IBD).

Stercoral Rectal Ulcers (Fig. 6)

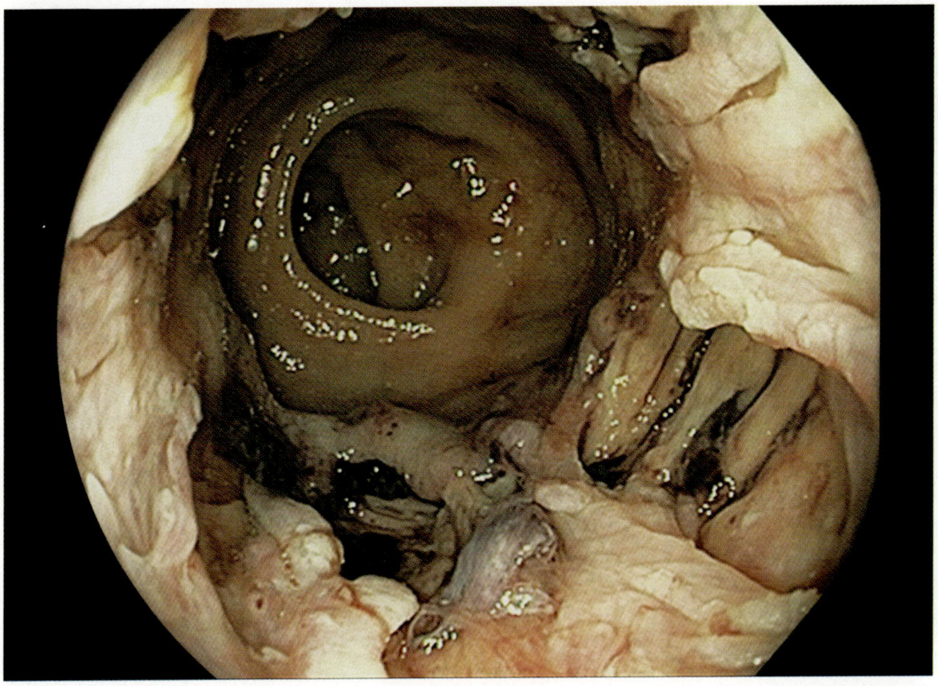

Fig. 6: Stercoral rectal ulcers: Large deep excavated ulcers approximately 2 cm in length extending up to muscularis layer in the rectum with smooth margins.

- Formed secondary to pressure effects on the rectal mucosa due to impacted hard stools following chronic constipation especially in bed ridden patients and intensive care unit (ICU) settings.
- Clinical presentation is usually in the form of lower GI bleed. Endoscopic therapy with or without rectal packing is required control the GI bleed.
- Treatment of constipation and removal of hard stools help treat and prevent these ulcers.

Crohn's Ileitis (Fig. 7)

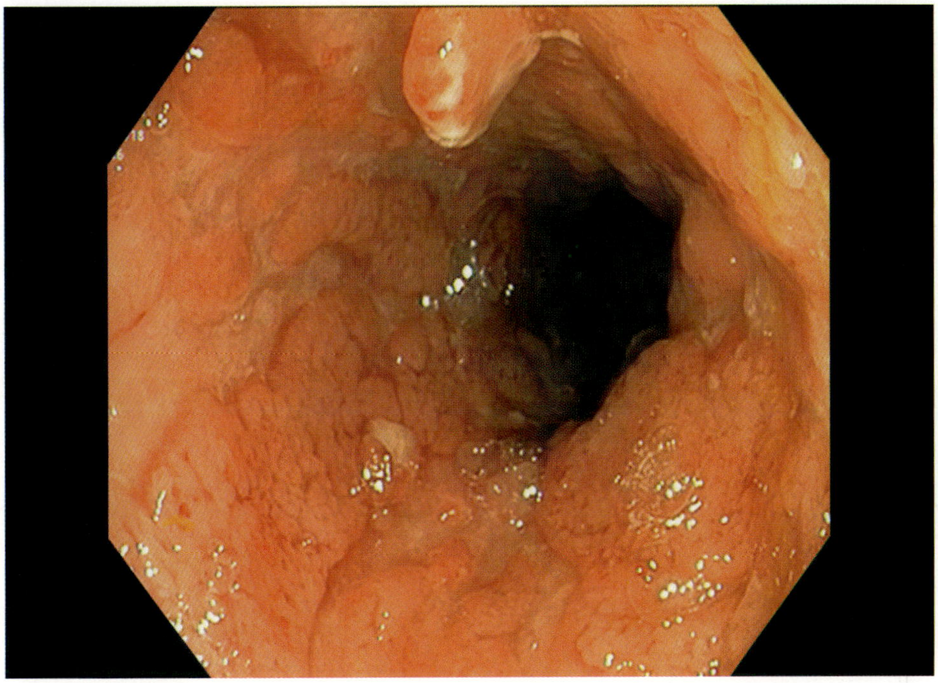

Fig. 7: Crohn's Ileitis: Deep longitudinal linear ulcers in the ileum with surrounding hypertrophied edematous mucosa—cobblestoning.

- Deep longitudinal linear ulcers with cobblestoning pattern seen in patients with Crohn's disease.
- Segmental involvement of ileum can occur with or without colonic involvement.

Perianal Fistula (Fig. 8)

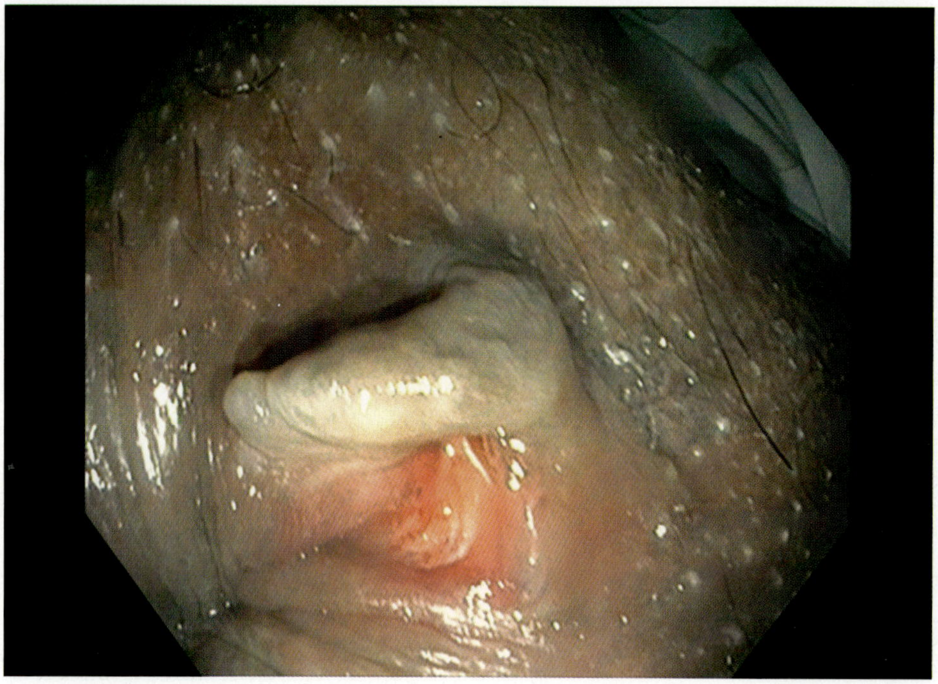

Fig. 8: Perianal fistula: Opening in the peri anal region in patient with Crohn's disease from a fistulous tract communicating with intestinal tract.

- Perianal fistula formation occurs in about 20–30% patients of Crohn's disease and commonly presents as purulent discharge from the fistulous opening.

Radiation Proctitis (Fig. 9)

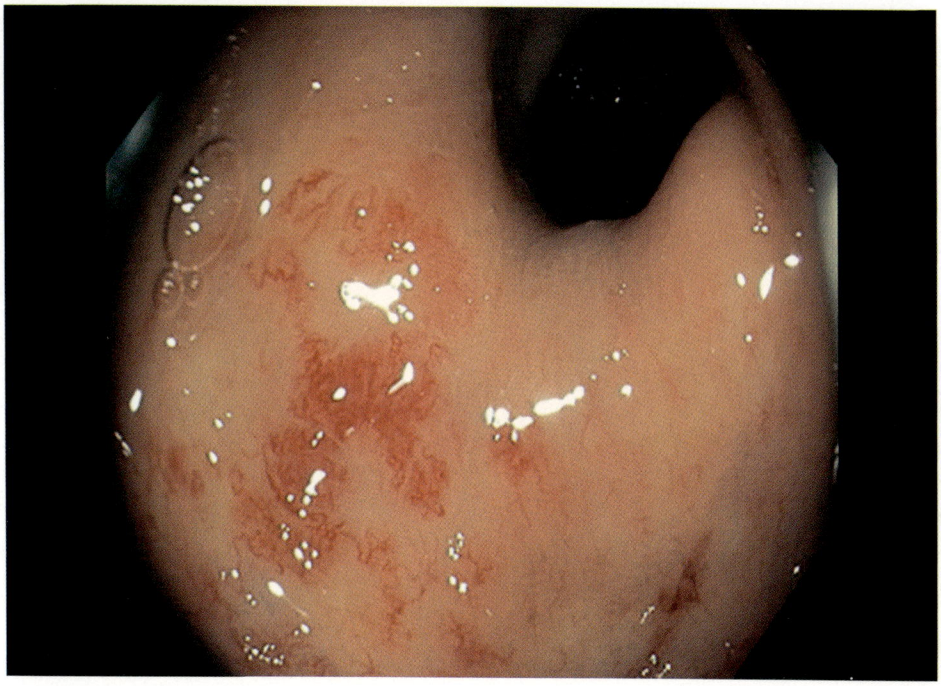

Fig. 9: Radiation proctitis: Rectal mucosal neovascularization causing telangiectasias seen in patients following radiation therapy.

- Presents as per rectal bleed. Past history of radiation therapy is present.
- Endoscopy shows multiple telangiectasias with friability and may bleed with spontaneously or on contact with scope.
- Treatment with fulguration using Argon plasma coagulation (APC) helps in controlling active bleed.

Ulcerative Colitis (Fig. 10)

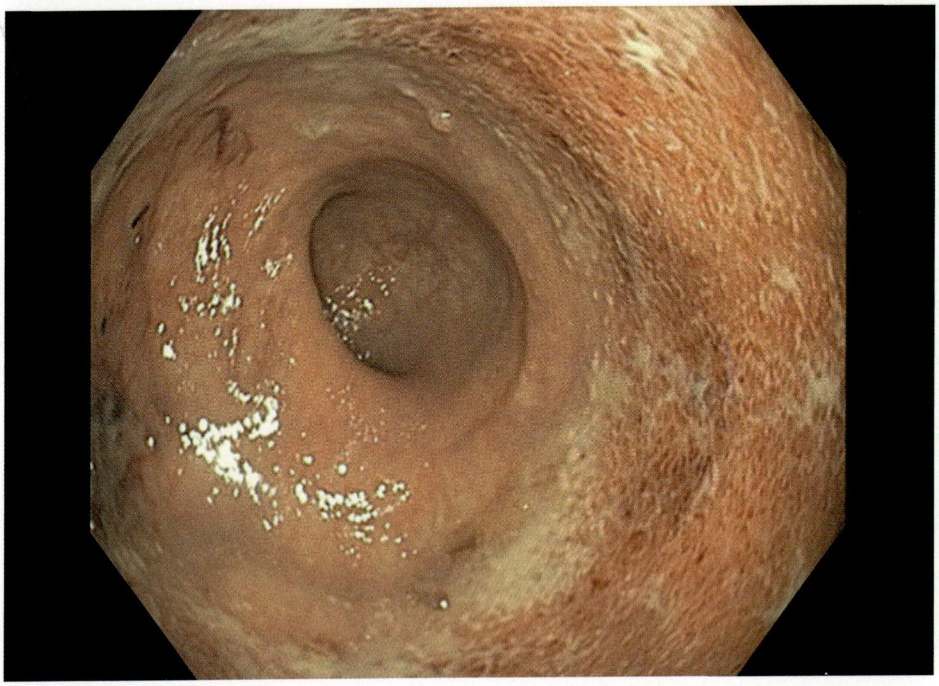

Fig. 10: Ulcerative colitis: Mucosa with continuous involvement with loss of vascular pattern, erythema and ulcerations with demarcation line between normal and diseased area.

- Represents other end of spectrum of IBD with continuous involvement of colonic mucosa from rectum to varying length of colon.
- Usually a demarcation line can be noted between involved and uninvolved mucosa.
- Various scoring systems are available for assessment of severity of disease.

DUODENAL LESIONS (FIGS. 11 TO 15)

Duodenal Nodule (Fig. 11)

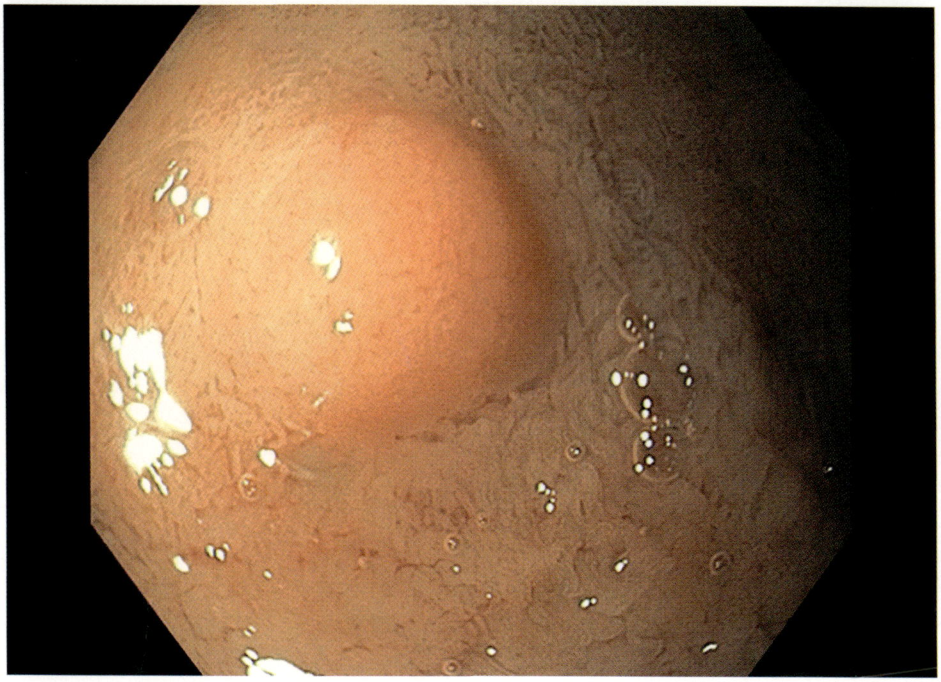

Fig. 11: Duodenal nodule: Subepithelial swelling/nodule with normal overlying mucosa—requires evaluation with EUS—possible D/D—GIST/NET/Carcinoid.

- Usually seen in the duodenal bulb, can be incidental finding or rarely may present as cause of GI bleed.
- It arises from subepithelial layer and requires endoscopic ultrasound (EUS) to determine layer of origin and determine further management.

Benign Duodenal Stricture (Fig. 12)

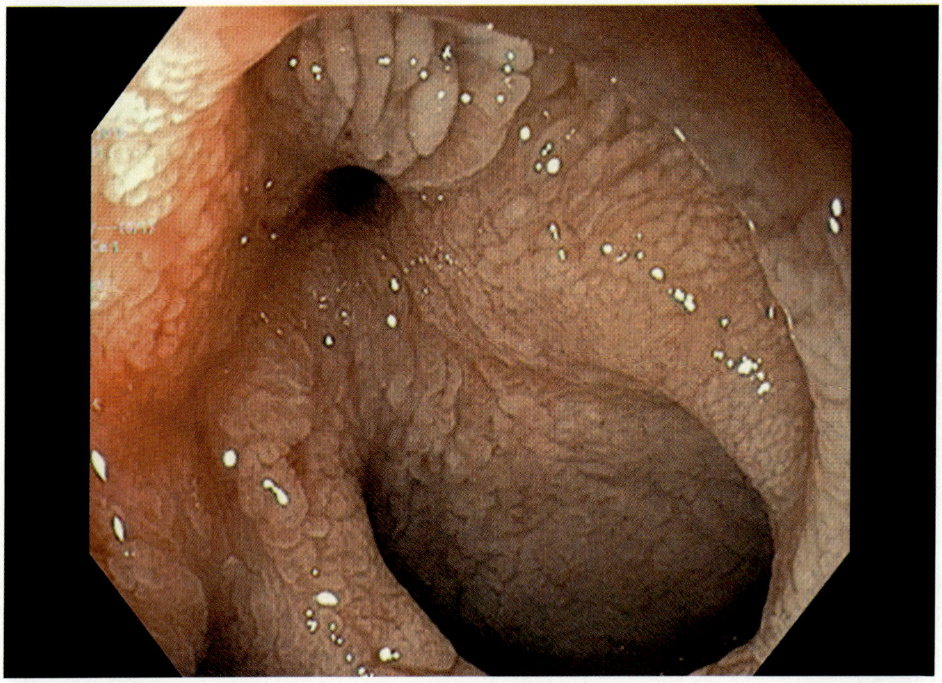

Fig. 12: Benign duodenal stricture: Pin head luminal narrowing with pseudodiverticulum formation—secondary to peptic ulcer disease.

- Duodenal stricture commonly presents with features of gastric outlet obstruction.
- Management can be done endoscopically by stricture dilatation or surgically.

Large Duodenal Ulcer (Fig. 13)

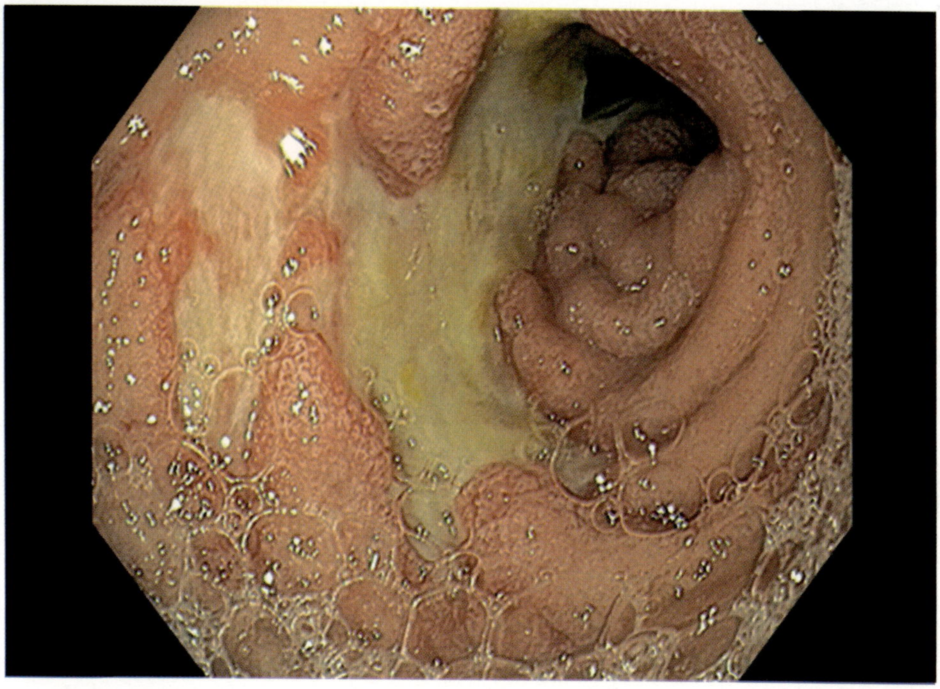

Fig. 13: Large duodenal ulcer—Clean-based large variegate duodenal ulcer extending from duodenal bulb into second part of duodenum.

- Duodenal ulcer bleed is the leading cause of upper GI bleed worldwide. Most duodenal ulcer bleed are managed with proton pump inhibitor (PPI) with or without endoscopic therapy depending upon the grading of duodenal ulcer.
- Eight weeks of high dose PPI therapy is required for adequate management of duodenal ulcer disease.

Periampullary Carcinoma (Fig. 14)

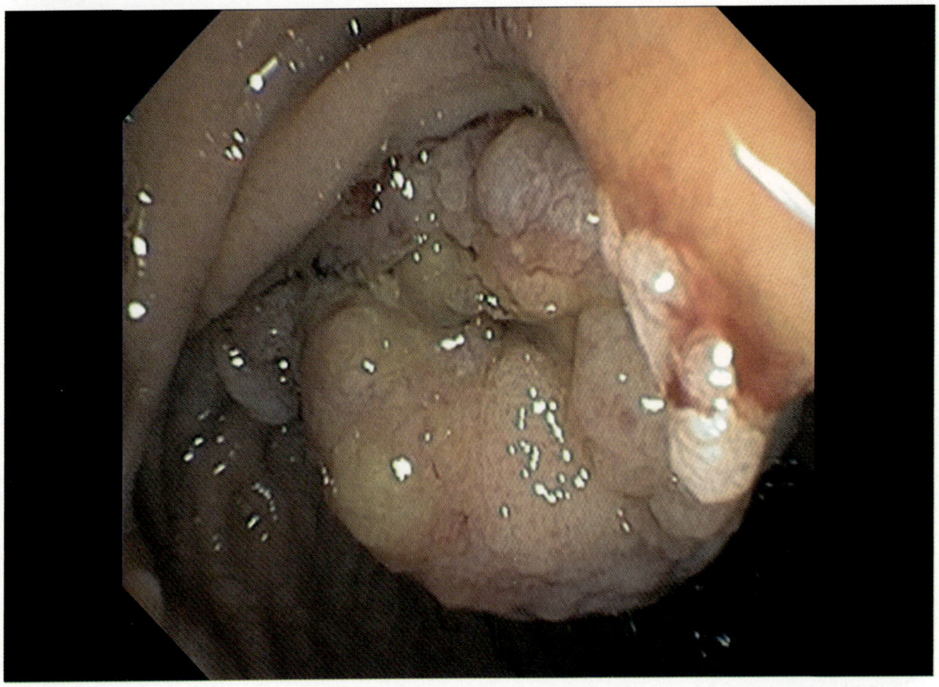

Fig. 14: Periampullary carcinoma: Ulceroproliferative growth in the ampullary region with bile flowing to the ampullary orifice.

- Periampullary carcinoma can present as painless obstructive jaundice.
- Palliative biliary stenting may be done in unresectable disease in cases of symptomatic obstructive jaundice.

Celiac Disease (Fig. 15)

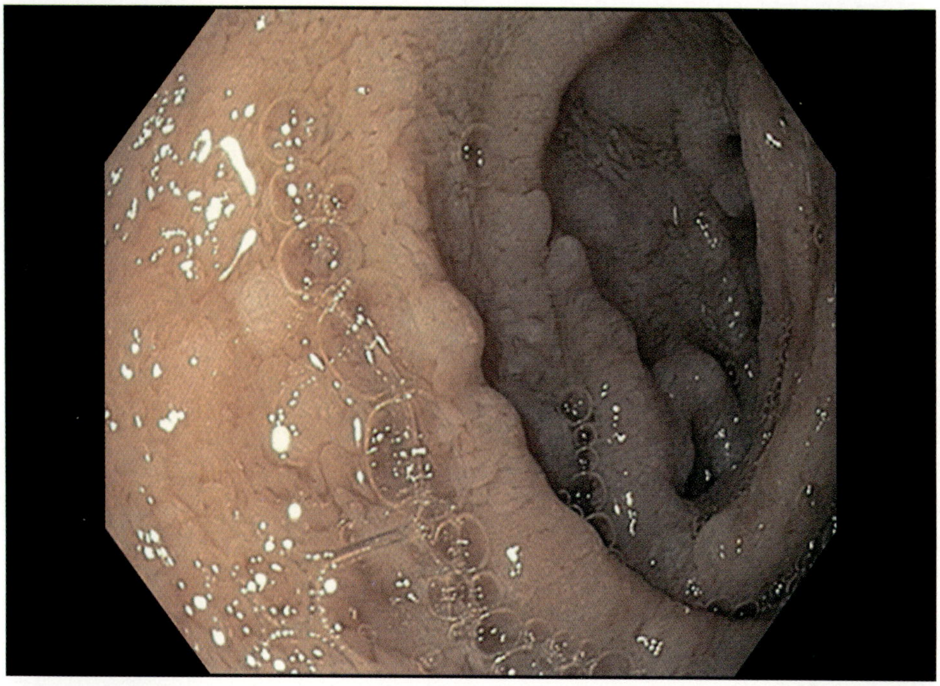

Fig. 15: Celiac disease: Scalloping of the mucosal folds in the second part of duodenum commonly seen in patient with celiac disease.

- Celiac disease occurs due to gluten hypersensitivity, with varying clinical presentation.
- Diagnosis is confirmed by endoscopic biopsies along with immunoglobulin A (IgA) anti-tissue transglutaminase (tTG) antibodies.

ESOPHAGEAL LESIONS (FIGS. 16 TO 27)

Esophageal Varices (Fig. 16)

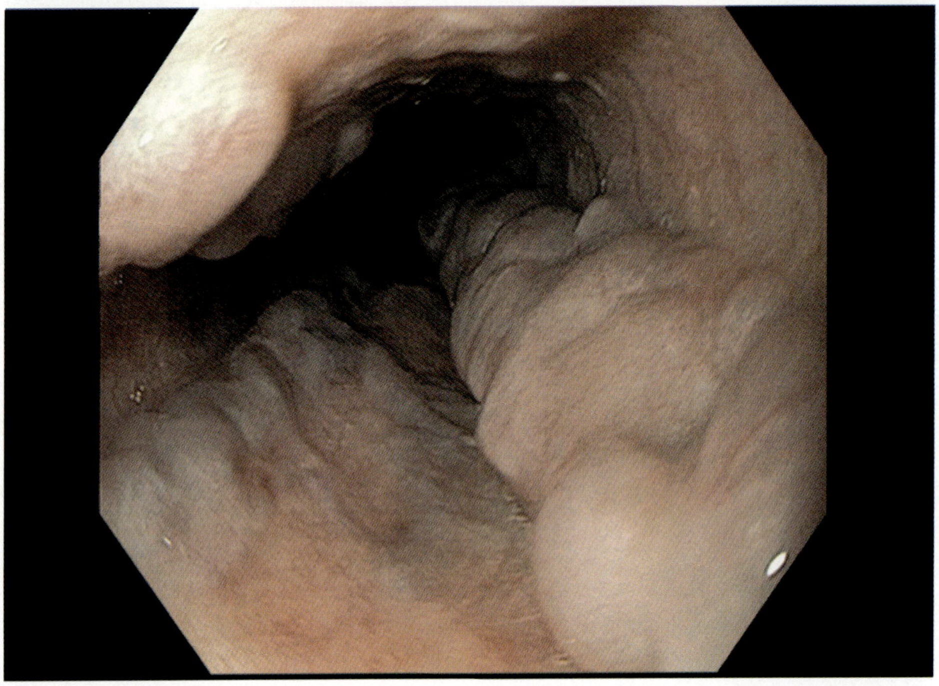

Fig. 16: Large esophageal varices: Three columns of dilated tortous venous columns running vertically.

- Esophageal varices is a common cause of upper GI bleed in patients with cirrhosis of liver.
- It is a marker of portal hypertension.

Esophageal Variceal Bleed (Fig. 17)

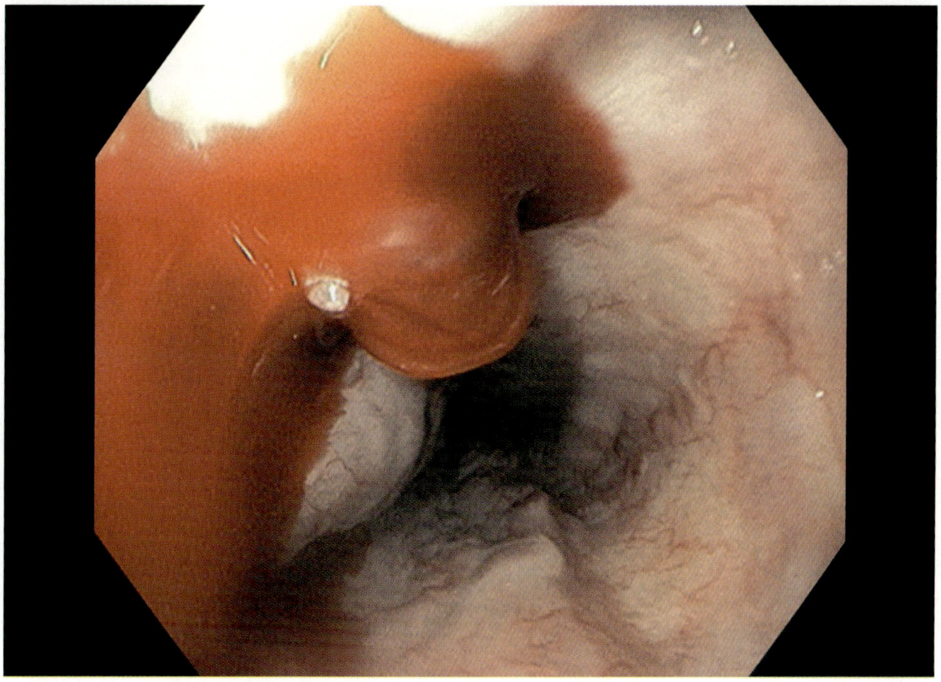

Fig. 17: Active bleed: Active spurt of bleed from variceal column.

- Esophageal variceal bleed can be life-threatening presenting as massive upper GI bleed and requires urgent endoscopic therapy (endoscopic variceal band ligation/sclerotherapy) to control the bleed along with adequate hemodynamic resuscitation and terlipressin/somatostatin.

Esophageal Candidiasis (Fig. 18)

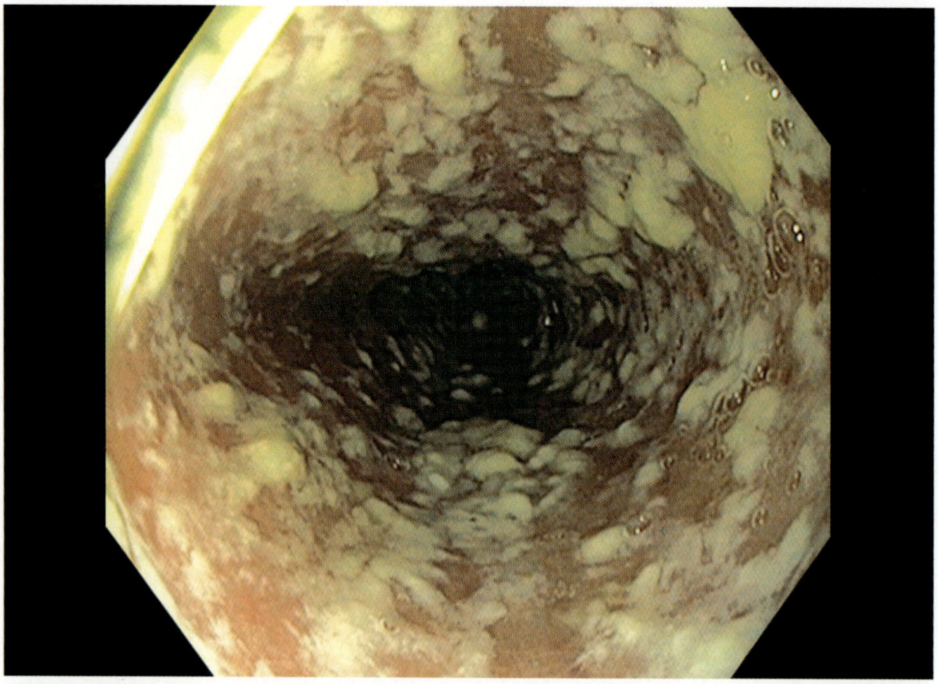

Fig. 18: Esophageal candidiasis: Curdy white plaques which are difficult to wash overlying the esophageal mucosa.

- Commonly seen in immunocompromised states/steroid therapy.
- It can present as dysphagia/odynophagia and requires adequate antifungal therapy.

Esophageal Fistula (Fig. 19)

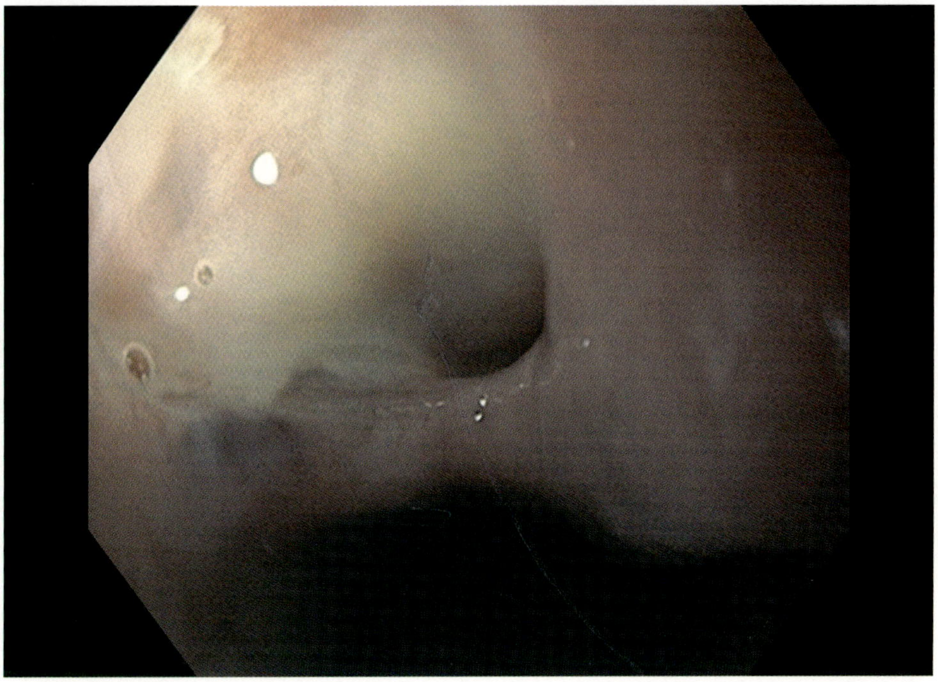

Fig. 19: Esophageal fistula: Defect in the esophageal wall with pus discharge (Communicating with mediastinum).

- Refers to defect in the esophageal wall communicating with the bronchial tree lumen or mediastinum.
- Tracheoesophageal fistula may be formed in patients with tuberculosis or post-traumatic/iatrogenic injuries.
- Common presentation may be coughing or features of aspiration pneumonia following intake of food.

Reflux Esophagitis (Fig. 20)

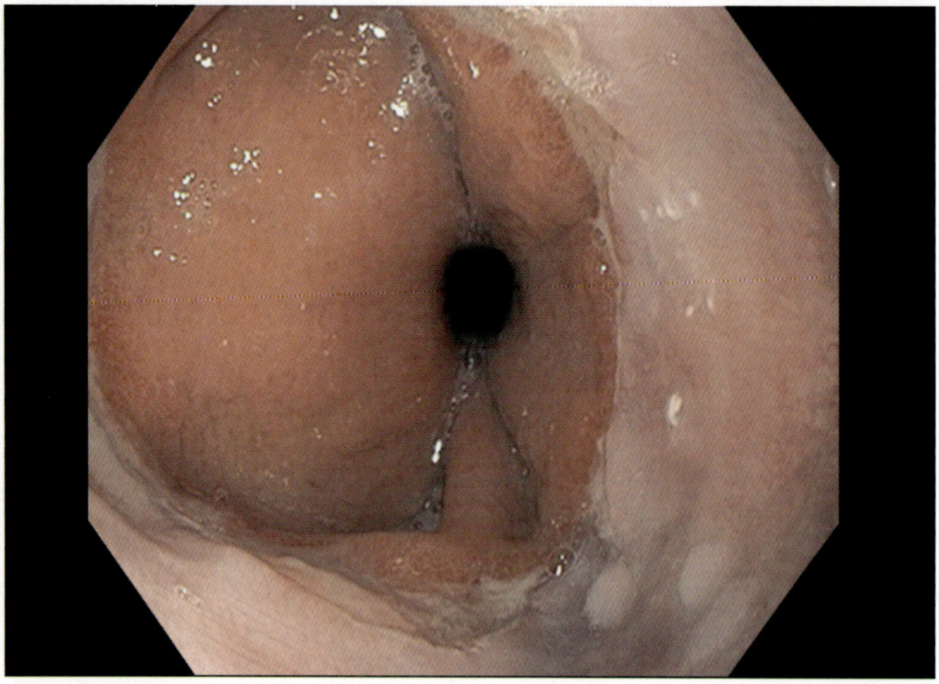

Fig. 20: Reflux esophagitis: Nonconfluent mucosal breaks at the Z line suggestive of reflux esophagitis.

- Reflux esophagitis is usually noted in patients with decreased lower esophageal sphincter (LES) tone resulting in reflux of gastric acid into esophageal lumen causing damage to esophageal mucosa to varying degrees.
- It commonly presents with features of dyspepsia. Esophageal ulceration may present as chest pain, odynophagia and rarely as GI bleed.

Hiatus Hernia (Fig. 21)

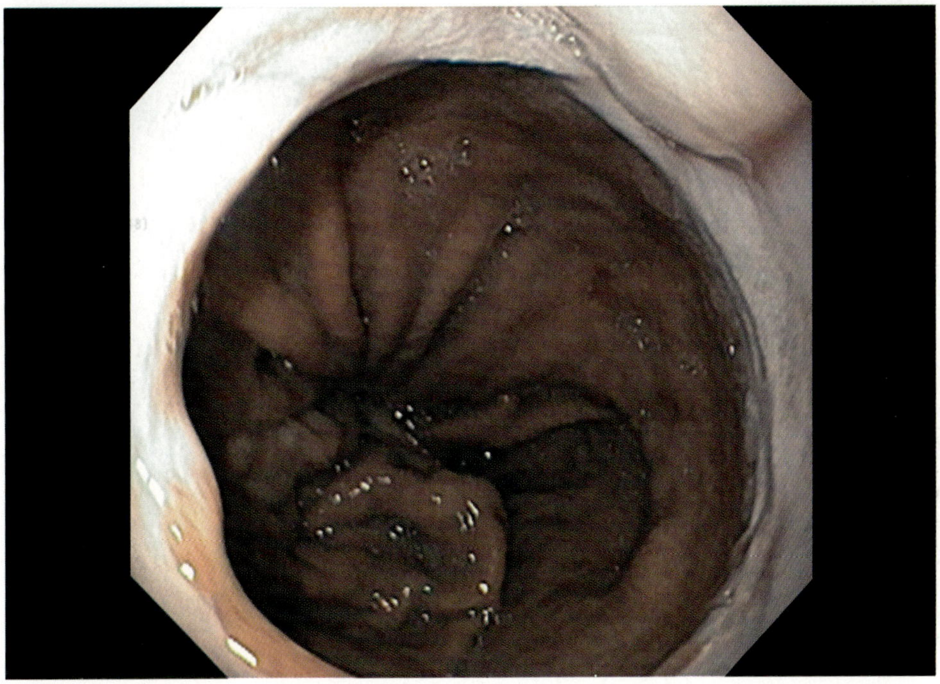

Fig. 21: Hiatus hernia: Hernia sac formed between the Z line and the diaphragmatic pinch.

- Hiatus hernia refers to formation of hernia sac at the level of esophageal hiatus on the diaphragm and is seen endoscopically as a sac forming between Z line and diaphragmatic pinch.
- Ulceration in the hiatal sac may present as a cause of obscure GI bleed which requires careful evaluation (known as Cameron ulcer).

Cameron Ulcer (Fig. 22)

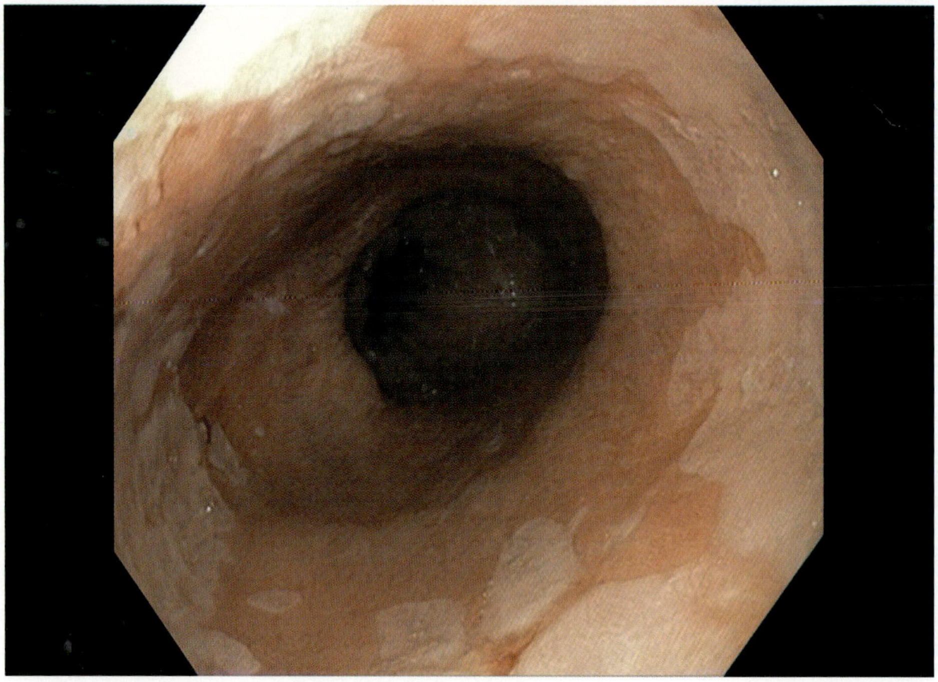

Fig. 22: Cameron ulcer: Linear clean-based ulcer in the hiatal sac seen at 3 o'clock position.

Barrett's Esophagus (Fig. 23)

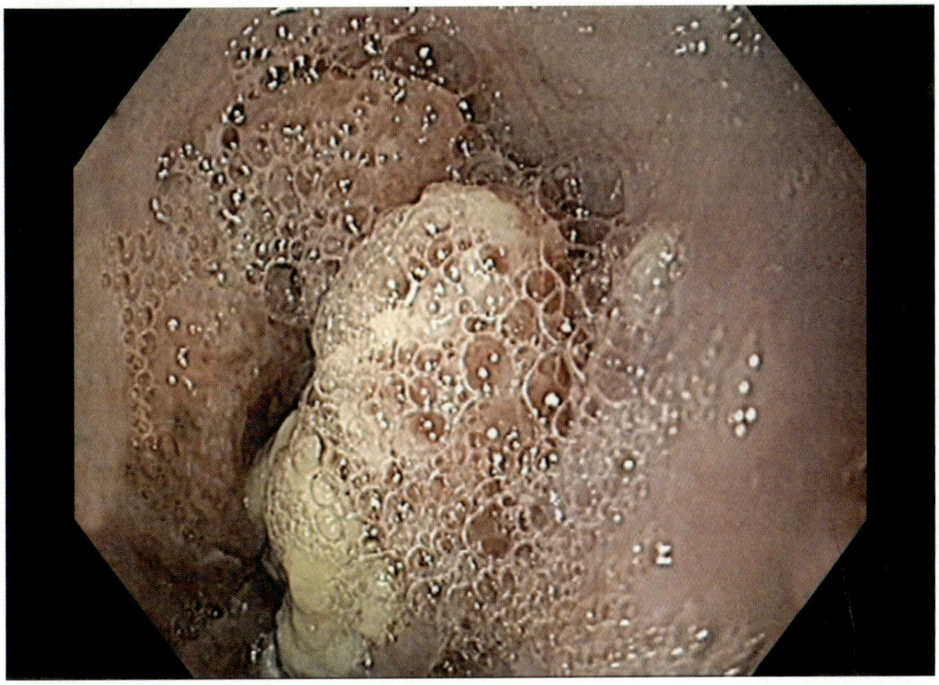

Fig. 23: Barrett's esophagus: Circumferential salmon-pink mucosa extending beyond the normal squamous cell epithelium with intestinal metaplasia.

- Barrett's esophagus refers to the intestinal metaplasia of the esophageal wall.
- Diagnosis is made by histological confirmation.
- It can be predecessor of esophageal adenocarcinoma and requires surveillance endoscopy to rule out dysplasia and malignancy.

Carcinoma Esophagus (Fig. 24)

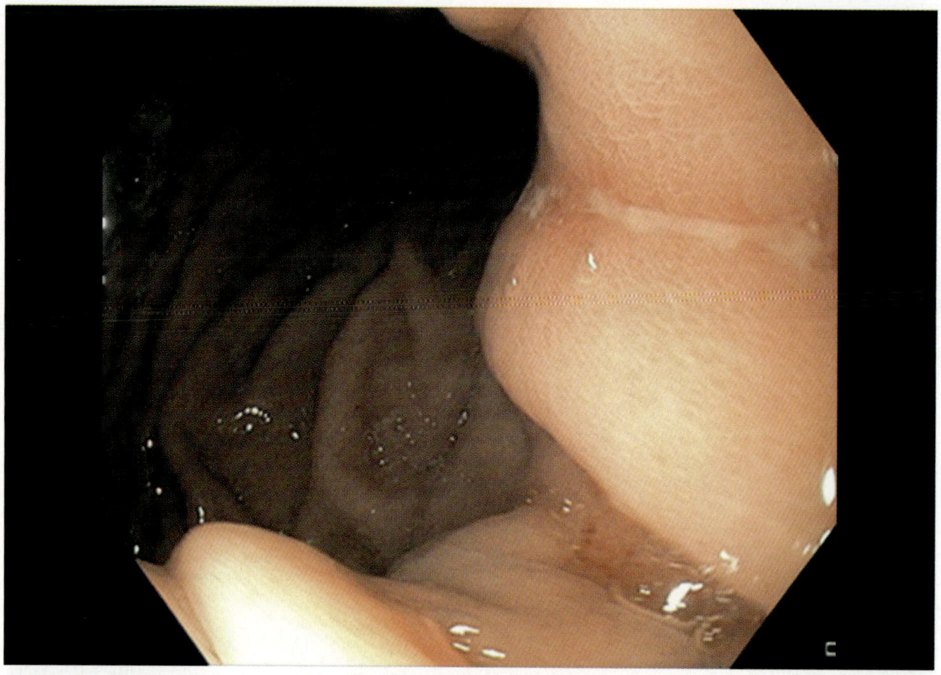

Fig. 24: Carcinoma esophagus: Ulceroproliferative growth in the esophagus causing luminal narrowing.

Esophageal Self-expanding Metal Stent (Fig. 25)

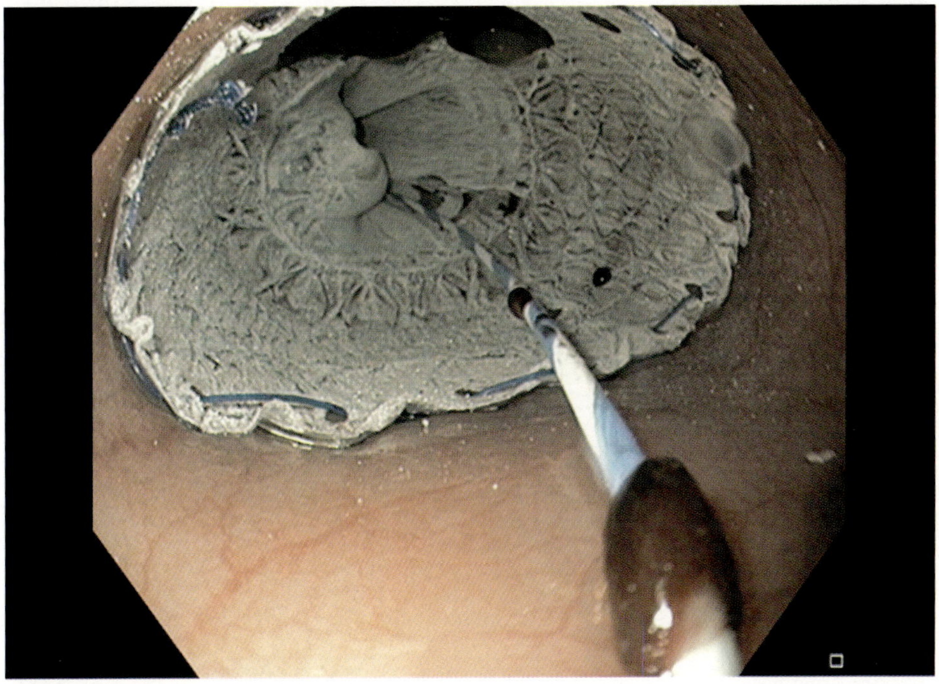

Fig. 25: Esophageal self-expanding metal stent (SEMS): Fully covered SEMS Tplaced in the esophagus in patients with malignant lesions in the esophagus.

- Fully covered self-expanding metal stent (SEMS) in patients with malignant lesions in the esophagus is placed in the esophageal lumen for palliation of dysphagia.

Benign Esophageal (Fig. 26)

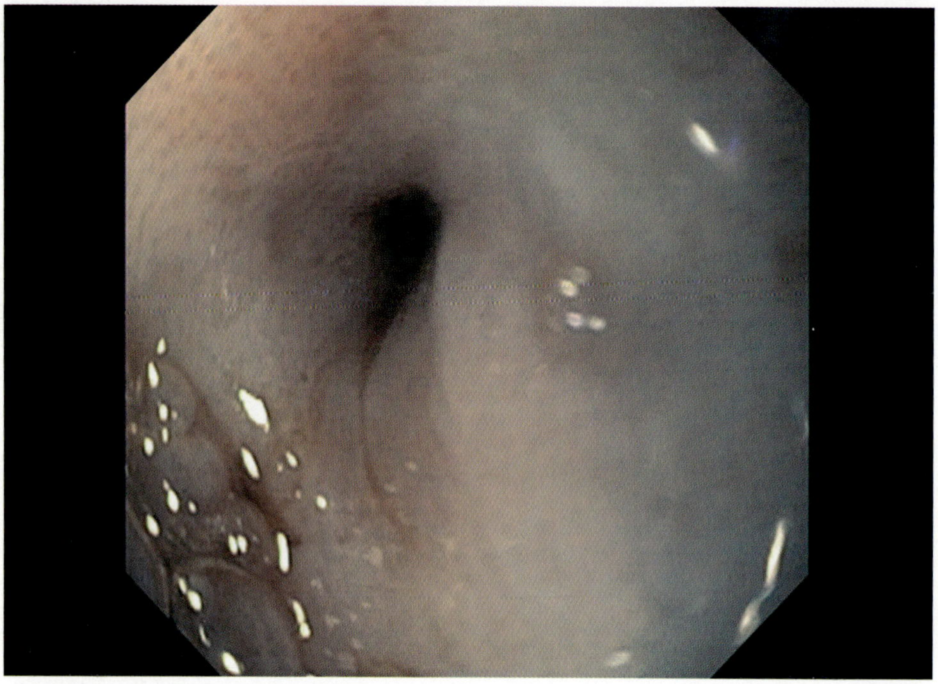

Fig. 26: Benign esophageal stricture: Smooth narrowing of the esophageal lumen at the lower end secondary to peptic stricture.

- Benign esophageal stricture can occur secondary to caustic ingestion or infections like tuberculosis, postradiation therapy or peptic esophageal disease.
- It can be managed with by endoscopic dilatation by bougie dilators (e.g. Savary-Gilliard dilators) or CRE balloon dilators.

Gastroesophageal Junction Carcinoma (Fig. 27)

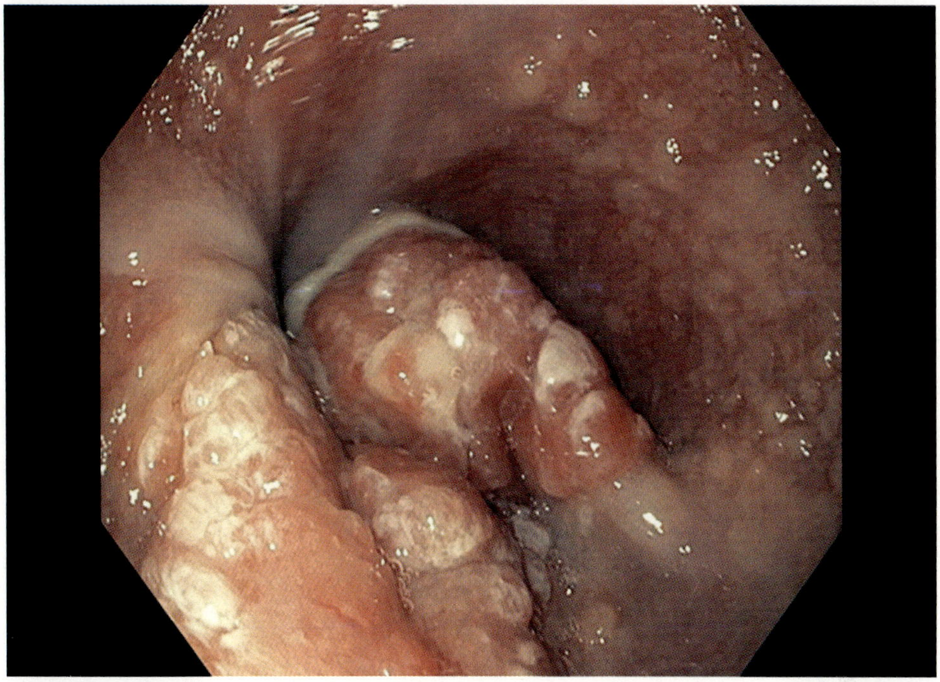

Fig. 27: Gastroesophageal (GE) junction carcinoma: Ulceroproliferative tumor at the lower end of esophagus extending into the cardia with friability.

- Gastroesophageal (GE) junction carcinoma refers tumors involving the GE junction (distal 3 cm of esophagus and proximal 2 cm of cardia of stomach).
- These can present with dysphagia or upper GI bleed.

STOMACH LESIONS (FIGS. 28 TO 35)

Fundal Varices (Fig. 28)

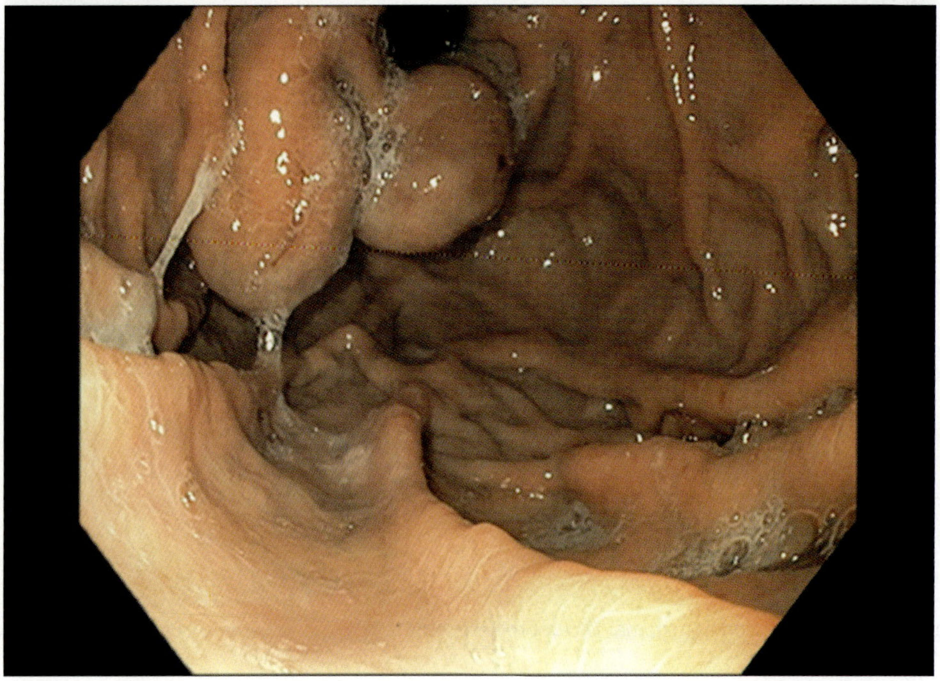

Fig. 28: Fundal varices: Submucosal venous channel in the stomach.

- Fundal varices refer to the submucosal venous channel seen as bulge in the fundus of the stomach.
- These can occur as continuation of esophageal varices or isolated gastric varices as single varix or bunch of varices.

Benign Gastric Ulcer (Fig. 29)

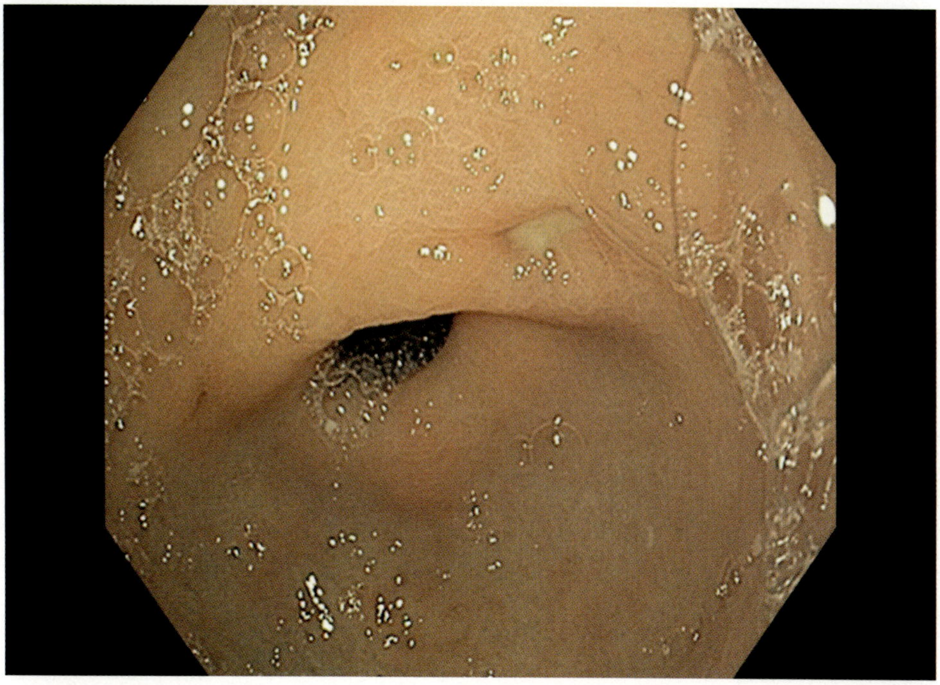

Fig. 29: Benign gastric ulcer: Clean-based ulcer in the antrum with sharp margins. No nodularity at the base of the ulcer.

- Gastric ulcer can present with dyspepsia or upper GI bleed.
- Common causes include drug induced, *Helicobacter pylori* related.
- Hemostatic endoscopic therapy may be required in active ulcer bleed followed by *H. pylori* eradication.

Gastric Antral Vascular Angioectasias (Fig. 30)

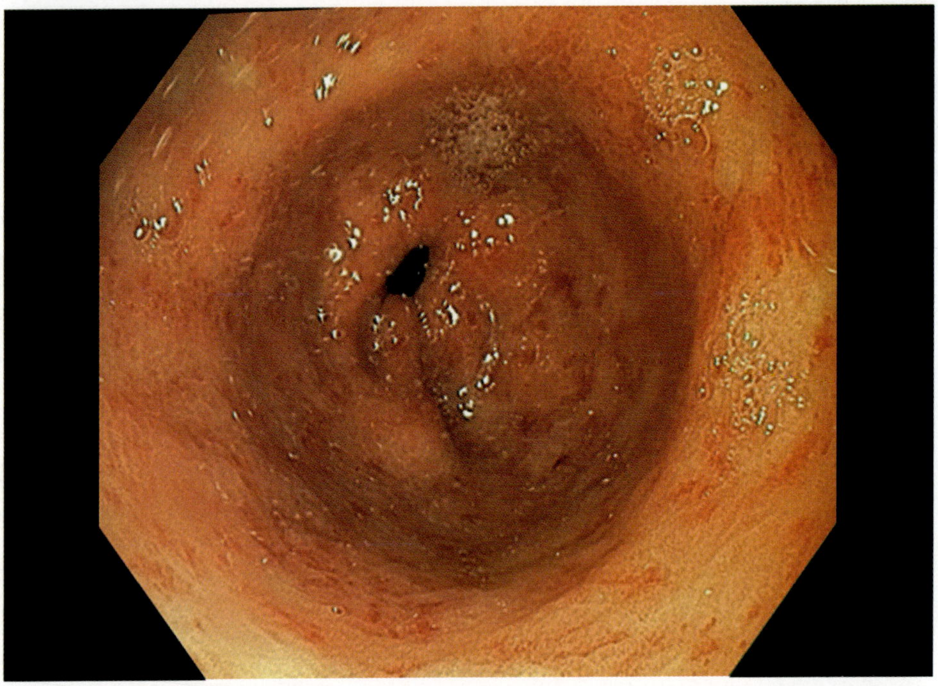

Fig. 30: Gastric antral vascular ectasias (GAVE): Vascular angioectasias in the gastric antrum secondary to chronic liver disease/chronic kidney disease CLD/CKD.

- Gastric antral vascular ectasias (GAVE) refers the vascular angioectasias which are abnormal small vessels which have friable walls and can bleed spontaneously.
- It can present as anemia or rarely melena. Active ooze can be managed by argon plasma coagulation (APC) fulguration.

Gastric Polyp (Fig. 31)

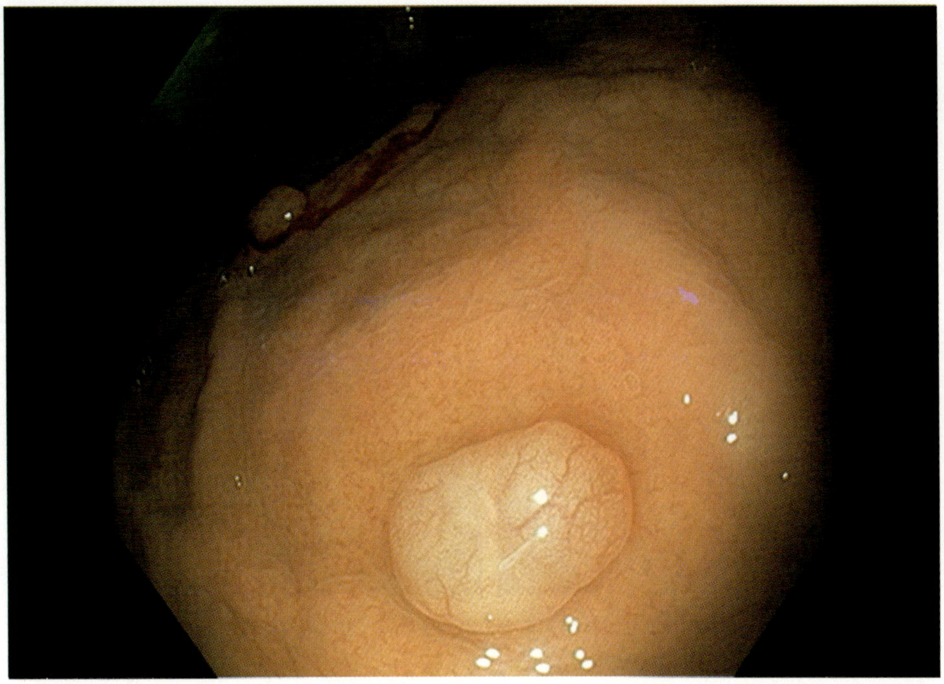

Fig. 31: Gastric polyp: 5 mm polyp with smooth mucosa above the surface of the stomach wall with fine lacy vessels—fundic gland polyp.

- Gastric polyps are frequently noted finding on endoscopic examination.
- Small sessile hyperplastic polyps are benign and can be associated with long-term PPI therapy.
- Hundreds of polyps can be noted in familial polyposis syndrome and require further evaluation.

Gastric Subepithelial Lesion (Figs. 32A and B)

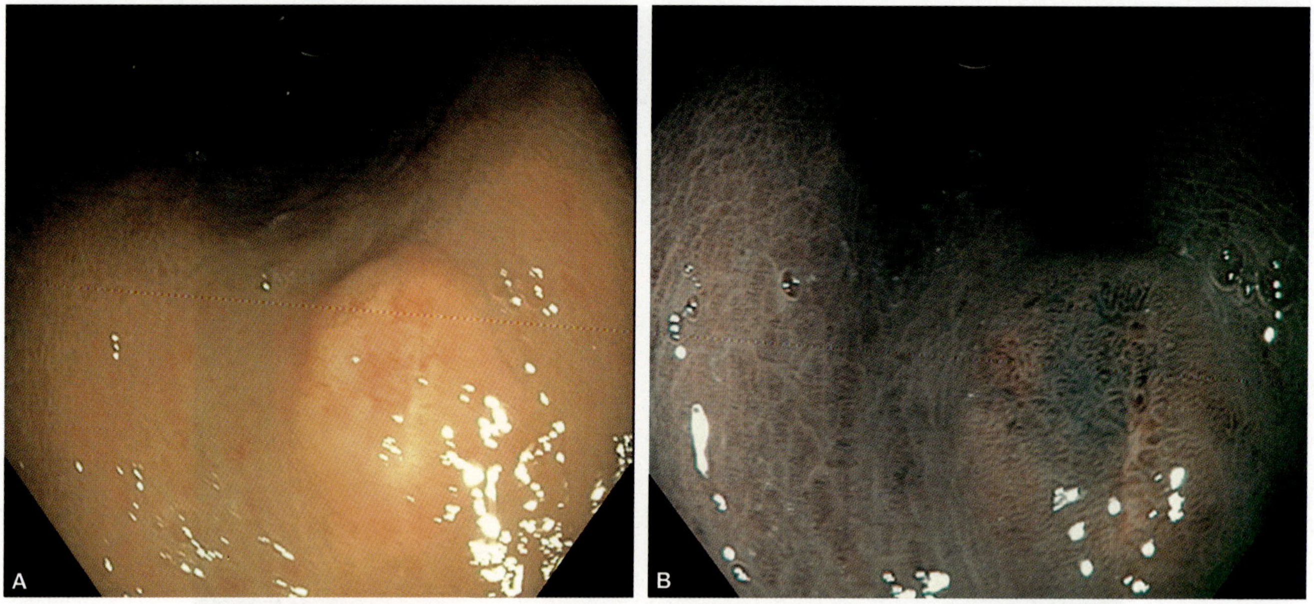

Figs. 32A and B: (A) Gastrointestinal stromal tumors (GISTs); (B) Narrow band imaging (NBI).

- 5 mm subepithelial lesion in the gastric body with central umbilication which shows end on capillaries on narrow band imaging (NBI) examination—neuroendocrine tumor of stomach.
- These can be incidental finding or present with GI bleed or paraneoplastic syndromes.
- Biopsies can help determine the nature of lesion and guide further therapy.

Gastric Cancer (Fig. 33)

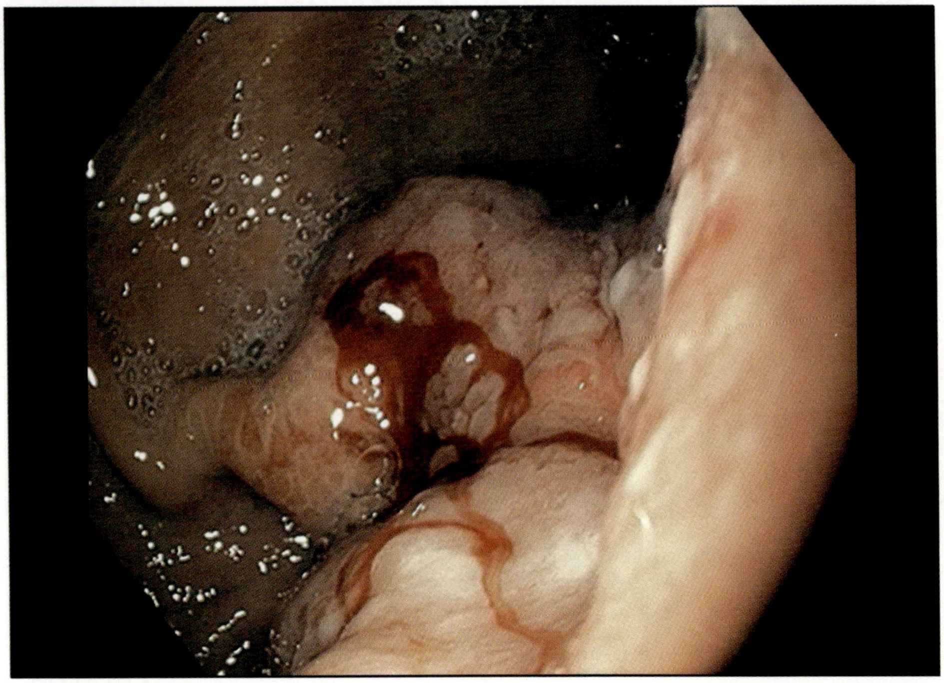

Fig. 33: Gastric cancer: Ulceroproliferative tumor in the gastric body with overlying ulceration and spontaneous ooze.

- Gastric cancer can present as a localized or diffuse involvement of the stomach.
- Ulceroproliferative tumors can have areas of necrosis/spontaneous oozing.
- Early gastric cancers can be diagnosed with careful endoscopic examination in suspect population groups by various image enhancement techniques.
- Further local staging can be done with help of EUS.

Linitis Plastica Stomach (Fig. 34)

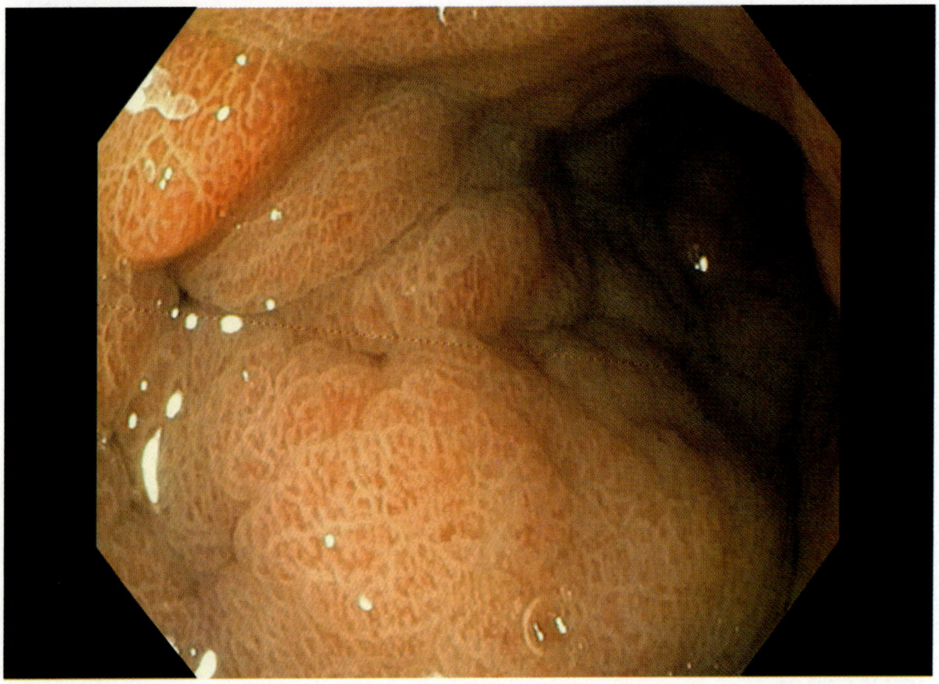

Fig. 34: Linitis plastica stomach: Hypertrophied gastric folds with lack of distensibility on insufflation.

- Linitis plastica refers to diffuse involvement of the stomach wall by invasive malignancy with thickened gastric folds reduced distensibility of the gastric lumen.
- Deep jumbo biopsies are warranted to ascertain the diagnosis.

Subepithelial GIST (Fig. 35)

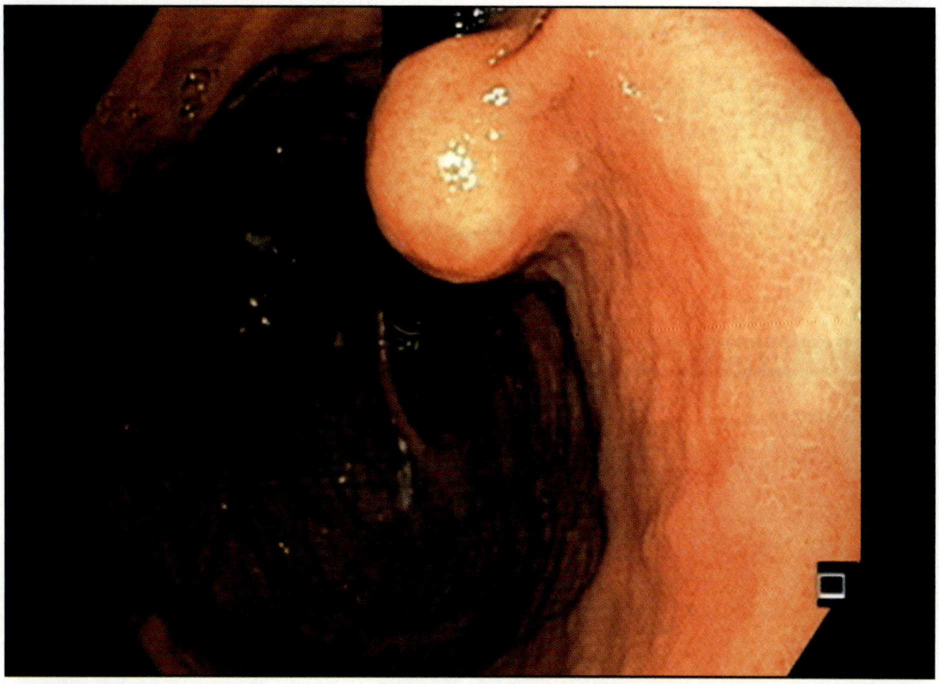

Fig. 35: Subepithelial gastrointestinal stromal tumor (GIST)—Subepithelial nodular lesion in the gastric wall with normal overlying mucosa suggestive of GIST.

- Subepithelial nodular lesions in the gastric wall with normal overlying mucosa suggestive of GIST.
- Subepithelial nodular lesions in stomach can be incidental finding or present as GI bleed.
- Evaluation with EUS to determine the nature of lesion followed by endoscopic or surgical treatment is required.

CHAPTER 12

Endoscopic and Radiological Images

BP Singh, Kaushal Madan

HEMATEMESIS AND SHOCK (FIGS. 1A TO C)

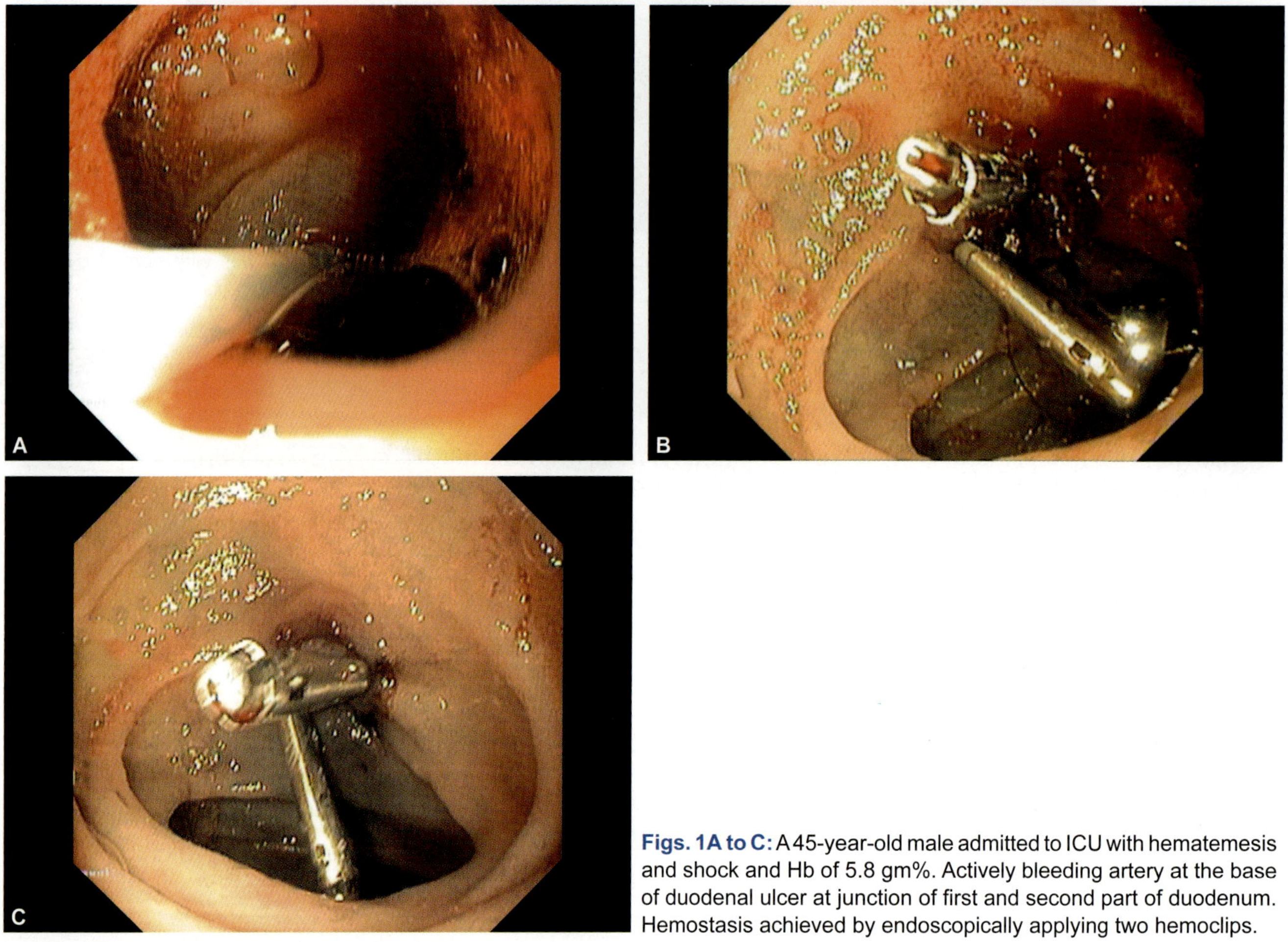

Figs. 1A to C: A 45-year-old male admitted to ICU with hematemesis and shock and Hb of 5.8 gm%. Actively bleeding artery at the base of duodenal ulcer at junction of first and second part of duodenum. Hemostasis achieved by endoscopically applying two hemoclips.

SIGMOIDOSCOPY WITH LARGE HEMORRHOIDS (FIGS. 2A AND B)

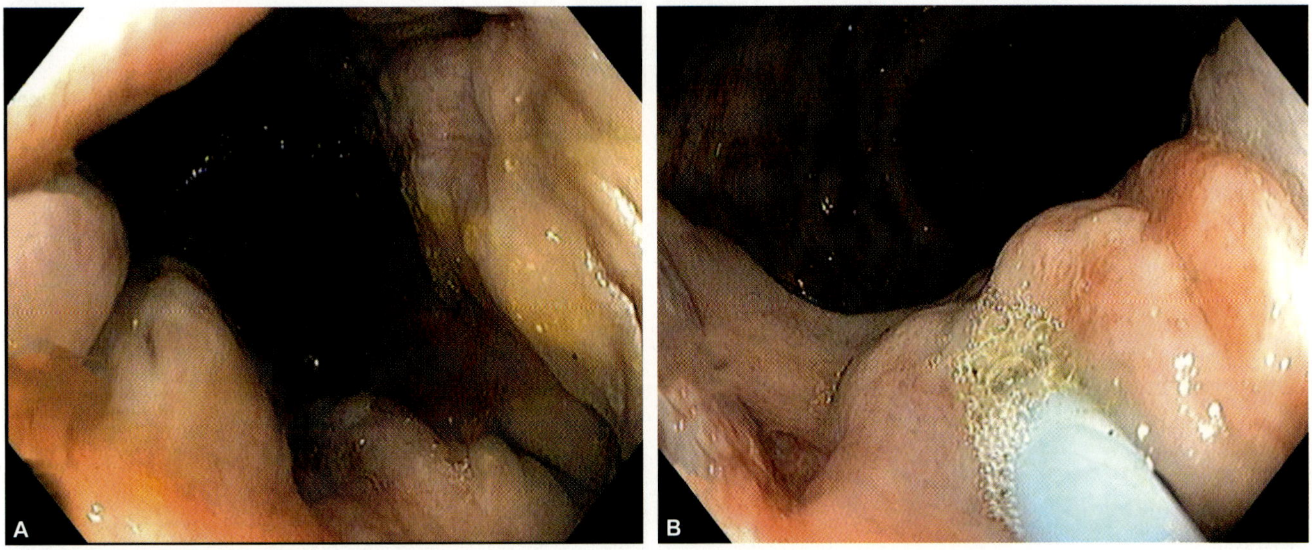

Figs. 2A and B: An 82-year-old male admitted in ICU and on ventilatory support for pneumonia with type 1 respiratory failure. On day 4 started having persistent bleeding PR. Sigmoidoscopy revealed large hemorrhoids—Injection sclerotherapy done with polidocanol 1%.

RECURRENT HEMATEMESIS (FIGS. 3A AND B)

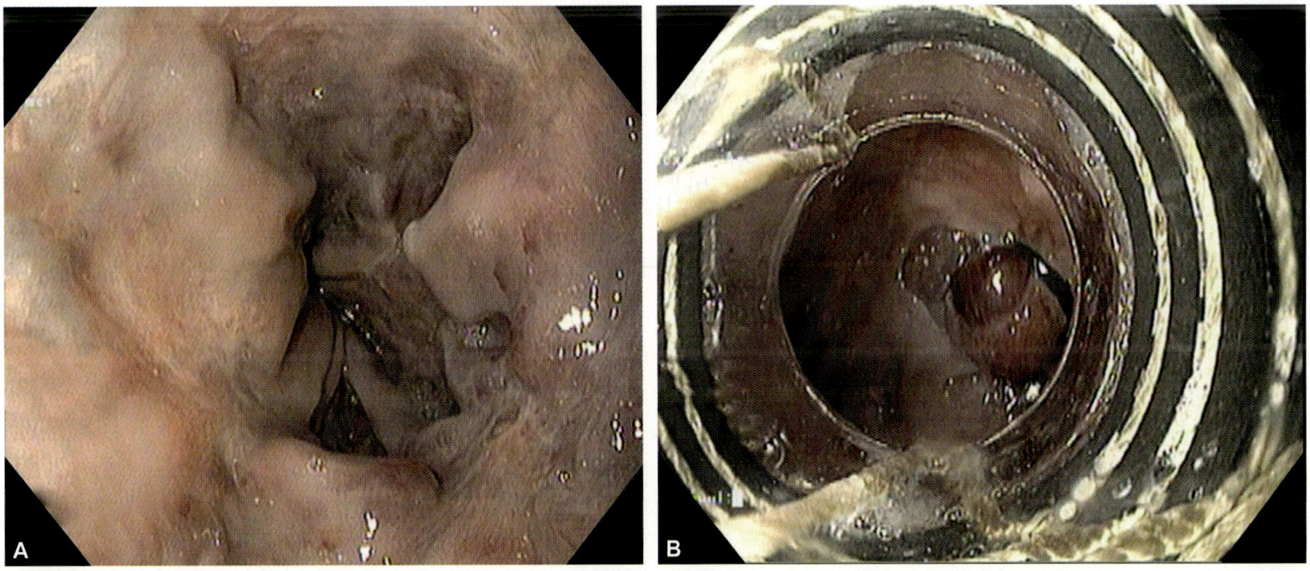

Figs. 3A and B: A 40-year-old patient with alcoholic cirrhosis admitted to ICU with recurrent hematemesis. Endoscopy revealed large esophageal varices with red colored signs: Endoscopic band ligation done.

FOOD BOLUS IN THE LOWER ESOPHAGUS (FIGS. 4A AND B)

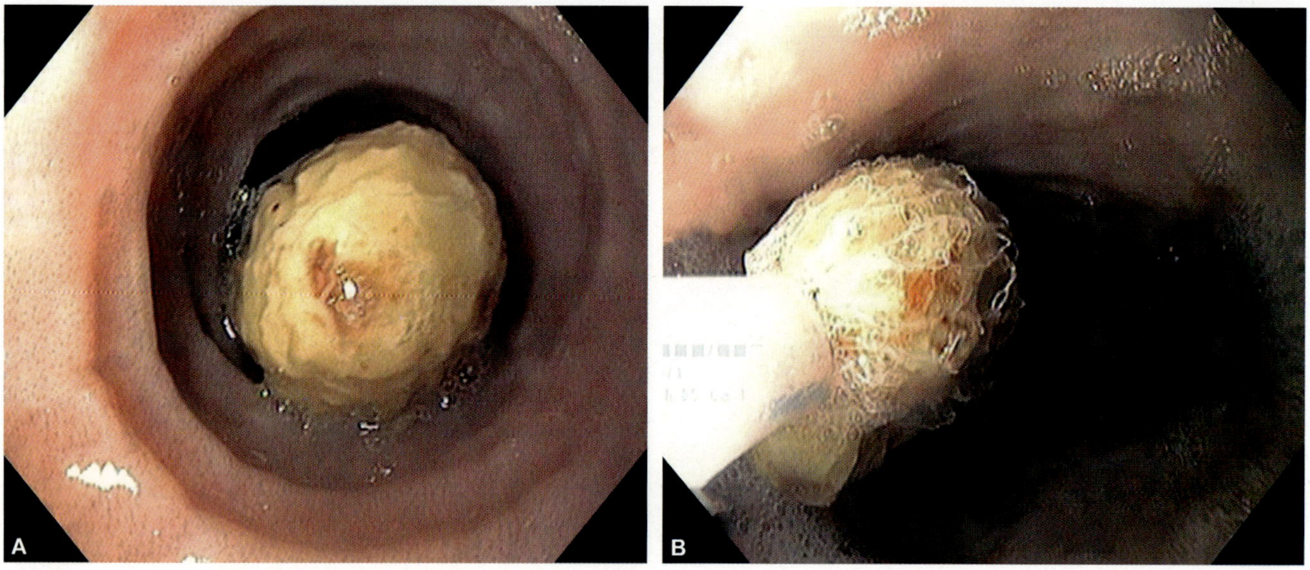

Figs. 4A and B: A 73-year-old lady presented with acute complete dysphagia with regurgitation of food, leading to aspiration. Upper gastrointestinal (UGI) endoscopy revealed a food bolus lodged in the lower esophagus due to a peptic stricture just above the gastroesophageal (GE) junction—Food bolus removed with Roth's net.

STAPLED HEMORRHOIDECTOMY (FIGS. 5A AND B)

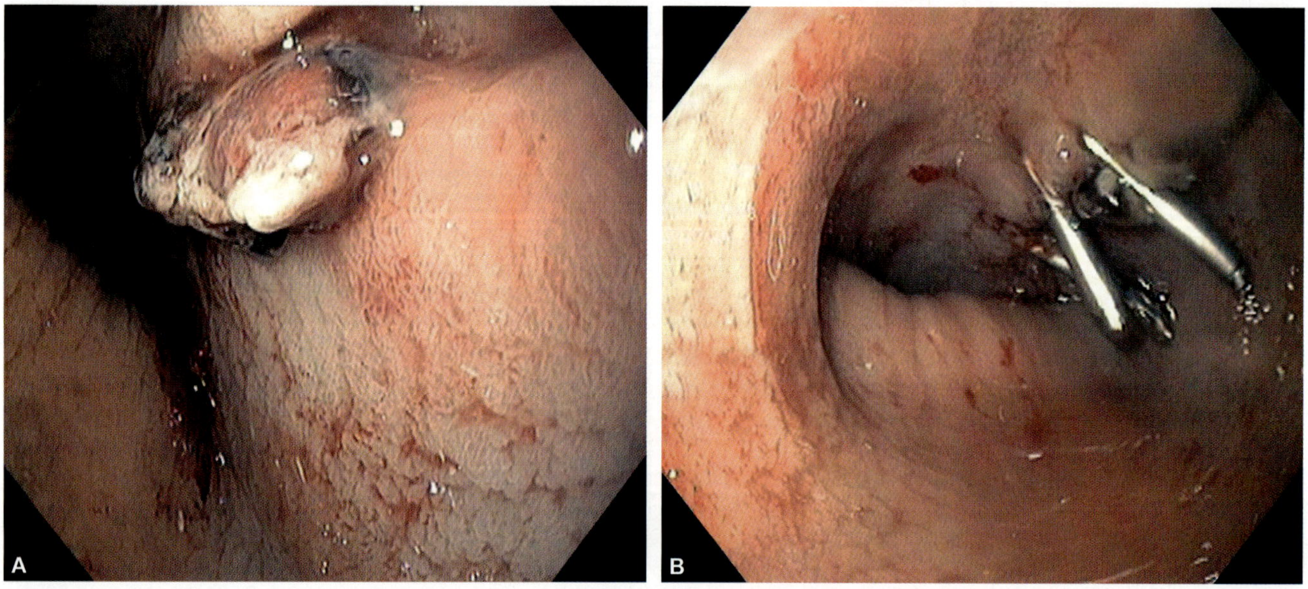

Figs. 5A and B: A 50-year-old male, after undergoing stapled hemorrhoidectomy, had hematemesis while he was in the postoperative ICU. UGI endoscopy revealed a deep Mallory Weiss tear with bleeding from the lower end of the tear. Hemostasis achieved with application of three hemoclips.

PERCUTANEOUS ENDOSCOPIC GASTROSTOMY (FIGS. 6A AND B)

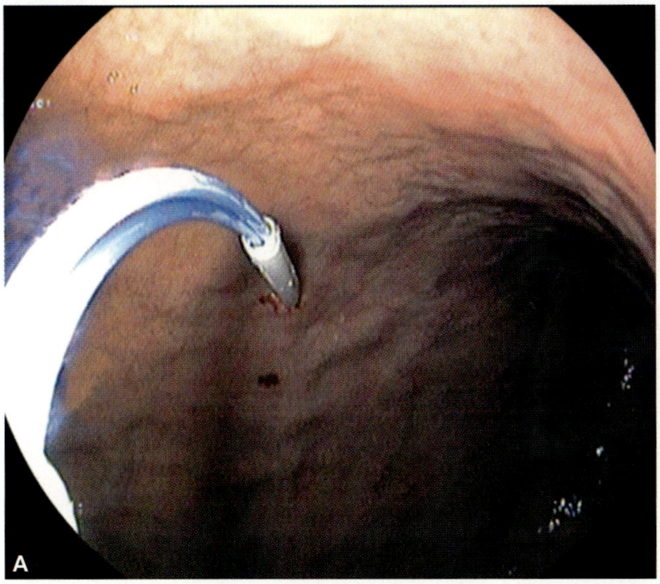

A

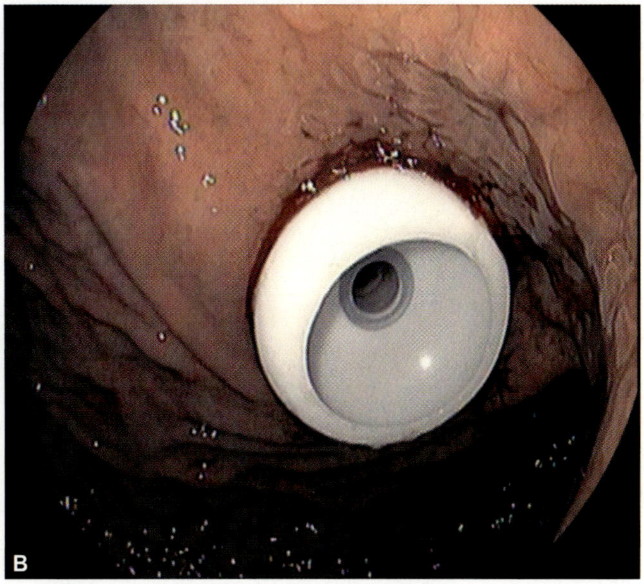

B

Figs. 6A and B: A 68-year-bedridden-old lady with multiple strokes, and transfer dysphagia: endoscopic placement of a percutaneous endoscopic gastrostomy (PEG) tube for long-term feeding—intragastric view of the bumper.

DILATED COMMON BILE DUCT IN MAGNETIC RESONANCE CHOLANGIOPANCREATOGRAPHY (FIG. 7)

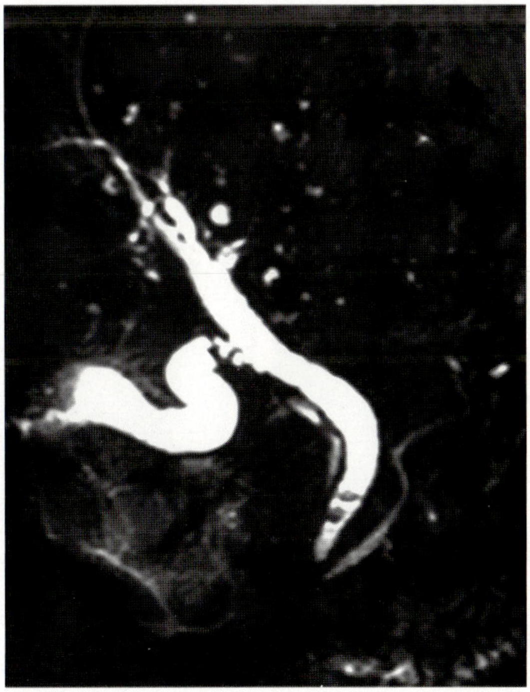

Fig. 7: A 30-year-old male was admitted with severe upper abdominal pain and high fever with chills and a bilirubin of 5.6 mg% suggestive of (s/o) cholangitis—magnetic resonance cholangiopancreatography (MRCP) revealed dilated common bile duct (CBD) of about 10 mm with two small filling defects in lower CBD (CBD stones).

RUPTURED HEPATOCELLULAR CARCINOMA (FIG. 8)

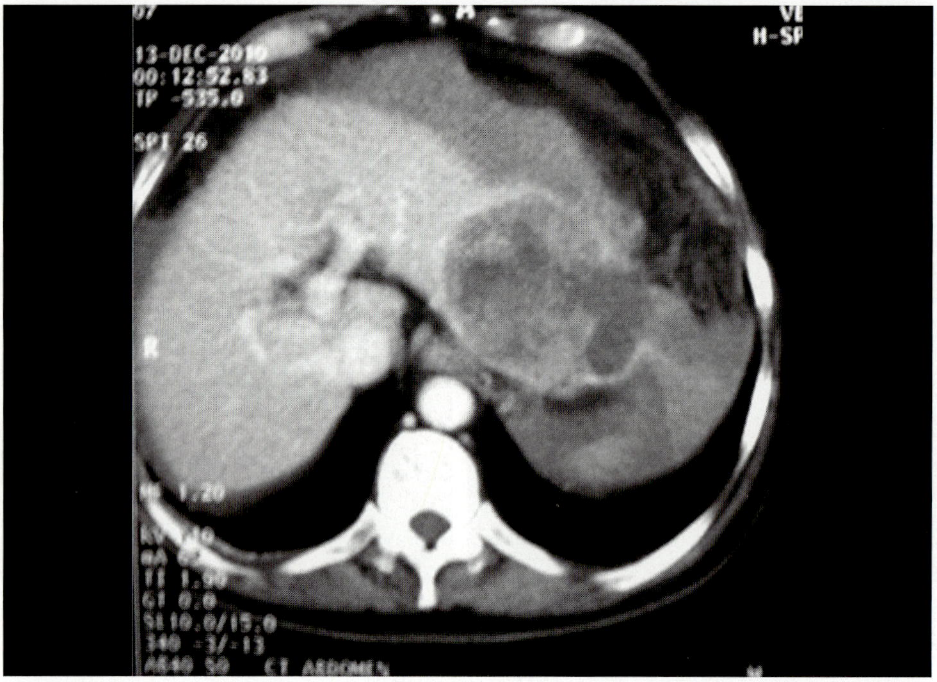

Fig. 8: A 55-year-old male who has chronic hepatitis B infection presented with acute abdomen, shock and Hb of 6.6 gm%. Triple phase contrast enhanced computed tomography (CECT) revealed a large left lobe space occupying lesion (SOL) with enhancement in arterial phase and wash out in delayed venous phase suggestive of hepatocellular carcinoma (HCC) with evidence of rupture and hemoperitoneum.

RUPTURED LARGE LIVER ABSCESS (FIGS. 9A AND B)

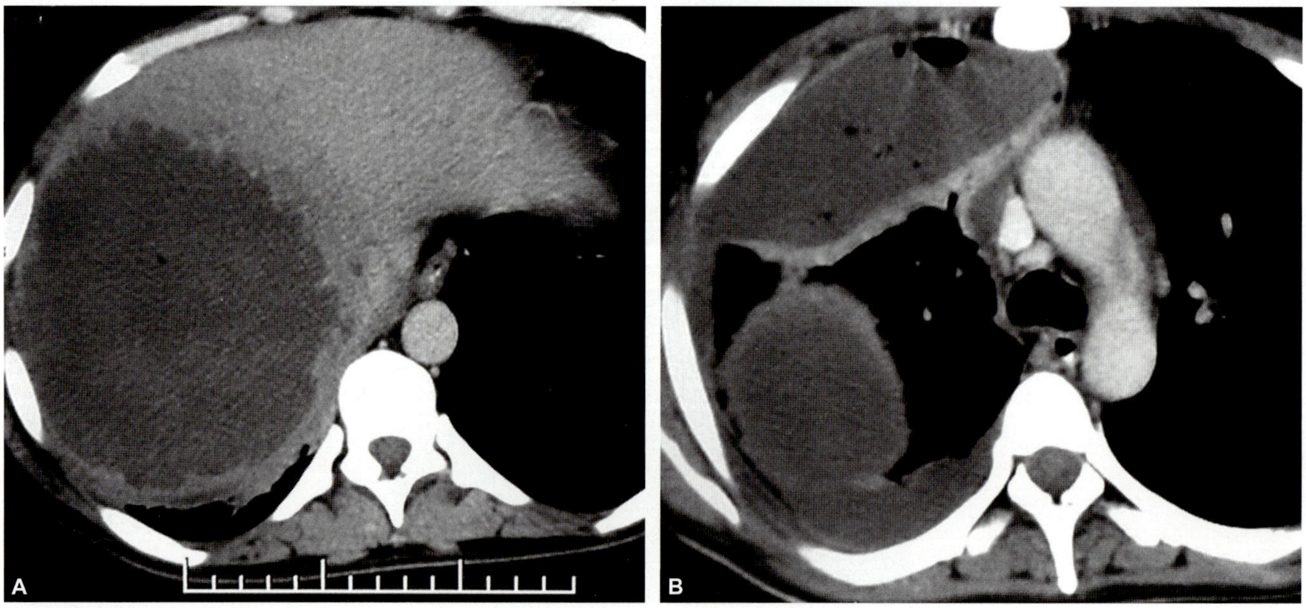

Figs. 9A and B: A 34-year-old male presented with high fever and pain upper abdomen for 1 week and admitted to ICU with worsening breathlessness over 2 days. CECT shows a large liver abscess in the right lobe with rupture in to right pleura, leading to right-sided empyema.

PANCREATITIS NECROSIS OF PANCREAS (FIG. 10)

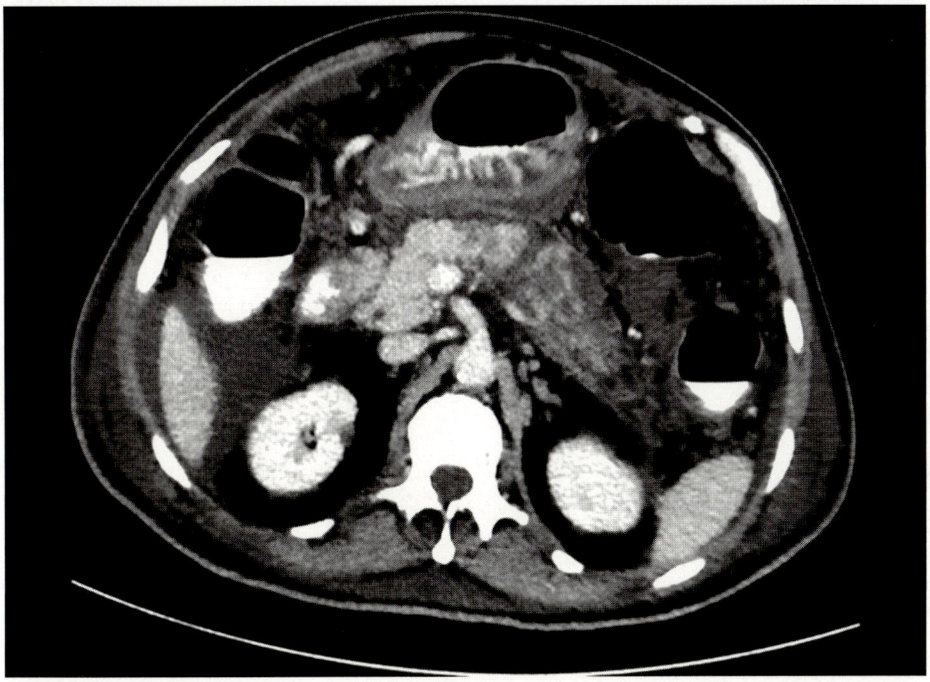

Fig. 10: A 52-year-old alcoholic male presented with acute abdomen with serum amylase of 1,400 and had persistent systemic inflammatory response syndrome (SIRS). CECT abdomen done after 72 hours of onset shows nonenhancing areas in the body and tail of pancreas s/o 33–50% necrosis, signifying severe pancreatitis with increased risk of local complications.

SECTION 5

Neurology

CHAPTER 13

Neuroimaging

Kapil Zirpe, Avinash Nanivadekar, Nivedita Shirol, Tripti Pareek, KD Rawool, Dhananjay Jadhav

CT MULTIPLANAR IMAGING (FIGS. 1A TO C)

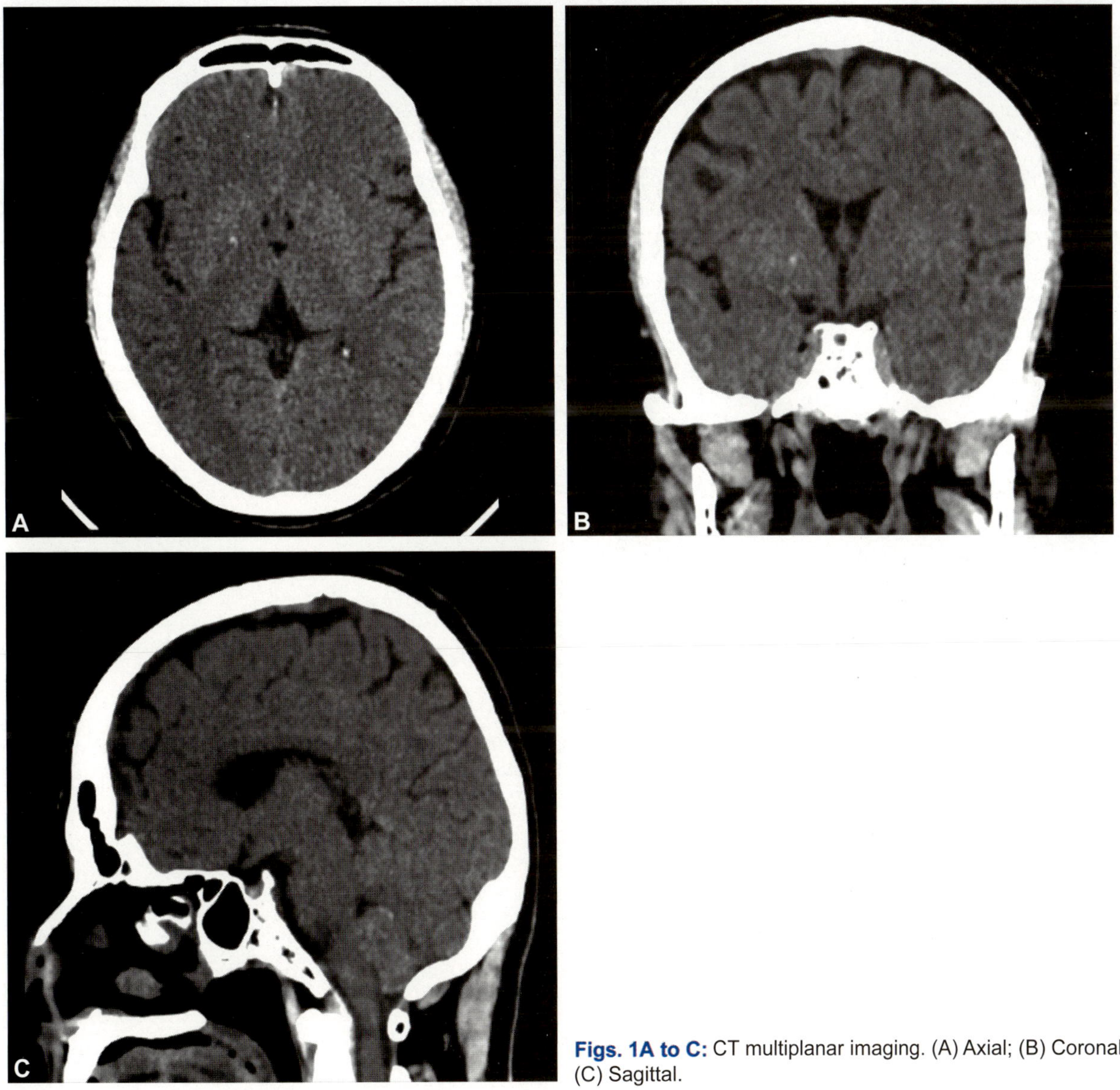

Figs. 1A to C: CT multiplanar imaging. (A) Axial; (B) Coronal; (C) Sagittal.

MRI MULTIPLANAR IMAGING (FIGS. 2A TO C)

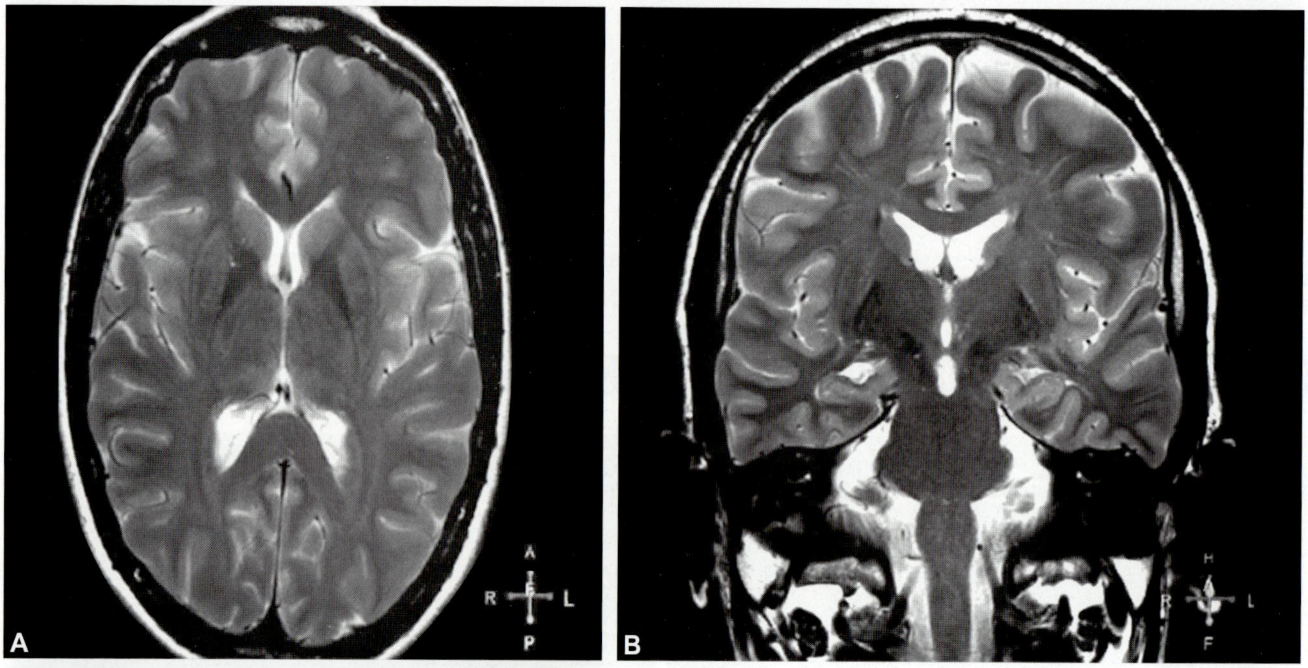

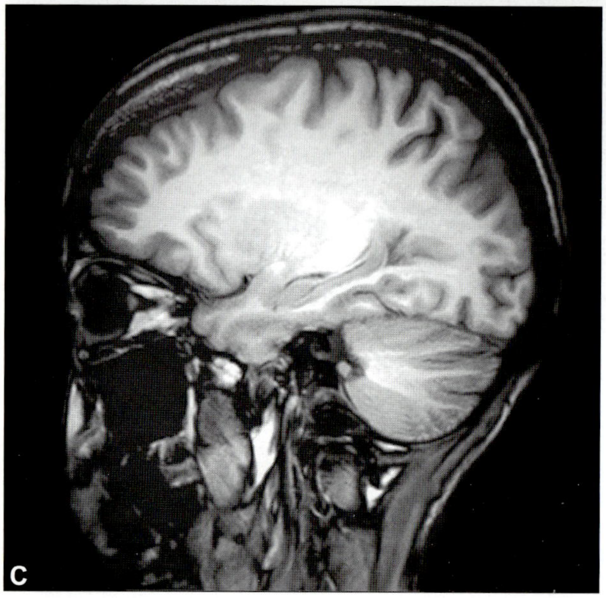

Figs. 2A to C: MRI multiplanar imaging. (A) Axial; (B) Coronal; (C) Sagittal.

POSTERIOR FOSSA BRAIN (FIGS. 3A AND B)

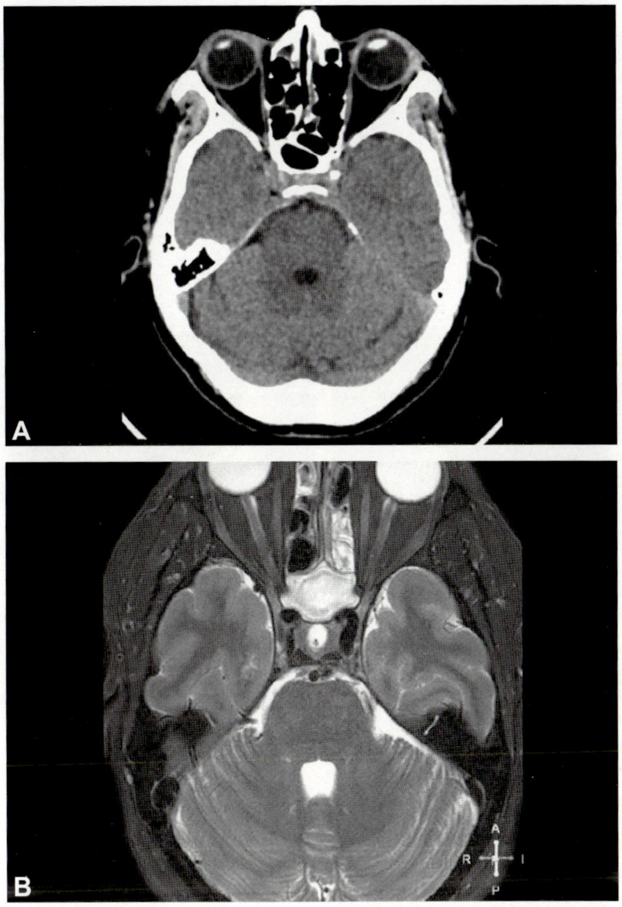

Figs. 3A and B: Posterior fossa brain.

NEUROTRAUMA AND STROKE IMAGING (FIGS. 4 TO 39)

Condition commonly encountered in neurotrauma:

- *Traumatic brain injuries*: Hematoma, contusion.
- *Stroke*: Hemorrhagic, ischemic, venous thrombosis.
- *Infections*: Meningitis, encephalitis, cerebritis, abscess.
- *Tumors*: Benign and neoplastic.
- *Miscellaneous*: Seizure disorders, metabolic, demyelinating disorders, and hypoxic brain injury.

Trauma: Situations

- Epidural (extradural) hemorrhage.
- Subdural hemorrhage.
- Hemorrhagic and nonhemorrhagic contusions.
- Axonal injuries.
- Cerebral edema.
- Herniations and midline shifts.
- Fractures.
- Hypoxic brain injuries.

Extradural Hemorrhage EDH (Figs. 4A to C)

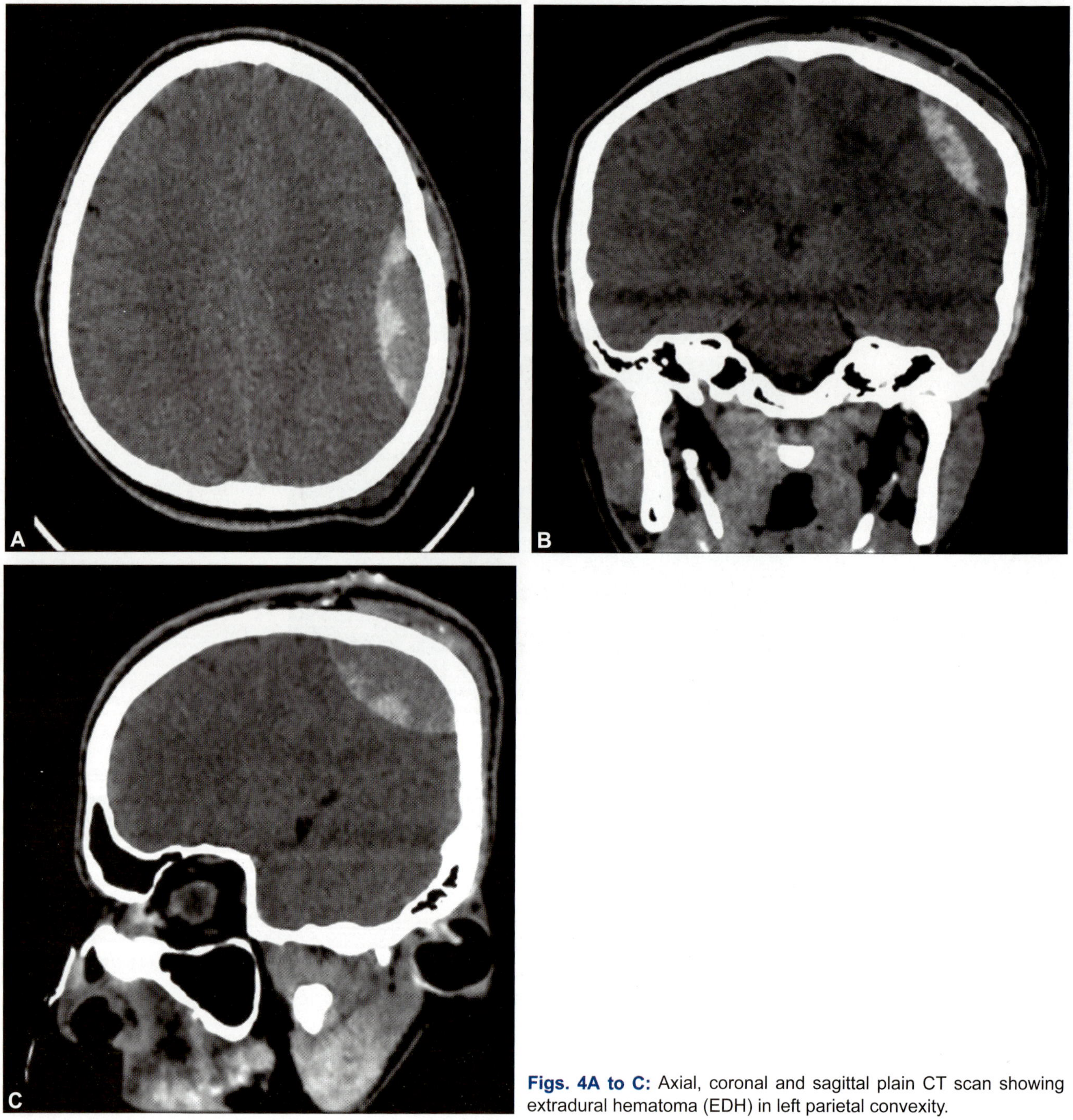

Figs. 4A to C: Axial, coronal and sagittal plain CT scan showing extradural hematoma (EDH) in left parietal convexity.

Frontoparietal Subdural Hemorrhage (Figs. 5A TO C)

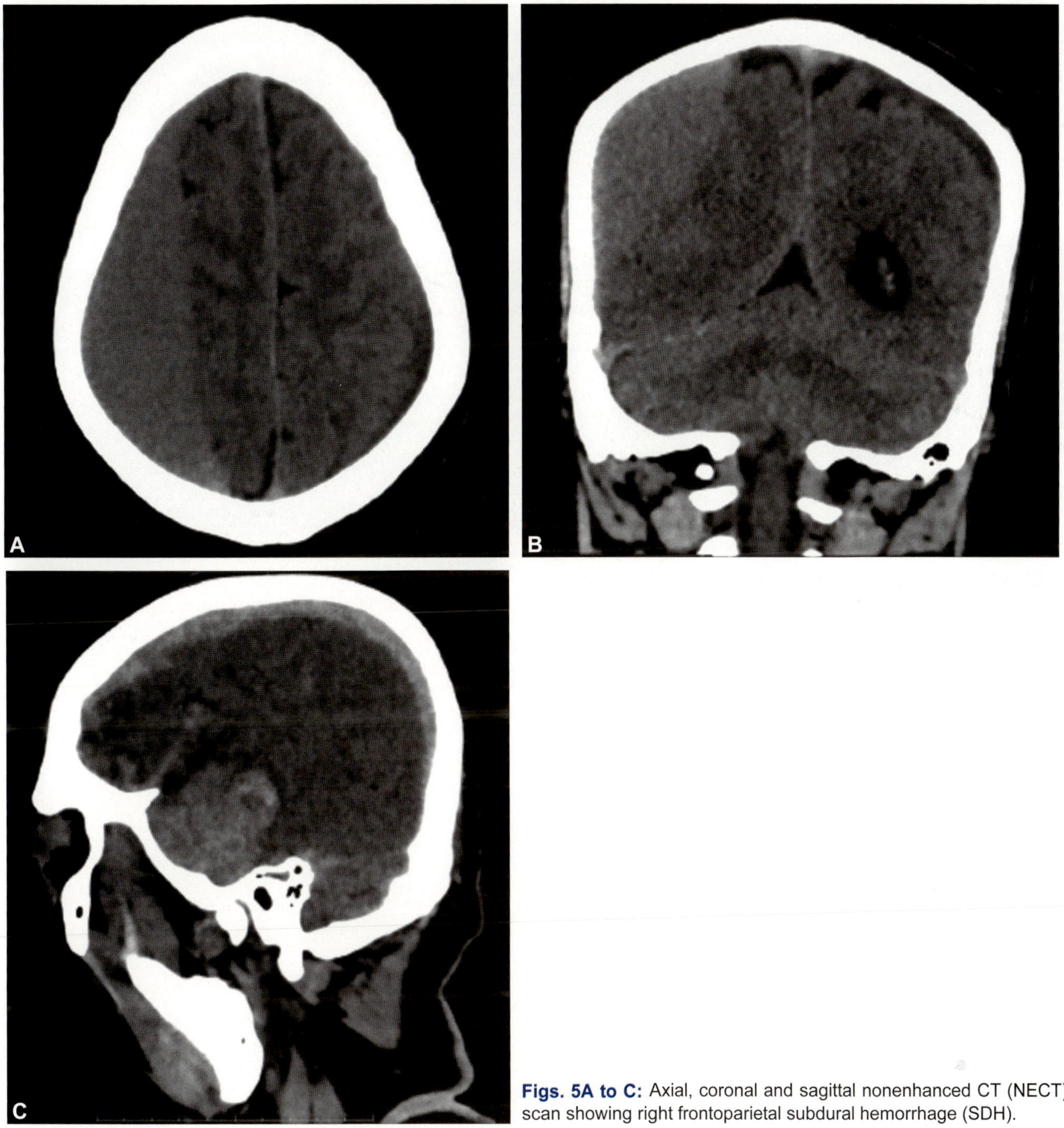

Figs. 5A to C: Axial, coronal and sagittal nonenhanced CT (NECT) scan showing right frontoparietal subdural hemorrhage (SDH).

Bilateral Subdural Collection with Blood Fluid Level (Figs. 6A to C)

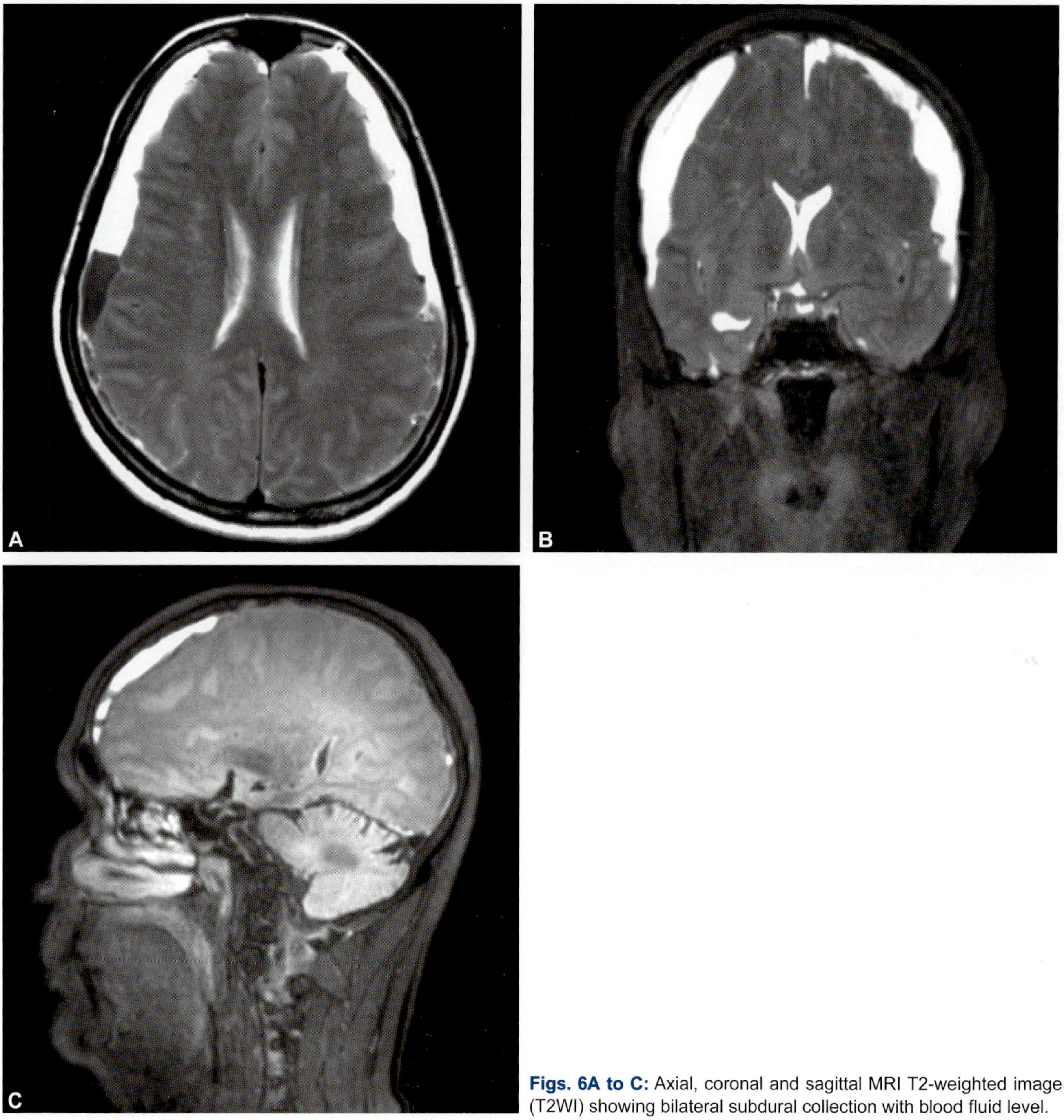

Figs. 6A to C: Axial, coronal and sagittal MRI T2-weighted image (T2WI) showing bilateral subdural collection with blood fluid level.

Subdural Collection in Left Frontoparietal Convexity (Figs. 7A to C)

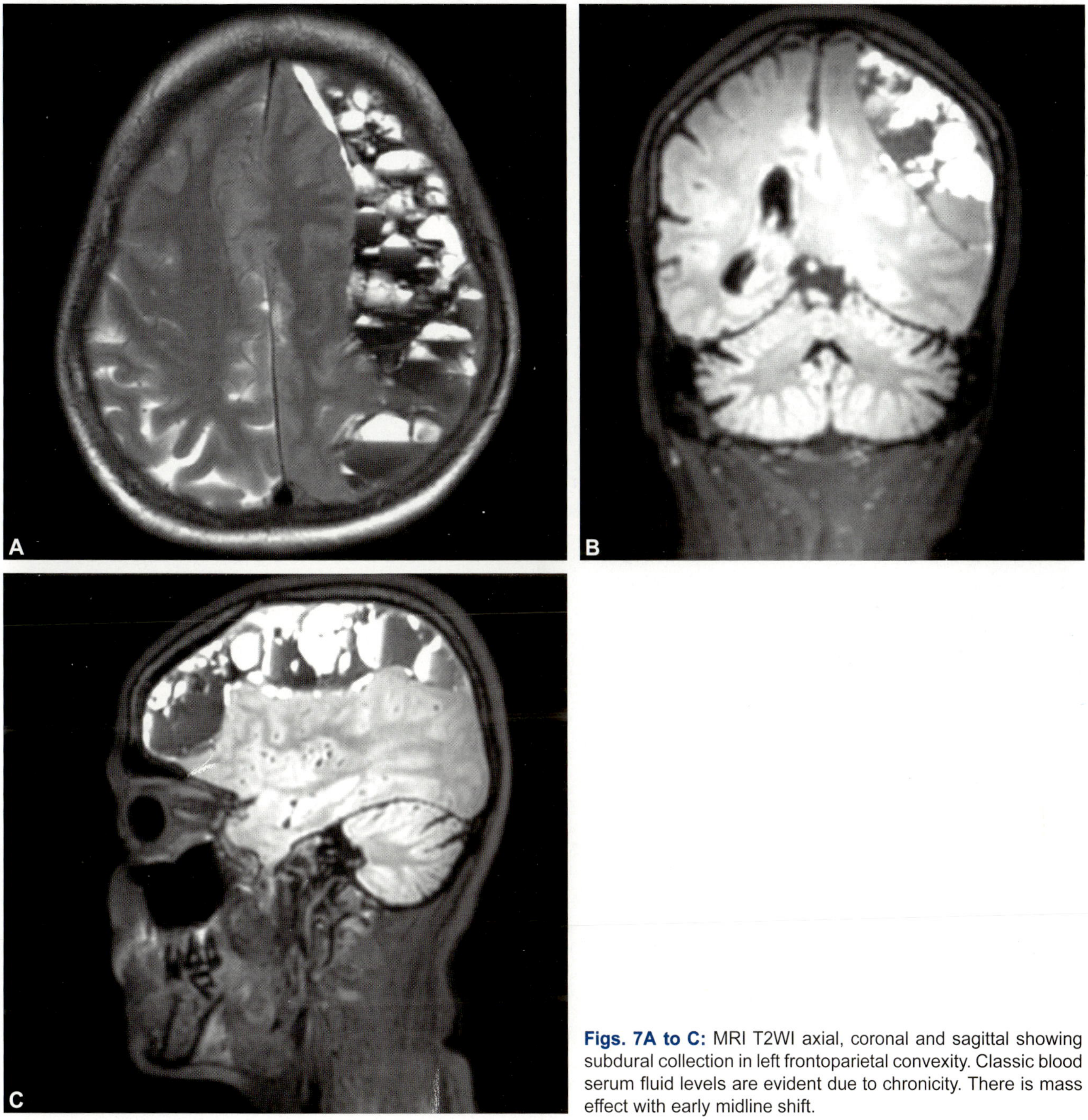

Figs. 7A to C: MRI T2WI axial, coronal and sagittal showing subdural collection in left frontoparietal convexity. Classic blood serum fluid levels are evident due to chronicity. There is mass effect with early midline shift.

Left Temporal Hemorrhagic Contusions (Figs. 8A to C)

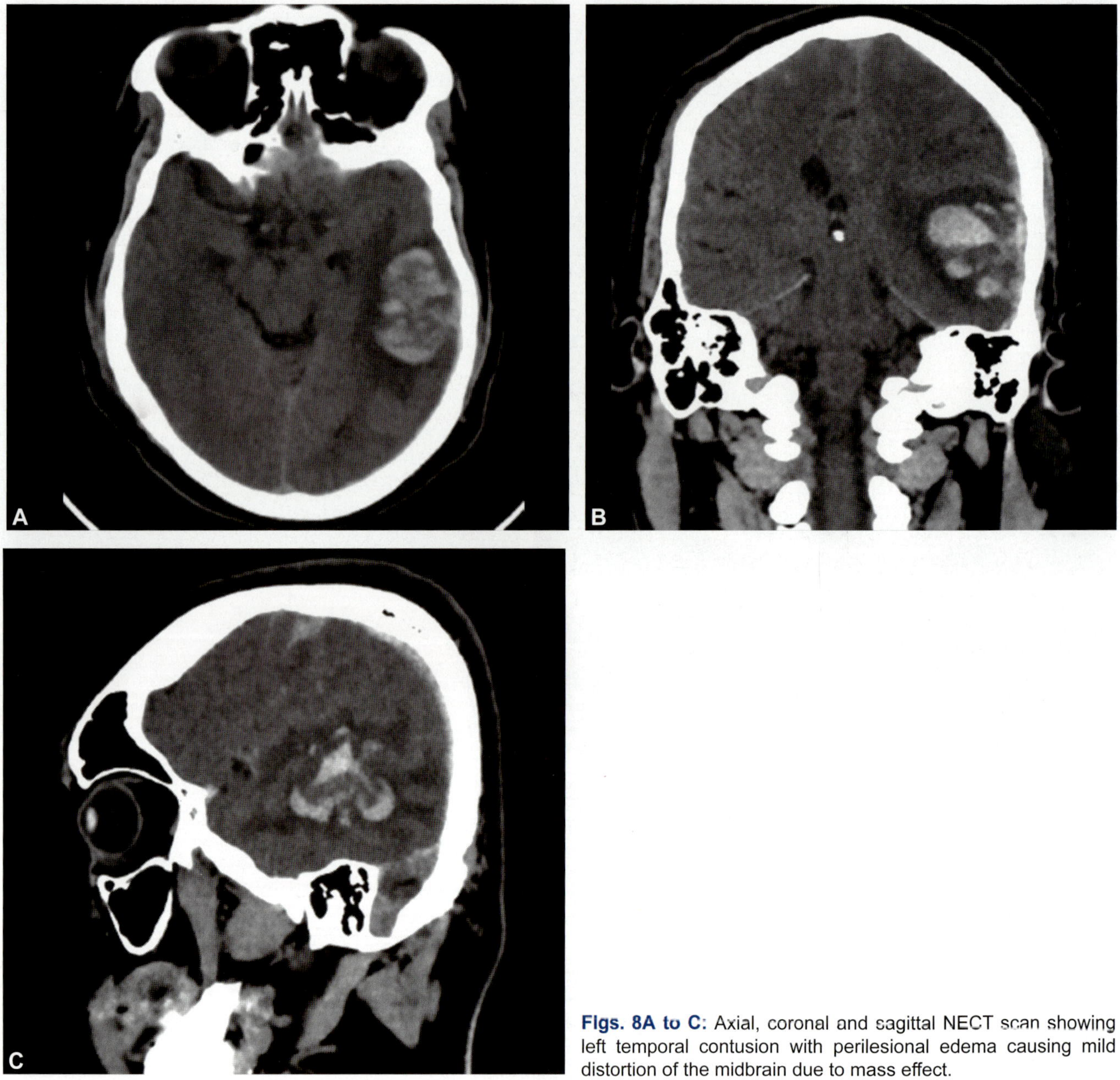

Figs. 8A to C: Axial, coronal and sagittal NECT scan showing left temporal contusion with perilesional edema causing mild distortion of the midbrain due to mass effect.

Bilateral Frontal Hemorrhagic Contusion (Figs. 9A to D)

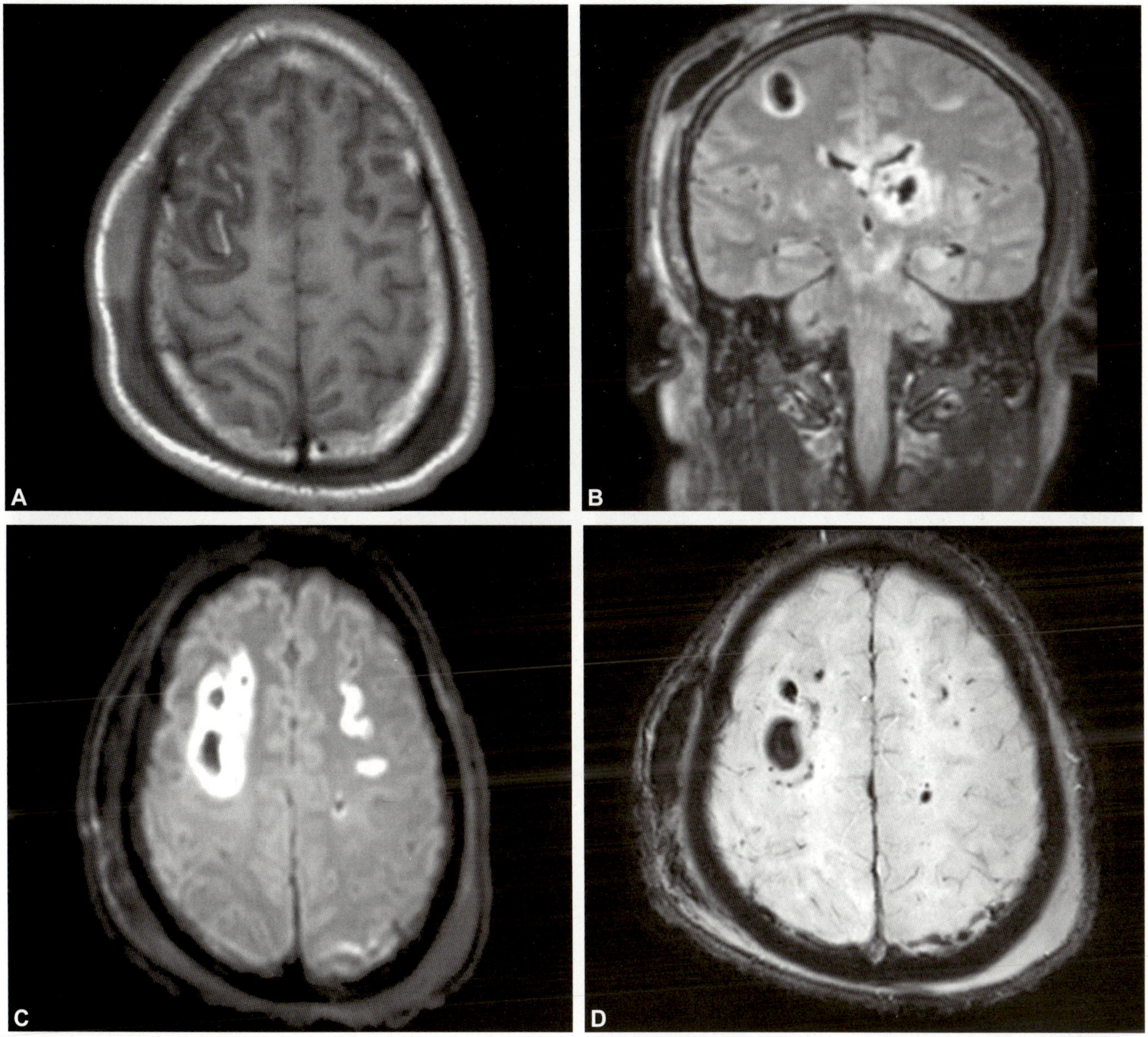

Figs. 9A to D: MRI of bilateral frontal hemorrhagic contusion perilesional edema. Diffuse axonal injuries (DAIs) are seen as tiny foci in the white matter.

Bilateral Subarachnoid (Figs. 10A to C)

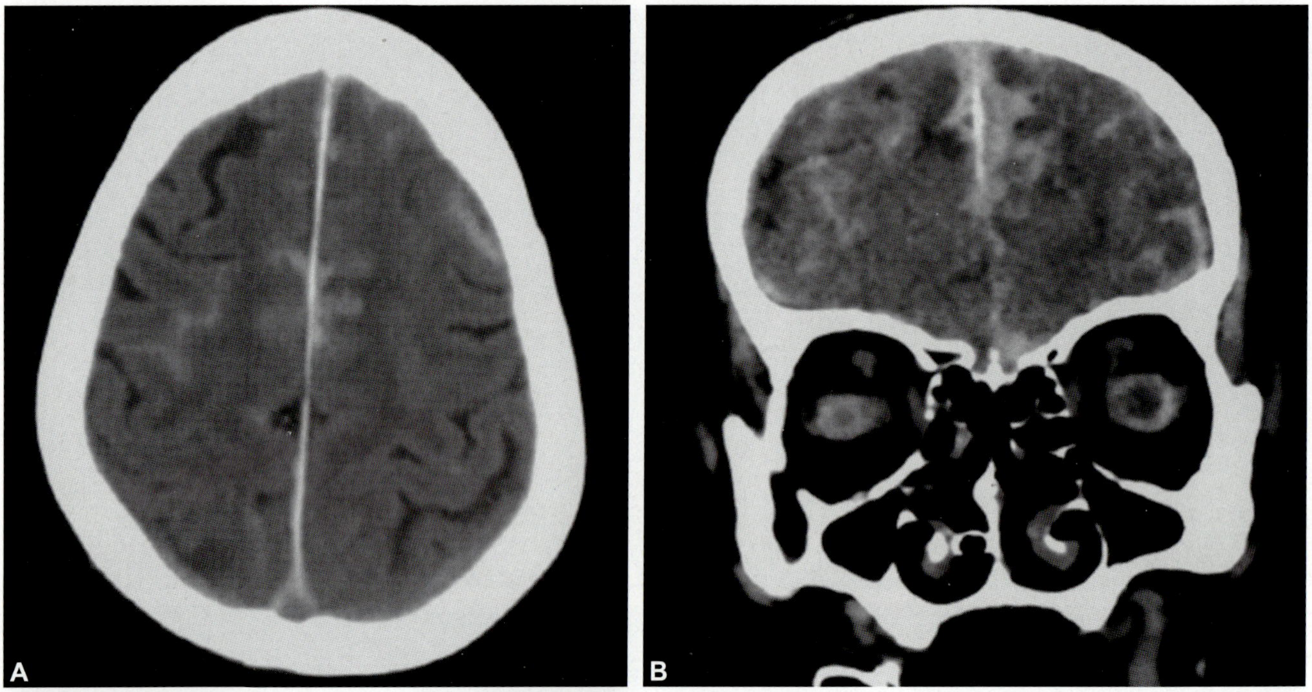

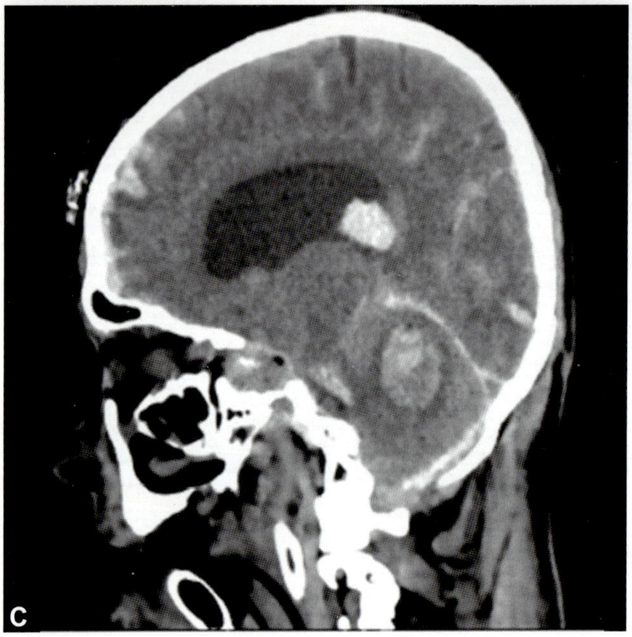

Figs. 10A to C: Axial, coronal and sagittal NECT scan showing bilateral subarachnoid hemorrhage (SAH) seen as hyperdense lesions replacing dark cerebrospinal fluid (CSF) over the sulci. The etiology is a bleed in the cerebellum seen on the sagittal reconstruction.

Right Frontoparietal Hemorrhage (Figs. 11A to C)

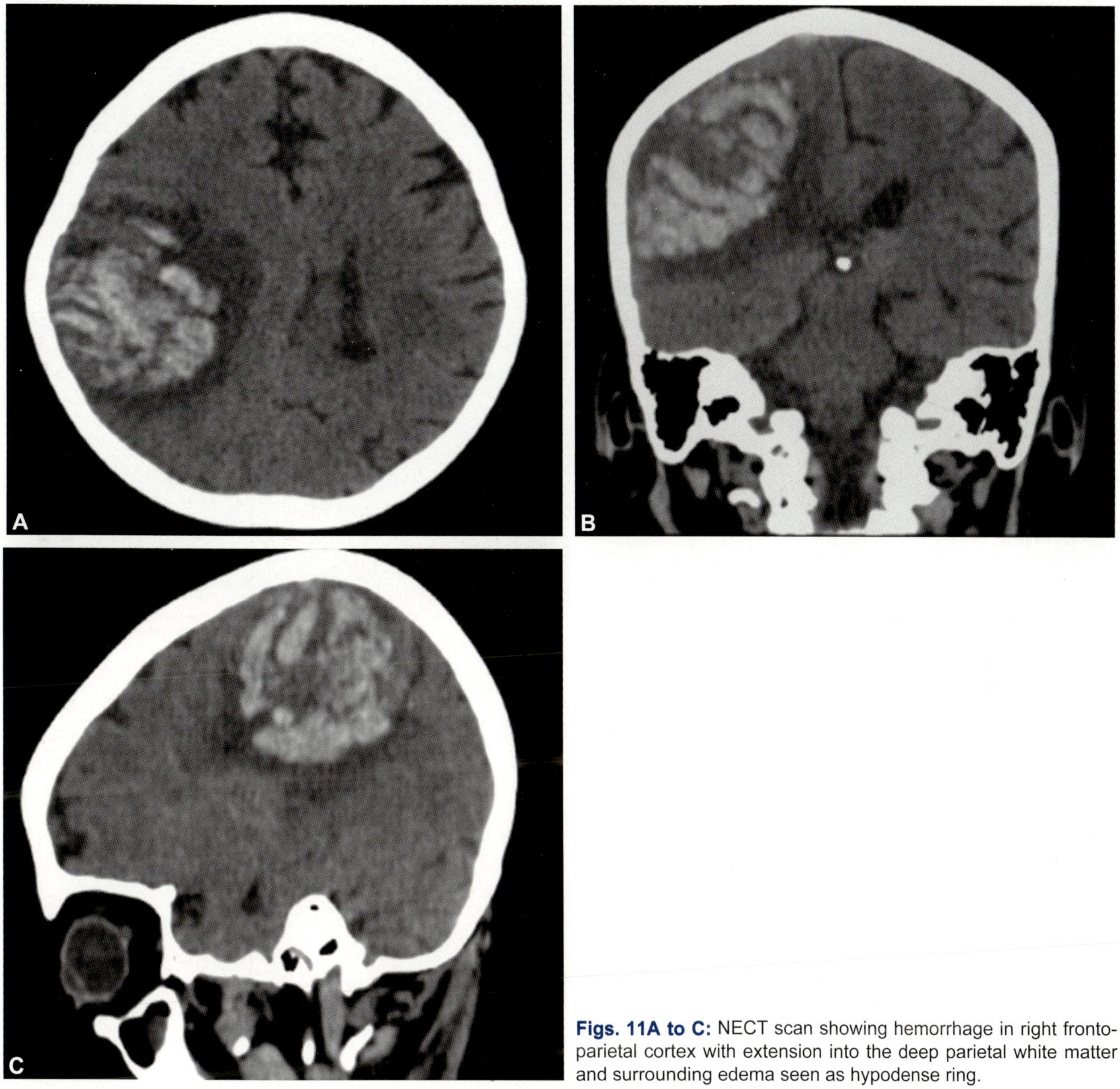

Figs. 11A to C: NECT scan showing hemorrhage in right fronto-parietal cortex with extension into the deep parietal white matter and surrounding edema seen as hypodense ring.

Left Frontoparietal Hemorrhage (Figs. 12A to C)

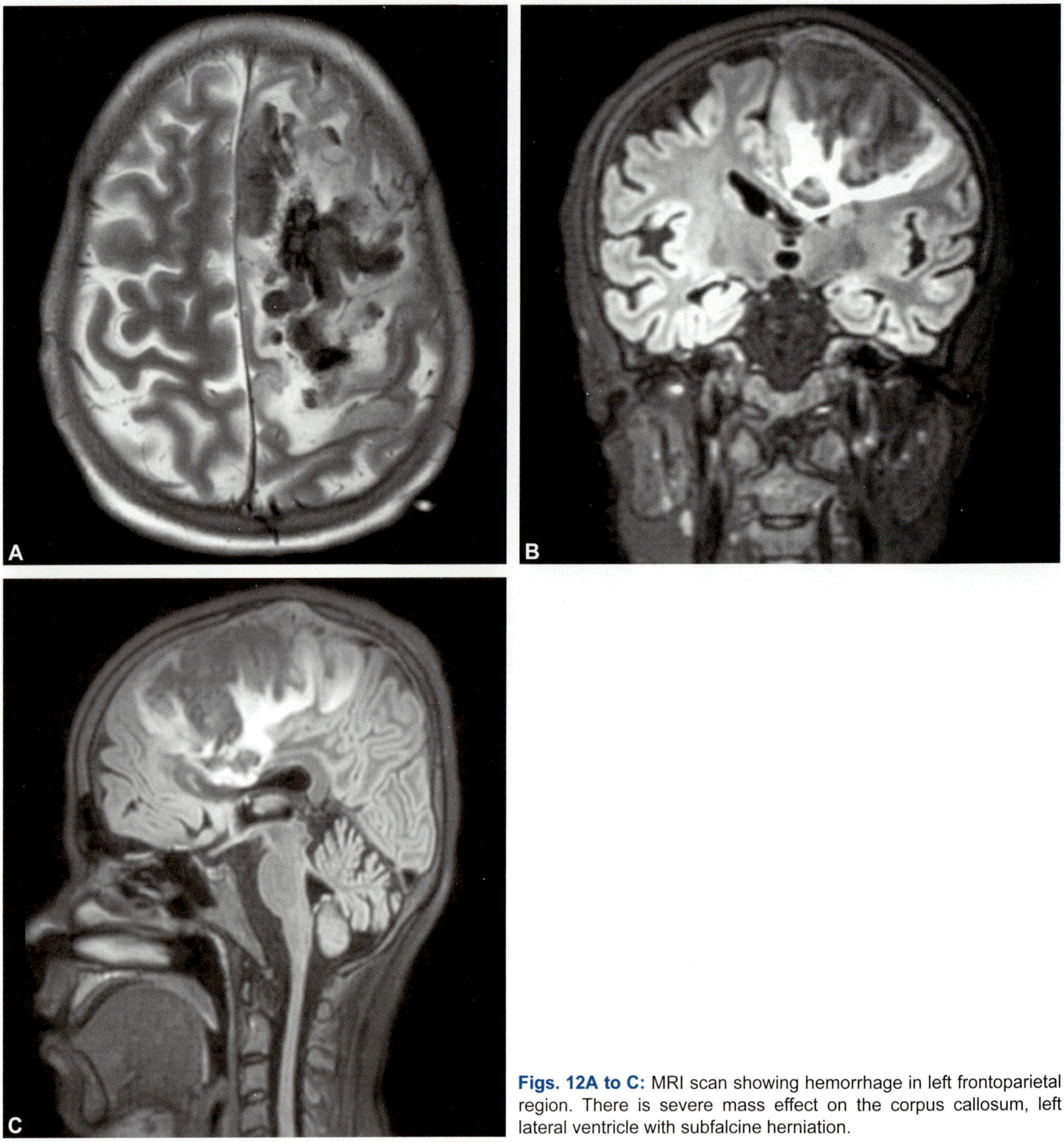

Figs. 12A to C: MRI scan showing hemorrhage in left frontoparietal region. There is severe mass effect on the corpus callosum, left lateral ventricle with subfalcine herniation.

Basal Ganglia Bleed CT and MRI (Figs. 13 and 14)

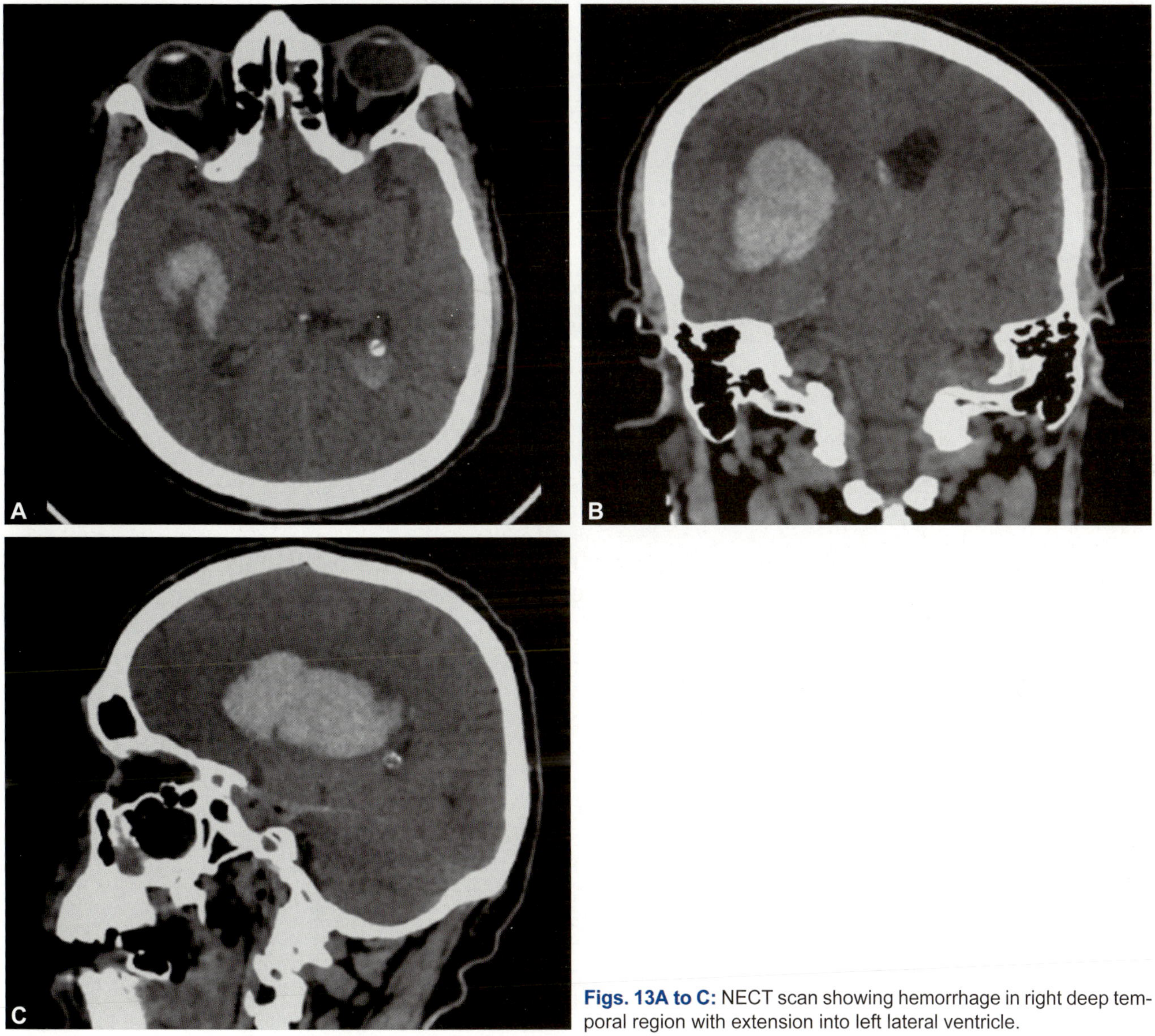

Figs. 13A to C: NECT scan showing hemorrhage in right deep temporal region with extension into left lateral ventricle.

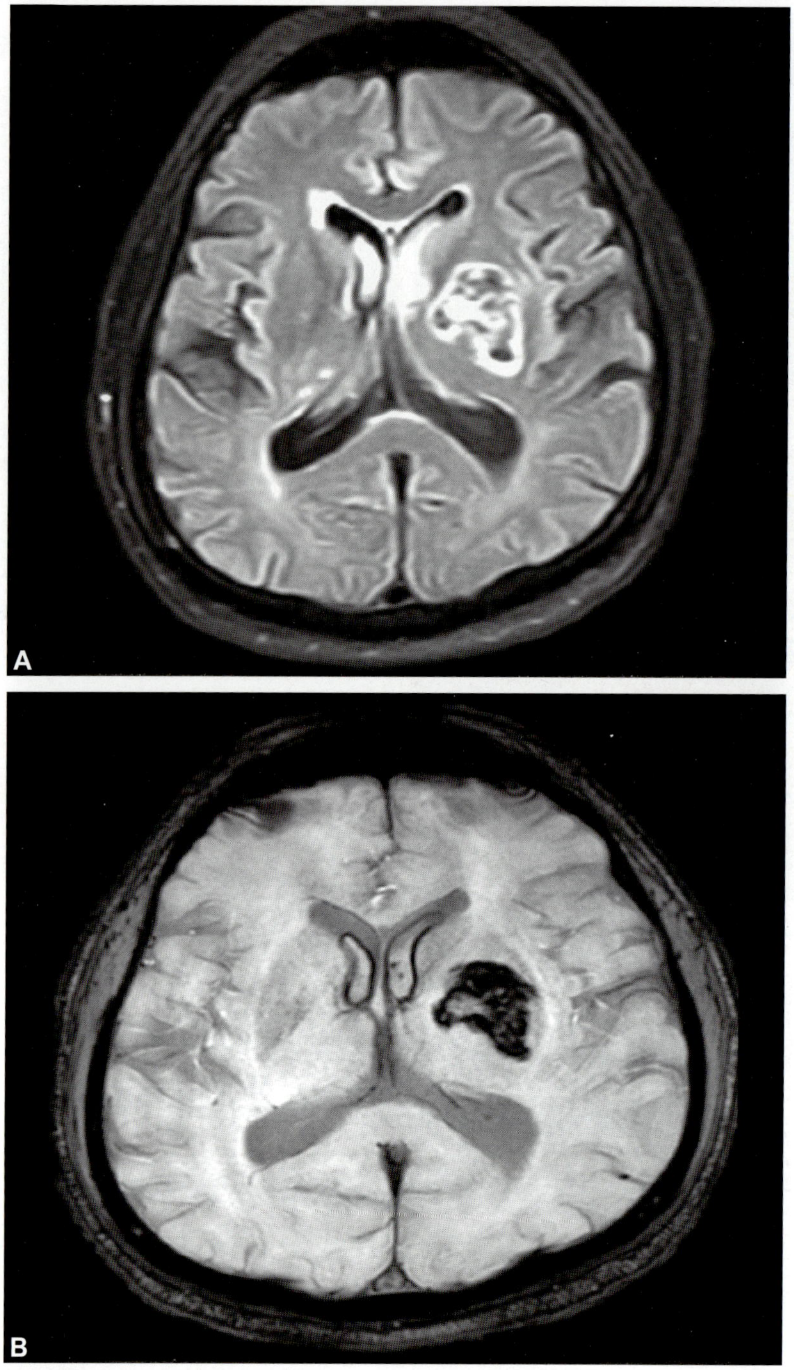

Figs. 14A and B: MRI scan showing hemorrhage in left basal ganglia region with intraventricular extension.

Intraventricular Hemorrhage CT and MRI (Figs. 15 to 17)

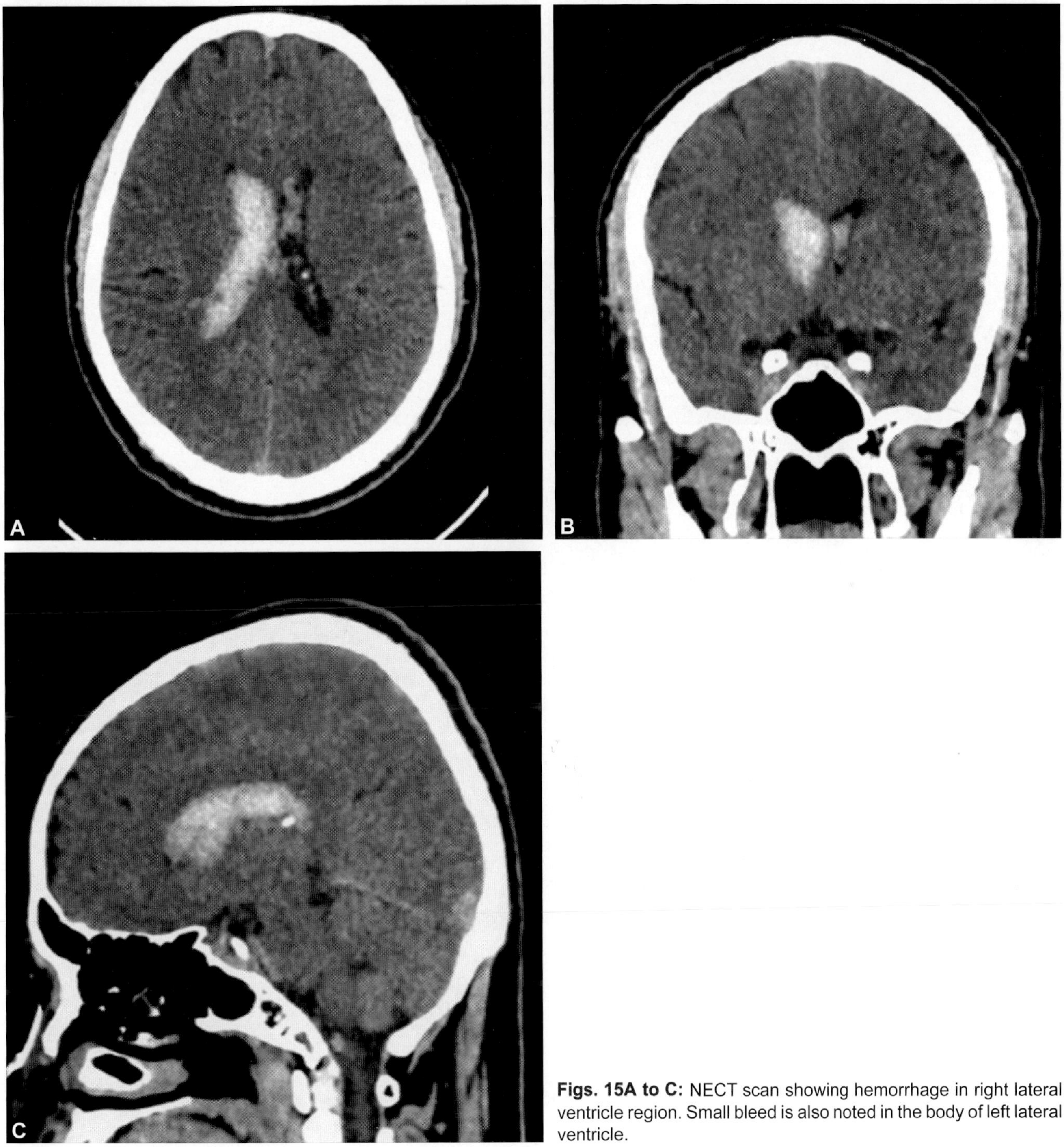

Figs. 15A to C: NECT scan showing hemorrhage in right lateral ventricle region. Small bleed is also noted in the body of left lateral ventricle.

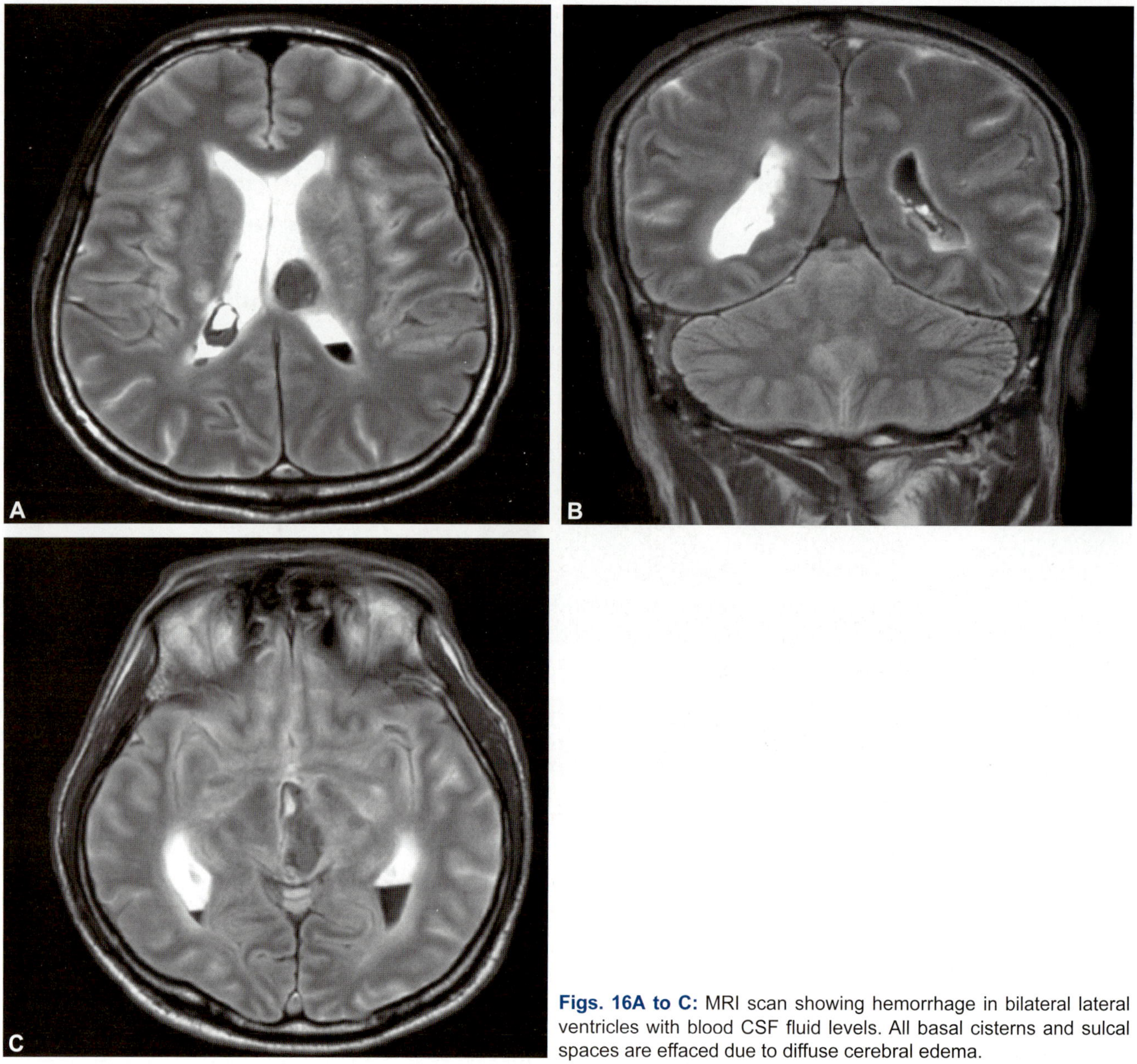

Figs. 16A to C: MRI scan showing hemorrhage in bilateral lateral ventricles with blood CSF fluid levels. All basal cisterns and sulcal spaces are effaced due to diffuse cerebral edema.

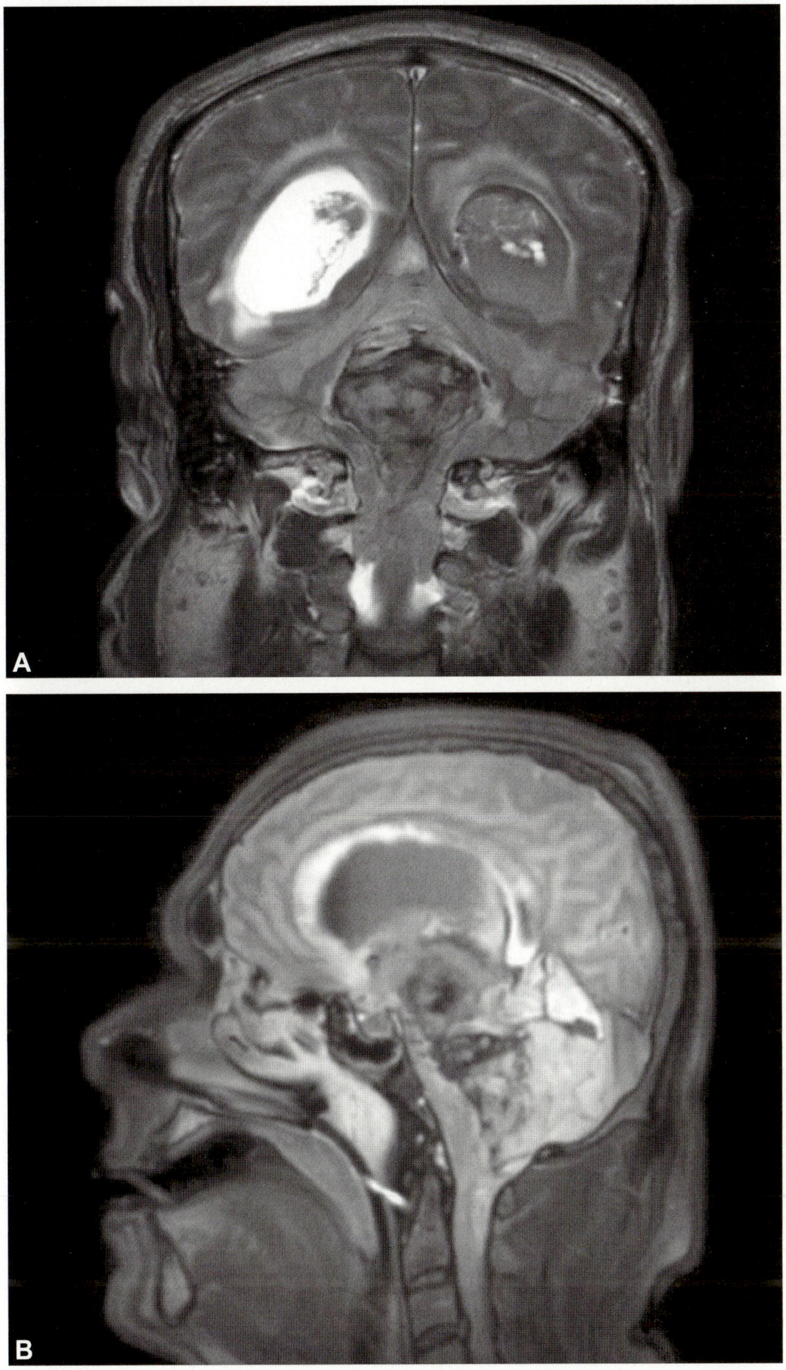

Figs. 17A and B: MRI scan showing extensive pan-ventricular hemorrhage. The epicenter of the bleed is a 4th ventricular mass. There is severe hydrocephalus associated with transforaminal herniation of tonsils.

Pontine Hemorrhage CT (Figs. 18A to C)

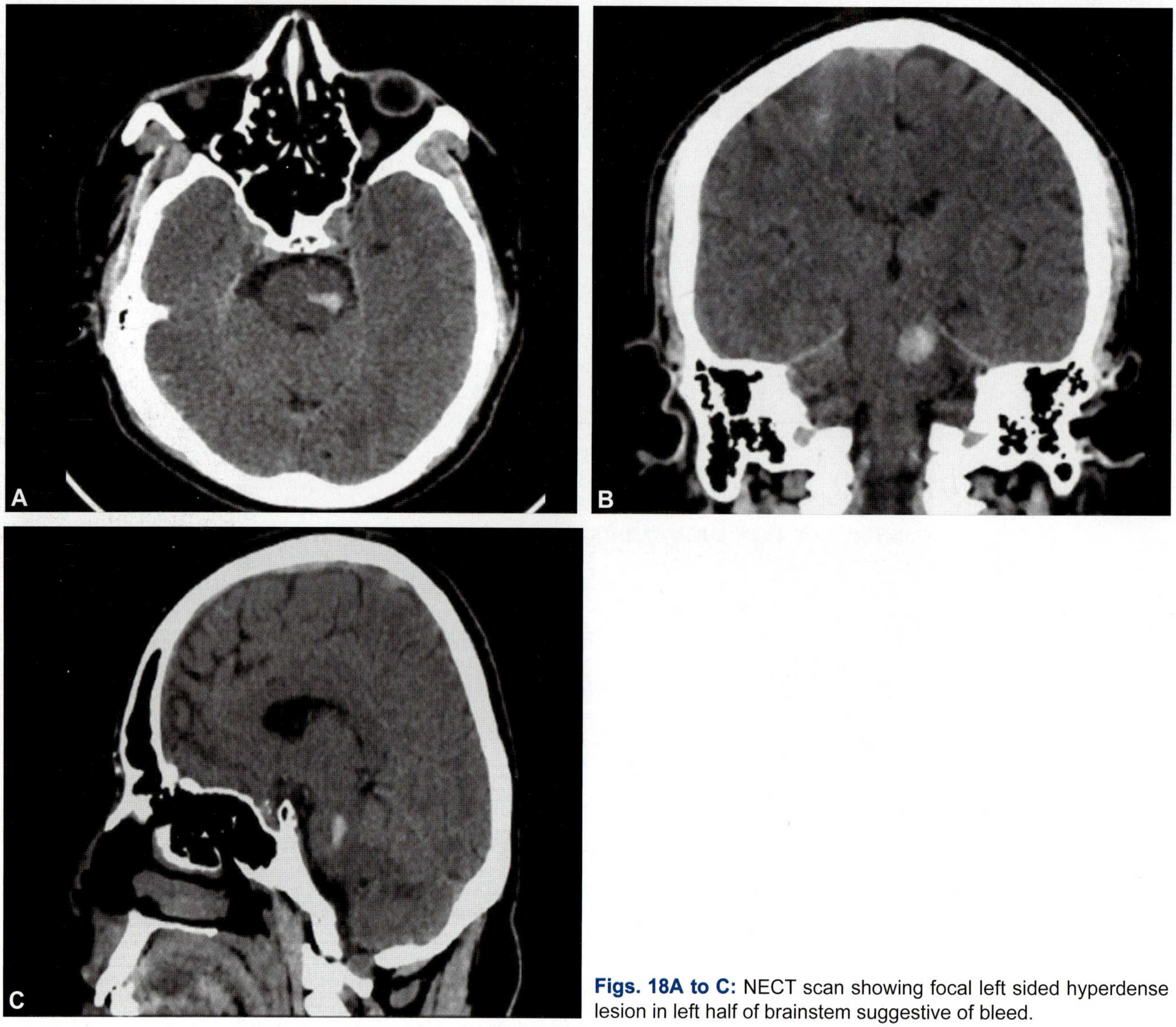

Figs. 18A to C: NECT scan showing focal left sided hyperdense lesion in left half of brainstem suggestive of bleed.

Pontine Hemorrhage MRI (Figs. 19 and 20)

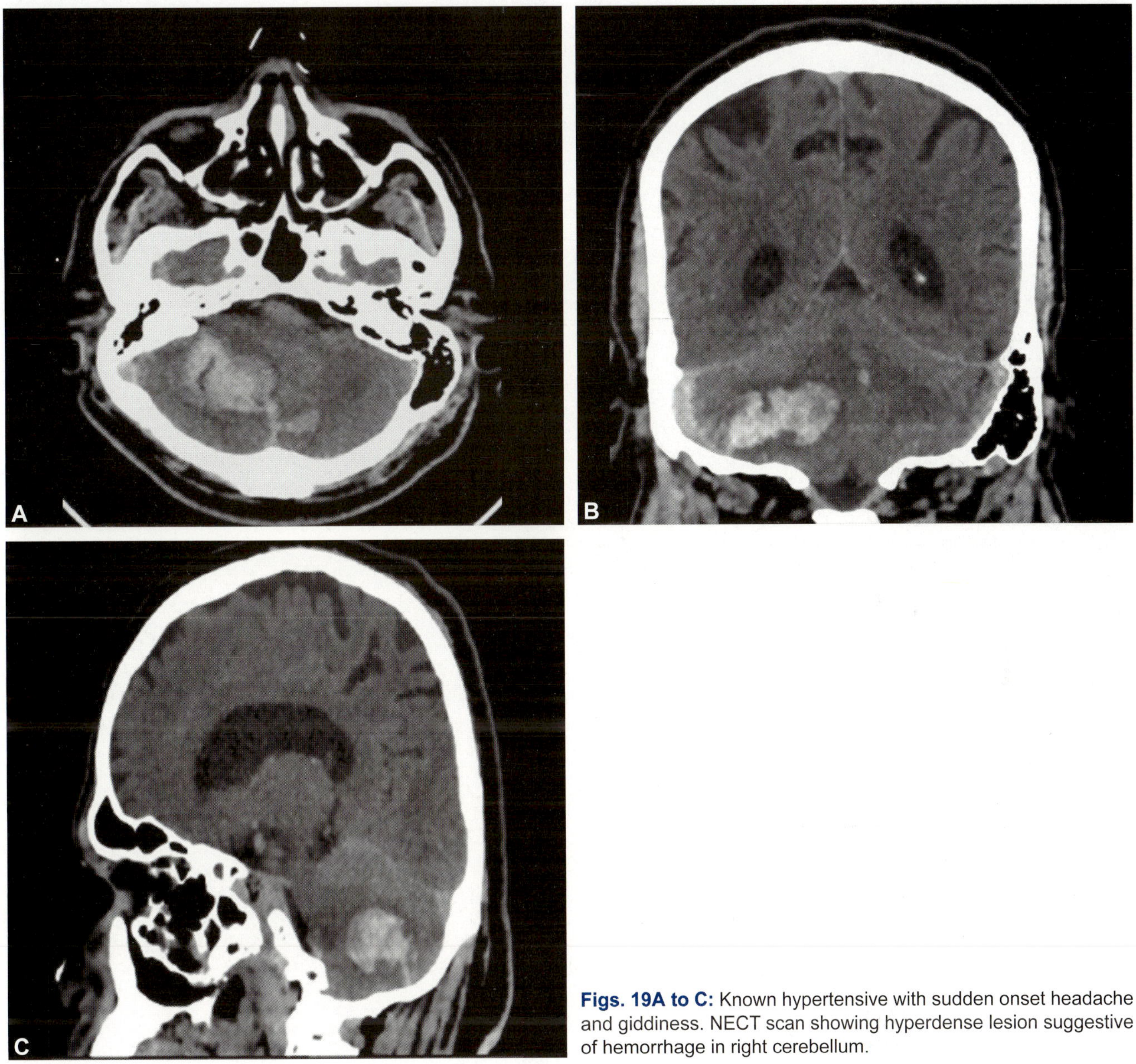

Figs. 19A to C: Known hypertensive with sudden onset headache and giddiness. NECT scan showing hyperdense lesion suggestive of hemorrhage in right cerebellum.

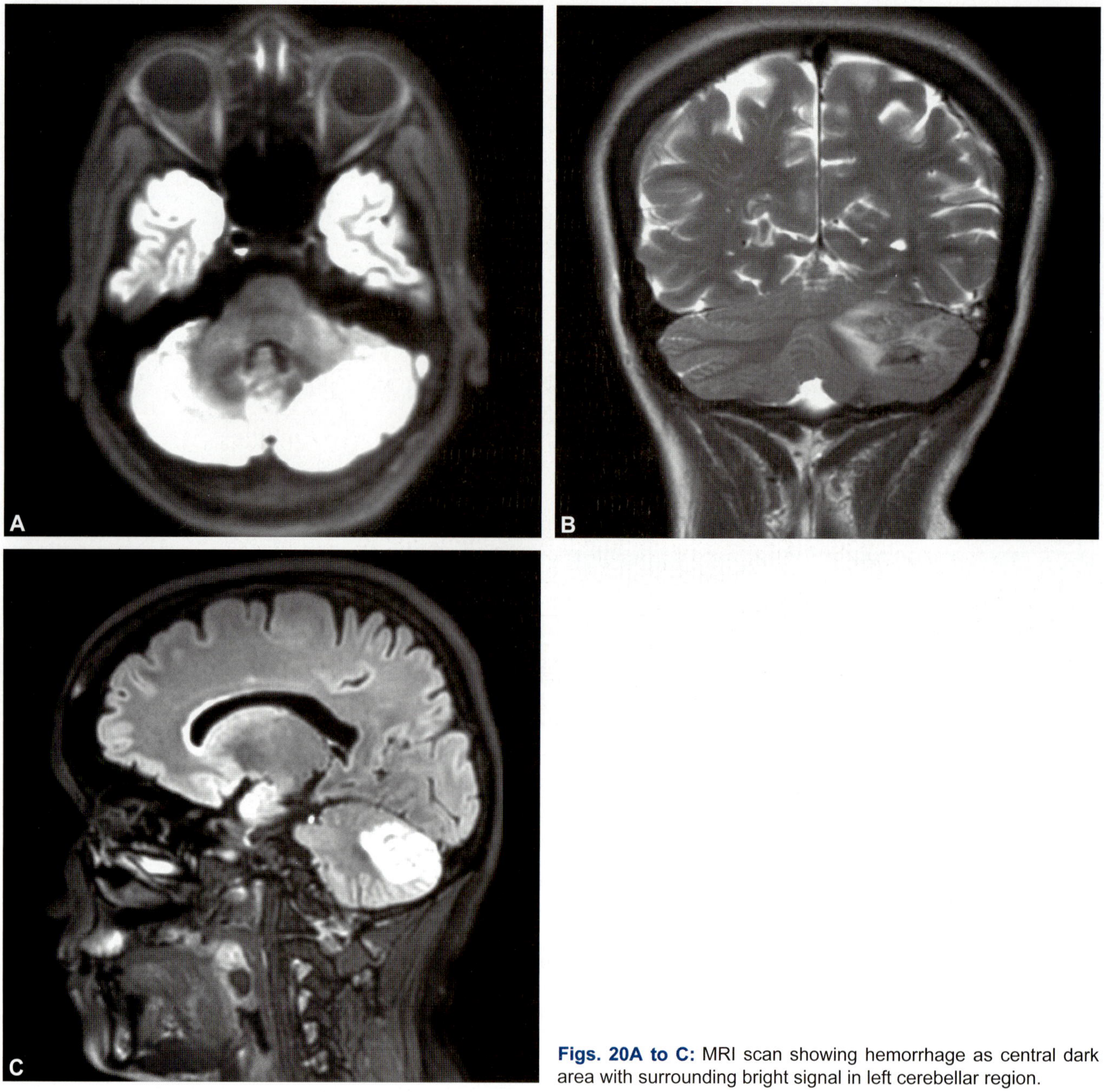

Figs. 20A to C: MRI scan showing hemorrhage as central dark area with surrounding bright signal in left cerebellar region.

Ischemic Stroke CT and MRI (Figs. 21 to 28)

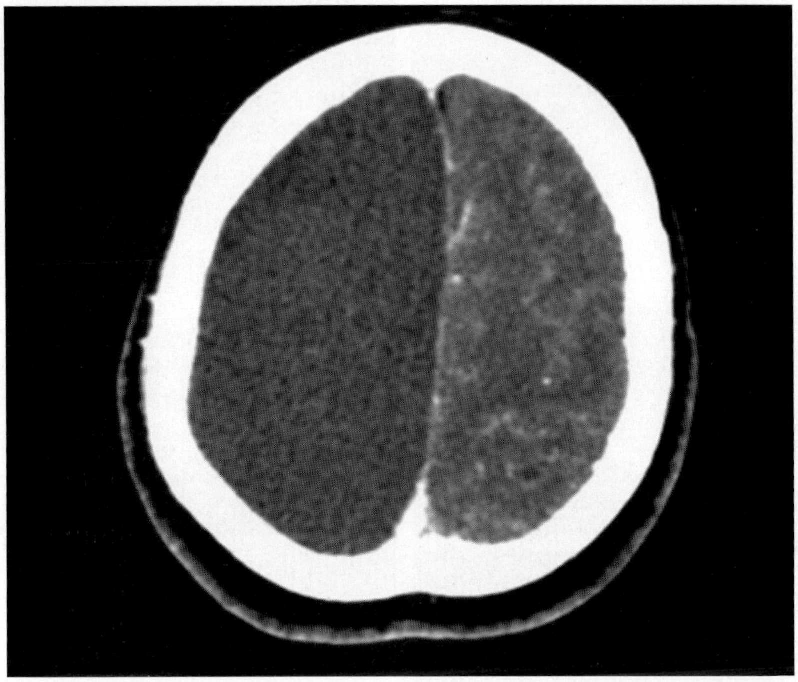

Fig. 21: Contrast-enhanced computed tomography (CECT) scan shows right anterior cerebral artery (ACA) and middle cerebral artery (MCA) infarct as hypodense cerebral hemisphere causing bowing of the falx to left.

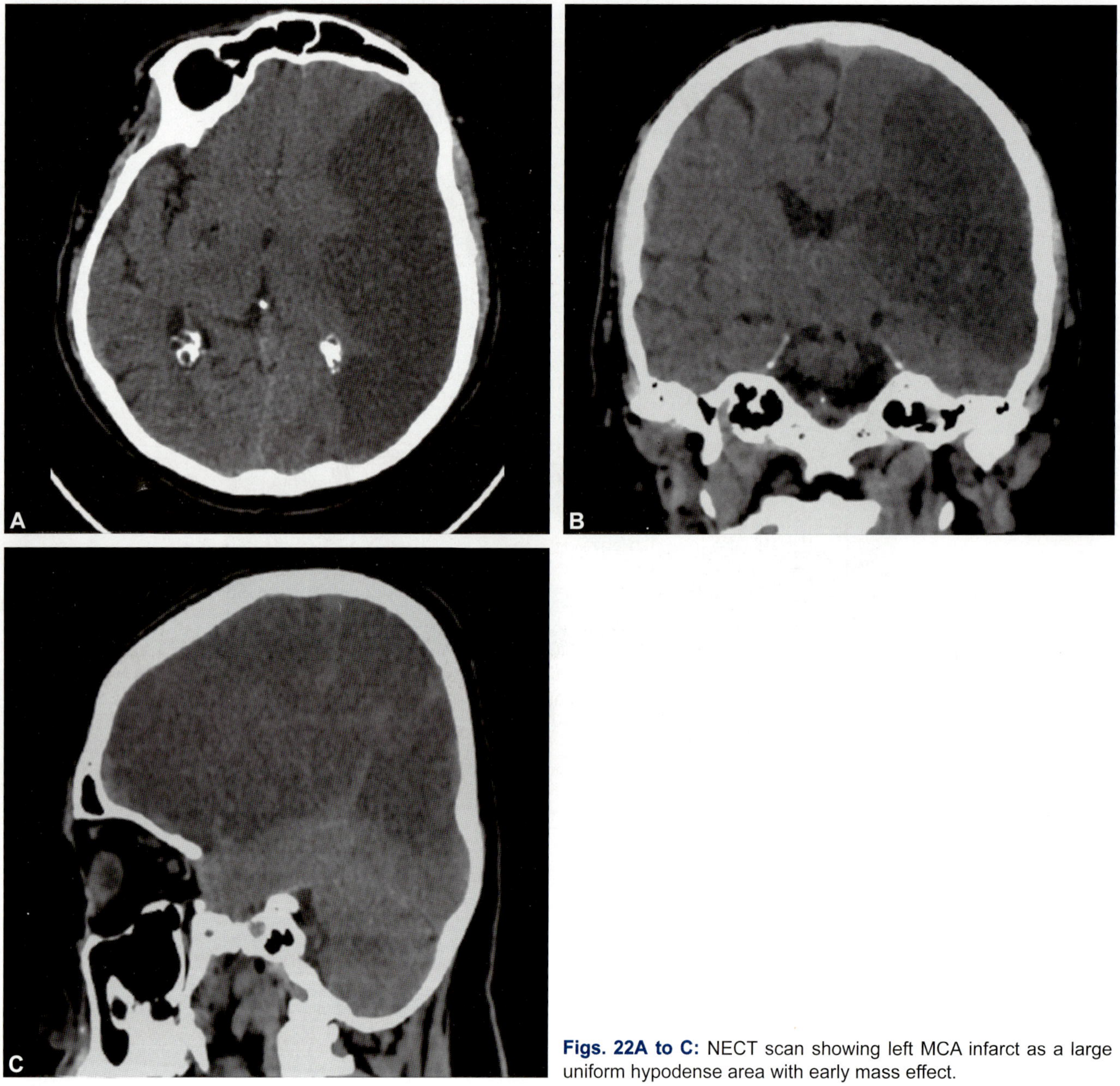

Figs. 22A to C: NECT scan showing left MCA infarct as a large uniform hypodense area with early mass effect.

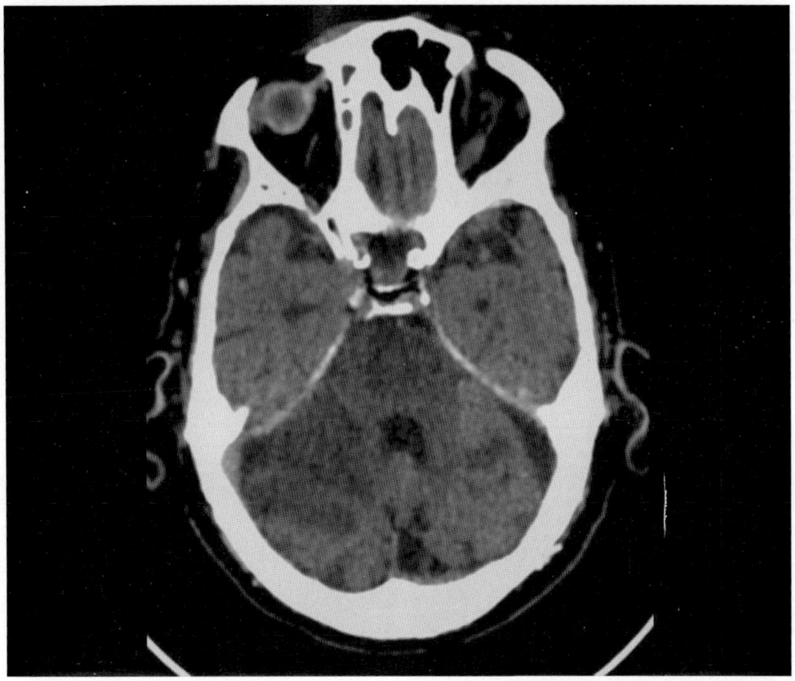

Fig. 23: NECT scan shows right posterior cerebral artery (PCA) infarct as hypodense areas in the pons, both cerebellar hemispheres, right more than left.

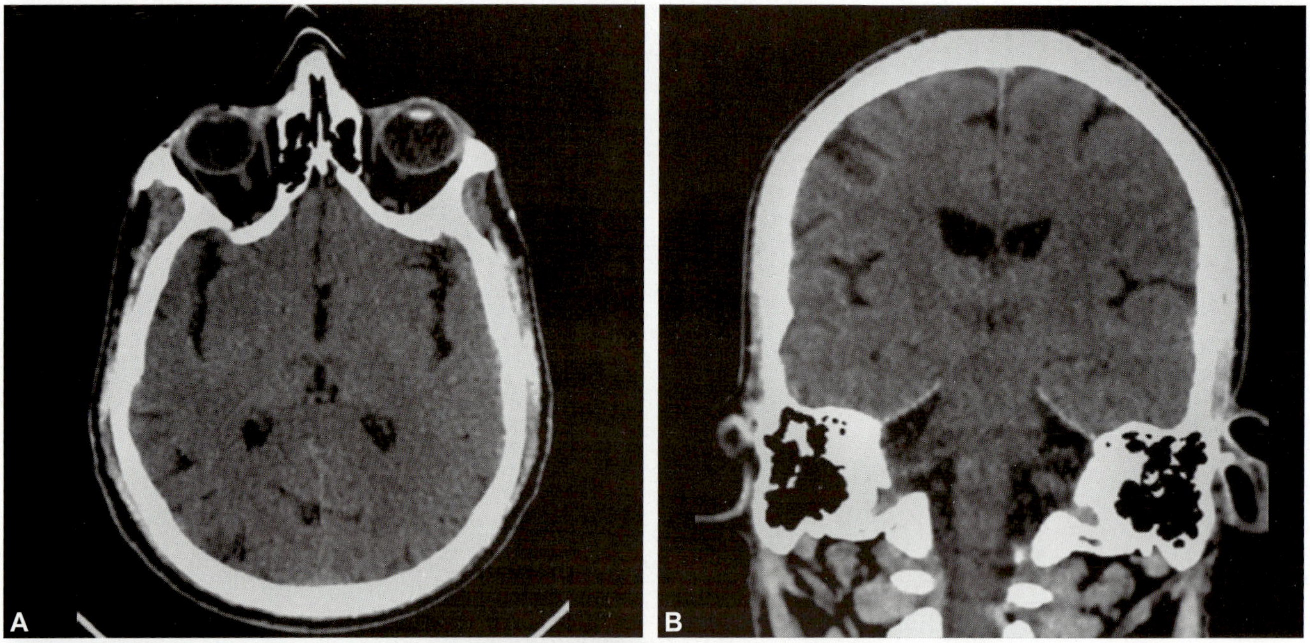

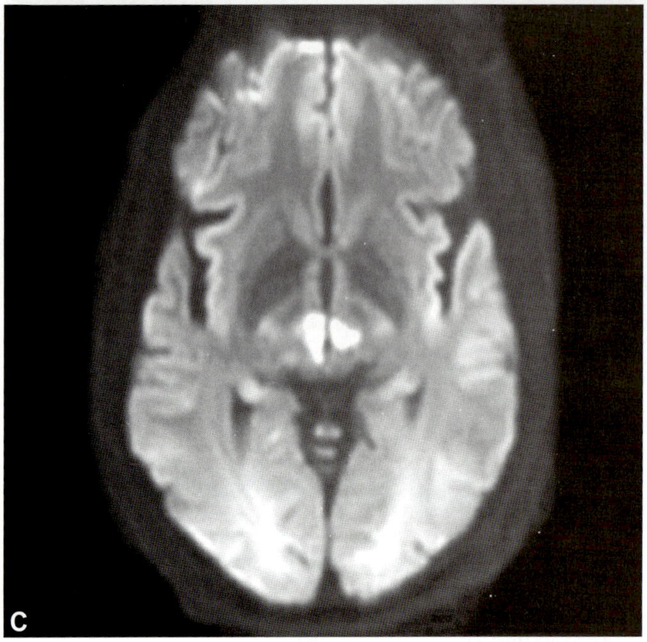

Figs. 24A to C: NECT and DW MR scan showing a hypodense lesion on CT and bright lesion on DW MRI in thalami. This is classic of artery of Percheron infarct.

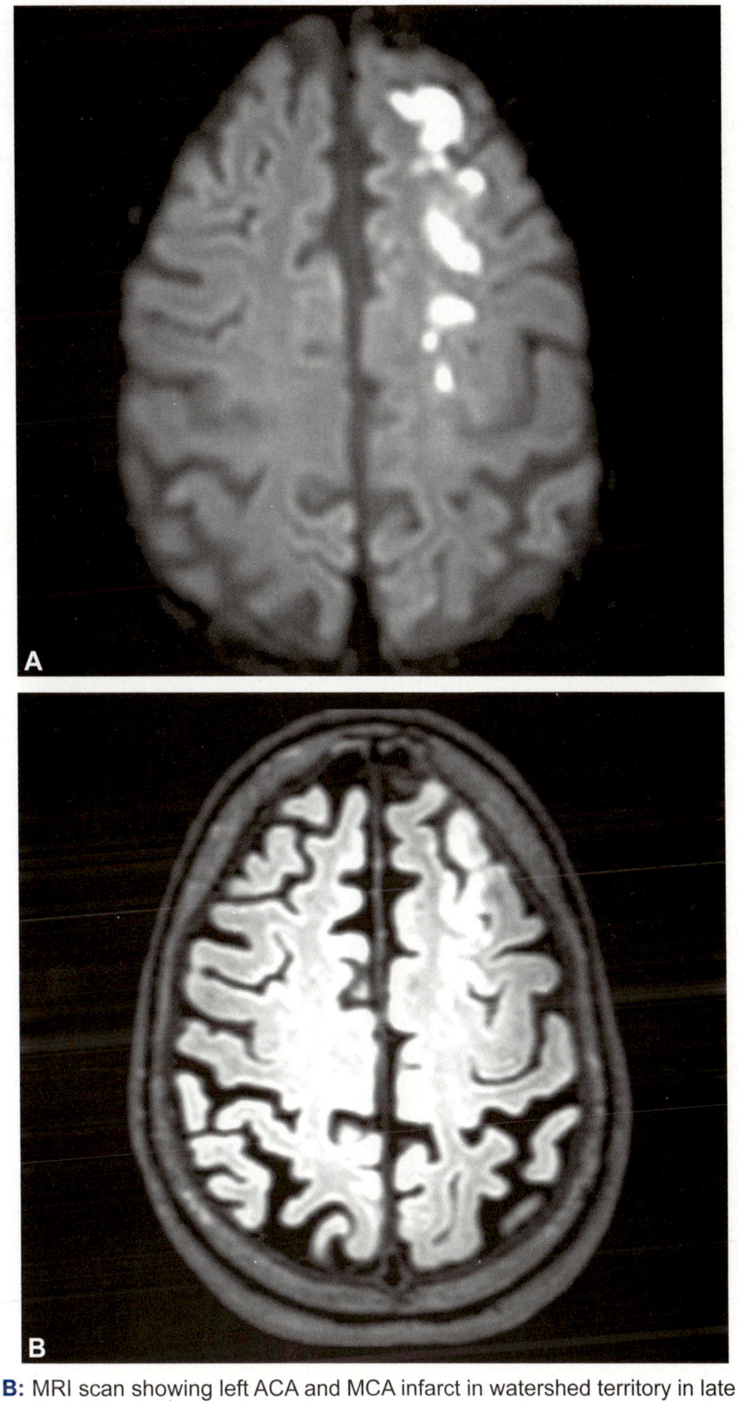

Figs. 25A and B: MRI scan showing left ACA and MCA infarct in watershed territory in late subacute stage.

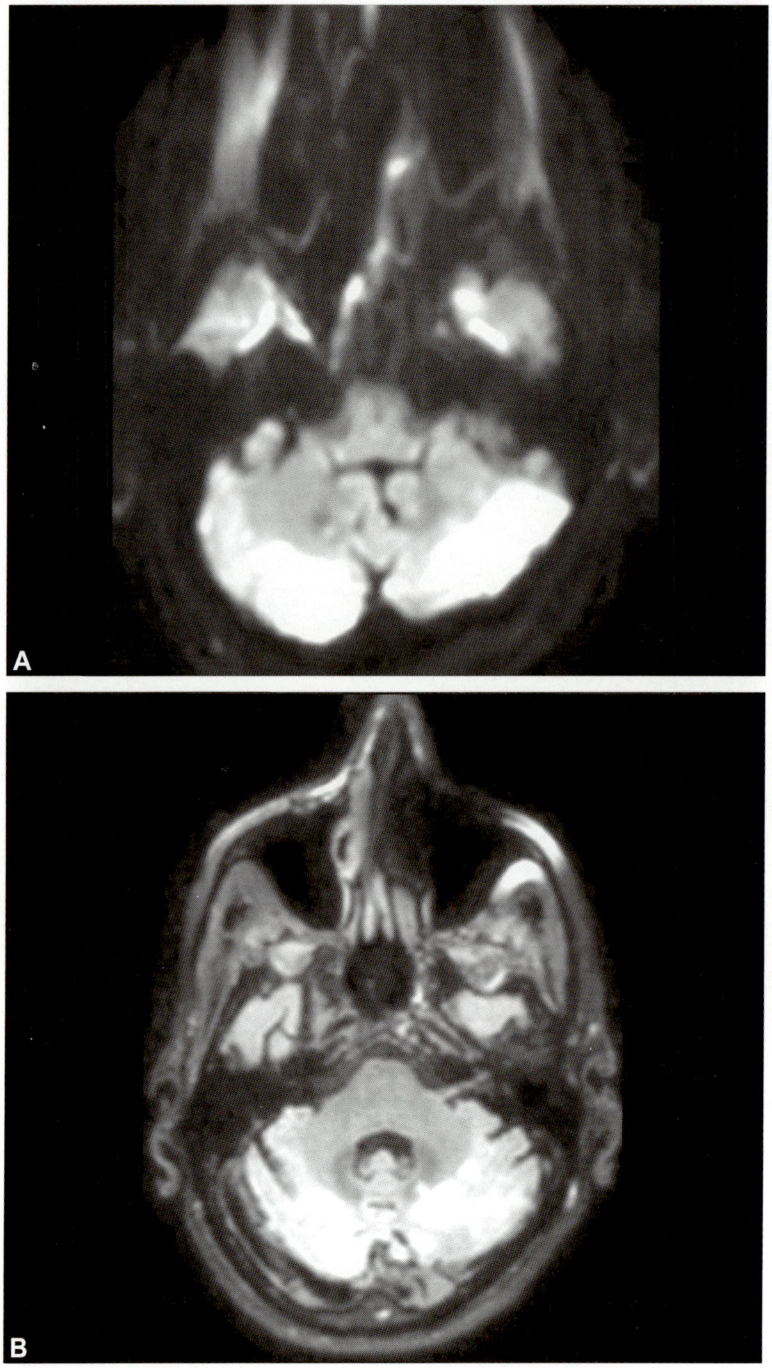

Figs. 26A and B: MRI scan showing bilateral posterior circulation infarct. The lesion is visible on the DW as well as fluid-attenuation inversion recovery (FLAIR) images due the subacute stage beyond 6–12 hours of the insult.

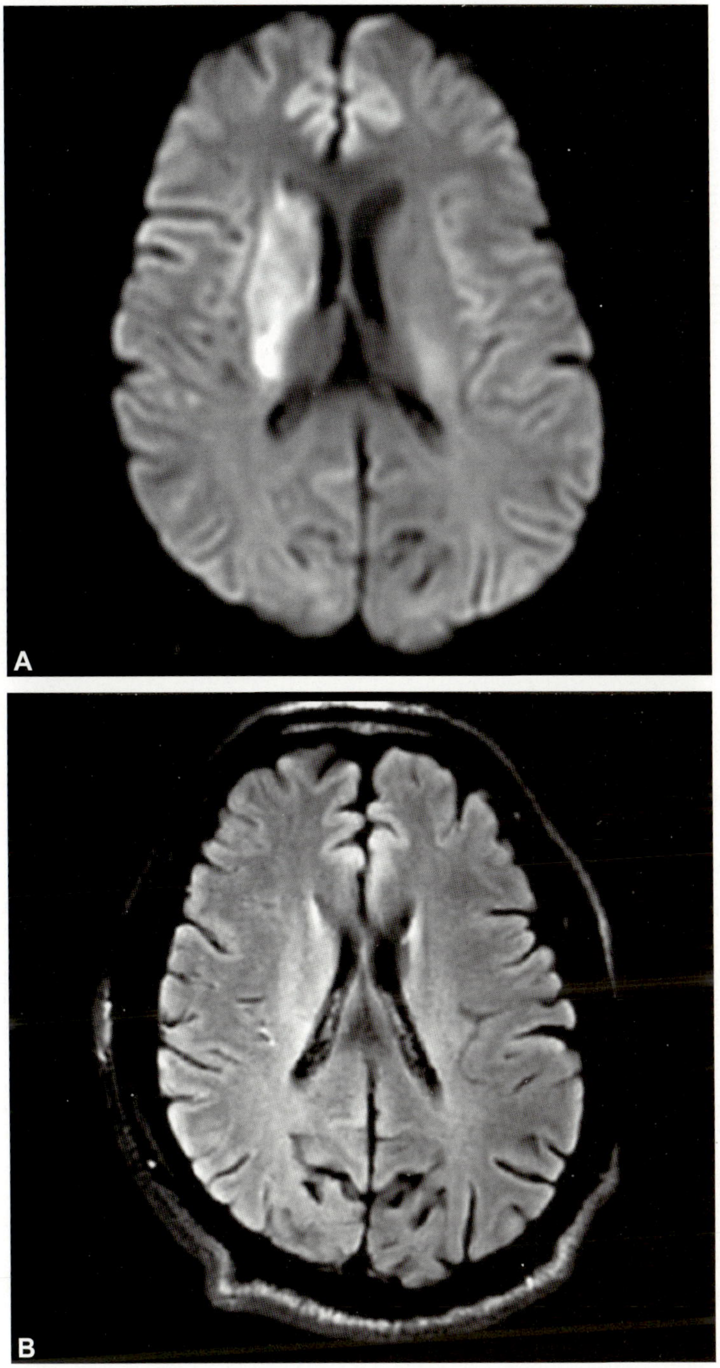

Figs. 27A and B: (A) DWI image showing infarct in acute stage; (B) FLAIR image is unremarkable.

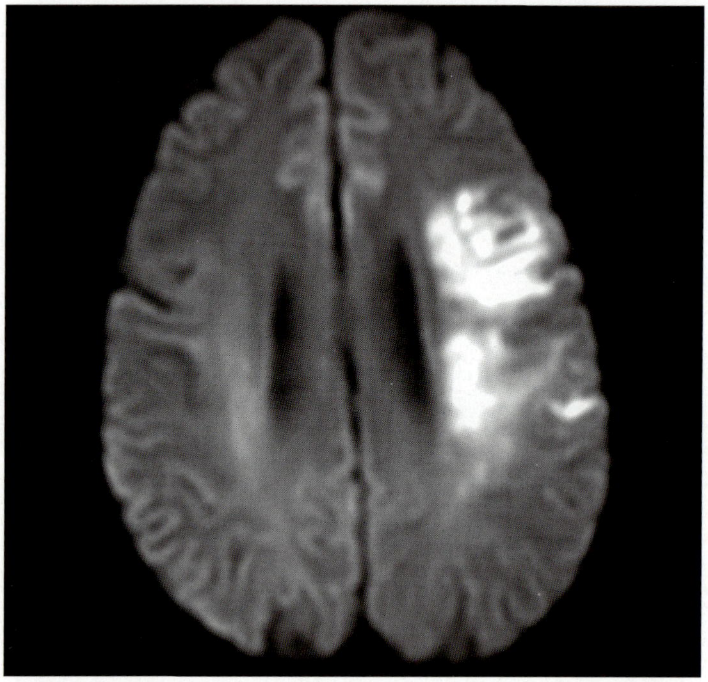

Fig. 28: MRI scan shows left MCA infarct extending into the white matter as well as the subcortical region.

Vascular Pathology (Figs. 29 to 39)

- Aneurysms.
- Dissection.
- Arterial occlusion.
- Venous sinus thrombosis.

All the above are usually associated with headache, unconsciousness, stroke like symptoms or seizures. Imaging plays a key role in the diagnosis as well as in planning the therapy.

Right Posterior Communicating Artery Aneurysm (Figs. 29A and B)

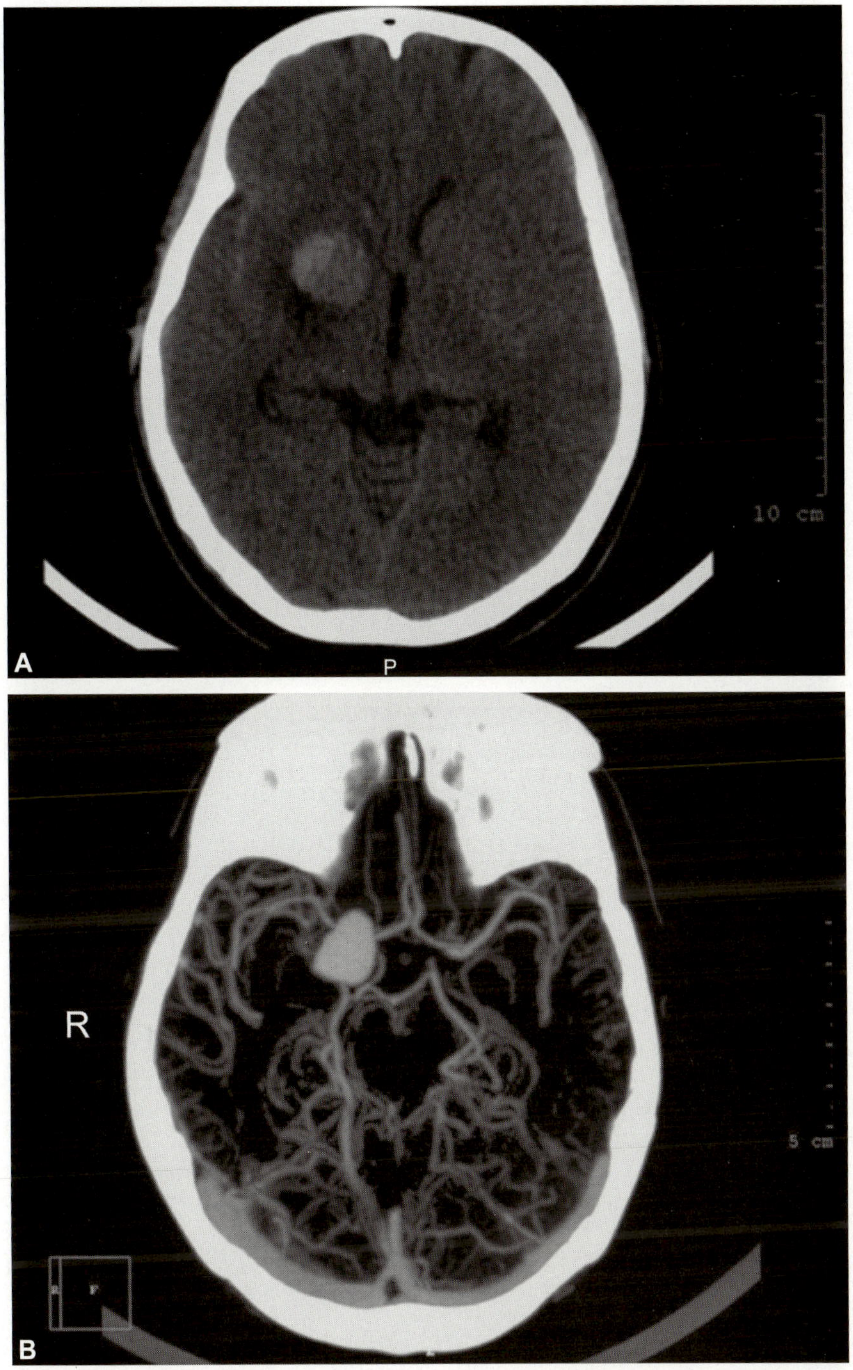

Figs. 29A and B: A 35-year-old female with thunderclap headache. Plain CT axial section with focal liquefying hematoma well defined with surrounding edema and mild compression of right lateral ventricle. Small focus of subarachnoid hemorrhage is noted as bright area in right sylvian fissure. Computed tomography angiography (CTA) reveals the aneurysm in A1 segment of anterior cerebral artery (ACA).

Liquefying Hematoma (Figs. 30A and B)

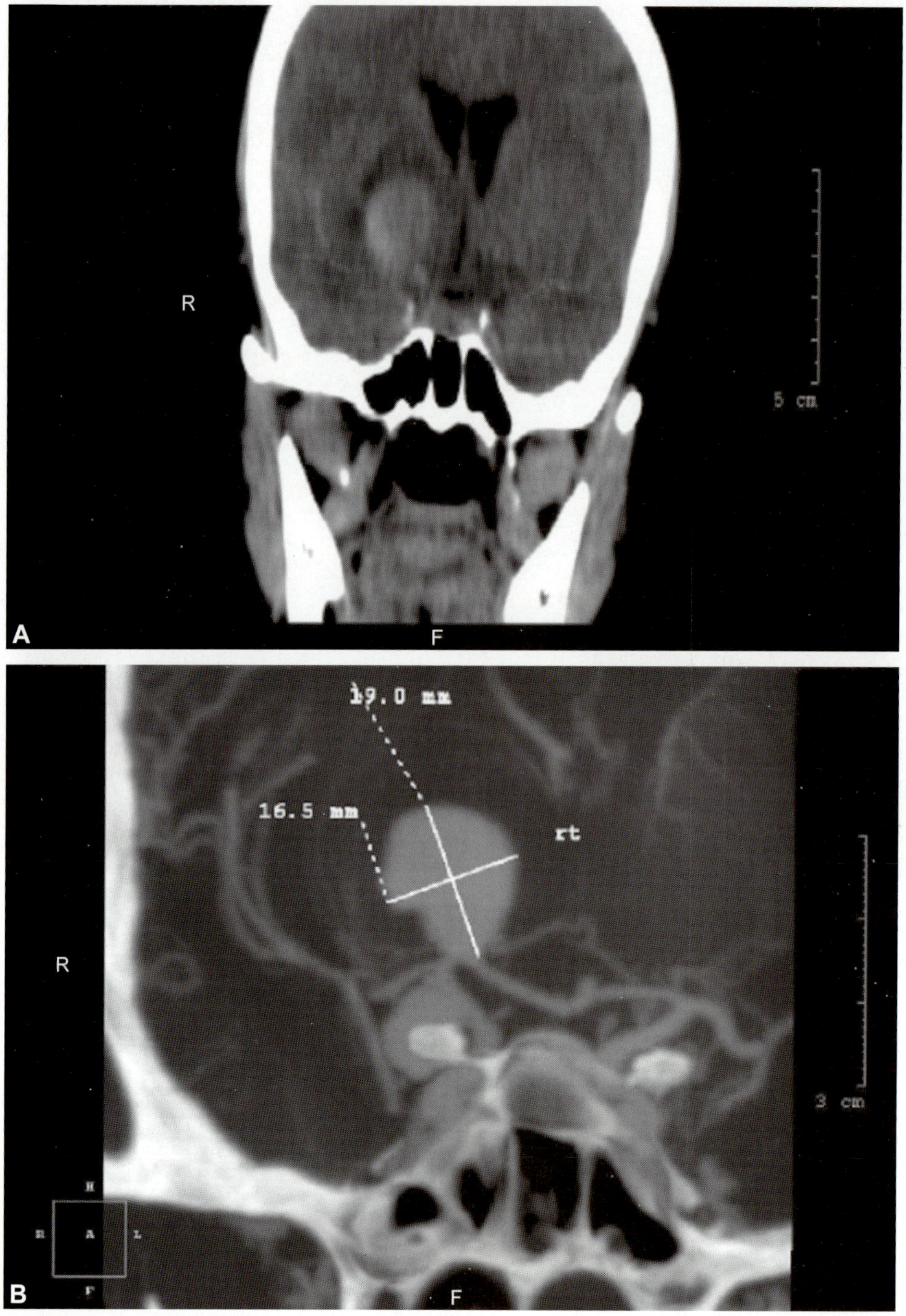

Figs. 30A and B: Plain CT coronal section with focal liquefying hematoma well defined with surrounding edema. CTA reveals two aneurysms, internal carotid artery (ICA) prebifurcation (posterior communicating) and A1 segment of ACA.

Anterior Communicating Artery Aneurysm (Figs. 31A to C)

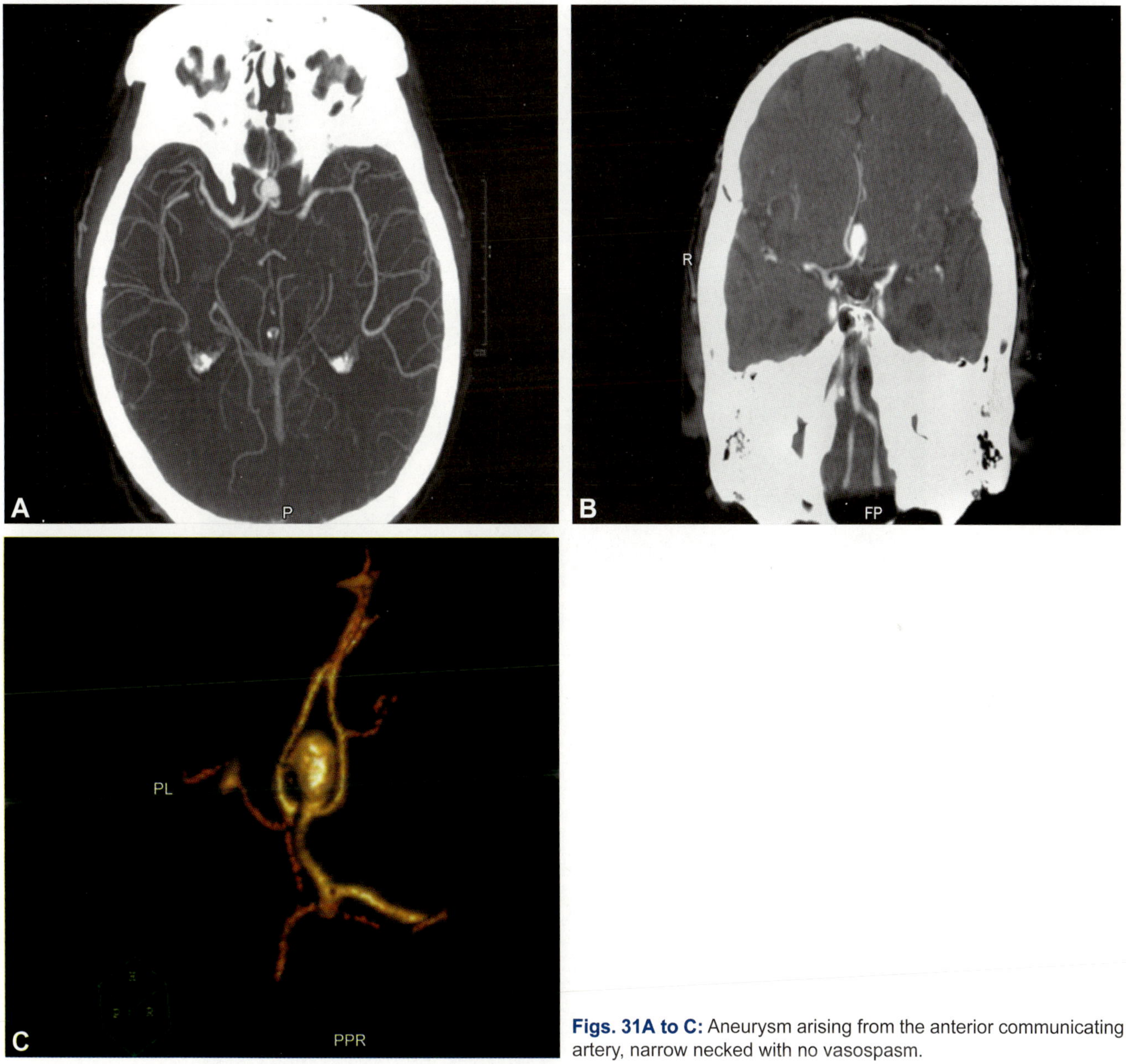

Figs. 31A to C: Aneurysm arising from the anterior communicating artery, narrow necked with no vasospasm.

Vertebral Artery Dissection (Figs. 32A to D)

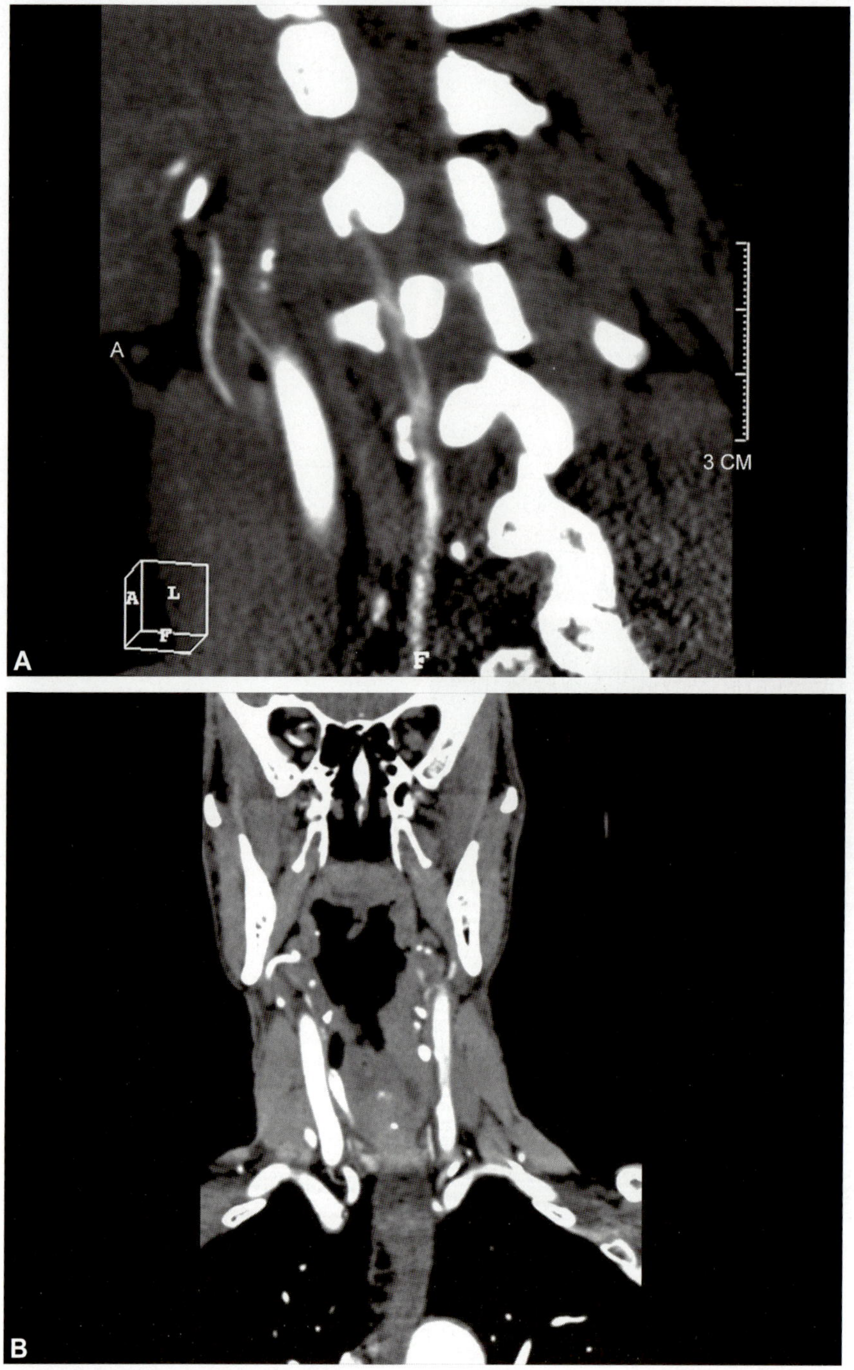

Figs. 32A and B: (A) Young 27-year-old male with history of neck impact CT angio reveals vertebral artery dissection as a linear filling defect within the poorly opacified left VA; (B) CT angio reveals left carotid artery dissection with central linear flap with associated arterial irregularity.

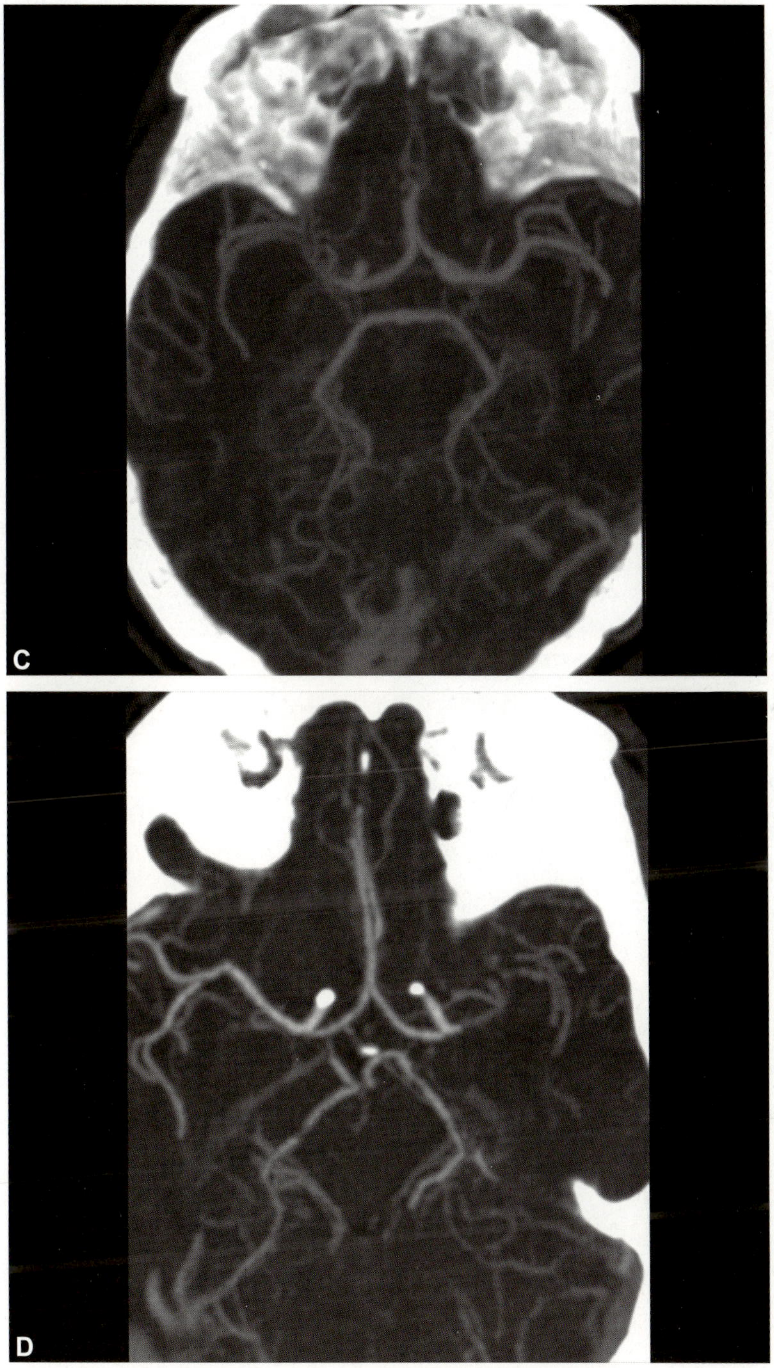

Figs. 32C and D: (C) CT angio shows right MCA occlusion; (D) CT angio shows left MCA occlusion.

Right Internal Carotid Artery Occlusion (Figs. 33A to C)

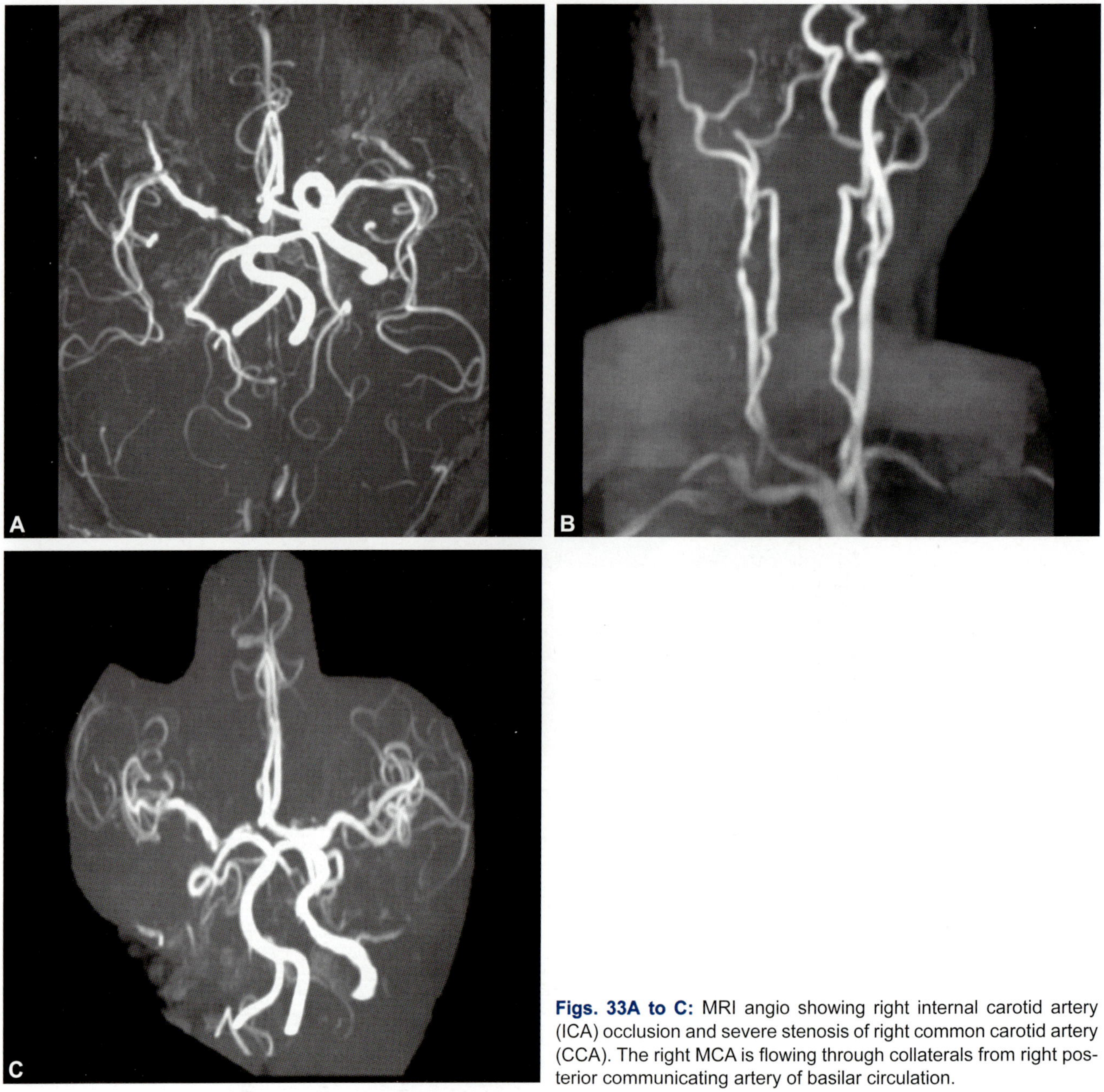

Figs. 33A to C: MRI angio showing right internal carotid artery (ICA) occlusion and severe stenosis of right common carotid artery (CCA). The right MCA is flowing through collaterals from right posterior communicating artery of basilar circulation.

Left Internal Carotid Artery Occlusion (Figs. 34A and B)

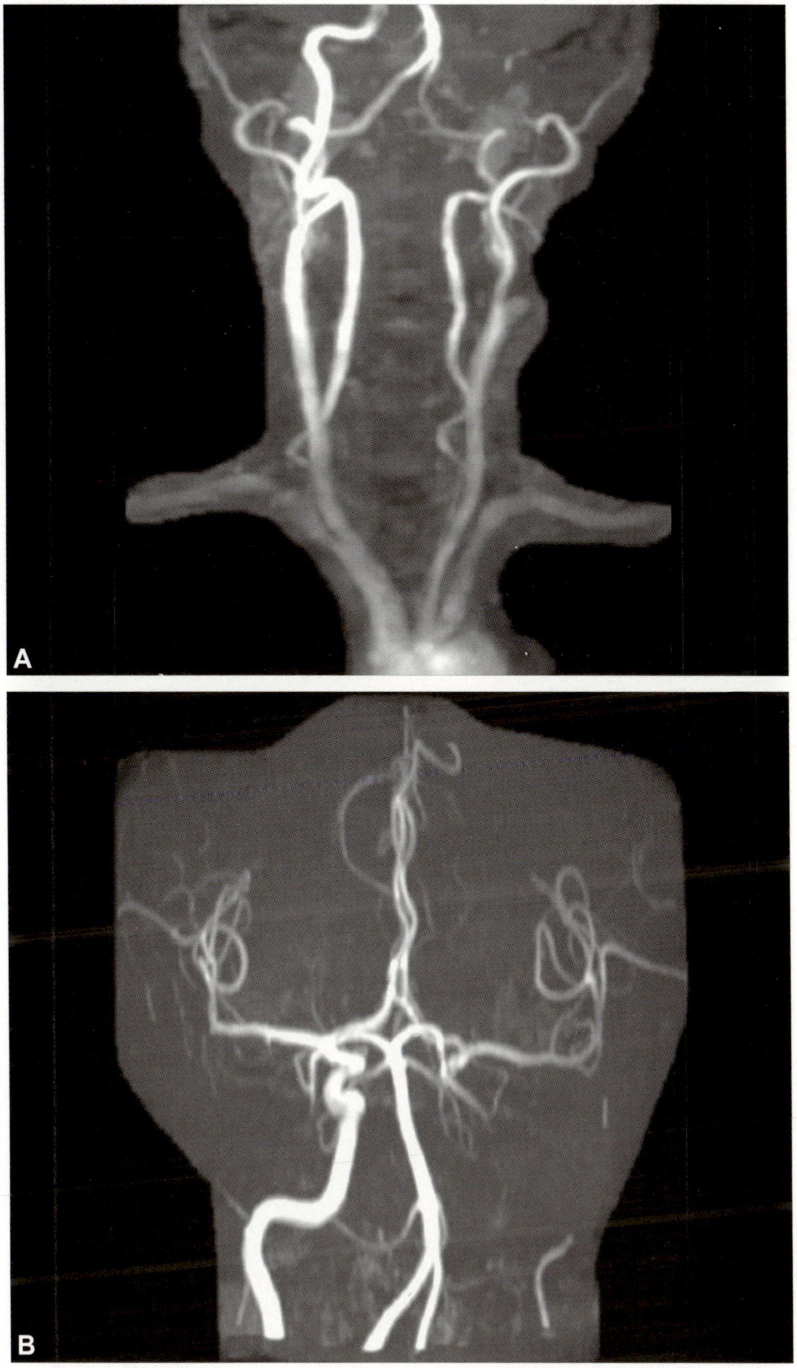

Figs. 34A and B: MRA through the circle of Willis shows left ICA occlusion from the carotid bifurcation. Left MCA is flowing through intracranial collaterals of anterior communicating artery from right ICA.

Bilateral Anterior Cerebral Artery Occlusion (Figs. 35A and B)

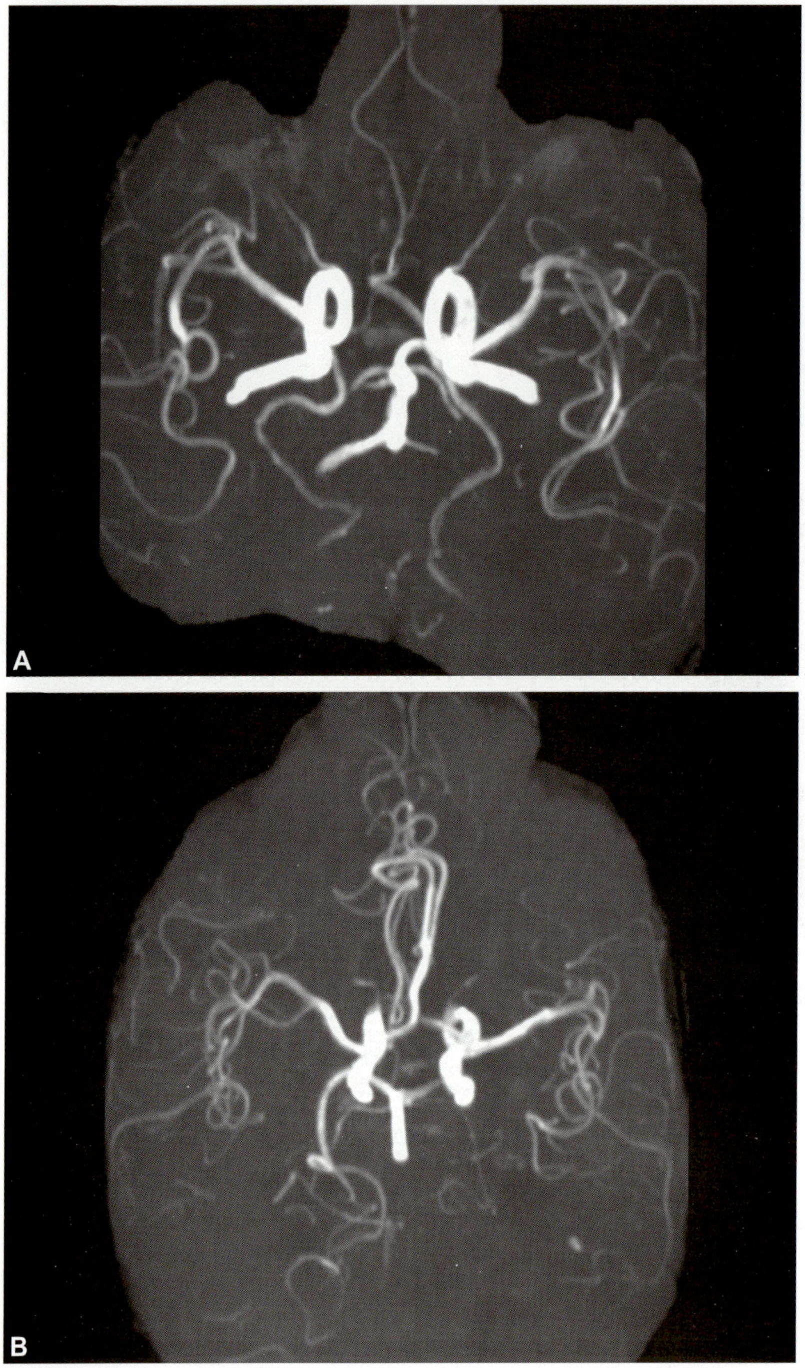

Figs. 35A and B: (A) MRI angio shows bilateral anterior cerebral artery (ACA) occlusion; (B) MRI angio shows left posterior cerebral artery (PCA) occlusion.

Left Transverse Sinus and Left Sigmoid Sinus Thrombus (Figs. 36A and B)

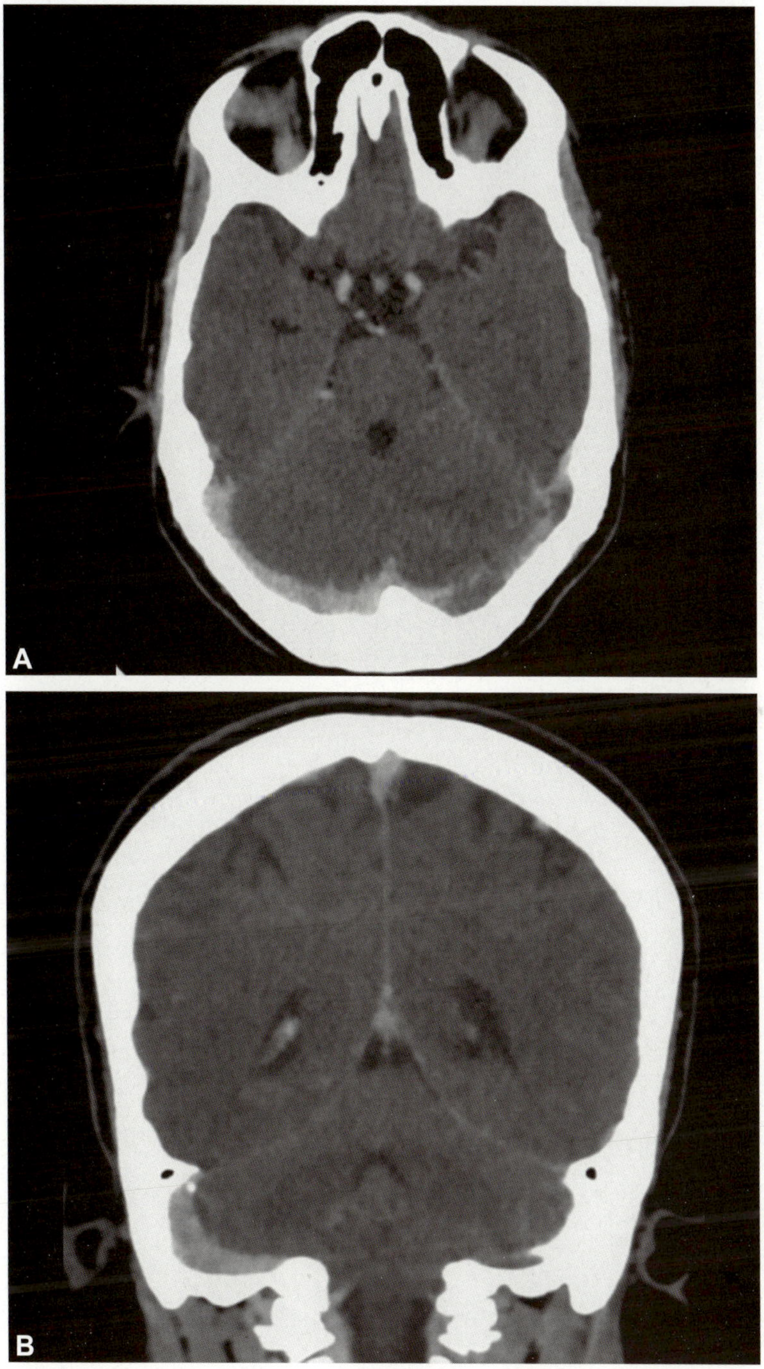

Figs. 36A and B: (A) CECT shows left transverse sinus thrombus as a filling defect as compared to a well-opacified right transverse sinus; (B) CECT shows extension of thrombosis into the left sigmoid sinus as compared to a well-flowing right sigmoid sinus.

Right Transverse Sinus and Internal Jugular Vein Thrombus (Figs. 37A and B)

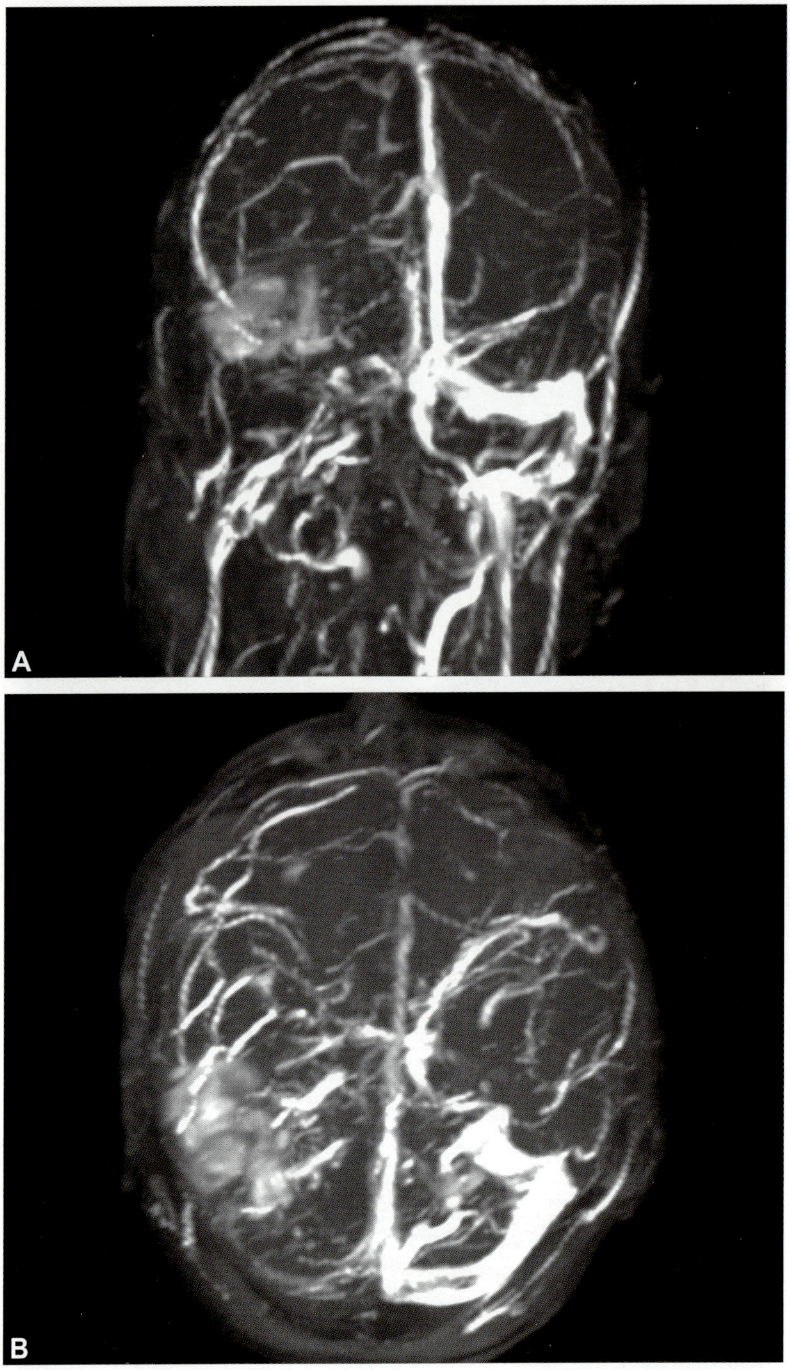

Figs. 37A and B: MR venogram showing nonfilling of right transverse, sigmoid sinus and internal jugular vein (IJV) due to thrombosis.

Left Internal Jugular Vein Thrombus (Fig. 38)

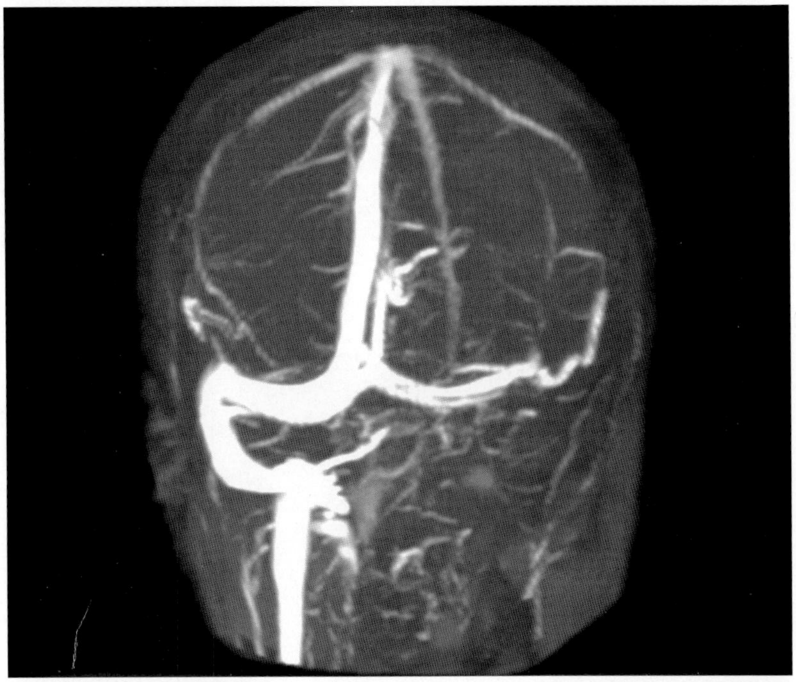

Fig. 38: MR venogram shows poor flow in left sigmoid sinus and IJV suggestive of thrombotic occlusion.

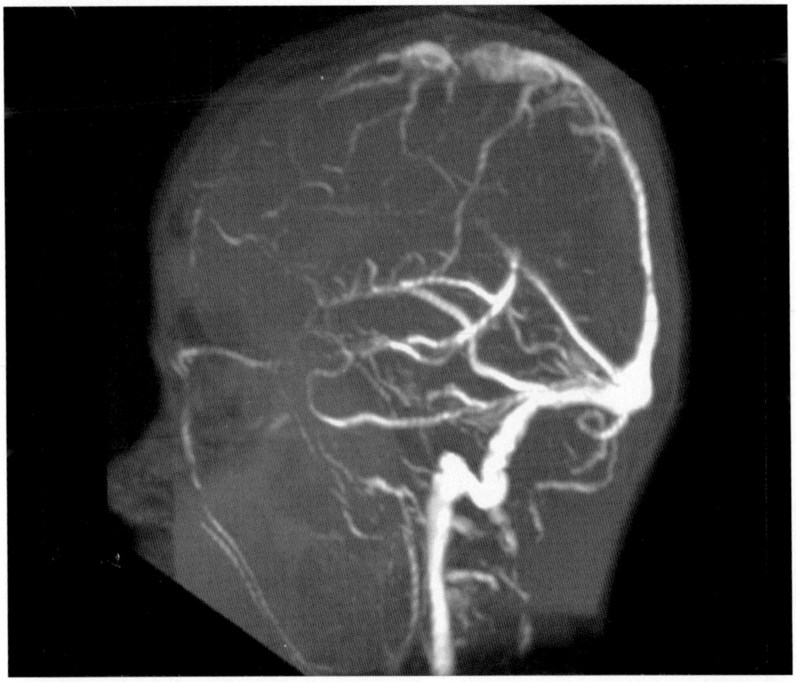

Fig. 39: MRI venogram shows poor flow in the anterior superior sagittal sinus suggestive of thrombosis.

RING ENHANCING LESIONS CT AND MRI (FIGS. 40 TO 42)

Tuberculoma in CT Scan (Figs. 40A and B)

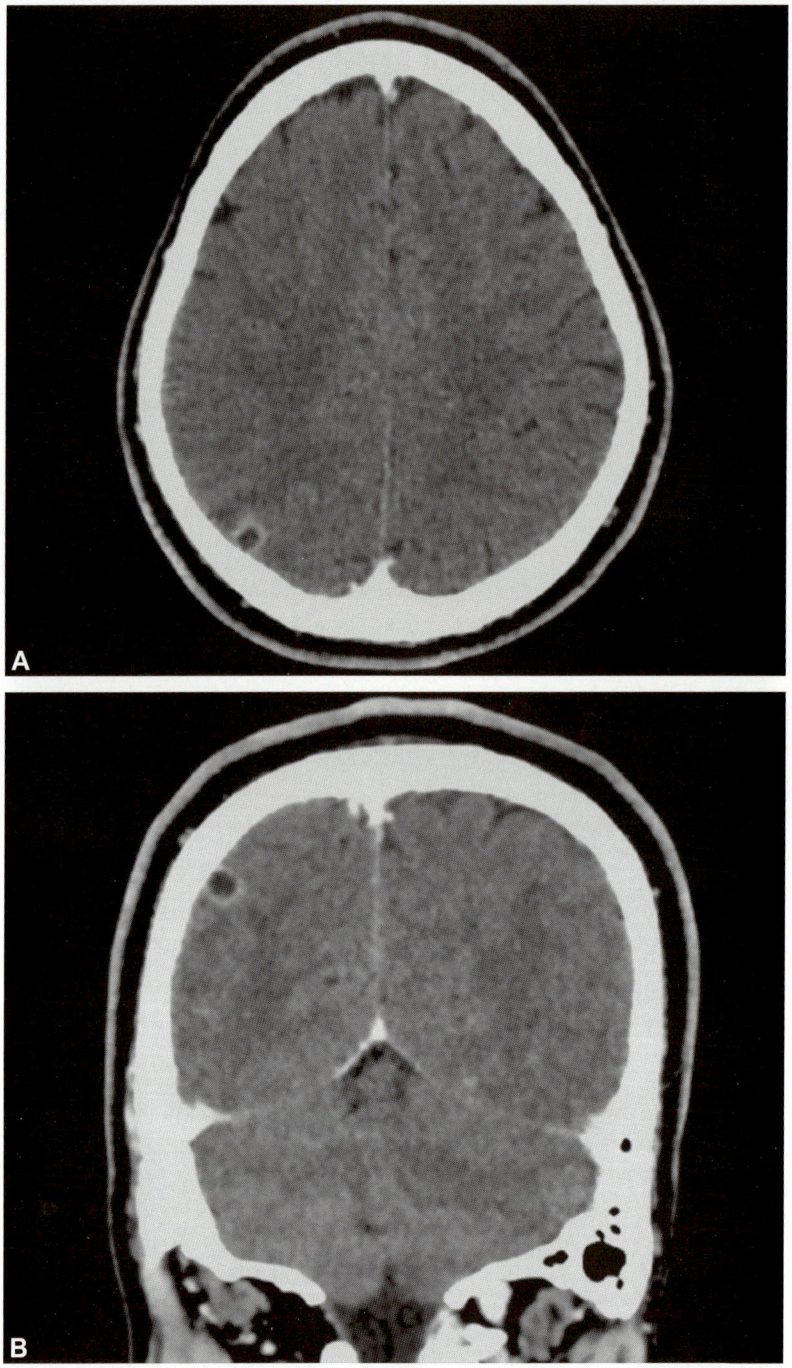

Figs. 40A and B: Postcontrast CT showing ring enhancing lesion in right parietal cortex suggestive of tuberculoma.

Tuberculoma (Figs. 41A to C)

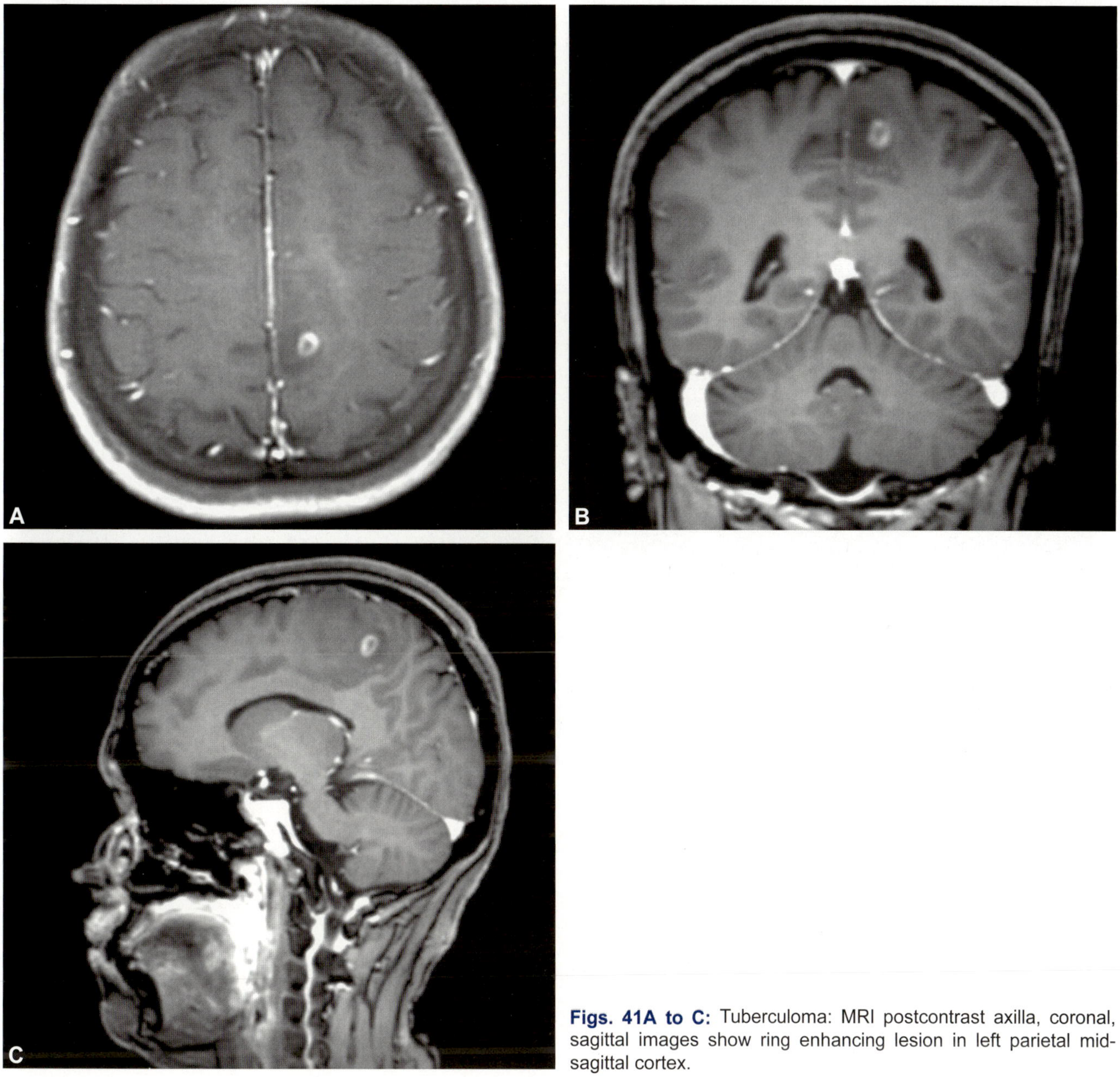

Figs. 41A to C: Tuberculoma: MRI postcontrast axilla, coronal, sagittal images show ring enhancing lesion in left parietal mid-sagittal cortex.

Calcified Granuloma (Figs. 42A to C)

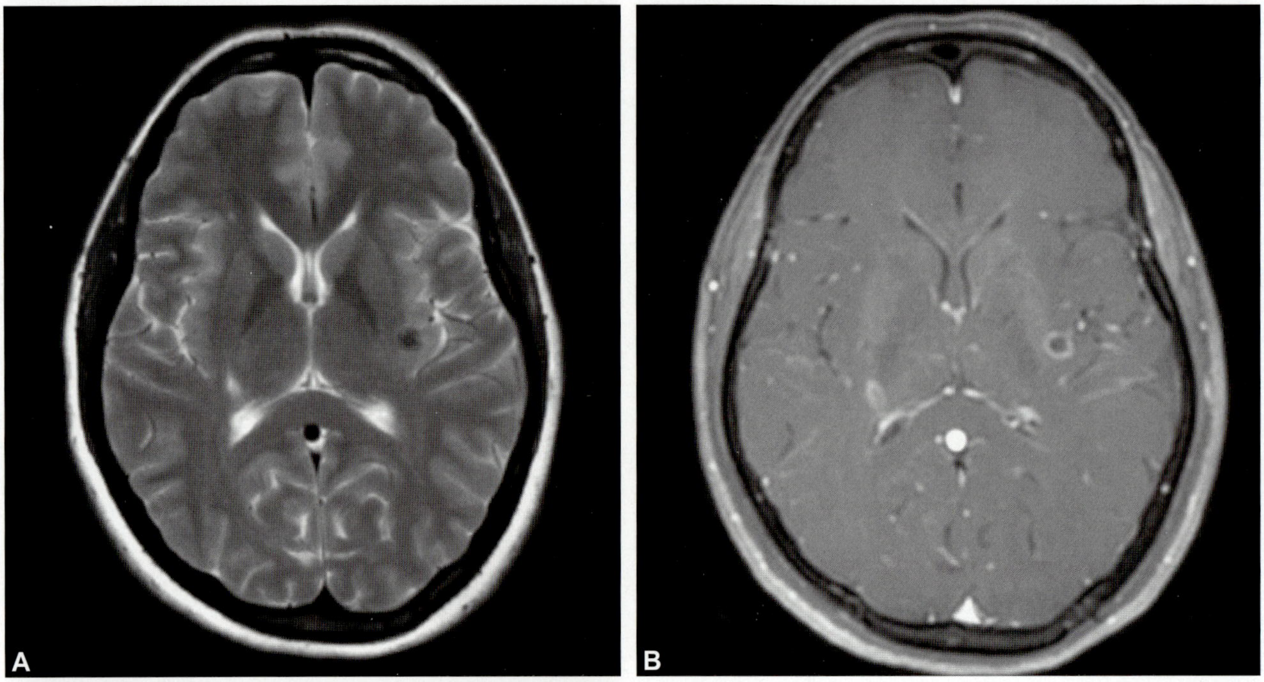

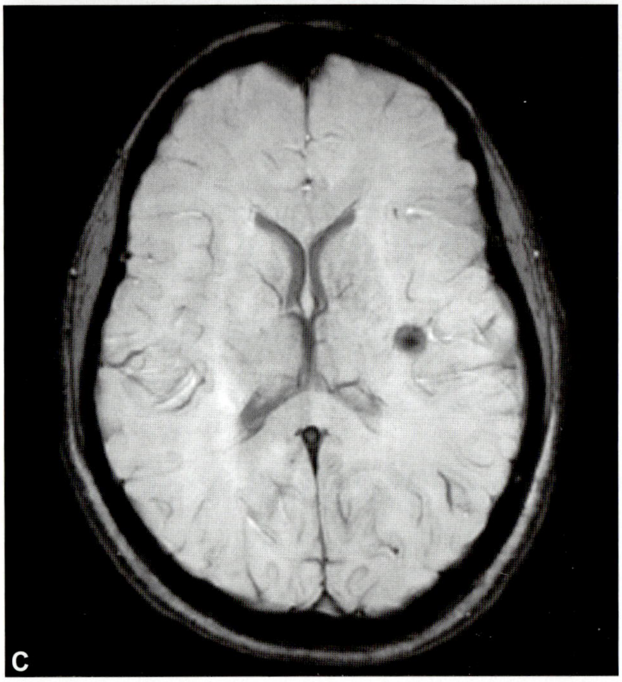

Figs. 42A to C: Contrast-enhanced magnetic resonance (CEMR): Left parietal calcified granuloma with ring enhancement, likely to be cysticercosis.

MENINGITIS (FIGS. 43A TO C)

Coronal MR noncontrast fluid-attenuated inversion recovery (FLAIR) image reveals hydrocephalus in frontal horns of lateral ventricle with transependymal CSF ooze.

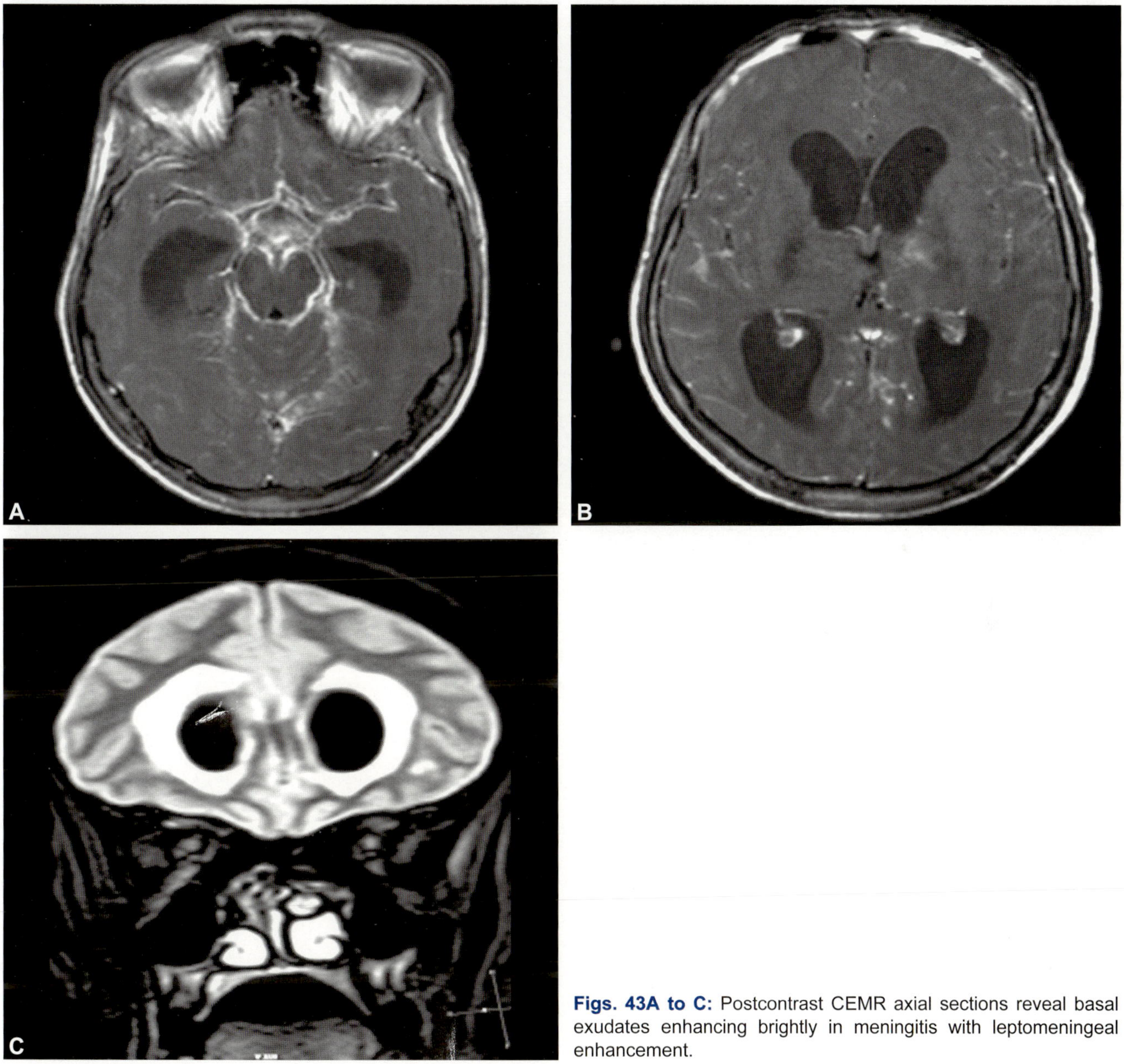

Figs. 43A to C: Postcontrast CEMR axial sections reveal basal exudates enhancing brightly in meningitis with leptomeningeal enhancement.

ENCEPHALITIS (FIGS. 44A TO C)

Periventricular CSF ooze is seen around the posterior horns of ventricles.

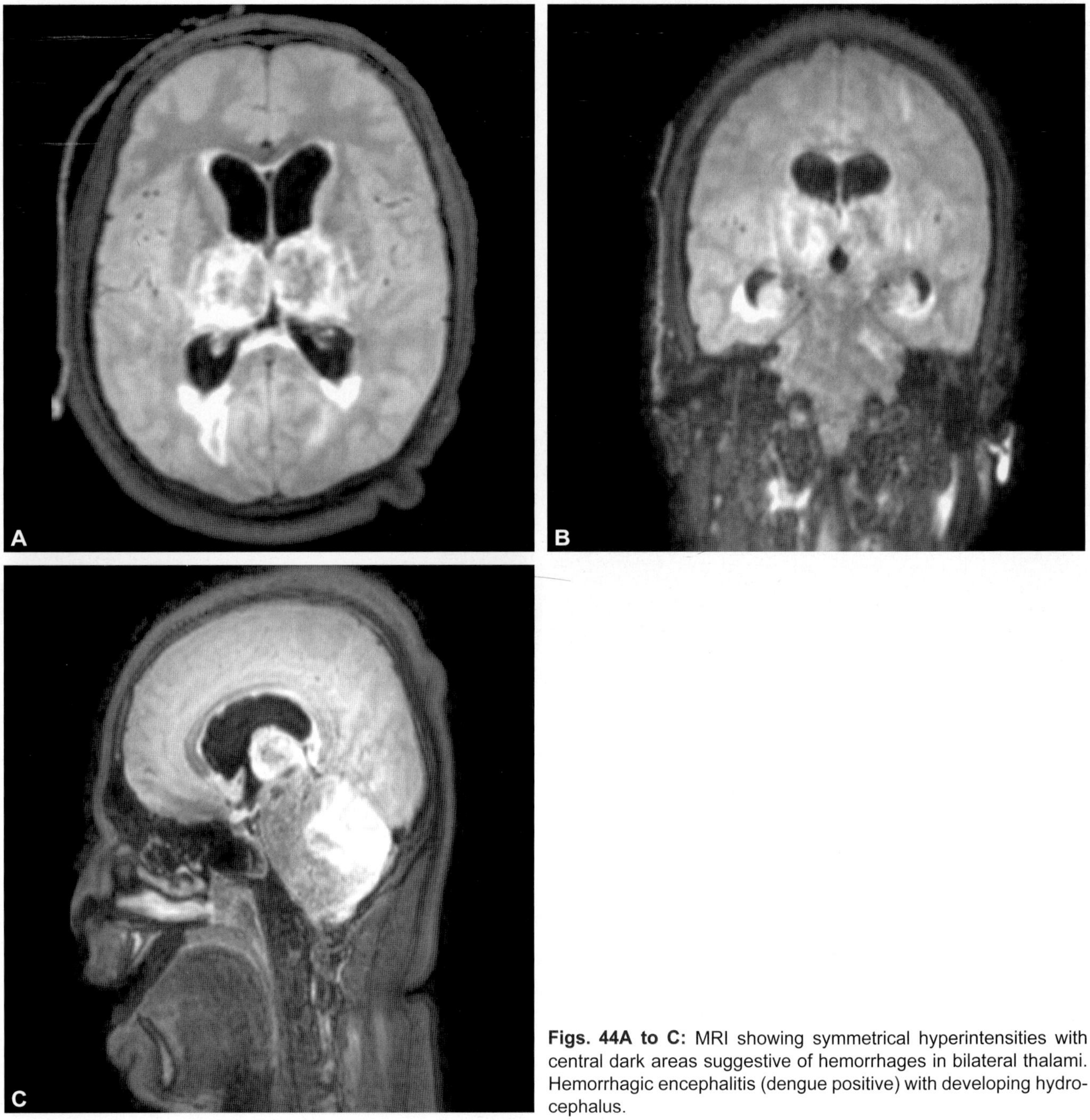

Figs. 44A to C: MRI showing symmetrical hyperintensities with central dark areas suggestive of hemorrhages in bilateral thalami. Hemorrhagic encephalitis (dengue positive) with developing hydrocephalus.

SPACE OCCUPYING LESIONS CT AND MRI (FIGS. 45 TO 50)

Meningioma (Figs. 45A and B)

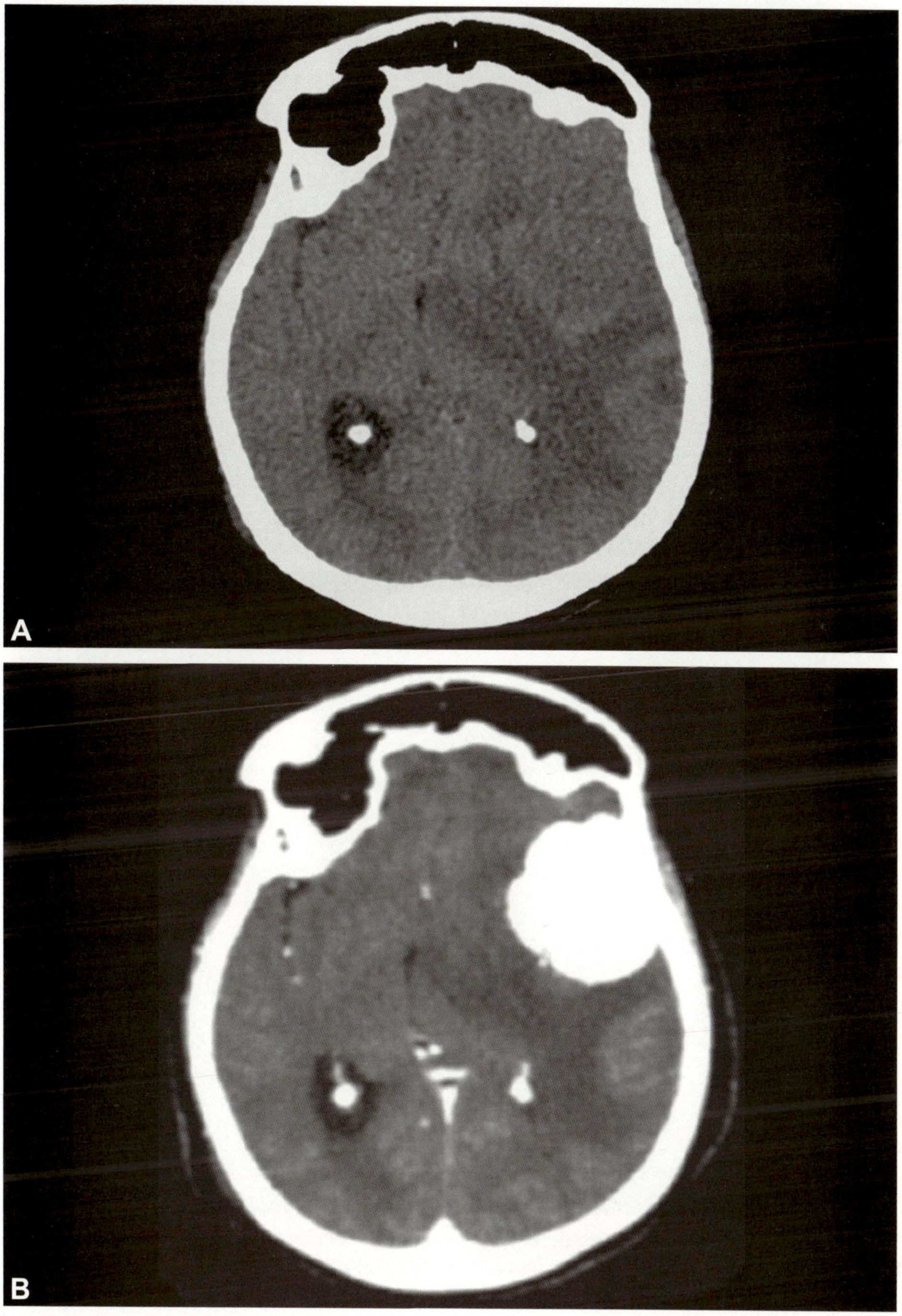

Figs. 45A and B: CECT: Intensely enhancing mass lesion in left frontotemporal cortex suggestive of a typical meningioma arising from the inner skull table.

Glioma (Figs. 46 and 47)

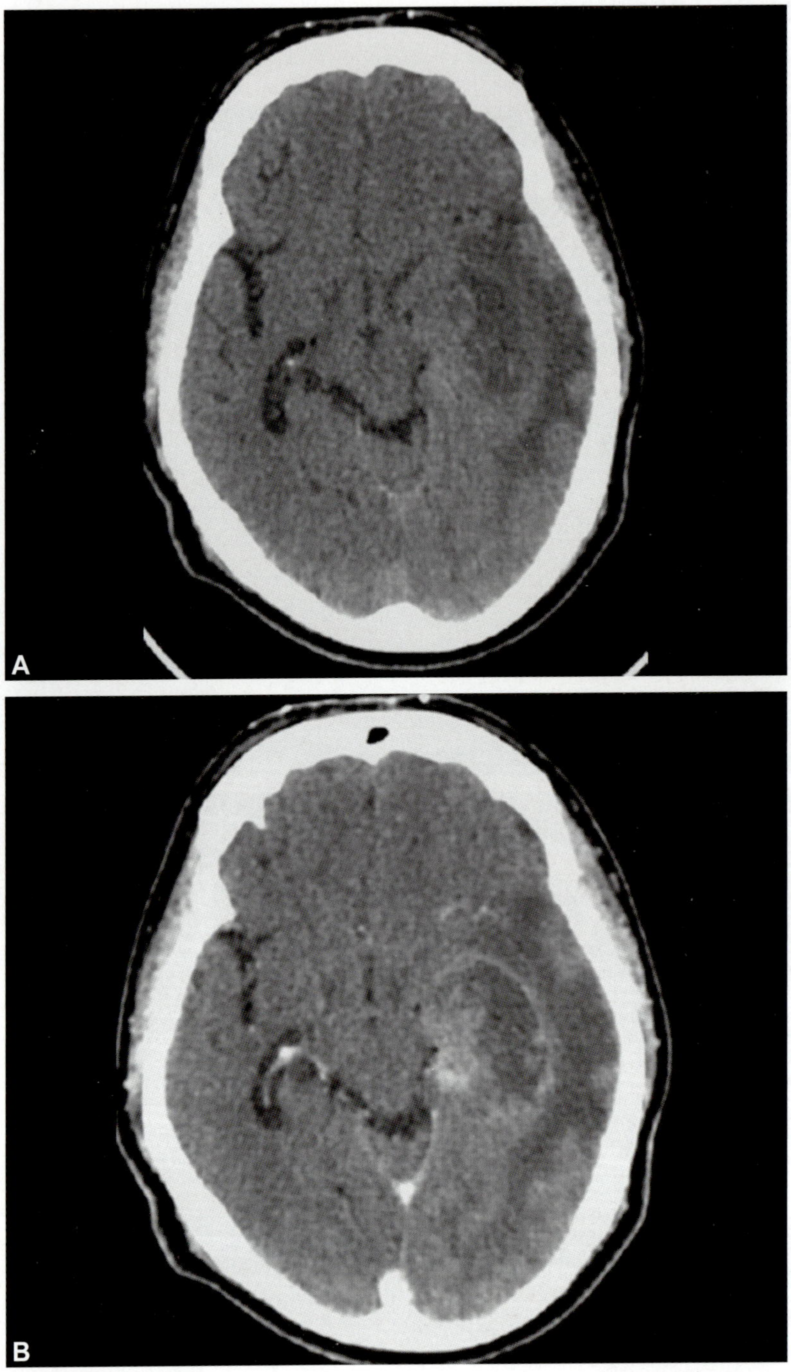

Figs. 46A and B: CECT: Hypodense lesion in left temporal lobe with mass effect on left temporal horn. Moderate compression of the left midbrain. Postcontrast enhancing mass in the medial temporal cortex suggestive of glioma.

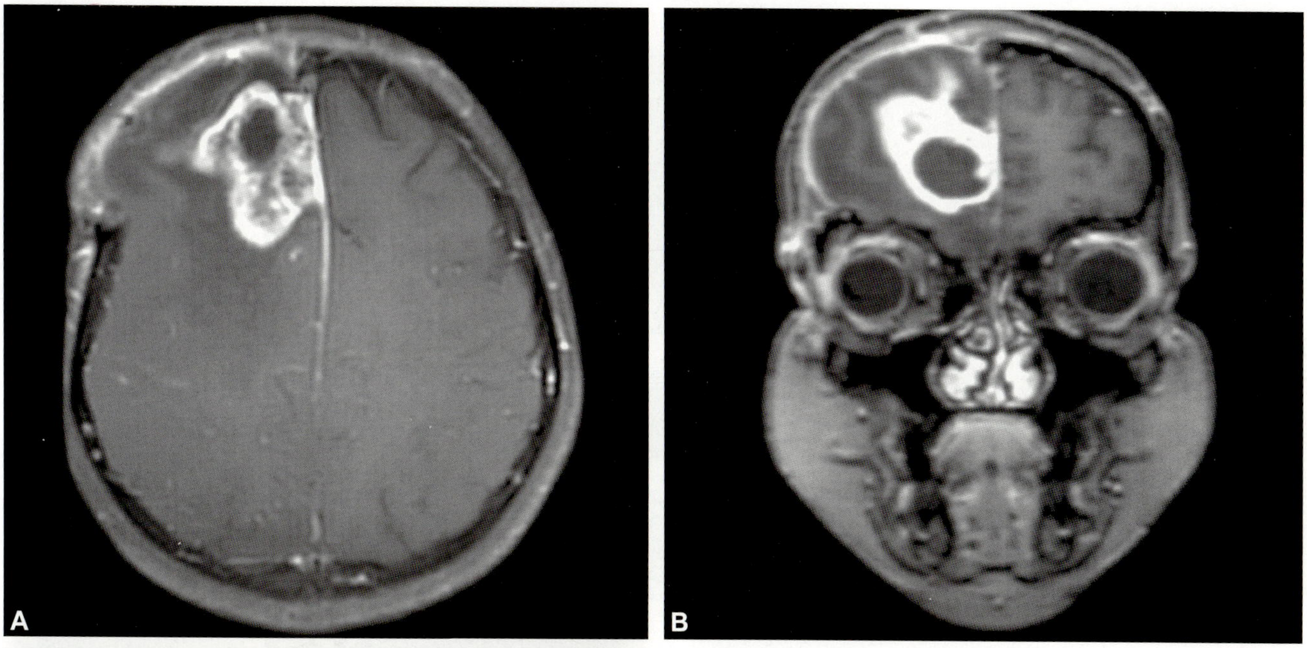

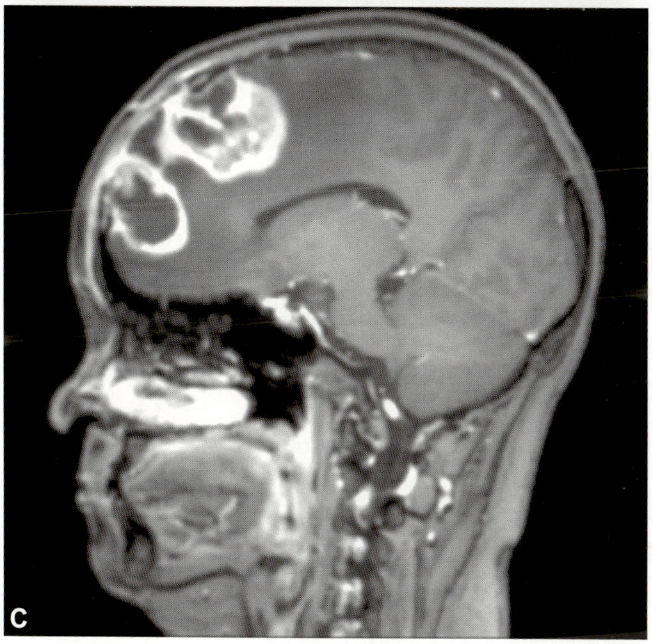

Figs. 47A to C: CEMR—postcraniectomy right frontal: Axial, coronal and sagittal postcontrast peripherally enhancing and centrally necrotic (Dark signal) lesion suggestive of glioma.

Vestibular Schwannoma (Figs. 48A and B)

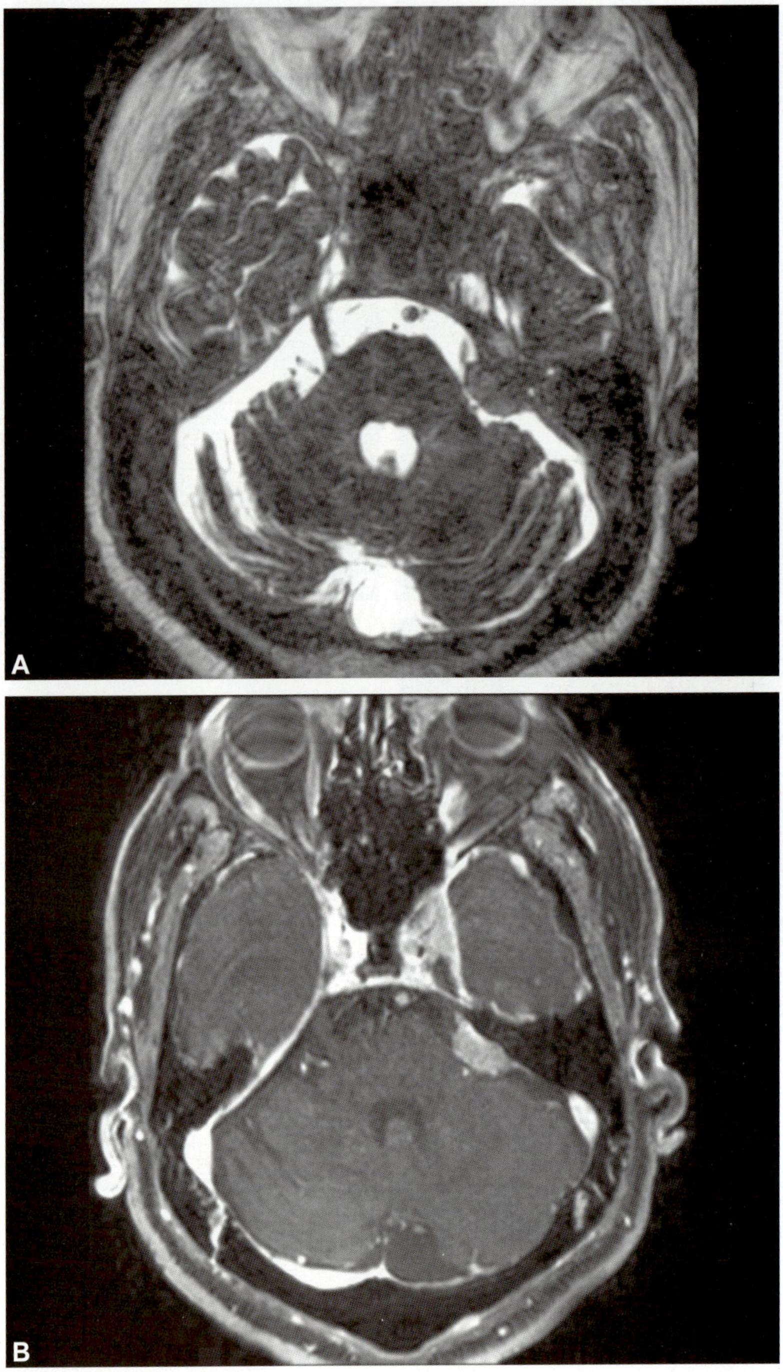

Figs. 48A and B: CEMR: Pre- and postcontrast study showing enhancing lesion in left cerebellopontine (CP) angle suggestive of vestibular schwannoma.

Multiple Meningiomatosis (Fig. 49)

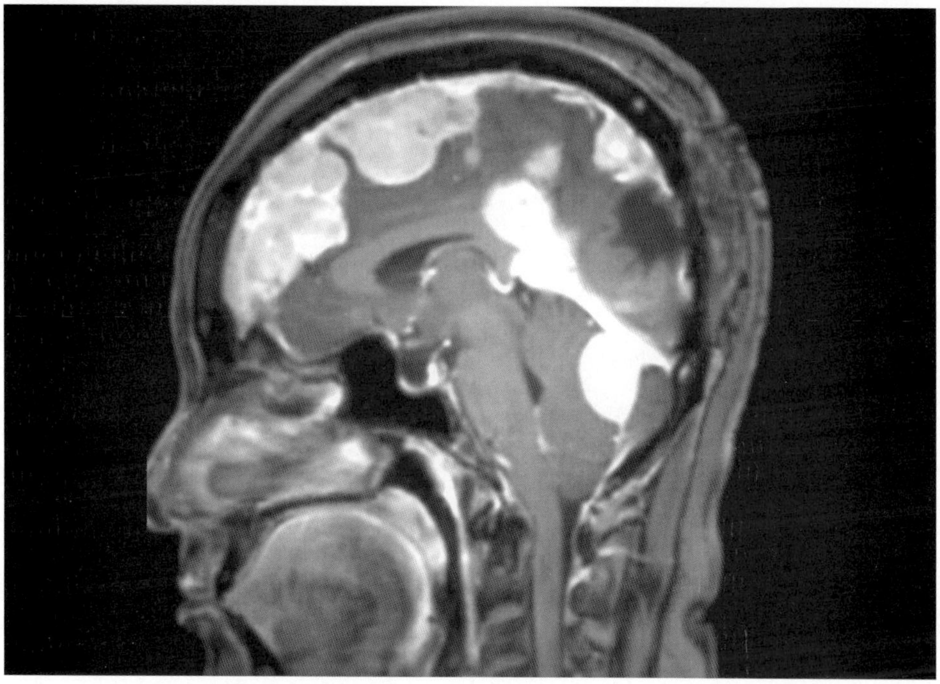

Fig. 49: CEMR: Study shows multiple meningiomatosis.

Pituitary Macroadenoma (Figs. 50A and B)

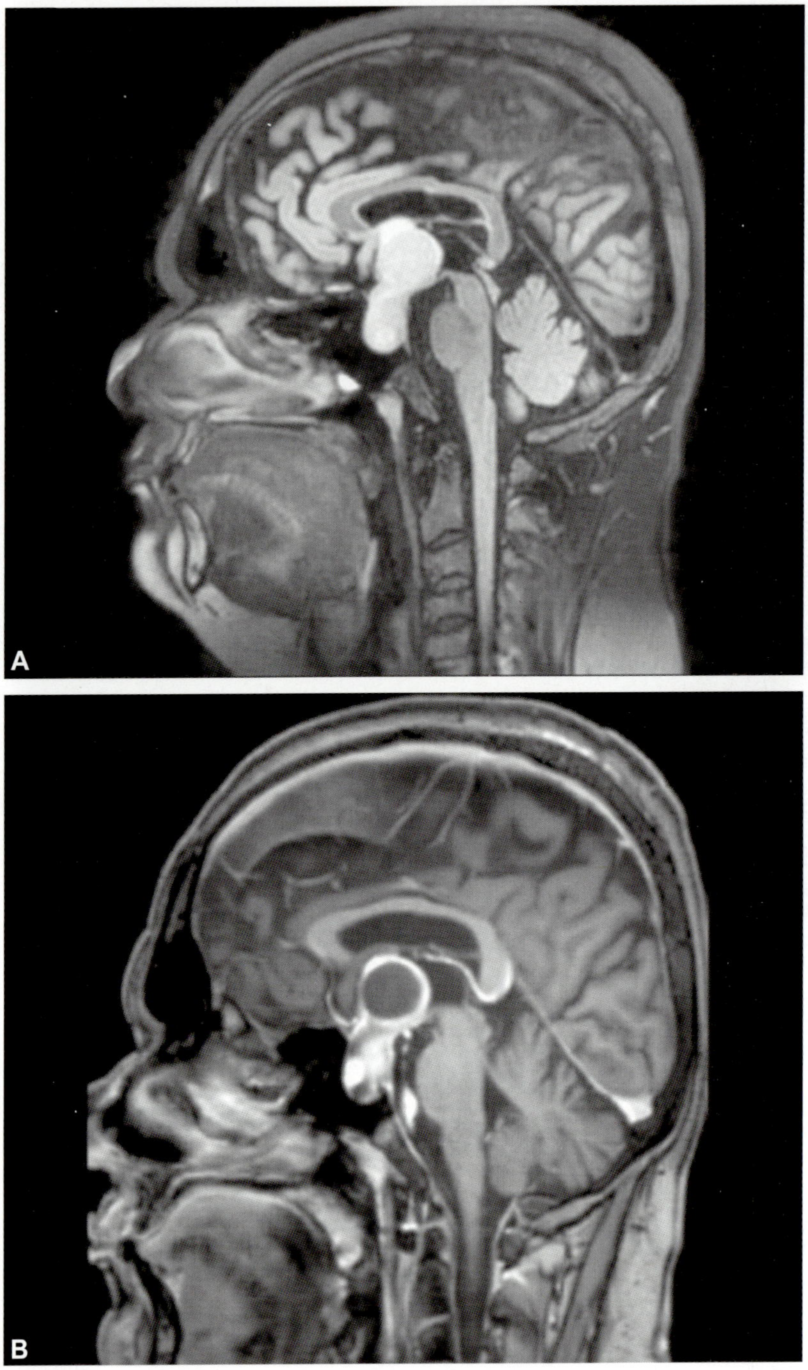

Figs. 50A and B: CEMR: (A) Pre; and (B) Postcontrast study showing lesion arising from pituitary gland suggestive of pituitary macroadenoma. The mass has a suprasellar necrotic as well as infrasellar sphenoid sinus extension.

HERPES SIMPLEX VIRUS ENCEPHALITIS (FIGS. 51A AND B)

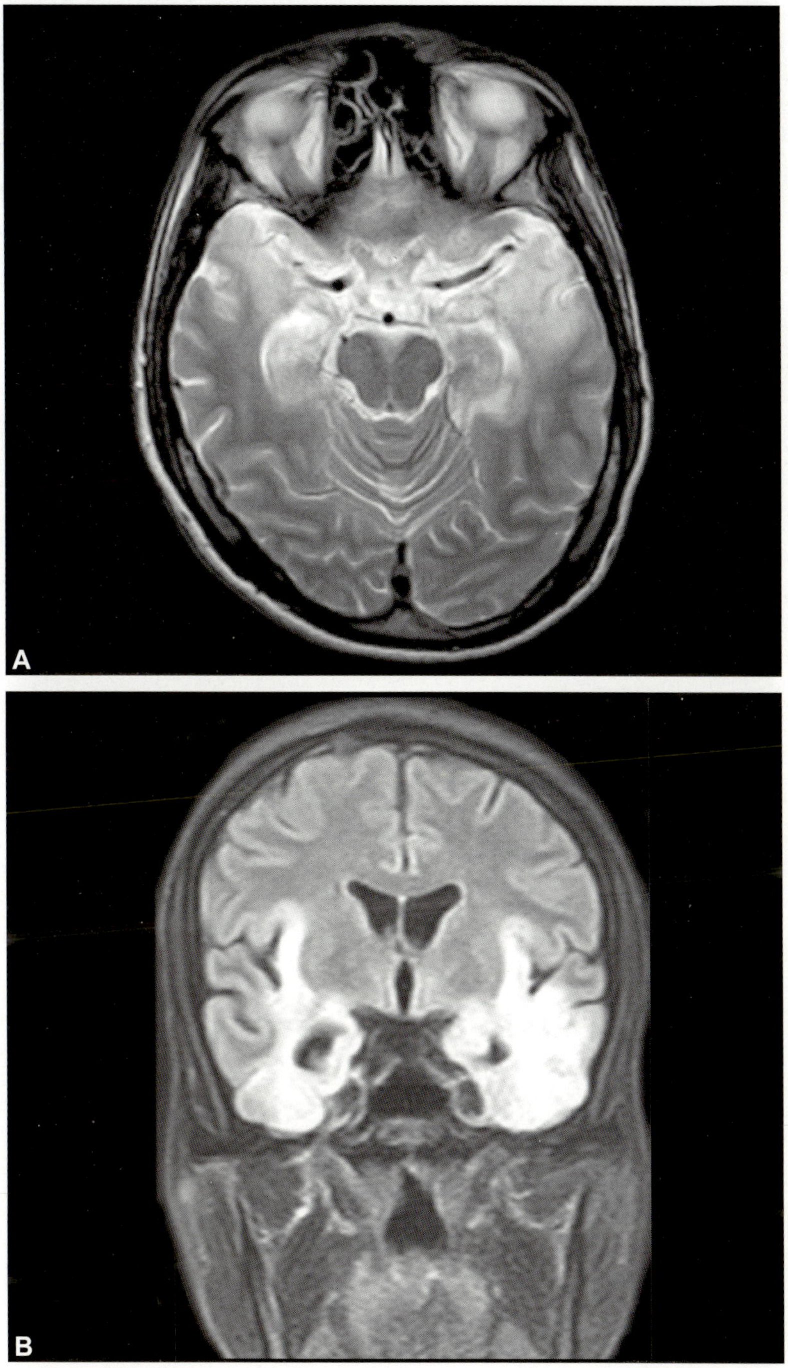

Figs. 51A and B: Herpes simplex virus (HSV) encephalitis affection of the bilateral symmetrical or asymmetrical temporal lobes and external capsule. The hallmark is noninvolvement of internal capsule.

Obstructive Hydrocephalus (Figs. 52A and B)

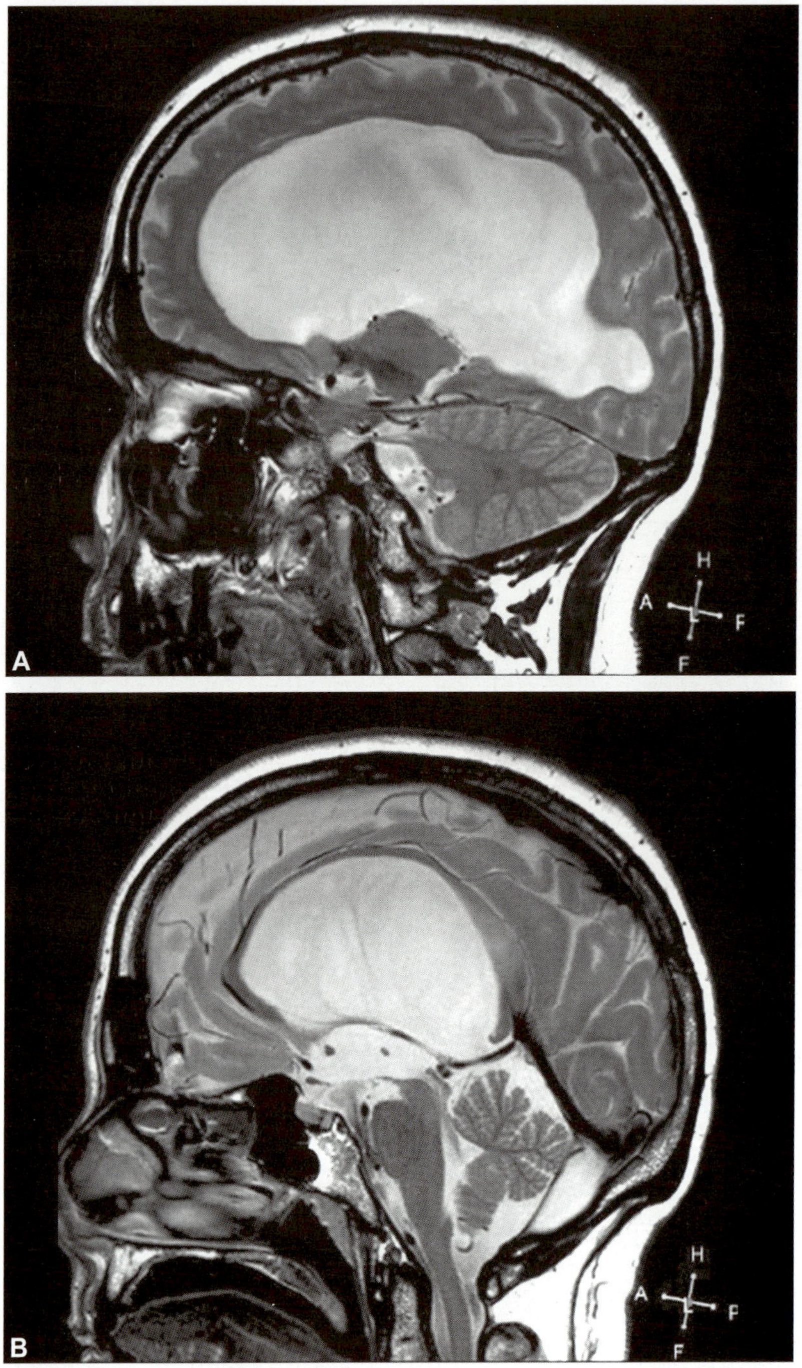

Figs. 52A and B: MRI sagittal: Hydrocephalus in lateral ventricles due to aqueductal stenosis. Normal appearance of 4th ventricle.

CHAPTER 14

Neuromonitoring and Neuroimaging

Harsh Sapra, Gaurav Kakkar

PTOSIS (FIG. 1)

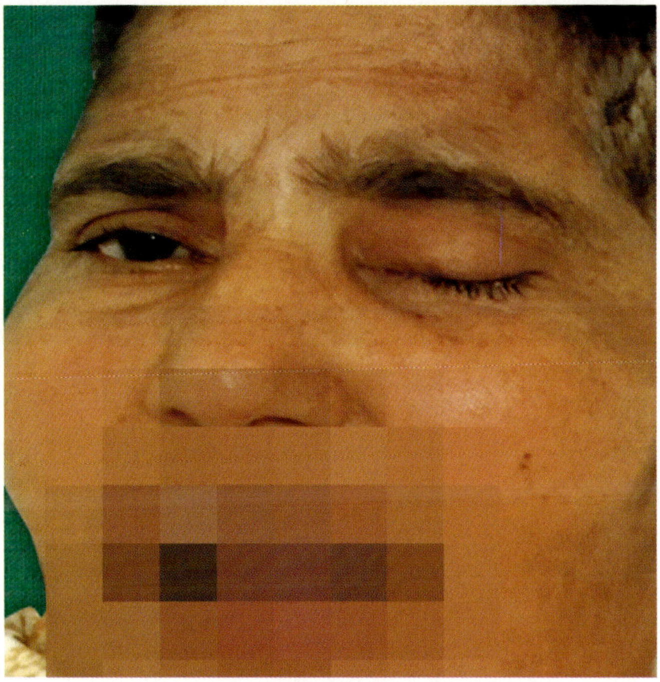

Fig. 1: Ptosis

- Drooping of the upper eyelid.
- Multiple causes, drugs, trauma, tumor, congenital, neuromuscular disorders, neurotoxins.
- Dysfunction of the muscle or the nerves supplying the muscles of the eyelid.
- In Horner's syndrome, cessation of the sympathetic supply causes ptosis, miosis and anhidrosis.

DECORTICATE POSTURE (FIG. 2)

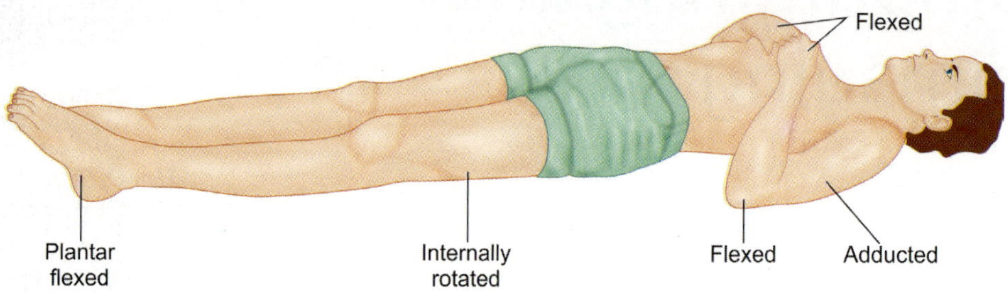

Fig. 2: Decorticate posture.

- Also called flexor posturing or decorticate rigidity.
- Caused by the facilitation of the rubrospinal tract and disruption of the corticospinal tract.
- Flexion of the upper limbs and extension of the lower limbs.
- Usually gets a motor score of 3 on the Glasgow coma scale (GCS).
- Commonly seen in damage to cerebral hemispheres, thalamus and internal capsule.

DECEREBRATE POSTURE (FIG. 3)

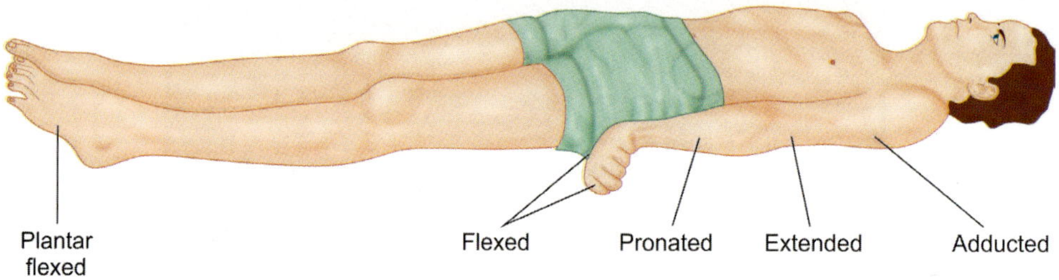

Fig. 3: Decerebrate posture.

- Also called extensor posturing or decerebrate rigidity.
- Indicative of brainstem damage below the red nucleus.
- Extension of the upper extremities especially elbows.
- Usually gets a score of 2 on the GCS.
- Commonly seen in pontine strokes.

EXTRADURAL OR EPIDURAL HEMATOMA (FIGS. 4A AND B)

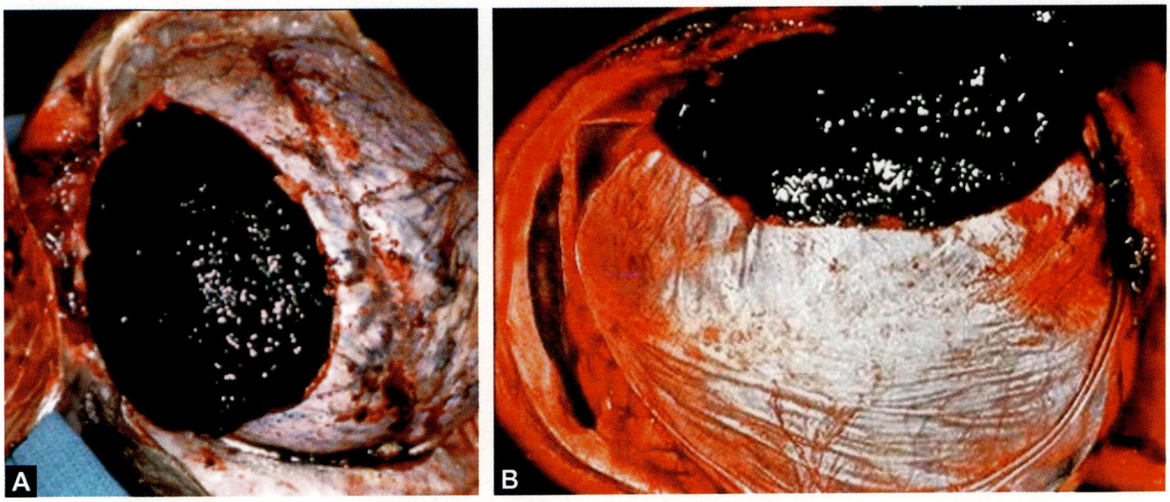

Figs. 4A and B: Extradural hematoma.

- Hematoma collection between the skull bone and dura.
- Life-threatening due to intracranial pressure (ICP) on the brain. Fatal in 15–20% cases.
- Expanding nature of the hematoma due to arterial bleed.
- The most common bleeder is the middle meningeal artery.
- Has a “lucid interval” after trauma before symptoms become evident.

ARTERIAL SUPPLY OF THE BRAIN (FIGS. 5A AND B)

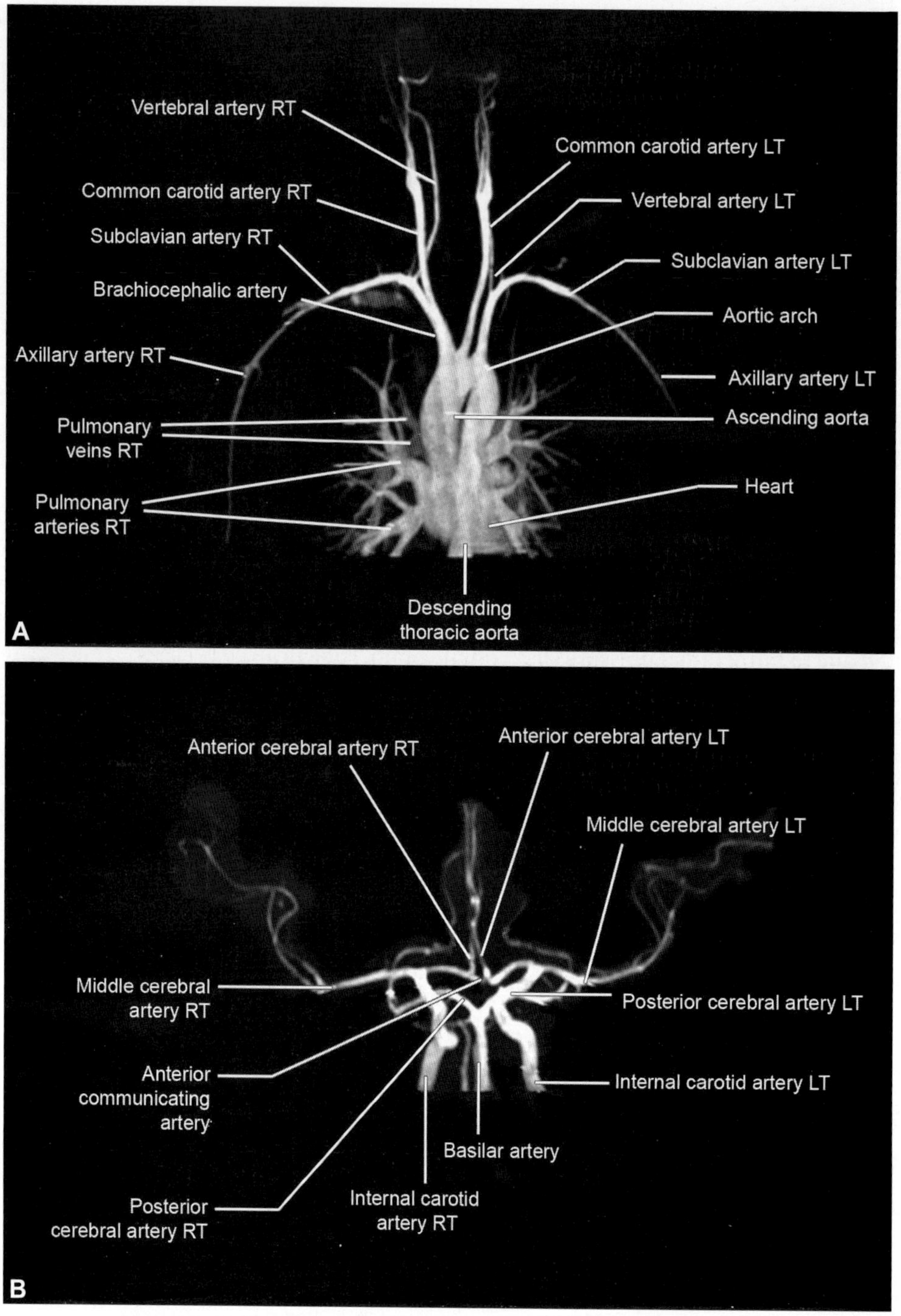

Figs. 5A and B: Arterial blood supply of the brain. (LT: Left; RT: Right)

- Is via the circle of Willis which is formed by the anastomosis of anterior and posterior circulations.
- Nature of the anastomosis preserves collateral flow in case of segmental ischemia.
- Middle cerebral artery comes off from the internal carotid and is outside the circle of Willis.

VENOUS DRAINAGE OF THE BRAIN (FIGS. 6A AND B)

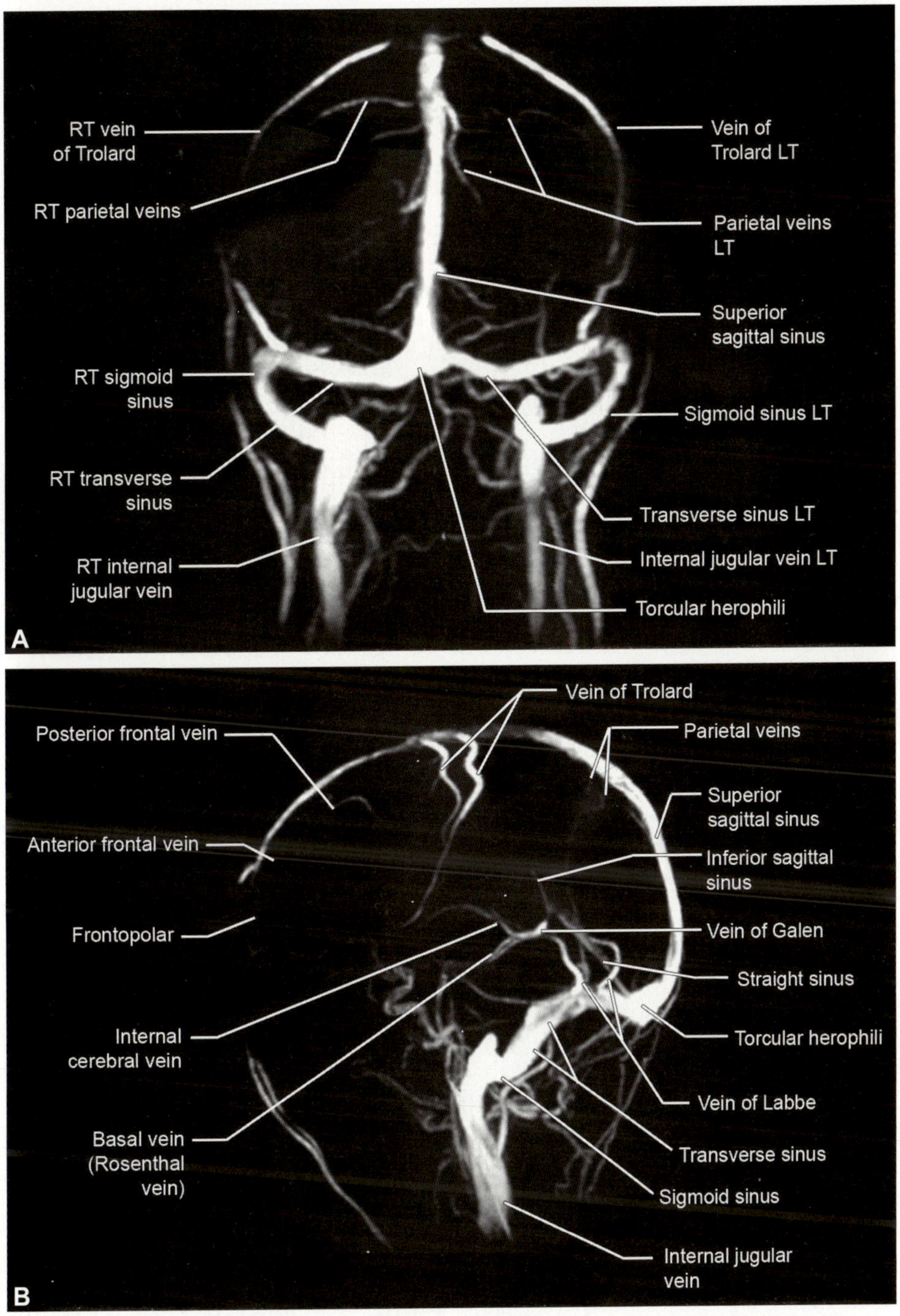

Figs. 6A and B: Venous drainage of the brain. (LT: Left; RT: Right)

- Cerebral veins drain into the dural sinuses.
- All dural sinuses eventually drain into the internal jugular veins.
- There are 11 dural venous sinuses in total.
- Dural venous sinuses are valveless system.
- Cerebral venous thrombosis requires a high index of suspicion and can be fatal.

CLIPPING OF INTRACRANIAL ANEURYSM (FIGS. 7A AND B)

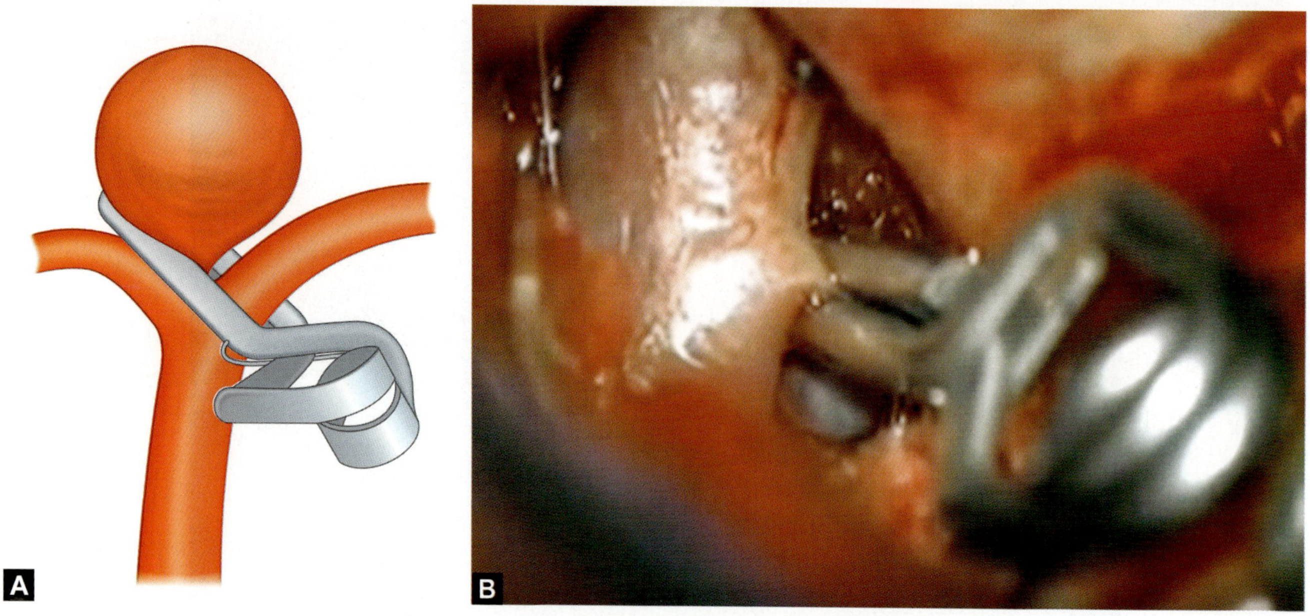

Figs. 7A and B: Clipping of intracranial aneurysm.

- Surgical invasive technique of putting a spring-loaded clip at the neck of the aneurysm.
- Has higher morbidity and mortality than intravascular coilings.
- More aneurysms are being coiled than clipped in the last decade onwards.

INTRACRANIAL ANEURYSM COILING (FIGS. 8A AND B)

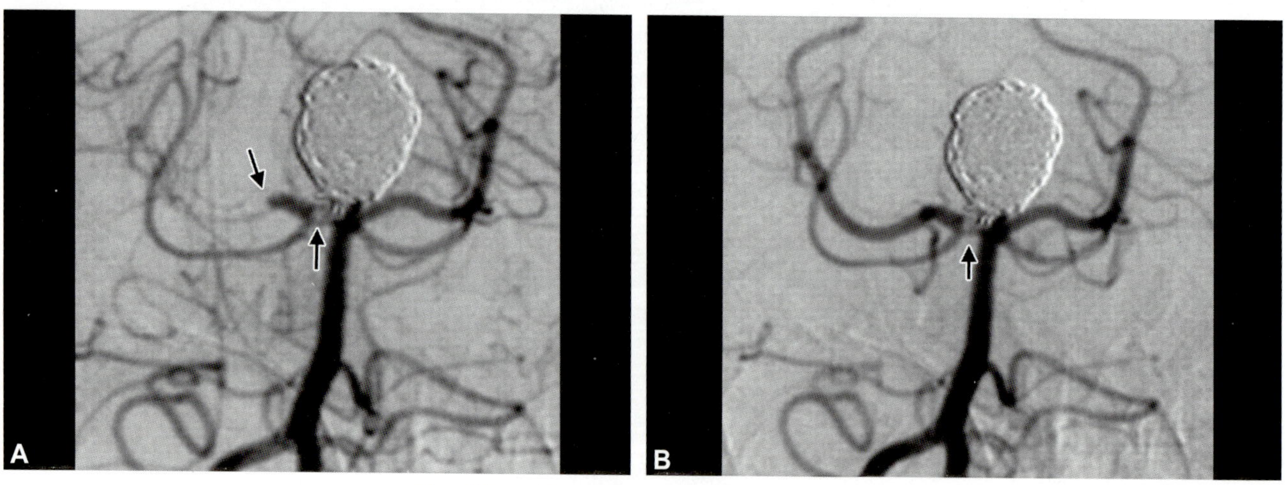

Figs. 8A and B: Intracranial aneurysm coiling.

- Minimally invasive intravascular treatment option for intracranial aneurysms.
- Practice changing treatment since the International Subarachnoid Aneurysm Trial (ISAT) in late 1990s.
- Less morbidity and mortality.
- Long-term outcome data is limited, can have problems of re-filling.

FLOW DIVERTER FOR INTRACRANIAL ANEURYSMAL COILING (FIGS. 9A AND B)

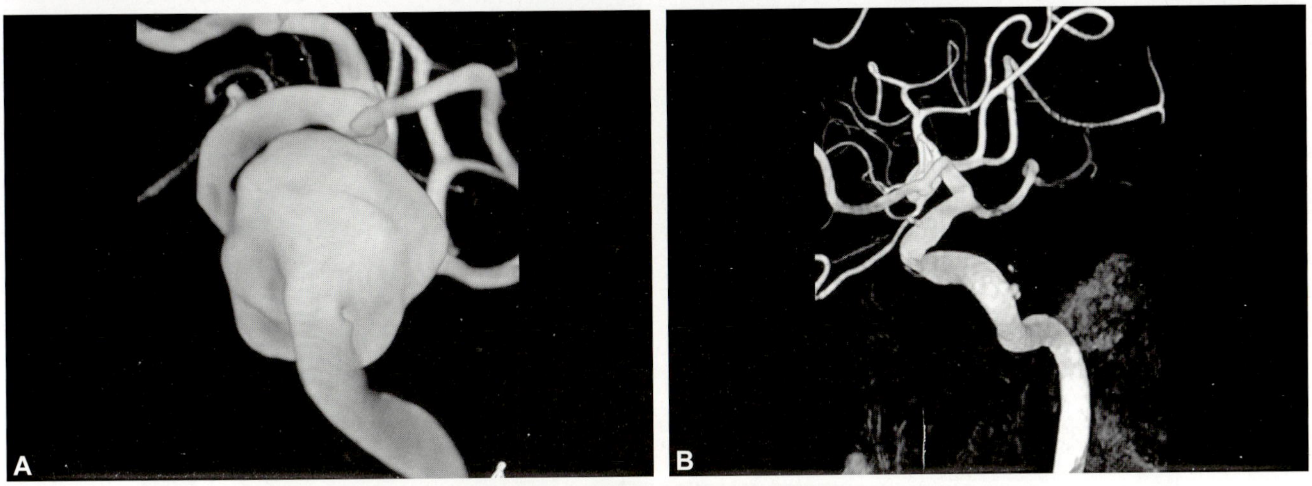

Figs. 9A and B: Flow diverter for intracranial aneurysmal coiling.

- Newer device in intervention radiology used for aneurysms with large neck.
- Based on the principle of diverting/reducing flow from the aneurysm to encourage stasis and eventual thrombosis.
- Few centers in the world currently perform due to cost and expertise.
- It has further reduced the number of aneurysms requiring open surgery/clipping.

CAROTID STENTING (FIGS. 10A AND B)

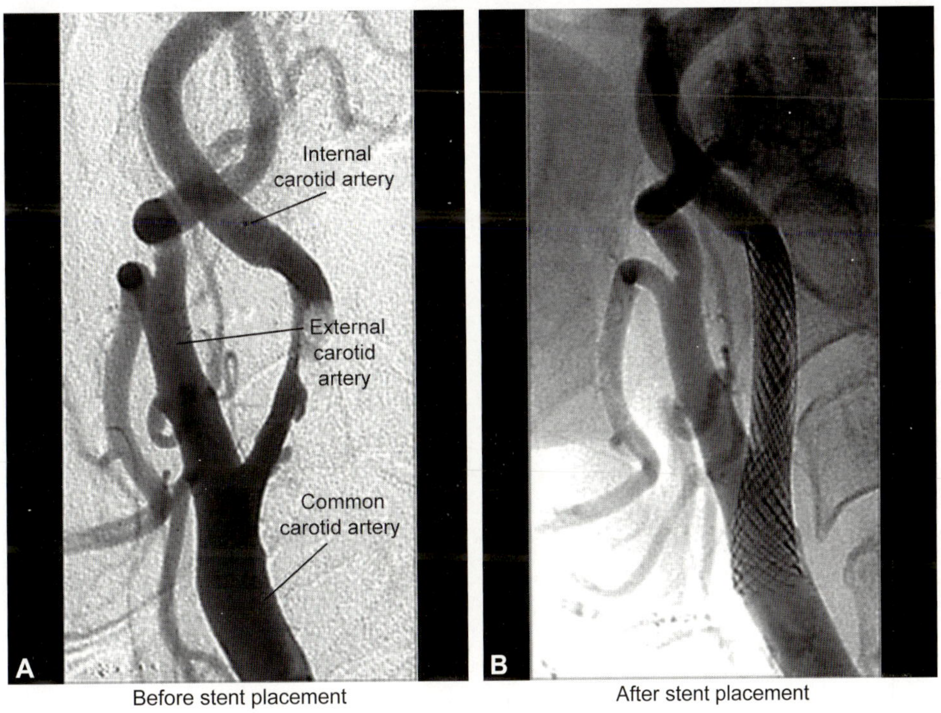

Figs. 10A and B: Carotid stenting.

- Endovascular intervention technique to treat carotid stenosis.
- Metal mesh stent inserted at the point of maximal stenosis.
- Used to treat or prevent thromboembolic strokes.
- Minimally invasive option to treat carotid stenosis than a surgically performed endarterectomy.

CT HEAD AND CT ANGIO: MIDDLE CEREBRAL ARTERY THROMBUS (FIGS. 11A AND B)

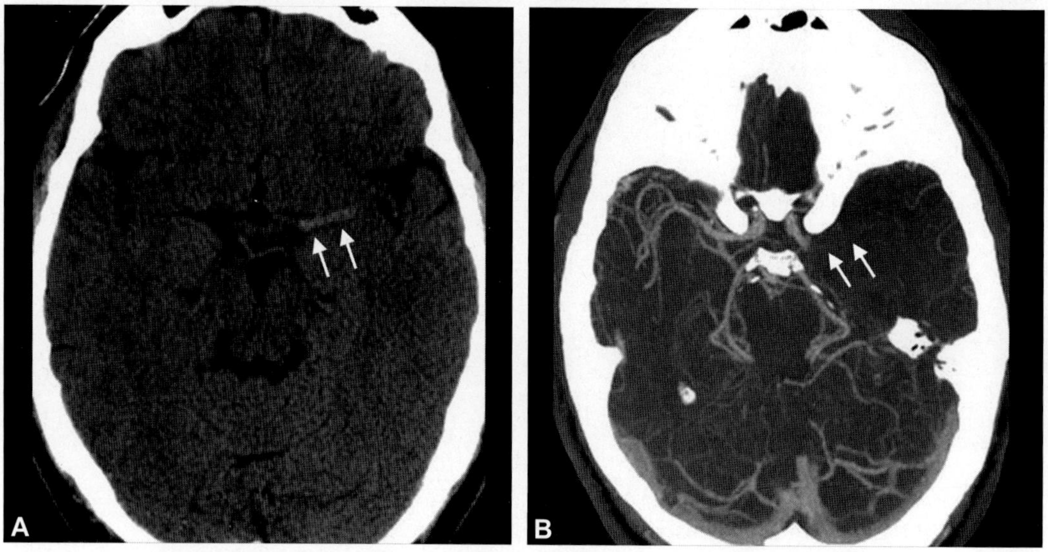

Figs. 11A and B: CT head and CT angio: Middle cerebral artery thrombus.

- The images show the classical left middle cerebral artery (MCA) "Dot Sign" due to the presence of a thrombus and the left MCA.
- Mechanical thrombectomy and bridging thrombolysis are the most effective treatment.
- The clinical outcomes are getting better with good mRS scores of at least 40% in the best reported studies.

INTRACRANIAL ANEURYSM ON PLAIN CT HEAD AND CEREBRAL ANGIOGRAPHY (FIGS. 12A AND B)

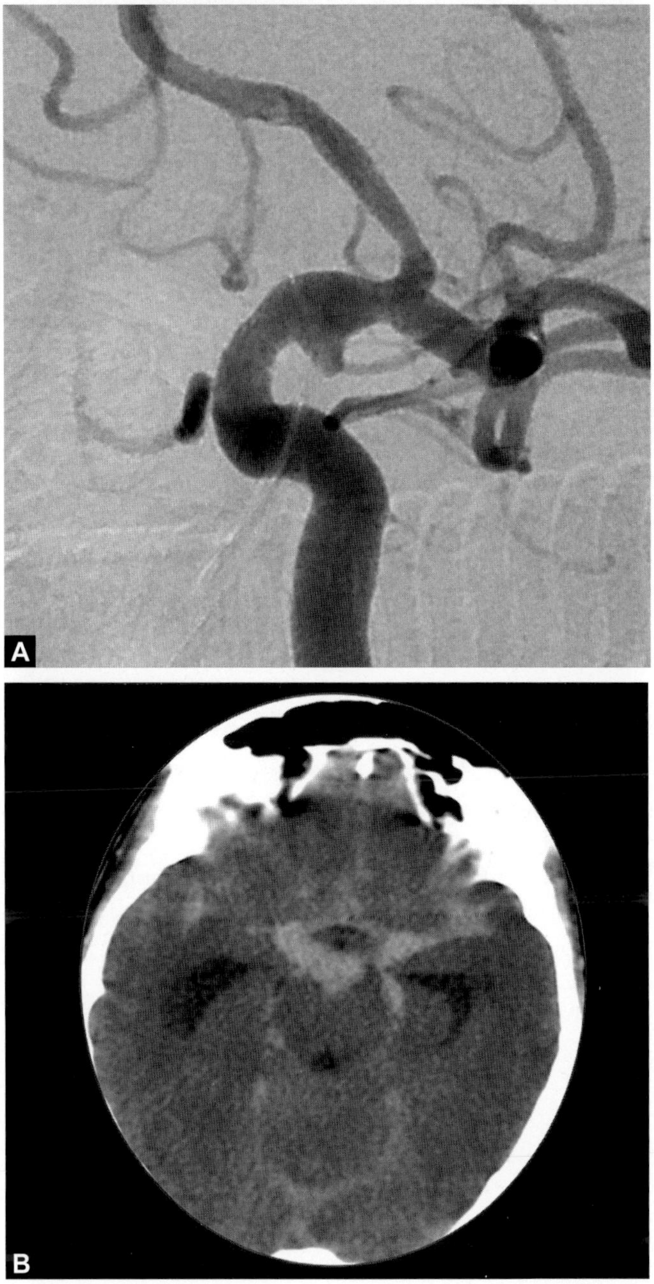

Figs. 12A and B: Intracranial aneurysm on plain CT head and cerebral angiography.

- The risk factors for poor outcome in subarachnoid hemorrhage (SAH) include female sex, World Federation of Neurological Surgeons (WFNS) grade 4, multiple aneurysms, posterior circulation aneurysms, low presenting Glasgow coma scale (GCS), delayed presentation and presence of major comorbidities.
- Tranexamic acid has shown some benefit in prevention of rebleeding only in aneurysms that are presenting late.
- Triple therapy and oral nimodipine are proven therapies for SAH management and are recommended by the American Stroke Association (ASA)/American Heart Association (AHA) guidelines.
- Angioplasty and IV milrinone are performed for vasospasm treatment.

CEREBRAL AV MALFORMATION (FIGS. 13A AND B)

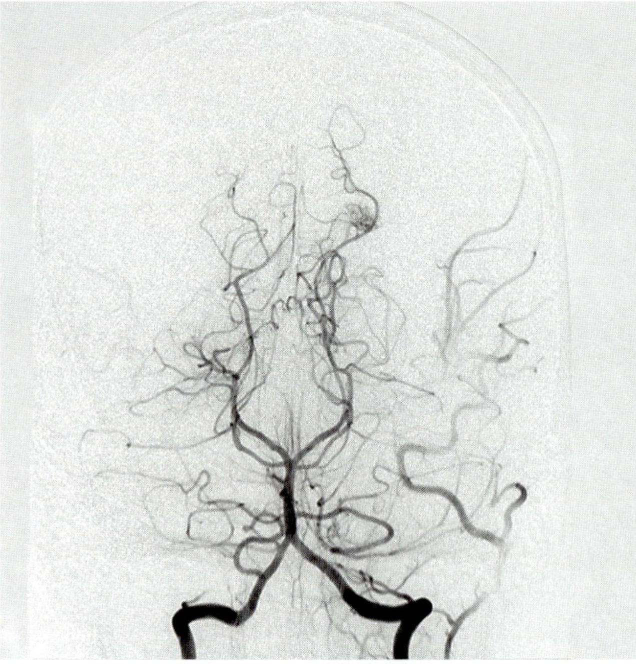

Fig. 13A: Cerebral AVM on a DSA of cerebral vessels.

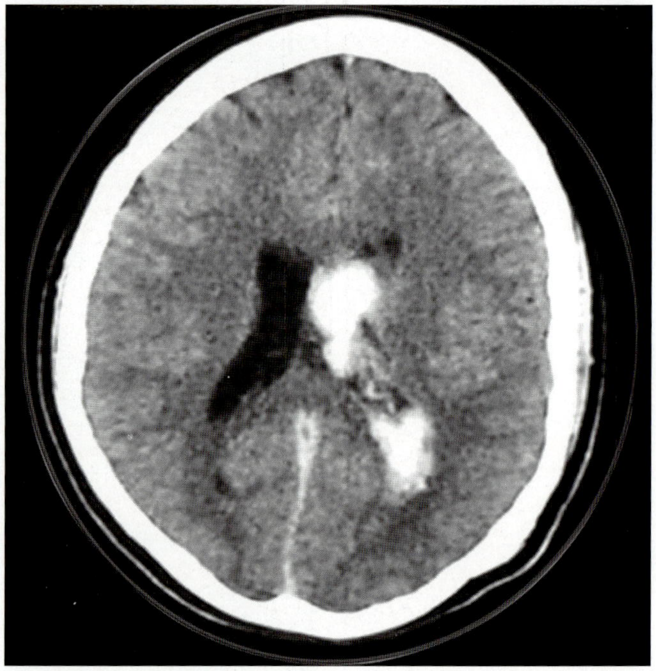

Fig. 13B: Cerebral hemorrhage on a CT head (Noncontrast) of the same patient with ventricular extension of the bleeding.

- Cerebral arteriovenous malformation (AVMs) are abnormal vascular connections between the arterial and venous circulations in the brain.
- Around 50% unfortunately present with hemorrhage and subsequent symptoms of hemorrhage, e.g. loss of consciousness, headache, seizures, etc.
- Gold standard diagnosis is usually with digital subtraction angiography (DSA) of the cerebral circulation, although CT and MRI can give initial clues.
- Treatment options are: Endovascular embolization with Glue/Onyx, open surgical excision or radiosurgery/Gamma Knife.

SPINAL AV FISTULA (FIGS. 14A AND B)

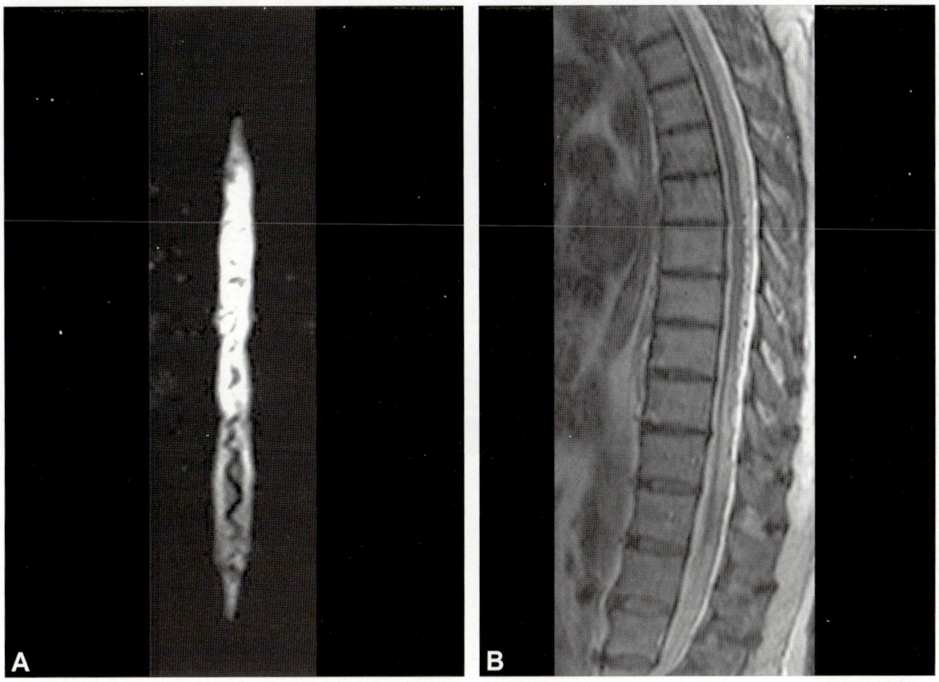

Figs. 14A and B: Spinal AV fistula.

- Classical cord edema with perimedullary dilated vessels typical of a dural AV fistula.
- Requires high index of suspicion and requires spinal DSA to confirm the diagnosis.
- Endovascular treatment is usually successful but symptomatic recovery may take time.

BRAIN ABSCESS (FIGS. 15A TO C)

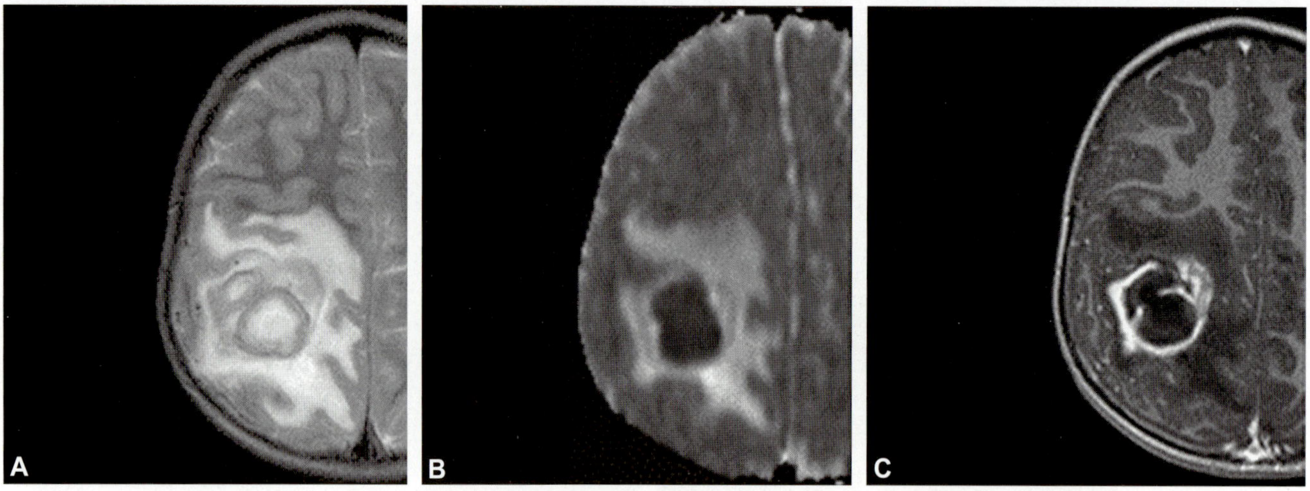

Figs. 15A to C: Brain abscess.

- Brain abscess is a neurological emergency warranting immediate surgery.
- Usual organisms are *Staphylococcus aureus*, Actinomyces, *Haemophilus* and Streptococci.
- Risk factors include: Endocarditis, nasal sinus infections, dental infections, etc.

MYCOTIC ANEURYSM (FIGS. 16A AND B)

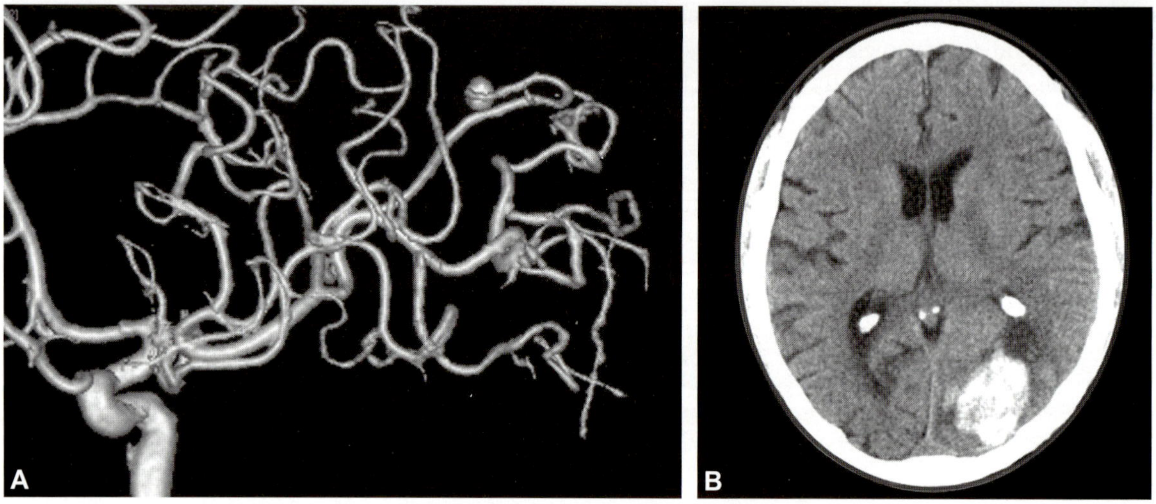

Figs. 16A and B: Mycotic aneurysm.

- Mycotic cerebral aneurysms are rare. They can present in patients with infective endocarditis and are difficult to diagnose unless a high index of suspicion is kept.
- *Streptococcus viridans* and *Staphylococcus aureus* are the usual causative organisms.
- Ruptured mycotic aneurysms should be treated with endovascular surgery as well whilst any corrective cardiovascular surgery should wait for the cerebral disease to stabilize unless there is evidence of Frank left heart failure.

CHRONIC SUBDURAL HEMATOMA (FIGS. 17A AND B)

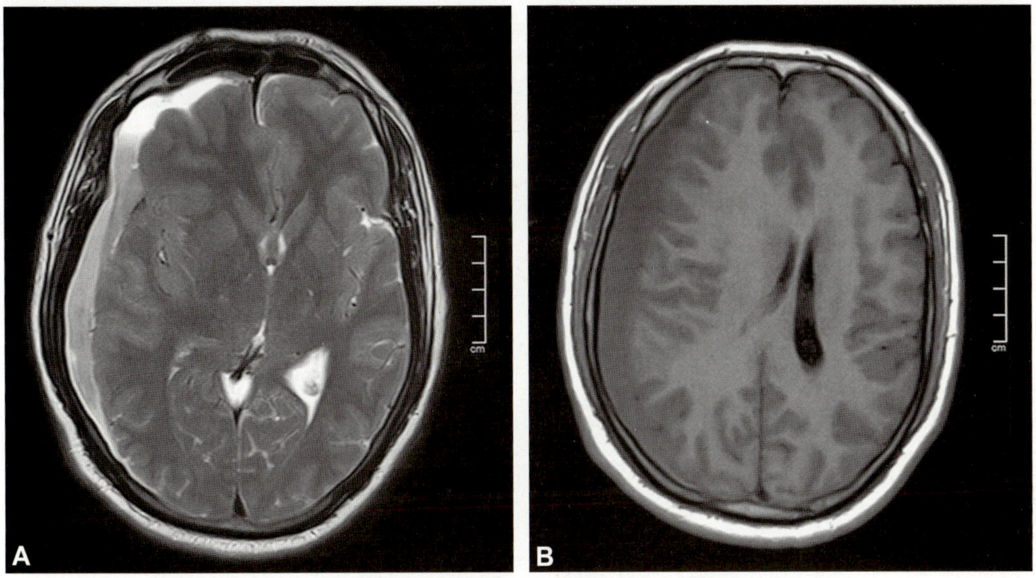

Figs. 17A and B: Chronic subdural hematoma.

- Liquefaction of clot resulting in hemoserous fluid.
- Usually result from tearing of bridging veins.
- Burr holes generally suffice, craniotomy is usually not required.

ACUTE SUBDURAL HEMATOMA WITH SKULL FRACTURE (FIGS. 18A AND B)

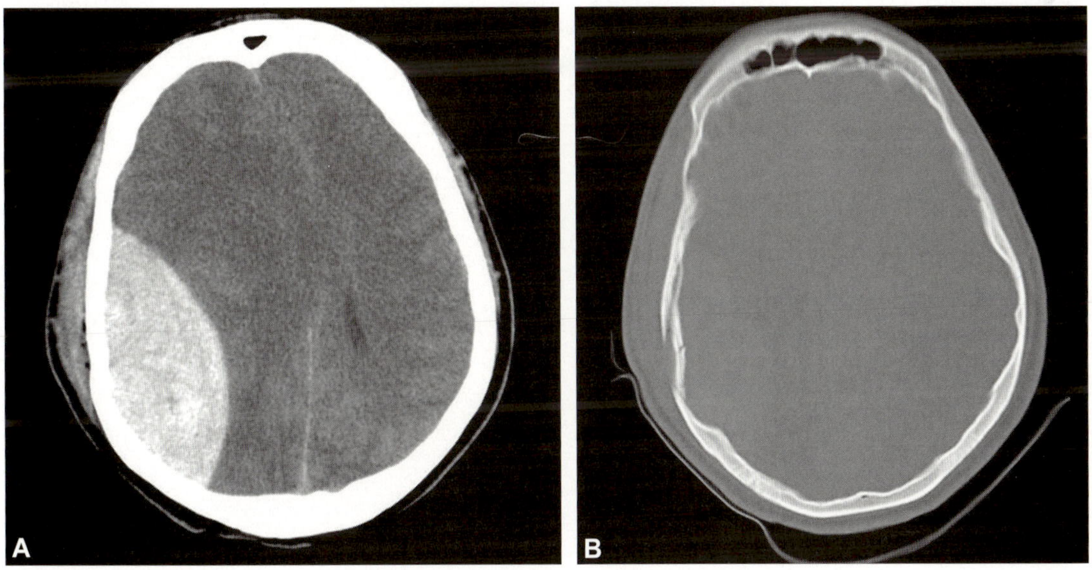

Figs. 18A and B: Acute subdural hematoma with skull fracture.

- Neurosurgical emergency.
- Lucid interval could be present.
- Usually arterial bleed from middle meningeal artery.

PNEUMOENCEPHALUS (FIG. 19)

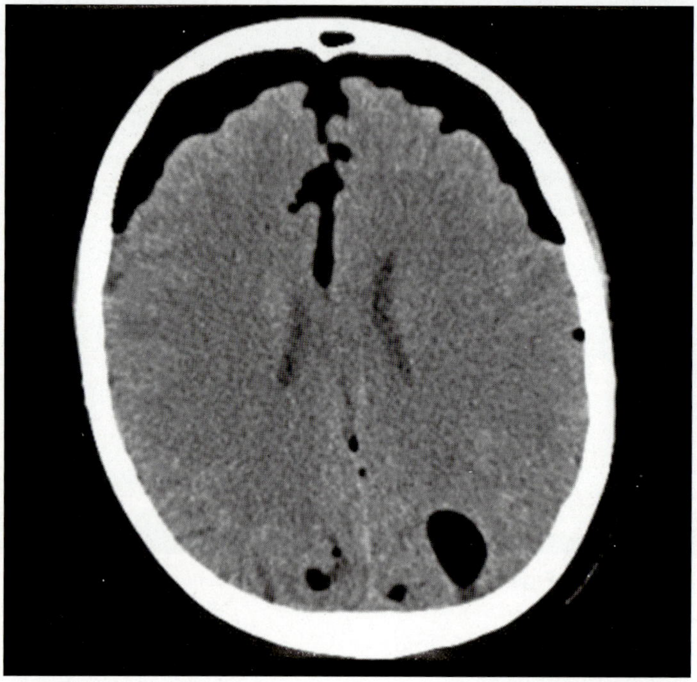

Fig. 19: Pneumoencephalus.

- Pneumoencephalus is a common finding after neurosurgical operations especially those involving the base of skull, pituitary or chronic subdurals.
- Risk factors include: hyperventilation, osmotherapy, barotrauma.
- Usually high flow oxygen is all that is required to denitrogenate the air and decompress the pneumoencephalus.
- "Mt Fuji" sign, if present, indicates urgent open decompression.

DECOMPRESSIVE CRANIECTOMY (FIG. 20)

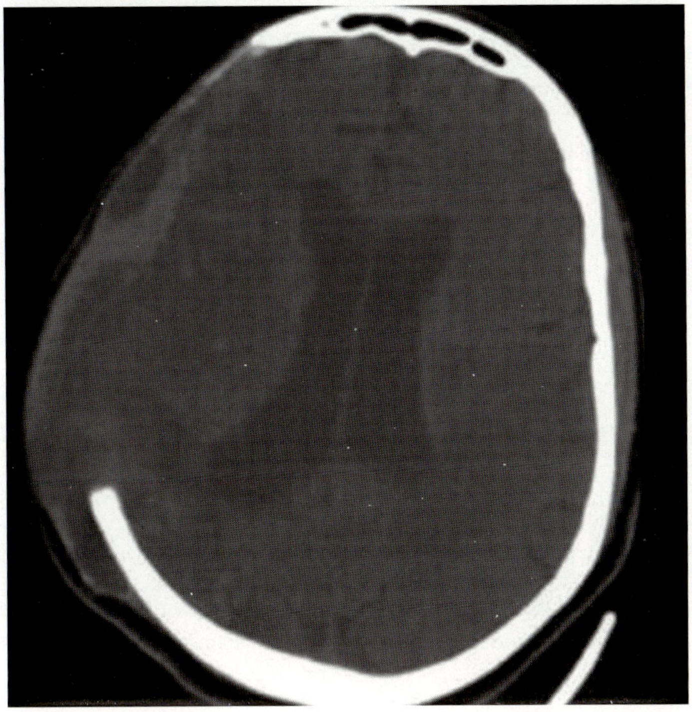

Fig. 20: Decompressive craniectomy—CT.

- Procedure of removal of the skull bone only to decrease intracranial pressure (ICP).
- Emergency procedure performed commonly post-traumatic head injury and stroke.
- Controversial as some recent trials show better survival but poor functional outcomes.
- Remains the mainstay of treatment where medical management of ICP is not performed due to nonmeasurement of ICP.
- Complications include bleeding, infection and risks in future surgery to replace the bony defect.

OPTICAL NERVE SHEATH DIAMETER (FIGS. 21A AND B)

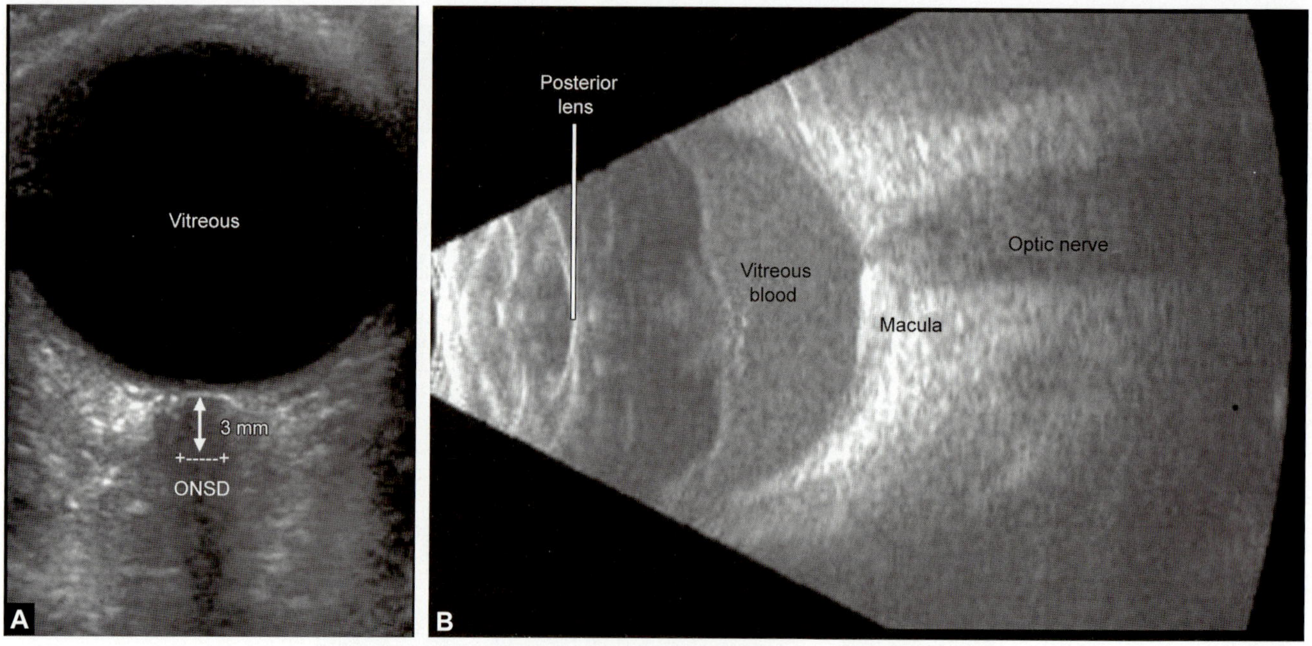

Figs. 21A and B: Optical nerve sheath diameter (ONSD).

- Noninvasive, bedside monitor of ICP.
- Noninvasive technique of using the USG to measure the optic nerve sheath diameter and diagnose raised ICP.
- Rapid and easily reproducible bedside test.
- Linear array USG transducer is used via closed eyelids on a supine patient.
- Optimal cut-off value of optical nerve sheath diameter (ONSD) for determining raised ICP is still unclear.
- Studies show a normal healthy ONSD range between 3.3 mm and 5.2 mm depending upon eyeball transverse diameter (ETD) and may be ethnicity.

INTRACRANIAL PRESSURE MONITORING PROBES (FIGS. 22A TO E)

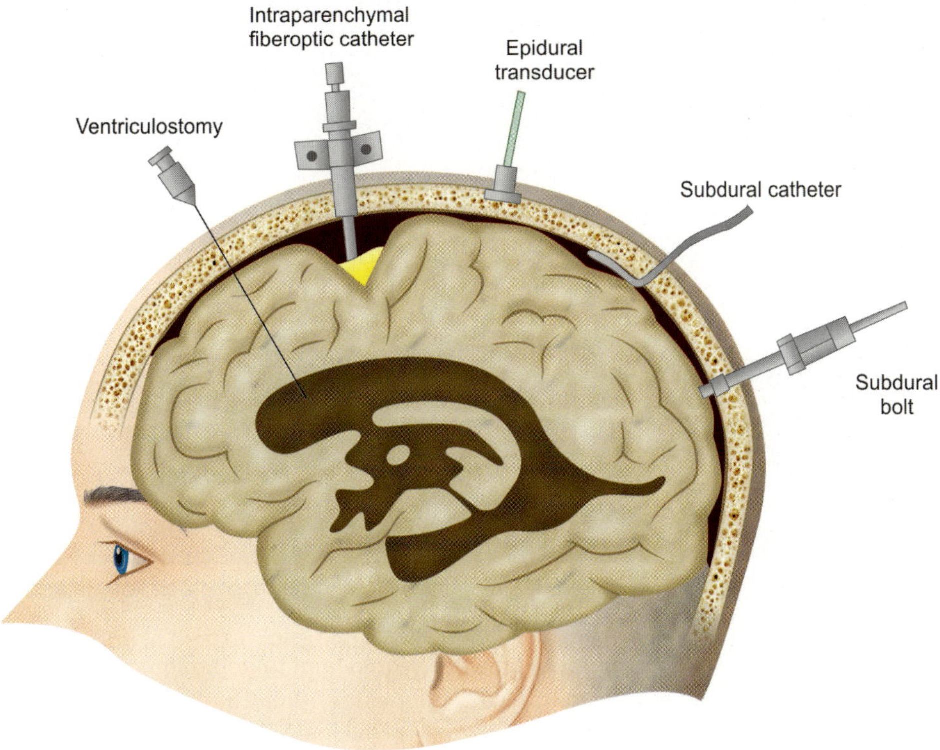

Fig. 22A: Intracranial pressure (ICP) probes.

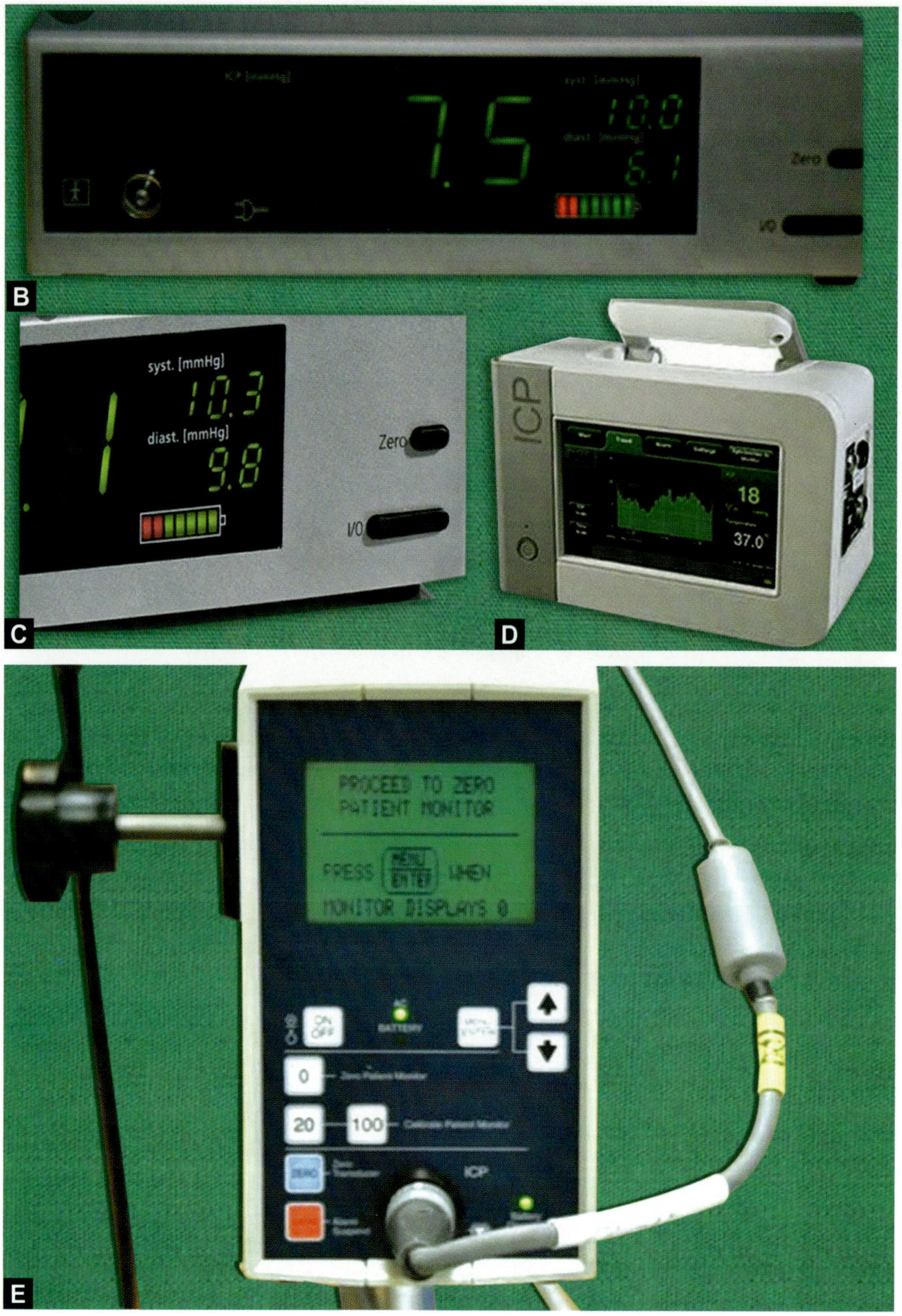

Figs. 22B to E: ICP monitoring probes monitors.

- Recommended technique for assessment and treatment of raised intracranial pressure (ICP).
- Can be intraventricular, intraparenchymal, subdural or extradural.
- Invasive procedure required under aseptic conditions for insertion of any of the probes.
- Treatment should be according to protocols to standardize ICP management.

EXTERNAL VENTRICULAR DRAIN (FIGS. 23A AND B)

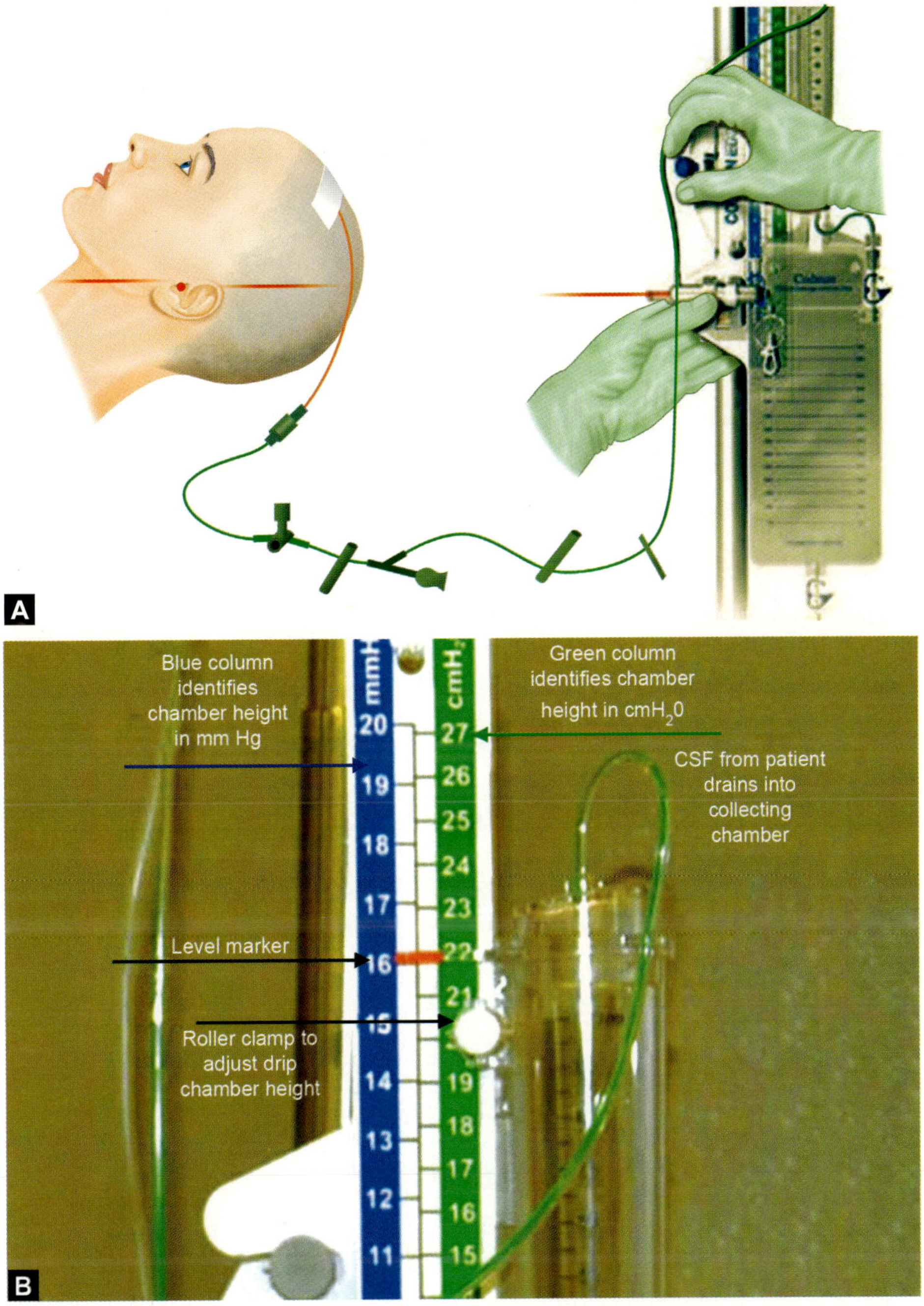

Figs. 23A and B: External ventricular drain (EVD).

- Drain inserted in the lateral ventricle of the brain at the level of the foramen of Monro.
- Most common therapeutic use is drainage of CSF to decrease the ICP.
- Also used to accurately monitor and measure the ICP.
- Invasive procedure requiring complete asepsis and training for optimal placement.
- Requires trained nursing staff to monitor and maintain asepsis.
- Complications include infection, ventricular hemorrhage and obstruction.

INTRACRANIAL PRESSURE WAVEFORM (FIGS. 24A AND B)

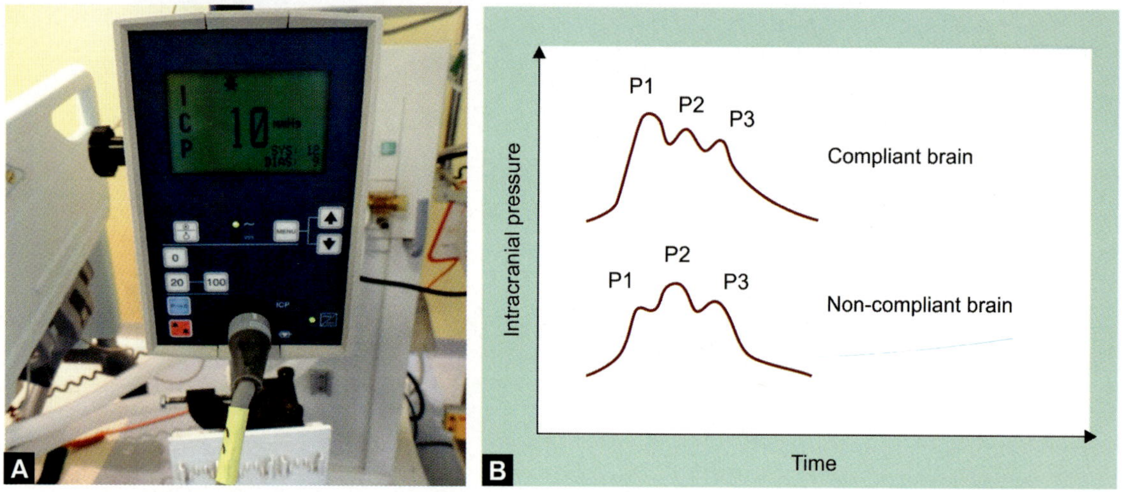

Figs. 24A and B: Intracranial pressure (ICP) waveforms.

- Graph of ICP waveform on X-axis trended with time over Y-axis.
- Modified arterial pressure waveform with three pressure tracings:
  - P1: Percussive wave resulting in the arterial pressure transmitting from the choroid plexus.
  - P2: Tidal wave generated from the compliance of the brain with varying amplitude.
  - P3: Represents the dicrotic notch due to the aortic valve closure.

LUNDBERG INTRACRANIAL PRESSURE WAVES (FIGS. 25A AND B)

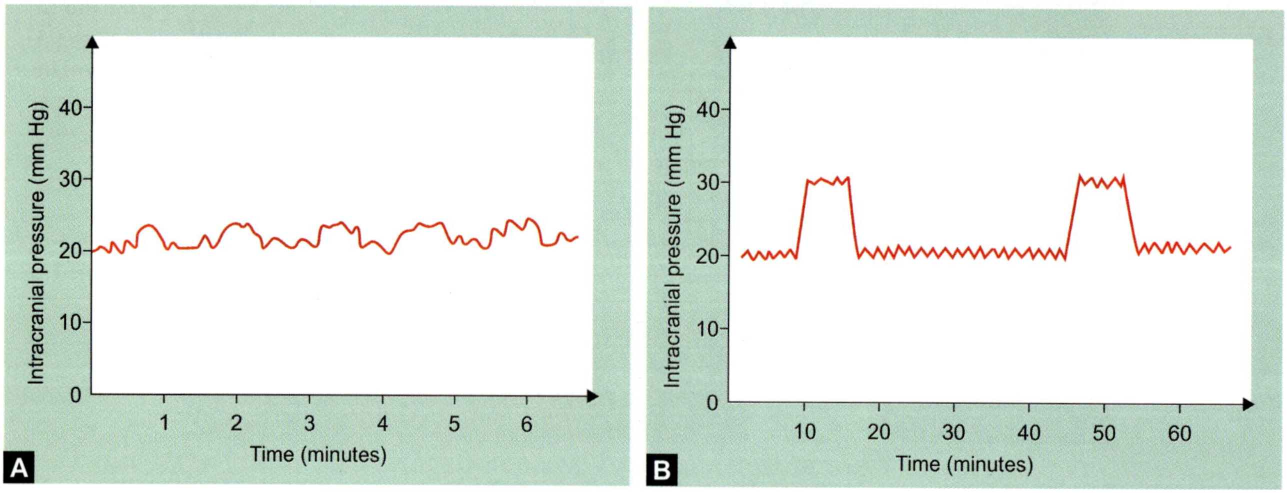

Figs. 25A and B: Lundberg waveforms.

- A waves are plateau waves with steep and sustained rise in ICP for 5–10 minutes.
- A waves are always pathological signifying raised ICP.
- B waves are oscillatory waves at a frequency of 0.5–2 waves/min.
- B waves are usually seen in vasospasm with increased middle cerebral artery velocity.
- C waves are oscillatory waves with a frequency of 4–8 waves/min seen in healthy subjects.

DIGITAL SUBTRACTION ANGIOGRAPHY SUITE (FIG. 26)

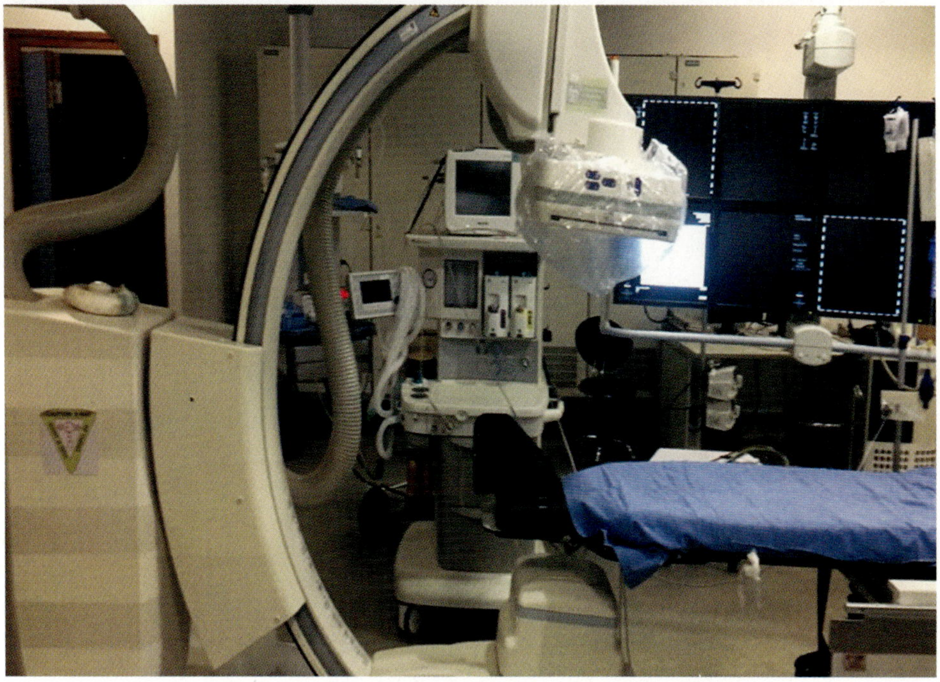

Fig. 26: Digital subtraction angiography (DSA) suite.

- Intervention neuroradiological suite with biplane imaging.
- Procedures performed include: Intracranial aneurysmal coiling, carotid stenting, stroke thrombectomy, and arteriovenous malformation (AVM) embolization.
- Radiation prone procedure area usually with a radiation free control room with slave monitors.
- Usually a remote site away from operating theaters necessitating trained staff and robust protocols to maintain safety.
- Increasing use due to growing interventional procedures.

BRAINSUITE OR INTRAOPERATIVE MRI (FIG. 27)

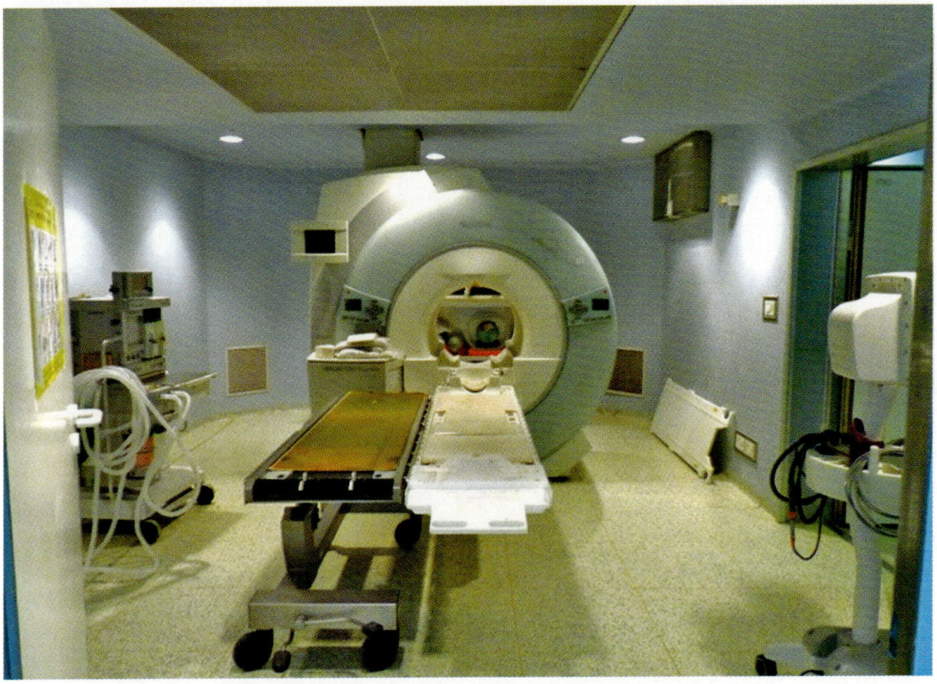

Fig. 27: BrainSuite or intraoperative MRI (iMRI).

- Combined name given to the neurosurgical operating theater which includes an intraoperative MRI (iMRI) and surgical operating navigation kit.
- Allows precision brain surgery to maximize output whilst minimizing damage to normal structure.
- Advanced and expensive set-up requiring major infrastructure and training.
- Reduces recurrence rates of lesions and improves patient safety.
- Cost and prolonged surgical duration are some of the downsides.

PORTABLE CT SCAN (FIGS. 28A TO C)

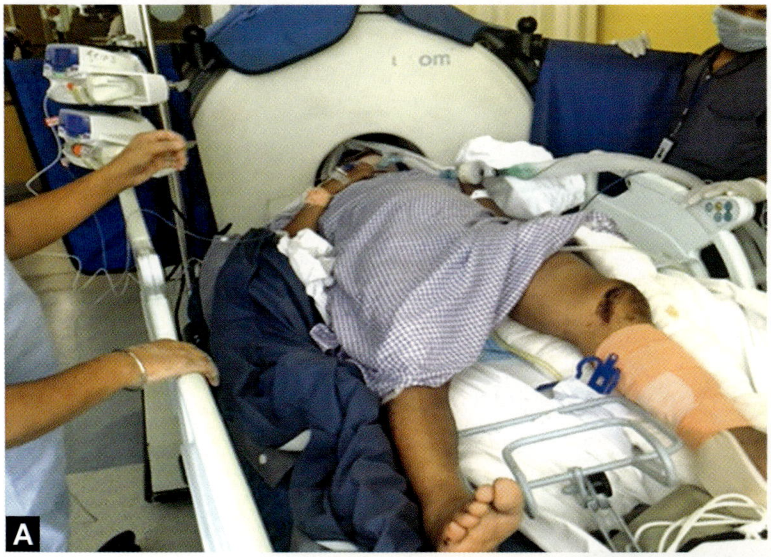

A

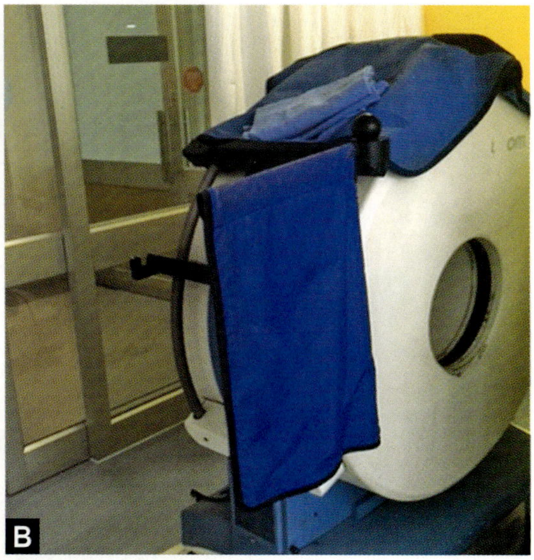

B

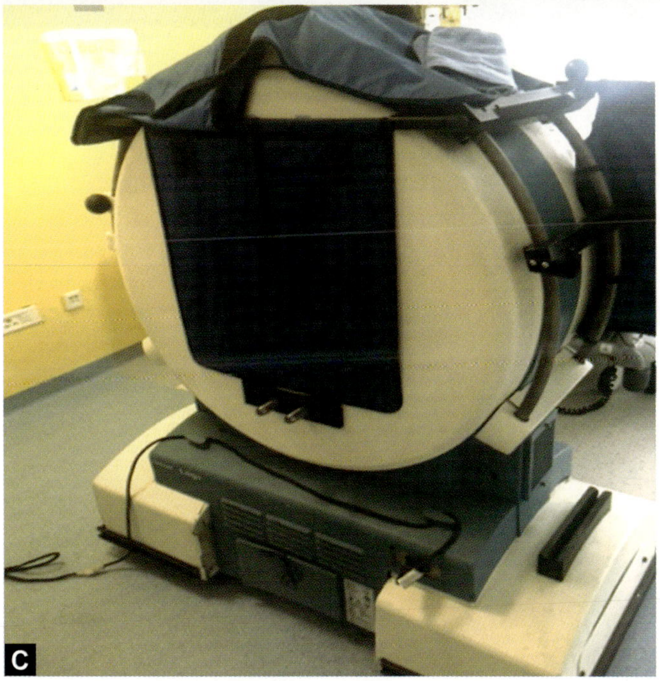

C

Figs. 28A to C: Portable CT scan.

- Portable computerized tomography machine to perform head scans in the ICU itself.
- Provides alternative to transferring critically ill patients for head CT.
- Feasible, portable, safe and provides good quality images promptly.
- Radiation safety must be ensured during the procedure.
- Costly and can only be justified in tertiary centers with higher turnovers.

O-ARM (FIG. 29)

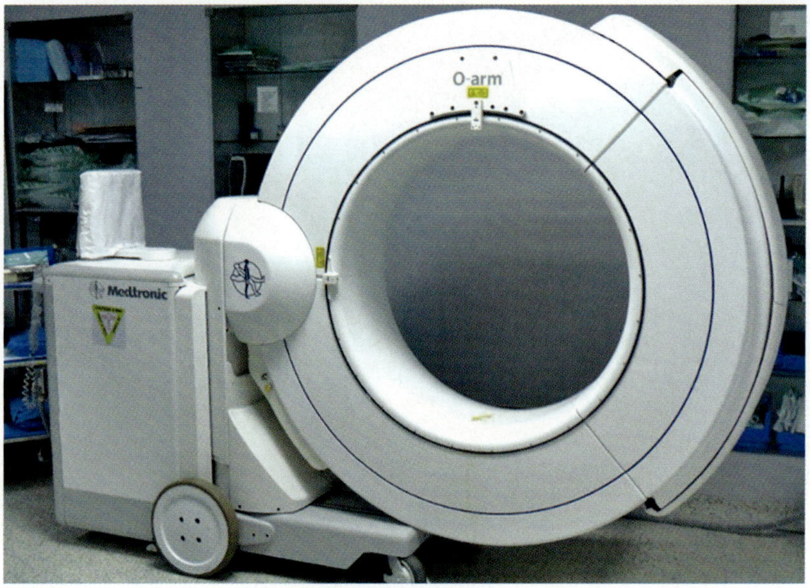

Fig. 29: O-arm.

- Intraoperative fluoroscopic visualization of the spine providing 3D imaging.
- Also provides real time stealth imaging and navigation during the spinal surgery.
- Facilitates safer and accurate spinal surgery through minimally invasive routes.
- Involves radiation exposure like CT scan thus robust radiation precautions required.
- Extensive training required to ensure safe and successful outcomes.

LUMBAR DRAIN (FIG. 30)

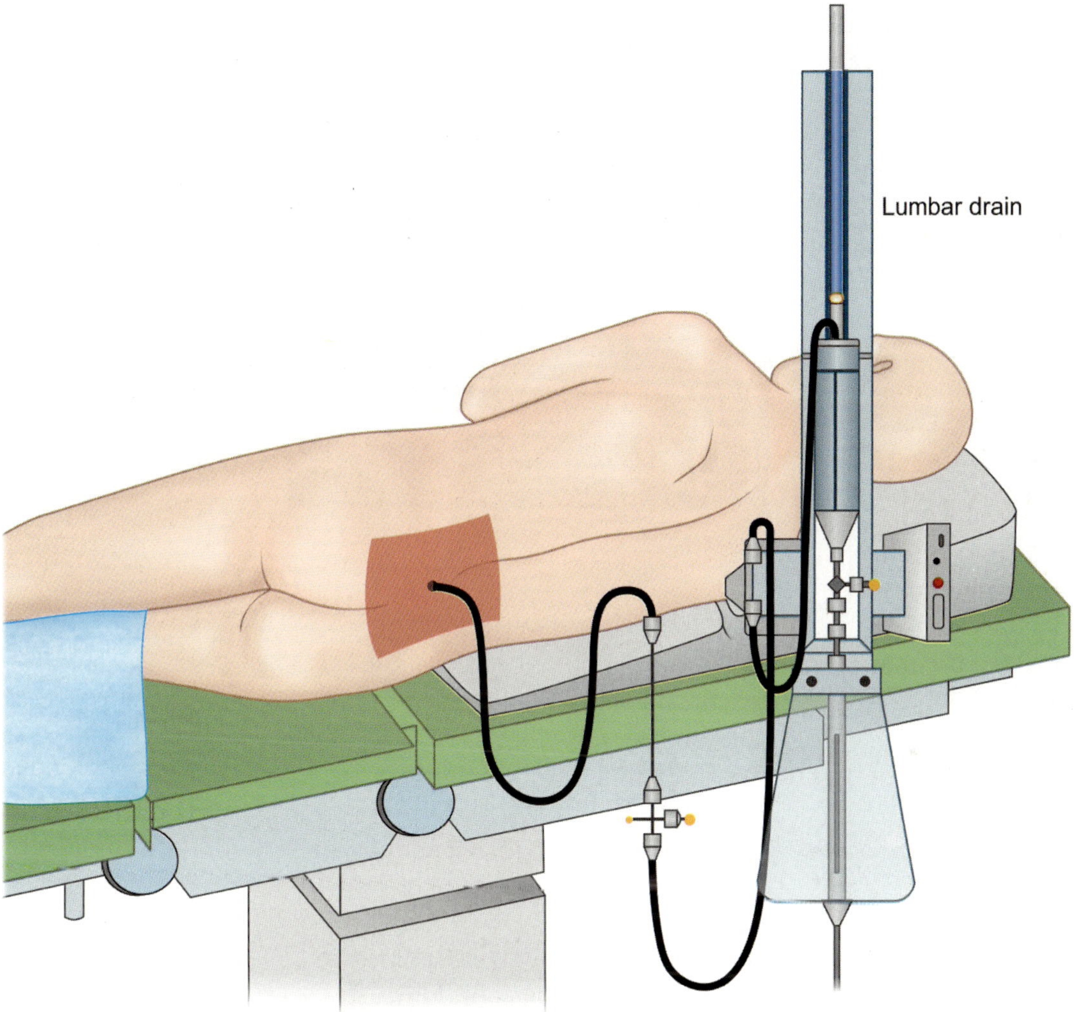

Fig. 30: Lumbar drain.

- Drain inserted in lumbar subarachnoid space usually L3/L4 or L4/L5 to drain cerebrospinal fluid (CSF).
- Indications include: Hydrocephalus evaluation and treatment, CSF analysis, CSF leakage, deliver medicines.
- Drainage is controlled by level of the drain, pressure or volume of the CSF.
- Sterile procedure and should be done with all aseptic precautions.
- Complications include infection, bleeding, worsening of neurological deficit, etc.

BISPECTRAL INDEX (FIG. 31)

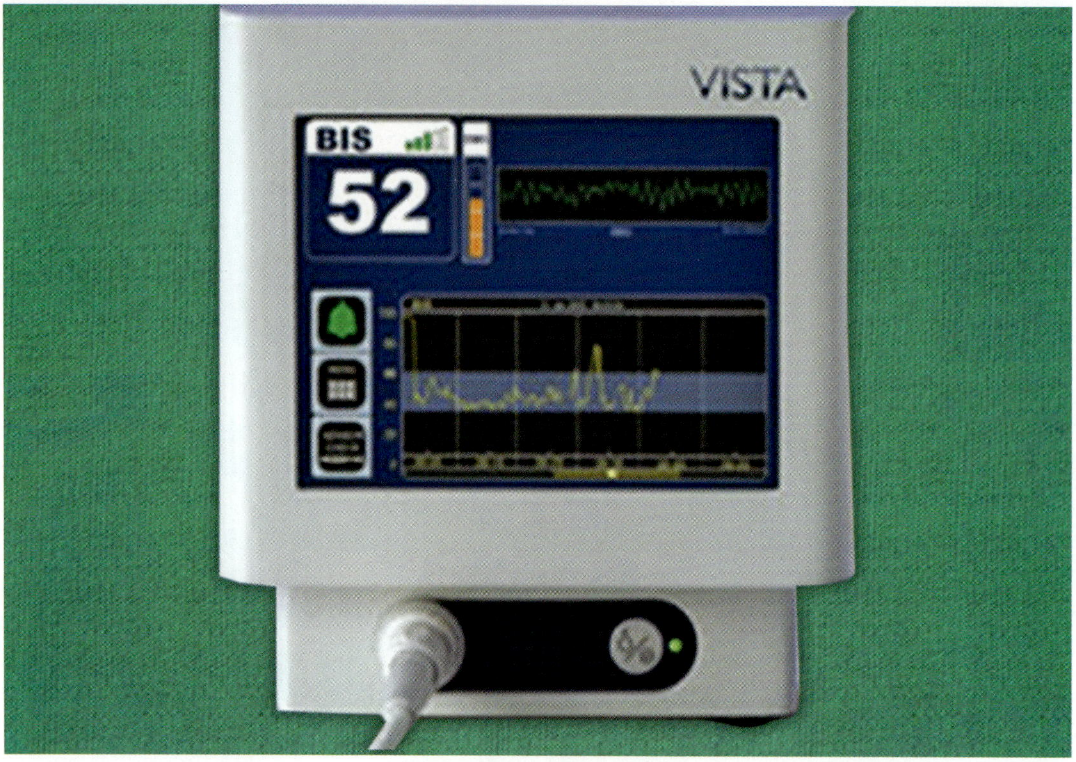

Fig. 31: Bispectral index (BIS).

- Most commonly used depth of anesthesia monitor and ICU sedation.
- Principle based on summated frontal electroencephalography (EEG).
- Does not prevent awareness although can be used to assess depth of anesthesia.

PATIENT-CONTROLLED ANALGESIA (PCA) PUMPS (FIGS. 32A TO C)

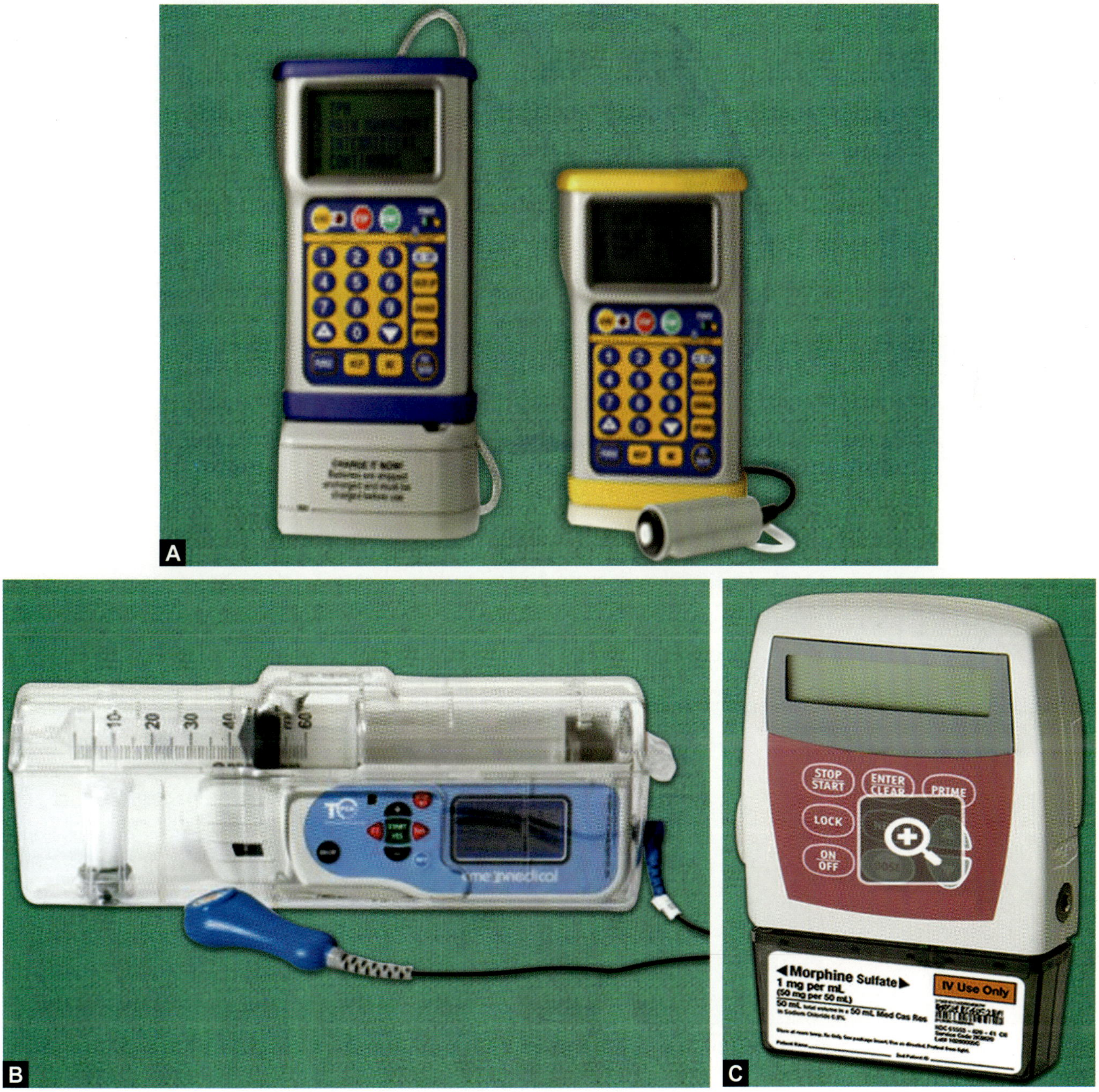

Figs. 32A to C: Patient-controlled analgesia (PCA) pumps.

- Safe mode of providing postoperative analgesia.
- Various pumps available.
- Safety profile established with robust protocols.
- Can be used with opioids like fentanyl, morphine or even remifentanil.

DEEP BRAIN STIMULATION IMAGES (FIGS. 33A TO D)

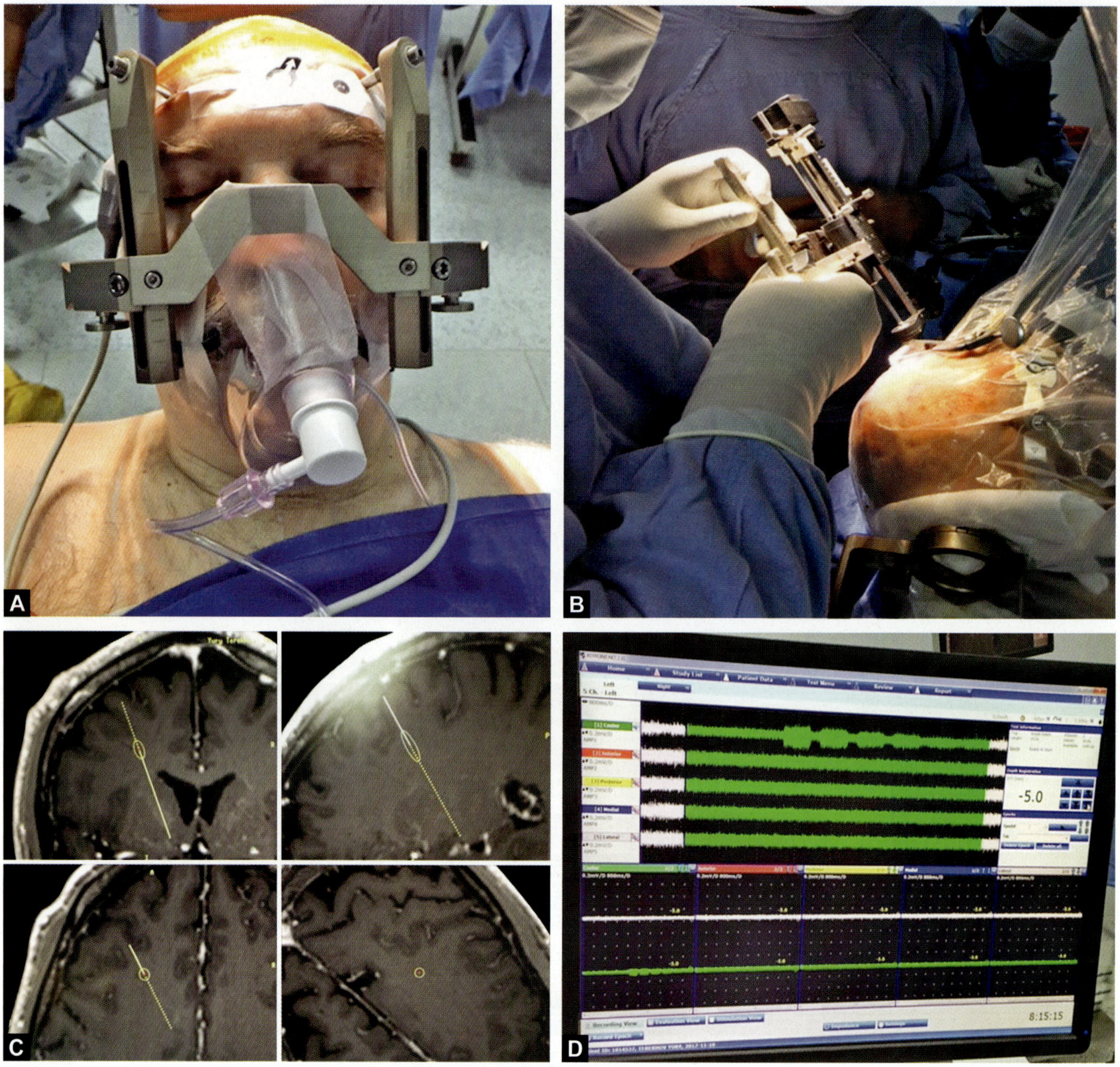

Figs. 33A to D: Deep brain stimulation images.

- A : Deep brain stimulation (DBS) with stereotactic frame *in-situ*.
- B : Insertion of stereotactic-guided electrode.
- C : MRI-guided stealth images displaying track.
- D : Stimulation screen at the time of electrode stimulation.

A NEAR INFRARED SPECTROSCOPY MONITOR (NIRS—MASSIMO) (FIG. 34)

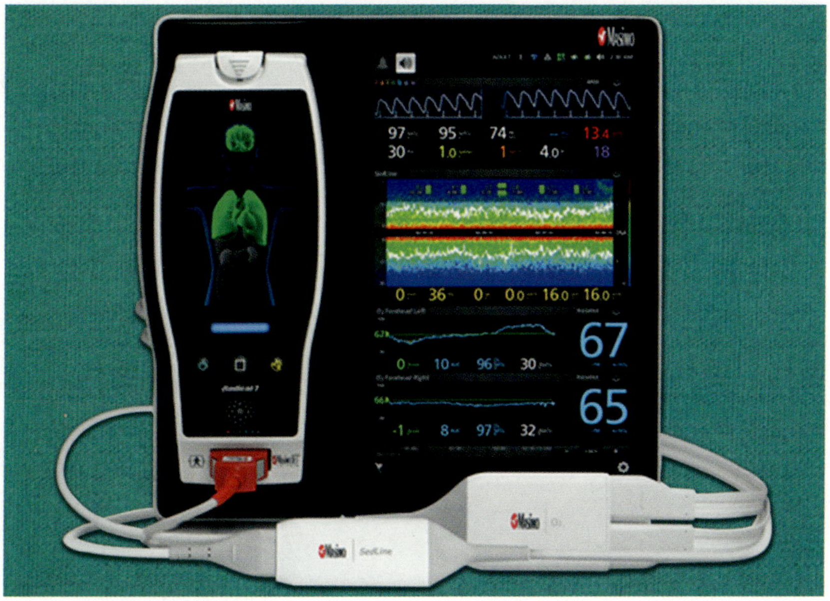

Fig. 34: A near infrared spectroscopy monitor (NIRS—Massimo).

- Near infrared spectroscopy.
- Used for monitoring cerebral oxygenation of both sides.
- Uses near infrared light for regional brain tissue oxygenation.
- Can compare brain tissue oxygenation of either hemispheres.
- Noninvasive monitor gives a numerical reading.

TRANSCRANIAL DOPPLER (FIG. 35)

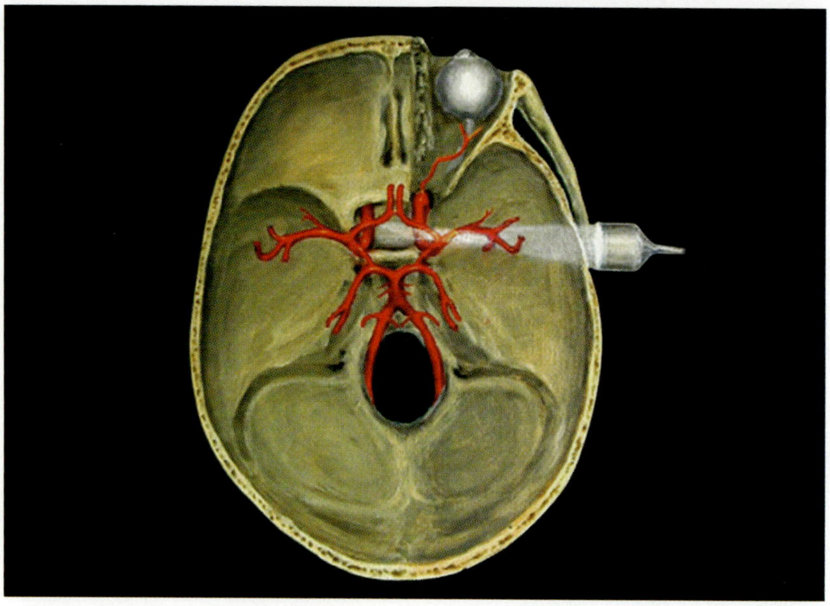

Fig. 35: Transcranial Doppler (TCD).

- Used to assess cerebral blood flow.

PORTABLE/WEARABLE NEW GENERATION TCD MACHINE (FIGS. 36A AND B)

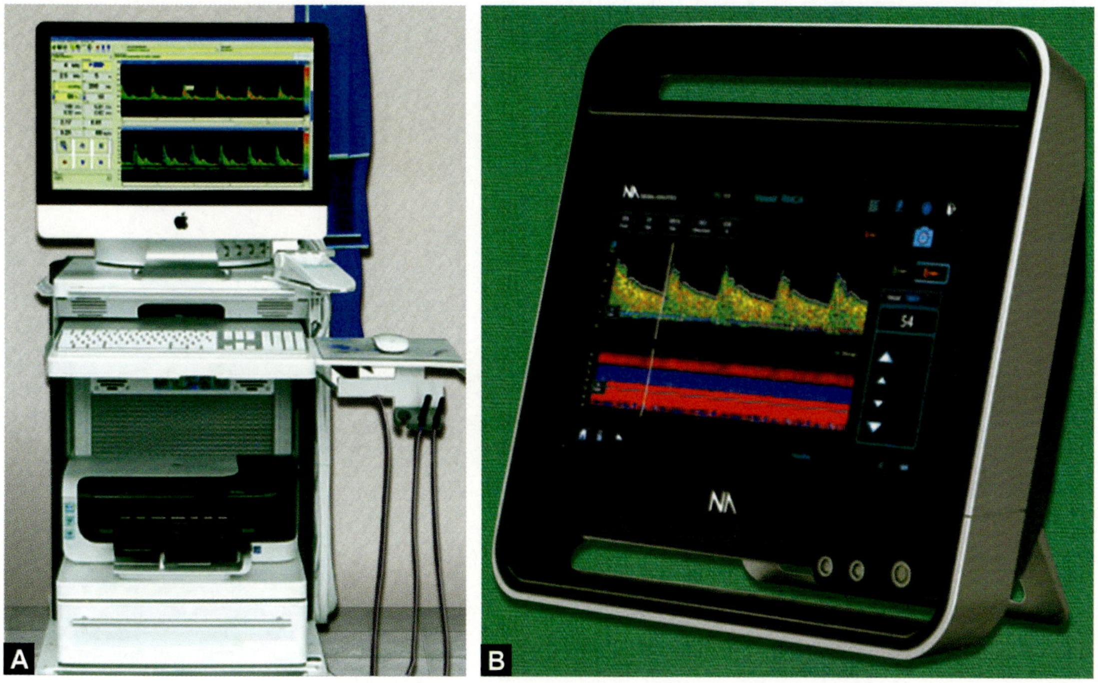

Figs. 36A and B: Portable/Wearable new generation TCD machine.

- Provides noninvasive, real time information of cerebral blood flow.
- Utilizes the Doppler shift mechanism for detection of tissue motion and blood flow.
- Most common use is for detection of vasospasm in subarachnoid hemorrhage (SAH).
- Also used for detection of right to left shunt and stroke thrombolysis evaluation.
- Newer machines have wearable and easy to use platforms for easy application.

PHRENIC NERVE STIMULATOR (FIGS. 37A AND B)

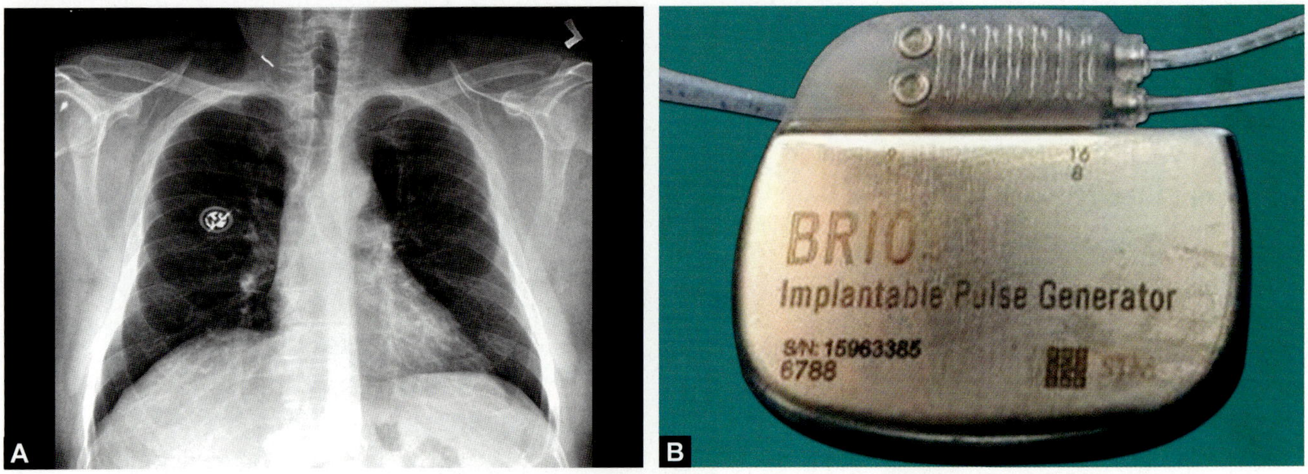

Figs. 37A and B: Phrenic nerve stimulator.

Indication: Diaphragmatic palsy, e.g. cervical spine injury.

- Also known as diaphragmatic pacing.
- Electrical stimulation of the phrenic nerve using a surgically implanted device.
- Helps in improving respiratory function and weaning in high cervical spinal injury patients.
- Can also be used in central sleep apnea and diaphragmatic paralysis.

TARGET CONTROLLED INFUSION PUMP (FIG. 38)

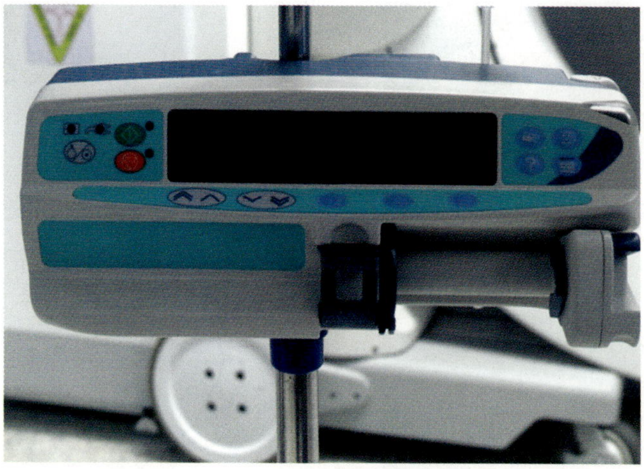

Fig. 38: Target controlled infusion (TCI) pump.

- Drug is given intravenously via a computer-driven pump.
- Principle is based on multicompartment pharmacokinetic models.
- Commonly used for total intravenous anesthetic (TIVA).
- Benefits from smooth induction, stable maintenance and a prompt recovery.
- Also used for ICU sedation, e.g. with propofol.

THROMBOELASTOGRAPHY (FIGS. 39A AND B)

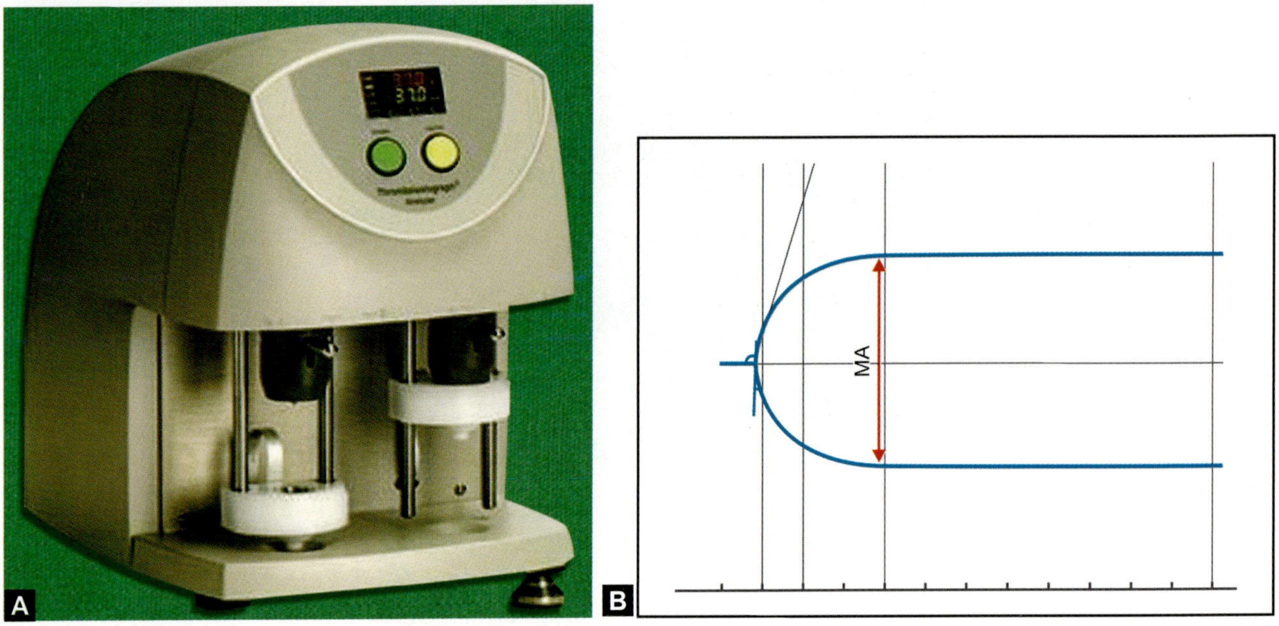

Figs. 39A and B: Thromboelastography (TEG).

- Point of care testing to check clotting.
- Provides real-time results during the intraoperative phase.
- Rationalizes the use of blood and blood products.

"PENUMBRA" SUCTION ASPIRATOR FOR MECHANICAL THROMBECTOMY (FIGS. 40A AND B)

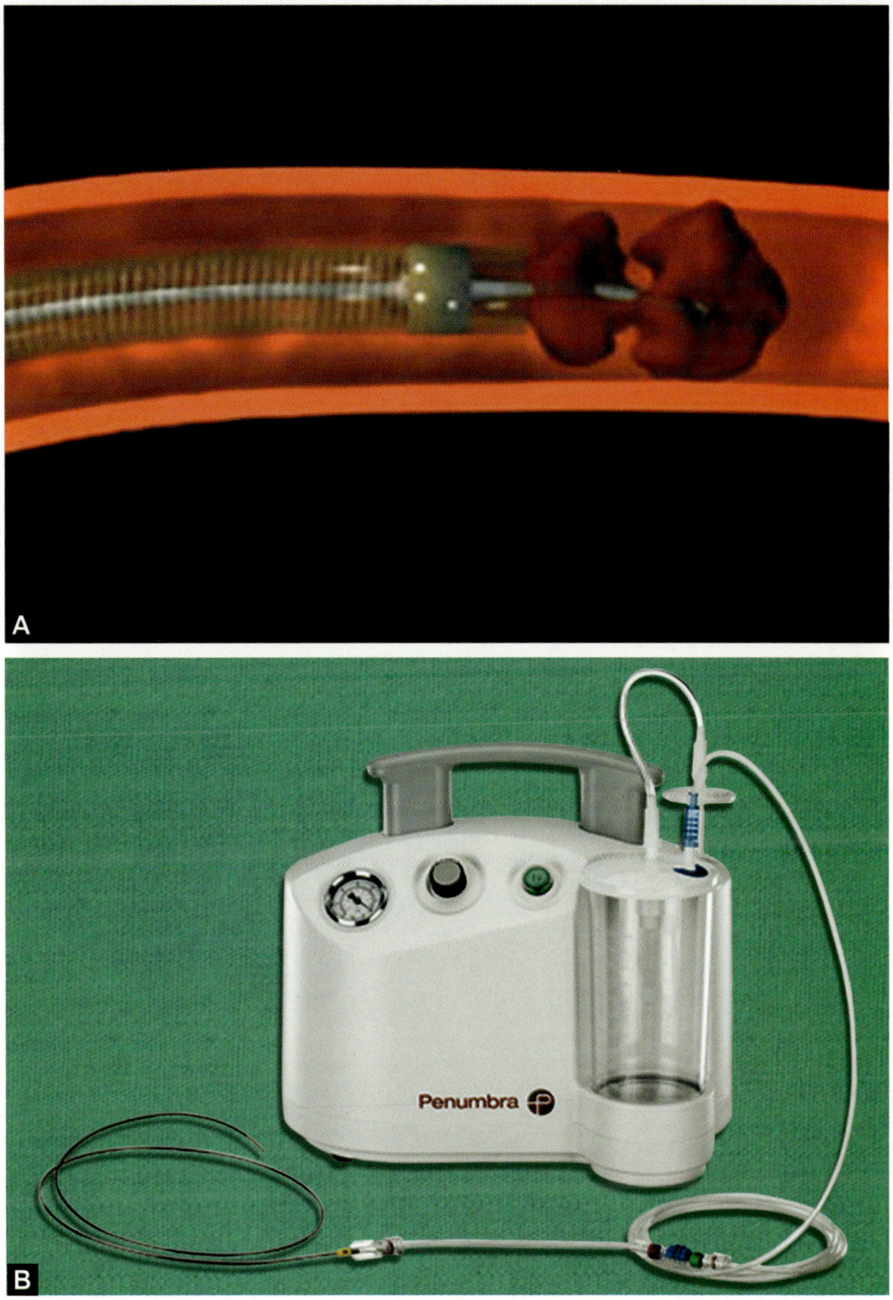

Figs. 40A and B: Penumbra suction aspirator for mechanical thrombectomy.

- Aspiration device used in mechanical thrombectomy.
- Improved thrombectomy results after replacing the first generation "Cork Screw" devices.
- Along with stent retriever devices, have revolutionized stroke service.

"SOLITAIRE" STENT RETRIEVER FOR MECHANICAL THROMBECTOMY (FIGS. 41A AND B)

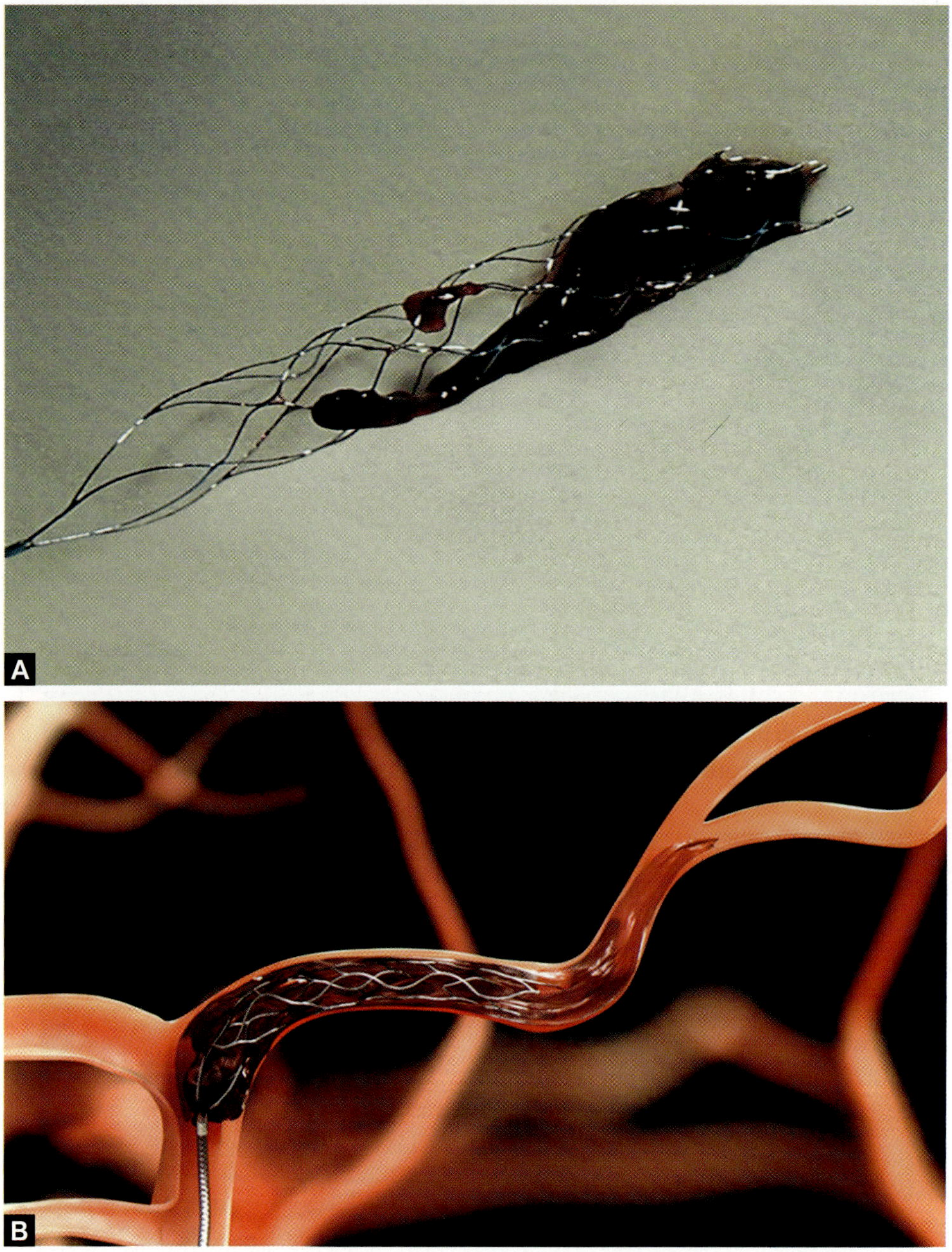

Figs. 41A and B: "SOLITAIRE" stent retriever for mechanical thrombectomy.

- Most promising mechanical thrombectomy devices.
- Latest studies have shown best results both radiologically and clinically.
- Allows early restoration of perfusion before complete clot evacuation.

MOTOR AND SENSORY EVOKED POTENTIAL (FIGS. 42A TO C)

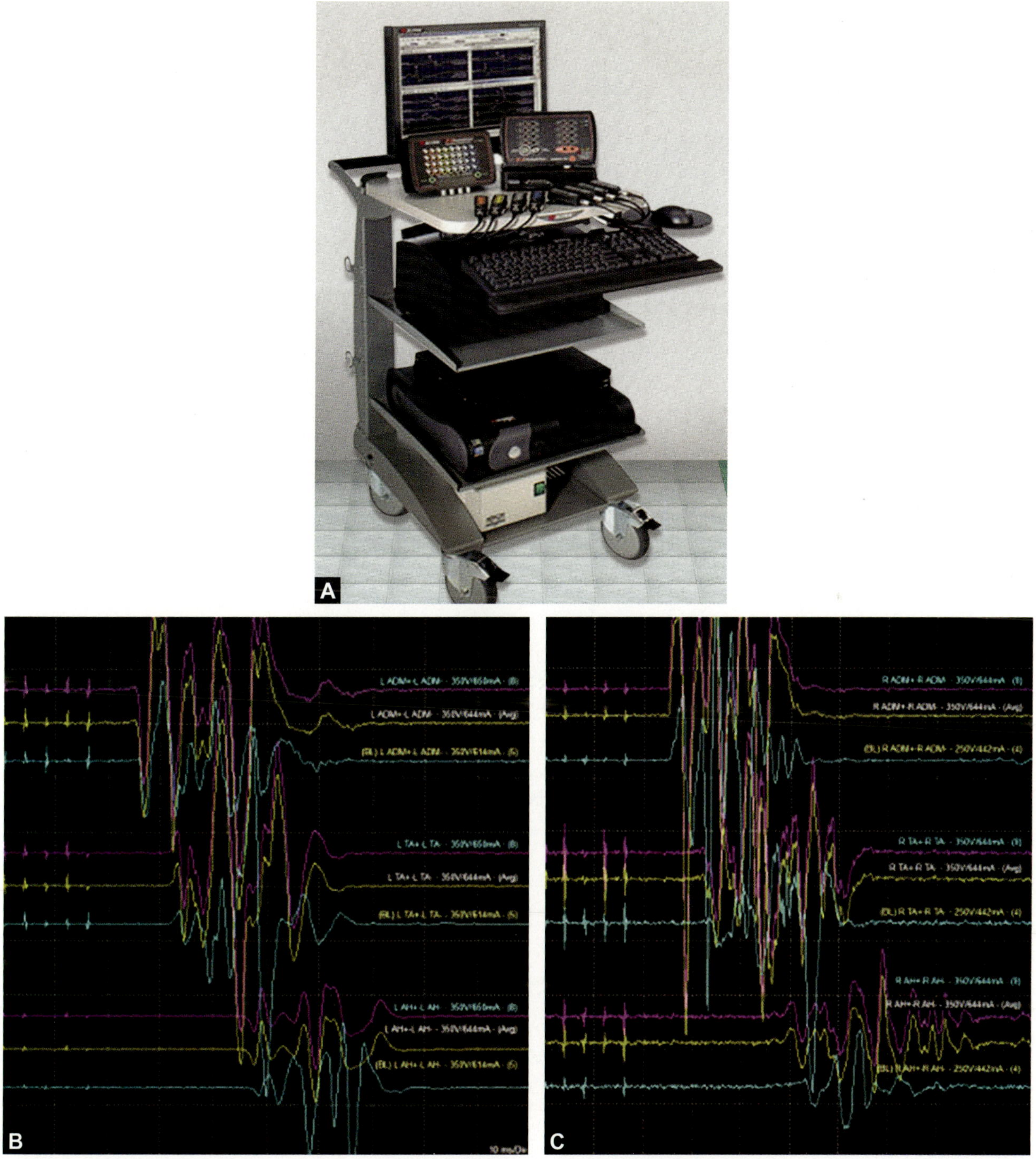

Figs. 42A to C: Motor and sensory evoked potential.

Indication: To assess the integrity of corticospinal and spinocerebellar pathways.

- Assess the somatosensory system functioning by using electrical stimulation of the peripheral nerves.
- Most commonly used in spinal surgery, e.g. scoliosis, vertebral fixation, etc.
- Also used in cranial surgery like skull base surgery, trigeminal decompression, etc.

ELECTROENCEPHALOGRAPHY (FIG. 43)

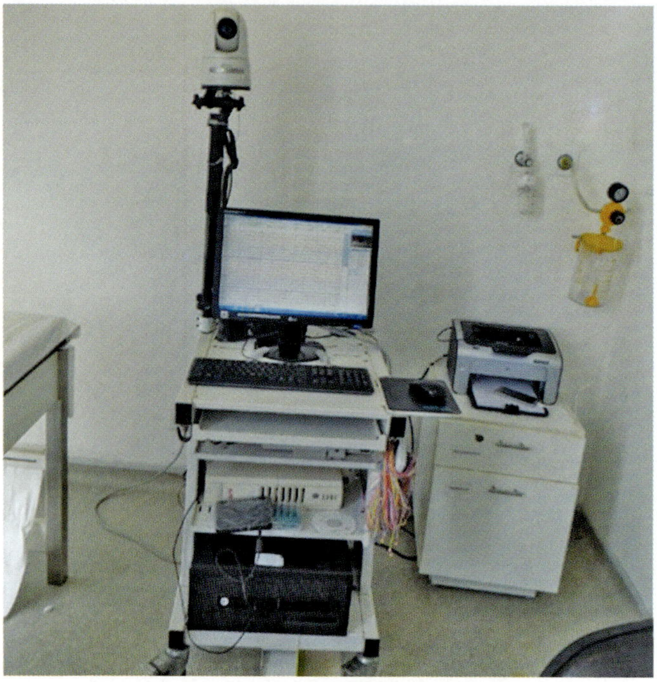

Fig. 43: Electroencephalography (EEG).

- Technique of recording the electrical activity of the brain via scalp electrodes.
- Used most commonly to diagnose various epilepsy disorders.
- Modified techniques are used in: Depth of anesthesia monitoring, brain perfusion, etc.
- Noninvasive, portable and quick technique.
- Limited by spatial resolution and time-dependent episodic capture.

CONTINUOUS OR VIDEO ELECTROENCEPHALOGRAPHY (CEEG/VEEG) (FIG. 44)

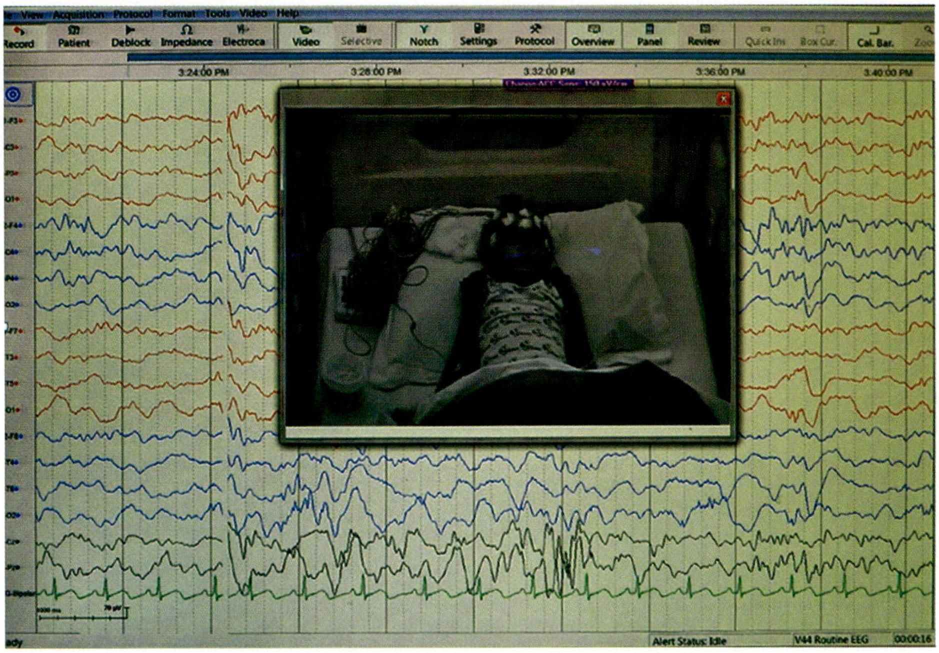

Fig. 44: Video electroencephalography.

- EEG along with simultaneous physical audio-visual recording of the patient.
- Helps identify electrical seizure activity with physical seizure episodes.
- Combined audio-visual process done within the hospital in an EEG laboratory.
- Determines the frequency, duration and severity of the seizures.
- Most useful in drug-resistant, status epilepticus and psychogenic seizures.

EEG: NORMAL AWAKE WITH BACKGROUND ALPHA WAVES (FIG. 45)

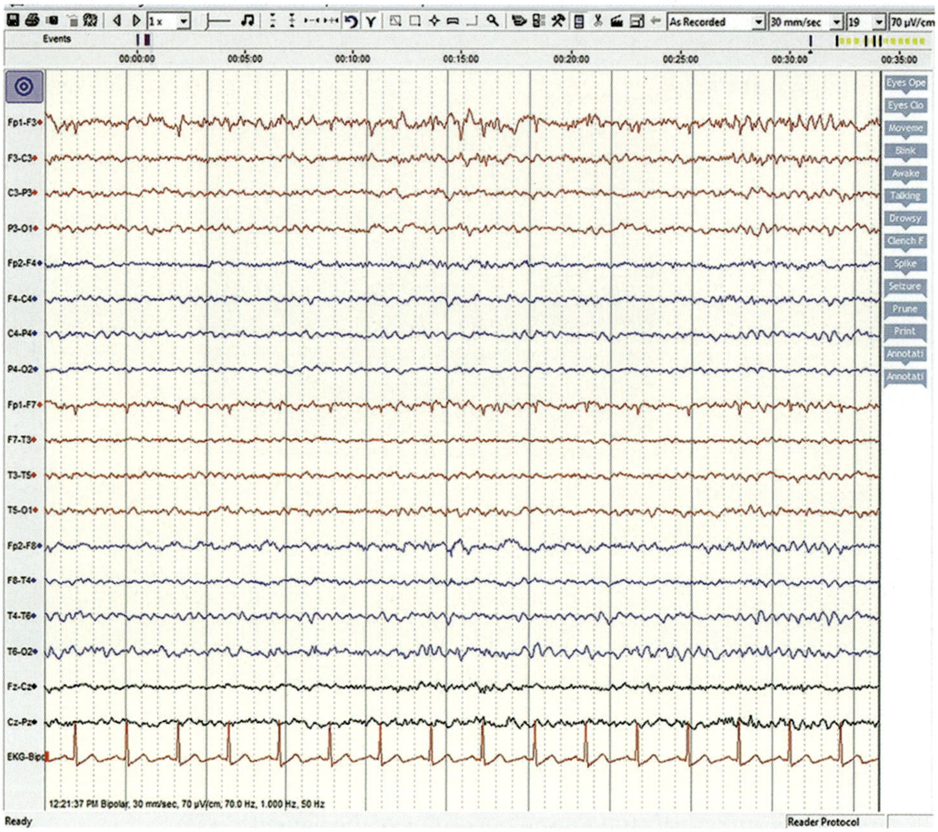

Fig. 45: EEG: Normal awake with background alpha waves.

- Shows normal EEG activity in awake patient.
- Alpha rhythm with frequency between 8 Hz and 13 Hz.

EEG: TONIC-CLONIC SEIZURES (FIG. 46)

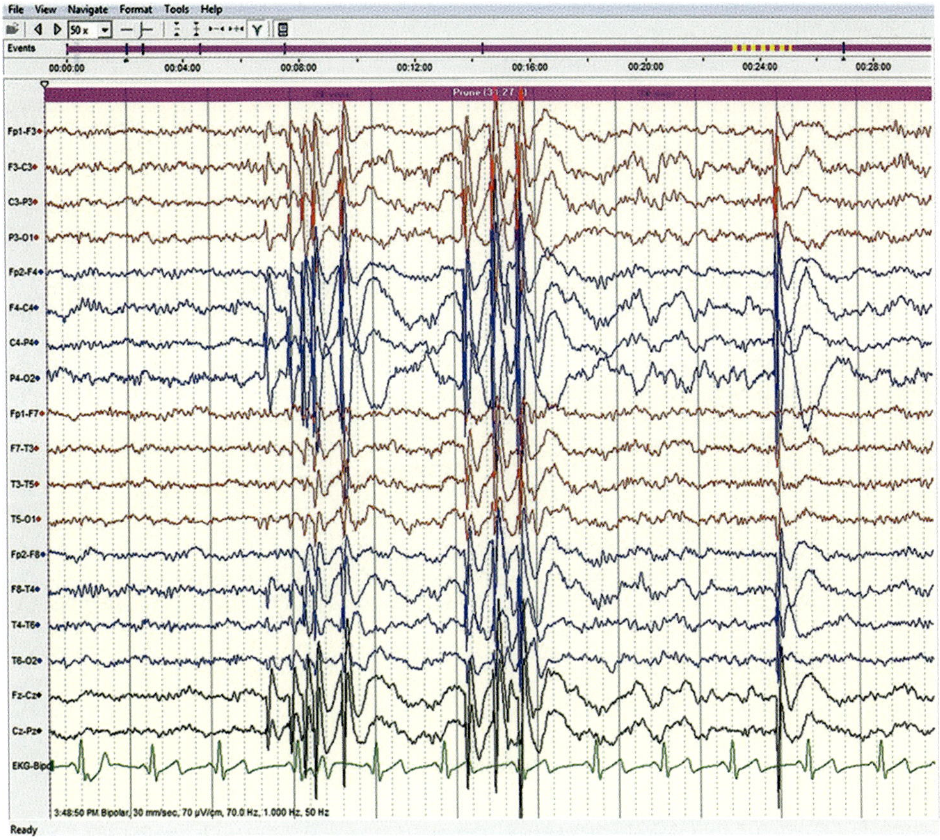

Fig. 46: EEG: Tonic-clonic seizures.

- EEG: Generalized tonic-clonic seizures.
- Spikes and slow waves alternating in both sides and all zones.

METABOLIC SYNDROME (FIG. 47)

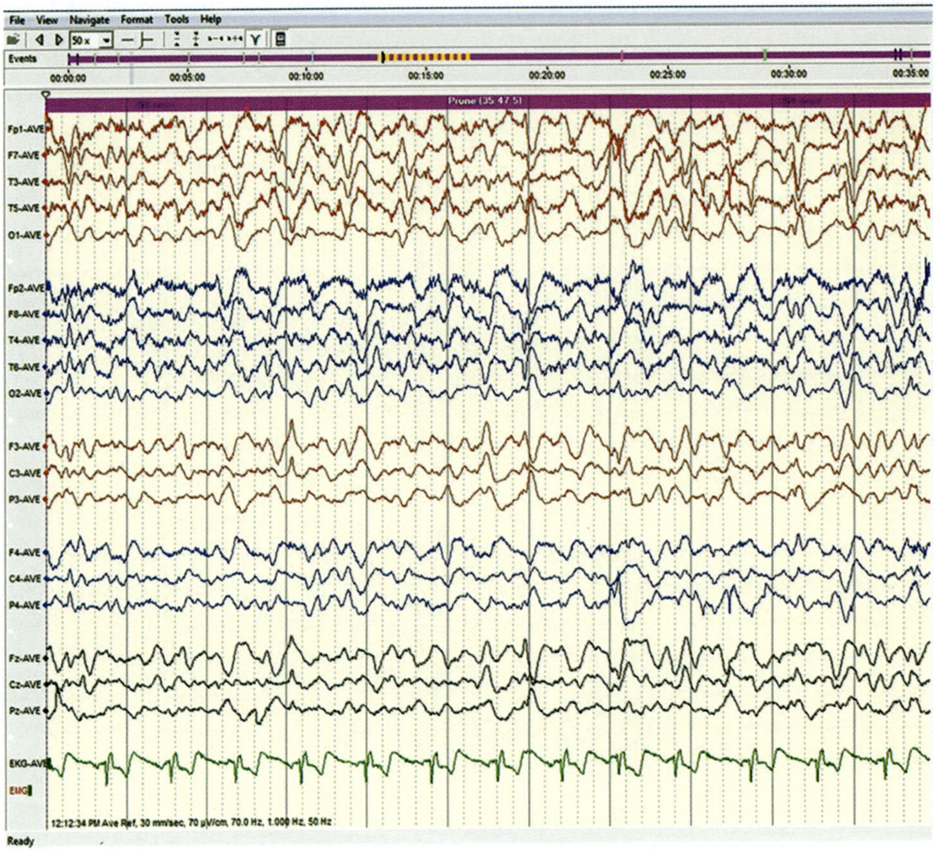

Fig. 47: Metabolic syndrome.

- EEG: Metabolic syndrome.
- Characteristic triphasic waves are seen.

EEG WITH PHOTIC DRIVE (FIG. 48)

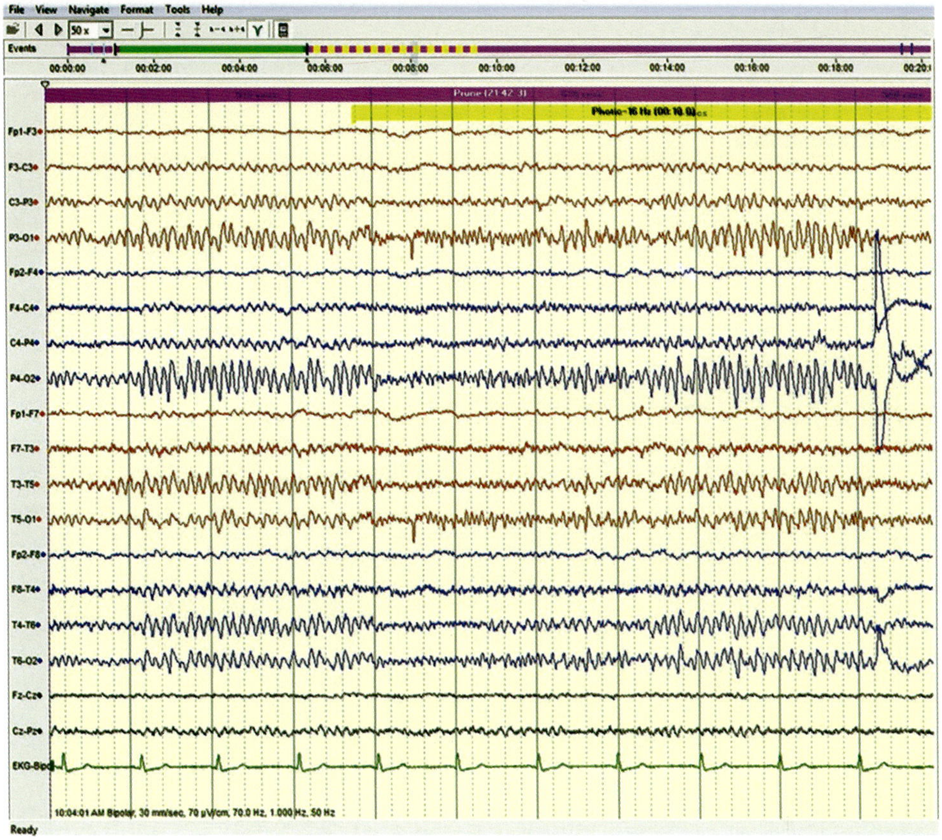

Fig. 48: EEG with photic drive.

- EEG: Photic drive seizure in an adult.
- Seizure activity at increased frequency of 8 Hz.

EEG WITH PERIODIC LATERALIZED EPILEPTIFORM DISCHARGES AND TRIPHASIC WAVES (FIG. 49)

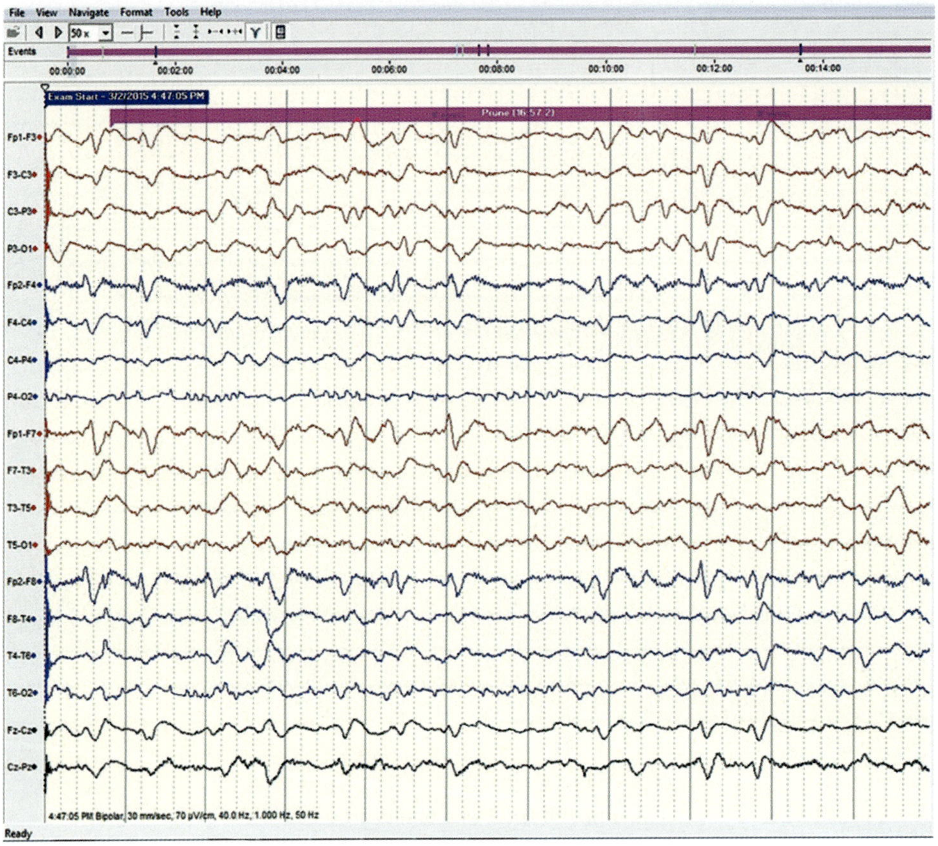

Fig. 49: EEG with PLEDs and triphasic waves.

- EEG showing periodic lateralized epileptiform discharges (PLEDs).
- Evidence of triphasic waves.

EEG WITH BURST SUPPRESSION (FIG. 50)

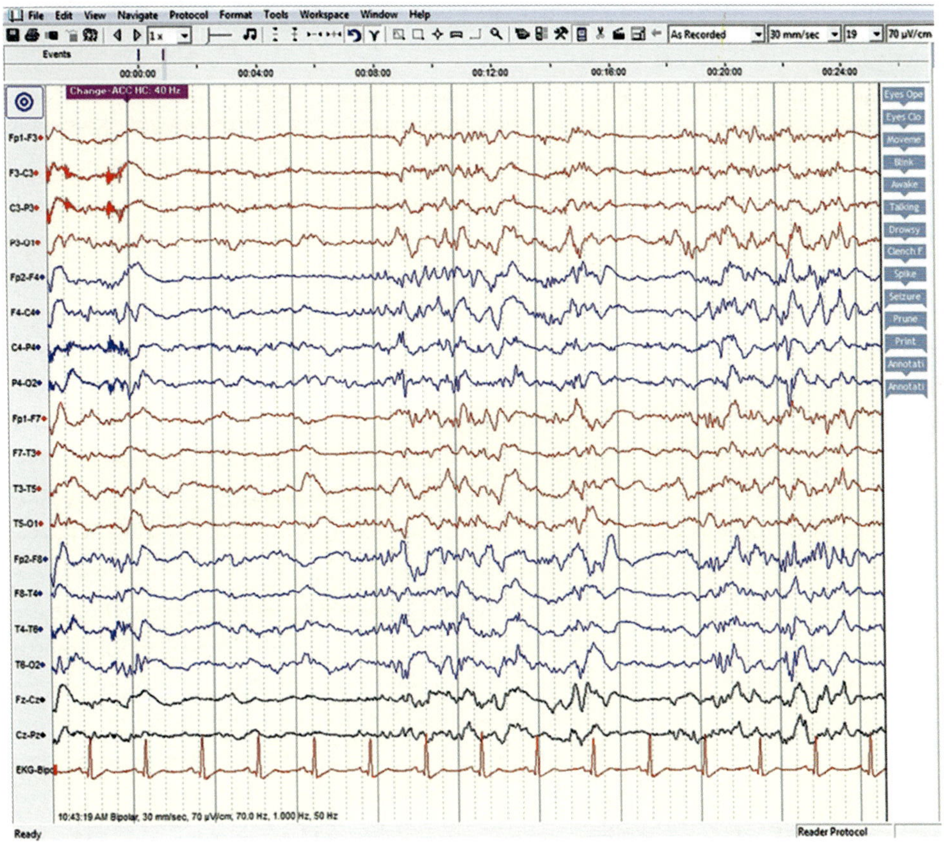

Fig. 50: EEG with burst suppression.

- EEG showing burst suppression in an adult comatose patient.
- Suppression lasting 4–5s and less than 10 mV.

EEG: ALPHA COMA (SHOWING NO ELECTRICAL ACTIVITY ABOVE 2 mV) (FIG. 51)

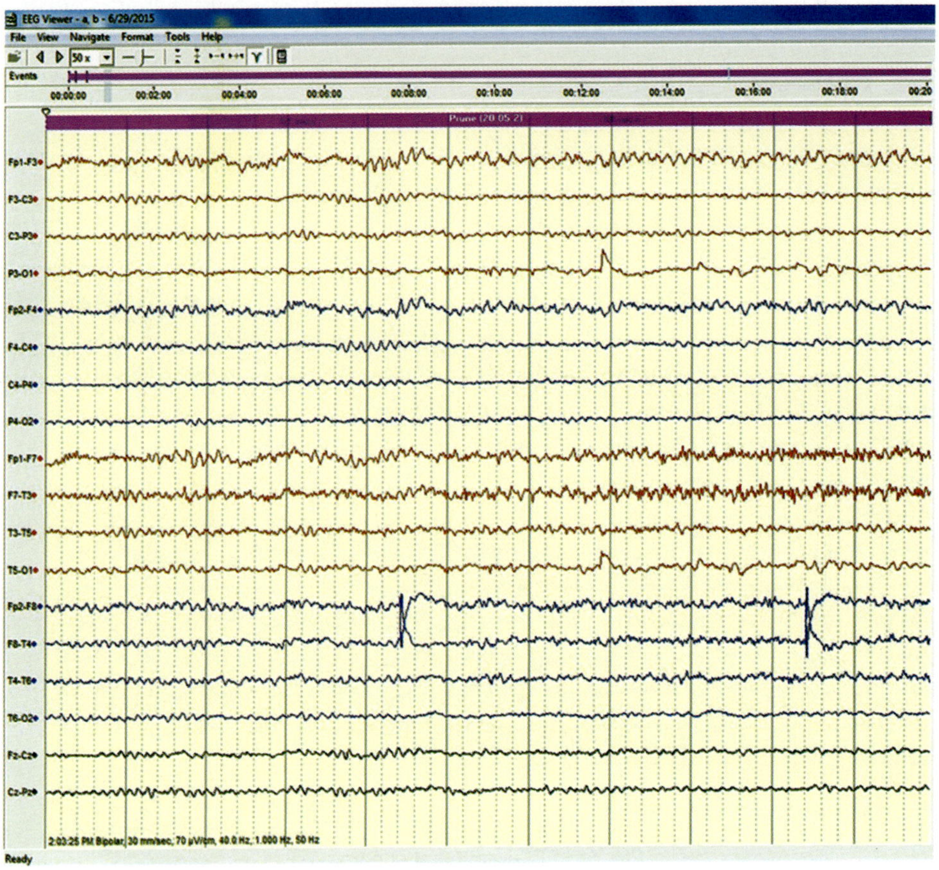

Fig. 51: EEG: Alpha coma (showing no electrical activity above 2 mV).

- EEG shows no activity above 2 mV.
- Demonstrative of alpha coma.

SECTION 6

Trauma

CHAPTER

15

Trauma Cases in ICU

Kapil Dev Soni, Atin Kumar, Amit Gupta

CHEST TRAUMA (FIG. 1)

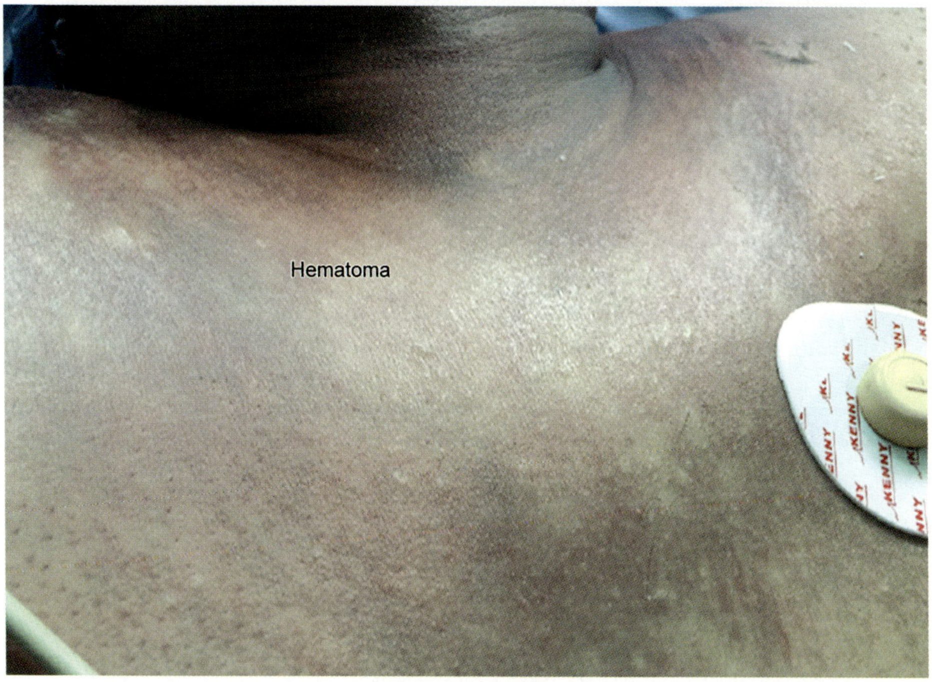

Fig. 1: Chest trauma.

- The patient sustained chest injury and left subclavian artery injury.
- The image illustrates big hematoma extending into the neck and upper chest.
- The patient got intubated due to shock and later recovered with resuscitation.
- Early resuscitation with hemorrhage control is the key.
- Frequent systematic physical examinations help to understand extent and severity of injuries.

PENETRATING INJURY TO CHEST (FIG. 2)

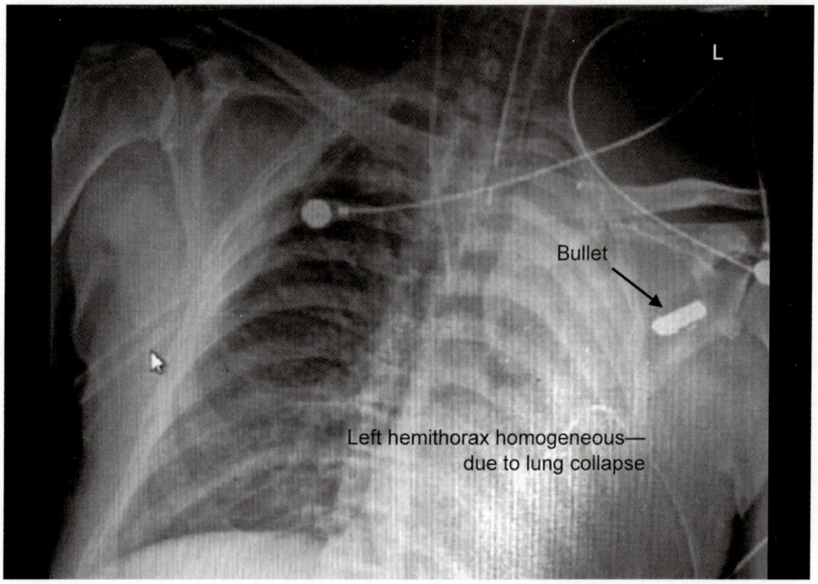

Fig. 2: Penetrating injury to chest.

- The patient sustained gunshot injury to left upper chest.
- The left lung is collapsed due to blood clot obstructing the left bronchi.
- Early bronchoscopic retrieval of clot is paramount to open the lung and avoiding ventilator-induced lung injury (VILI) to other healthy lung, if patient is on mechanical ventilator.

ACUTE RESPIRATORY DISTRESS SYNDROME FOLLOWING MAJOR TRAUMA (FIG. 3)

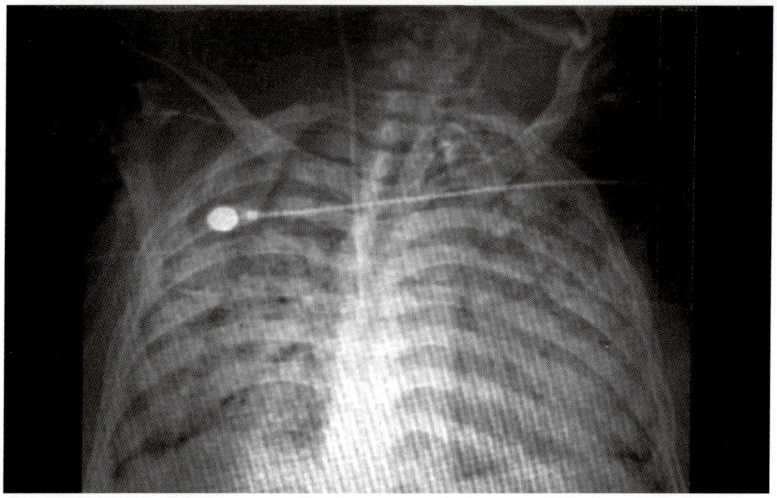

Fig. 3: Acute respiratory distress syndrome following major trauma.

- The patient developed acute respiratory distress syndrome (ARDS) following polytrauma.
- Ventilate these patients with lung protective strategies. In refractory ARDS prone ventilation can be considered.
- Supportive care and judicious fluids is the key during optimization and stabilization phase.
- Measurement of transpulmonary pressure helps in better adjustment of positive end-expiratory pressure (PEEP).

DYNAMIC HYPERINFLATION (FIG. 4)

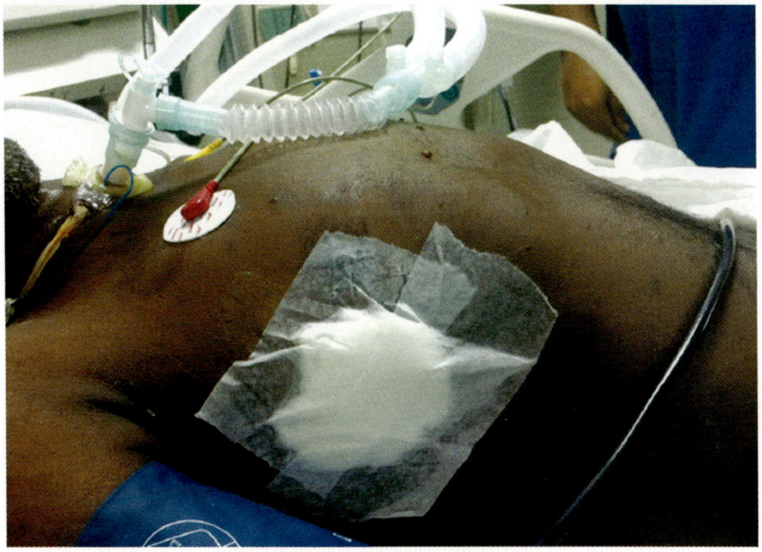

Fig. 4: Dynamic hyperinflation.

- Patient developing dynamic hyperinflation due to auto-PEEP.
- Past history of chronic obstructive pulmonary disease (COPD).
- Needs immediate disconnection from ventilator, if hemodynamically unstable or in cardiac arrest.
- Low tidal volume, low respiratory frequency, increased inspiratory-expiratory (IE) ratio and appropriate extrinsic PEEP minimize dynamic hyperinflation.

INTRA-ALVEOLAR HEMORRHAGE (FIG. 5)

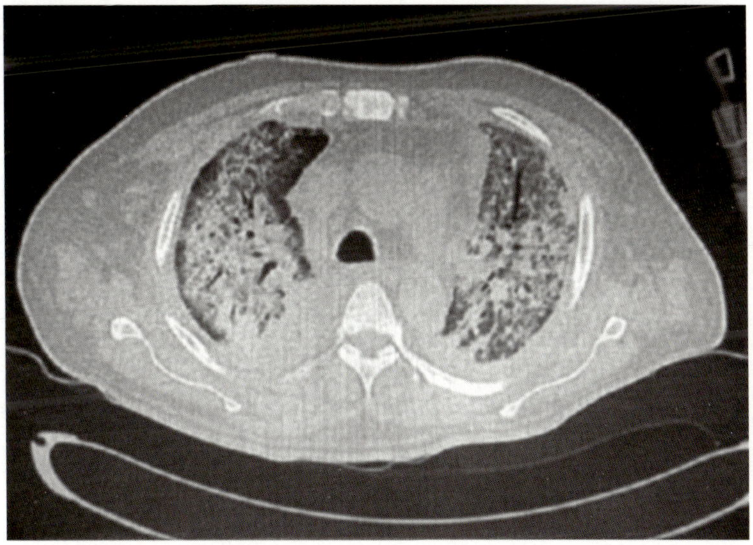

Fig. 5: Intra-alveolar hemorrhage.

- Patient developed intra-alveolar hemorrhage following a major trauma.
- Needed supportive care and correction of coagulopathy.
- Embolization of actively bleeding vessel can be considered in certain situations.

TRACHEAL INJURY (FIG. 6)

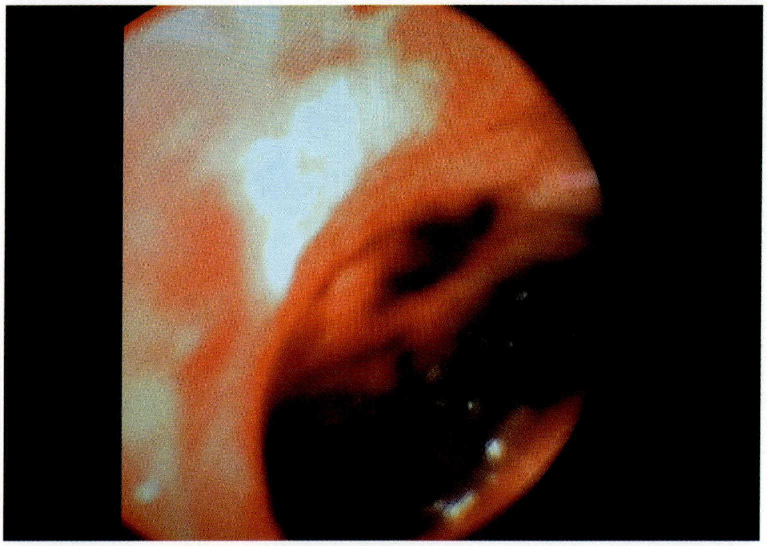

Fig. 6: Tracheal injury.

- Patient had tracheal injury and developed considerable air leak.
- Required repair of the rent.
- Tracheal stenting or bypass of the injured segment could not be achieved with standard intubation.

ABDOMINAL COMPARTMENT SYNDROME (FIG. 7)

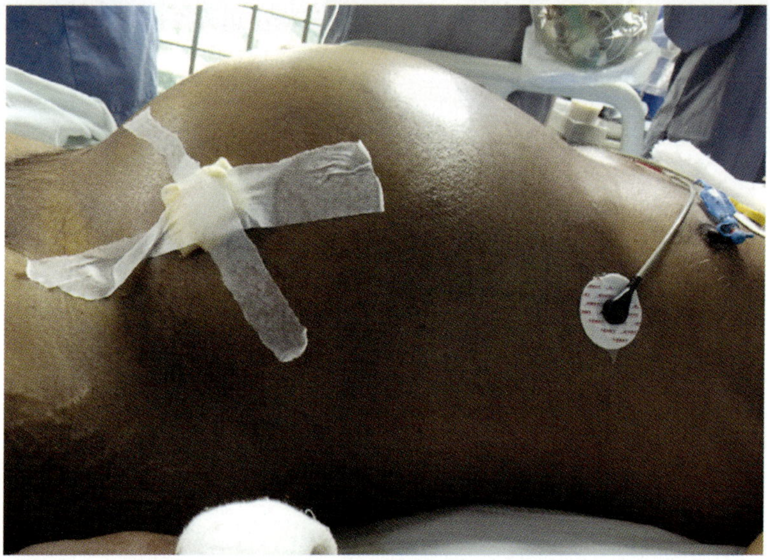

Fig. 7: Abdominal compartment syndrome.

- Patient developed intra-abdominal hypertension followed by abdominal compartment syndrome (ACS).
- Needed placement of abdominal drain along with supportive measures such as paralysis, gastric evacuation, rectal evacuation, and continuous monitoring of intra-abdominal pressure (IAP).
- Therapy should be guided by IAP monitoring for ACS.

TONGUE HEMATOMA (FIG. 8)

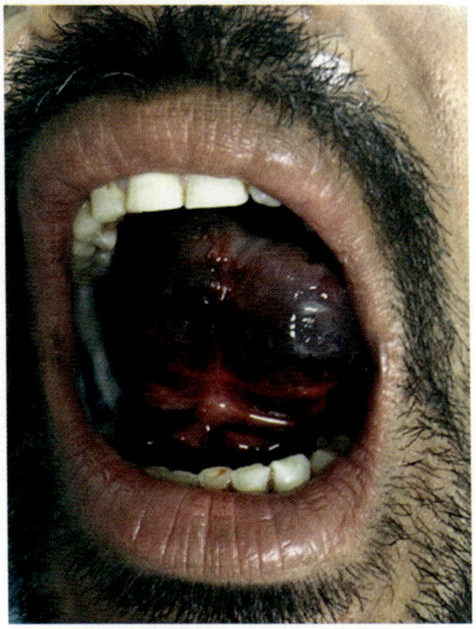

Fig. 8: Tongue hematoma.

- Patient developed large tongue hematoma due to a direct injury.
- Needed prophylactic intubation due to potentially threatened airway.
- With progressive edema, the tongue may be pushed back and obstruct the opening of trachea.

OBSTRUCTED ENDOTRACHEAL TUBE (FIG. 9)

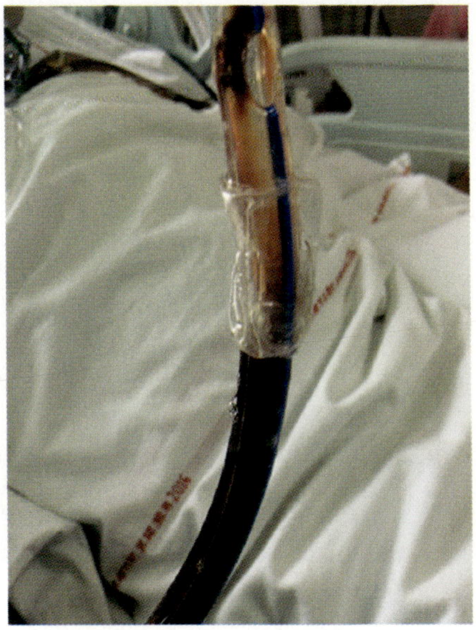

Fig. 9: Obstructed endotracheal tube.

- Patient had bilateral chest injury and hemoptysis.
- Endotracheal tube got obstructed from blood clot and needed replacement.

AMPUTED ISCHEMIC STUMP (FIG. 10)

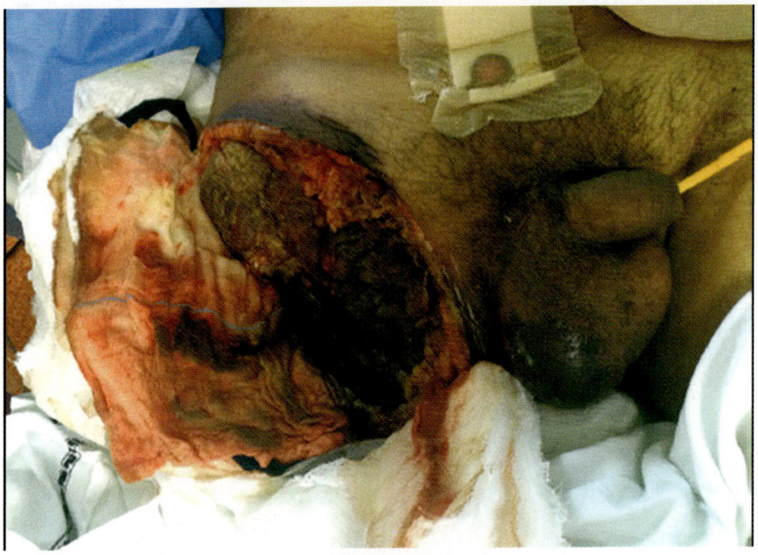

Fig. 10: Amputed ischemic stump.

- The patient sustained right lower limb crush injury and underwent amputation.
- However, the stump became ischemic and had to be further debrided.
- The muscles look avascular and congested.
- A source of infection.

INADVERTENT PLACEMENT OF RYLE'S TUBE (FIG. 11)

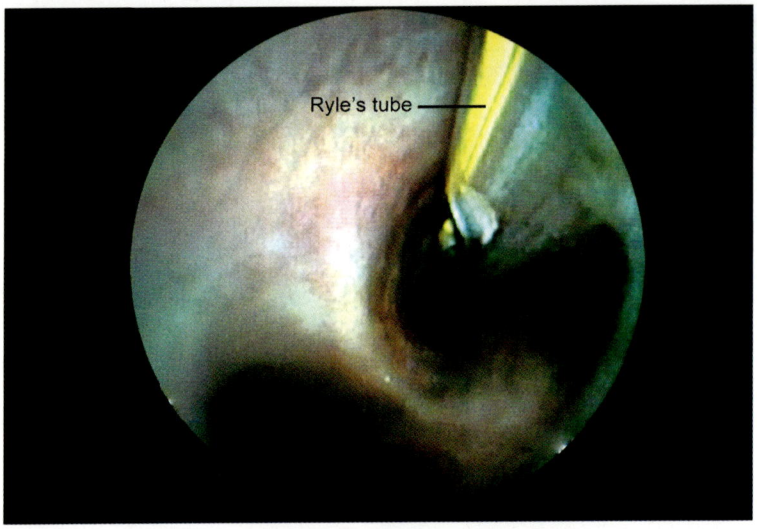

Fig. 11: Inadvertent placement of Ryle's tube.

- An inadvertently placed Ryle's tube was seen during a bronchoscopy procedure.
- Fortunately, Ryle's tube was on continuous drainage and did not caused aspiration, though it led to loss of tidal volume. Clinical signs alone sometime do not confirm correct placement.
- Chest X-ray post-Ryle's tube insertion is mandatory.

TRAUMATIC BRONCHOPLEURAL FISTULA (FIG. 12)

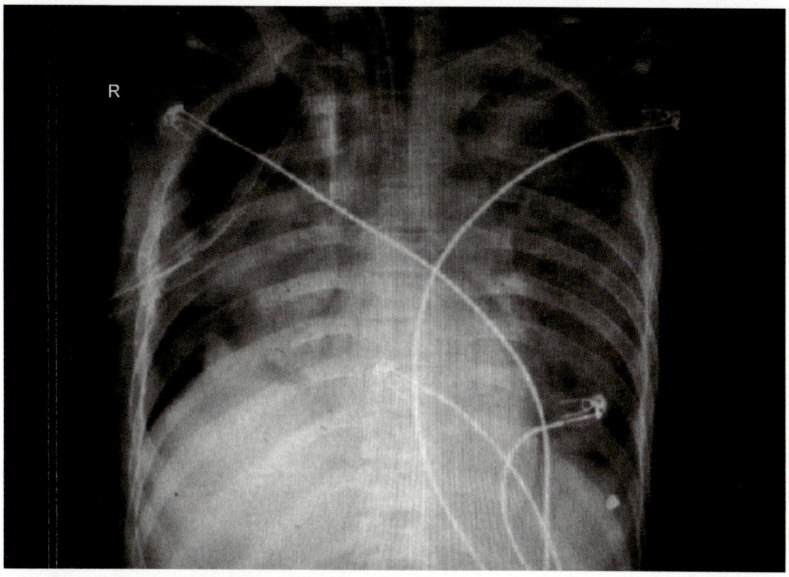

Fig. 12: Traumatic bronchopleural fistula.

- The patient, case of thoracic injury and had sustained multiple rib fractures.
- The image illustrates presence of bronchopleural fistula and collapsed right lung in spite of insertion of two chest tubes.
- Patient needed thoracotomy.

ARTERIAL INSUFFICIENCY IN RIGHT FOOT (FIG. 13)

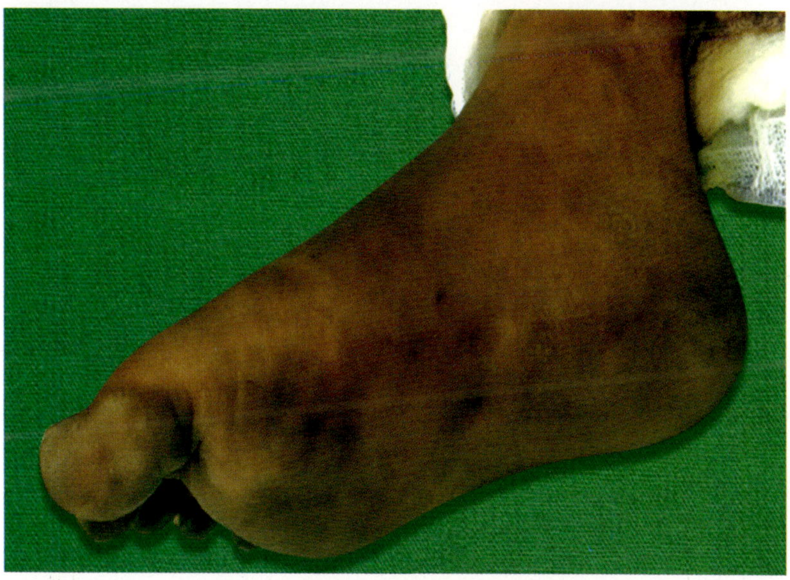

Fig. 13: Arterial insufficiency in right foot.

- The patient developed arterial insufficiency shown as cyanosed limb following an injury to the right leg.
- Immediate exploration was done to restore vascularity.

CELLULITIS OF THE UPPER LIMB (FIG. 14)

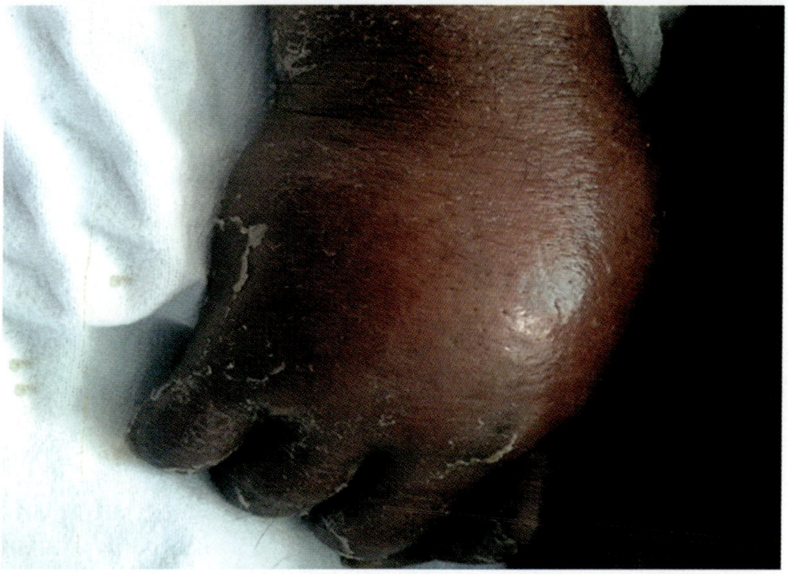

Fig. 14: Cellulitis of the upper limb.

- The patient developed cellulitis following an injury to upper limb.
- Evident as inflamed and painful swelling over the hand.
- Appropriate antibiotics were administered.

SEPTIC EMBOLI (FIG. 15)

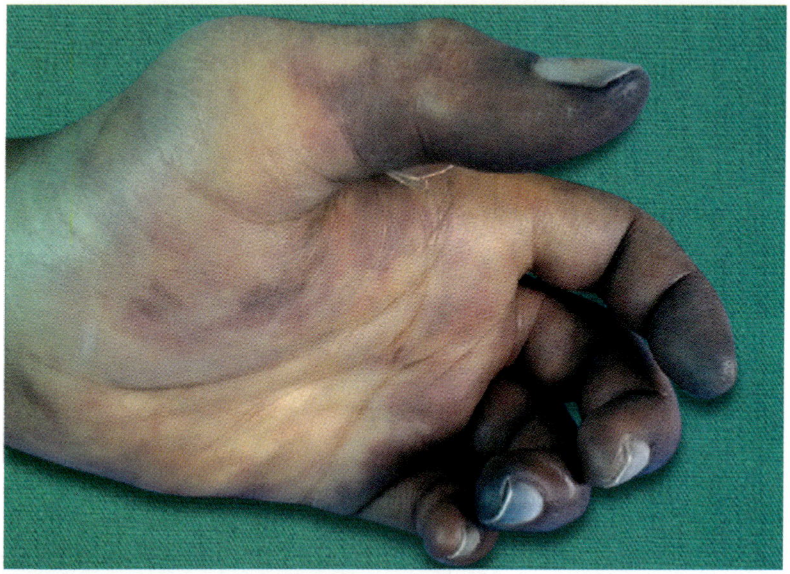

Fig. 15: Septic emboli.

- Patient developed septic shock and Gram-negative bacteremia following polytrauma.
- The image demonstrates septic emboli evident as digital ischemia.
- Source control is the key for survival.

COMPLETE TRACHEAL SEPARATION FOLLOWING A NECK INJURY (FIG. 16)

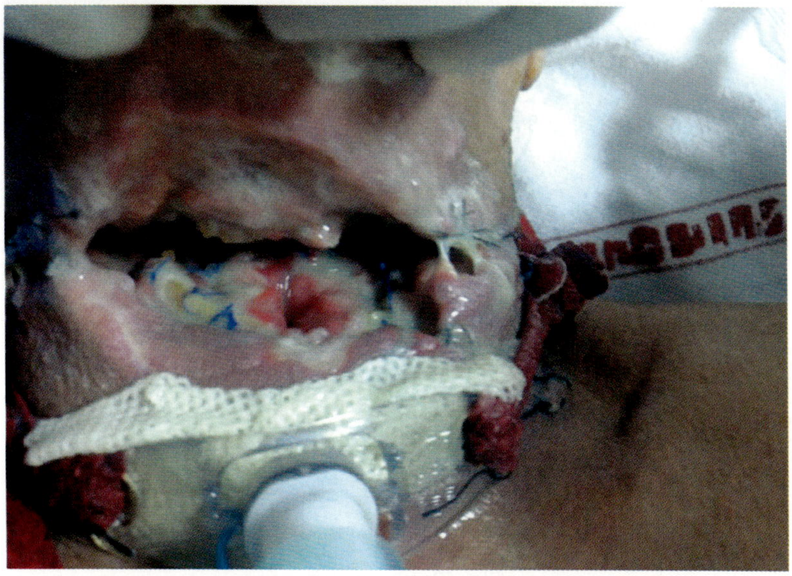

Fig. 16: Complete tracheal separation following a neck injury.

- The image shows complete tracheal separation following a neck injury.
- The patient needed tracheostomy and cervical esophagostomy.

FUNGAL INFECTION OF THE SURGICAL WOUND (FIG. 17)

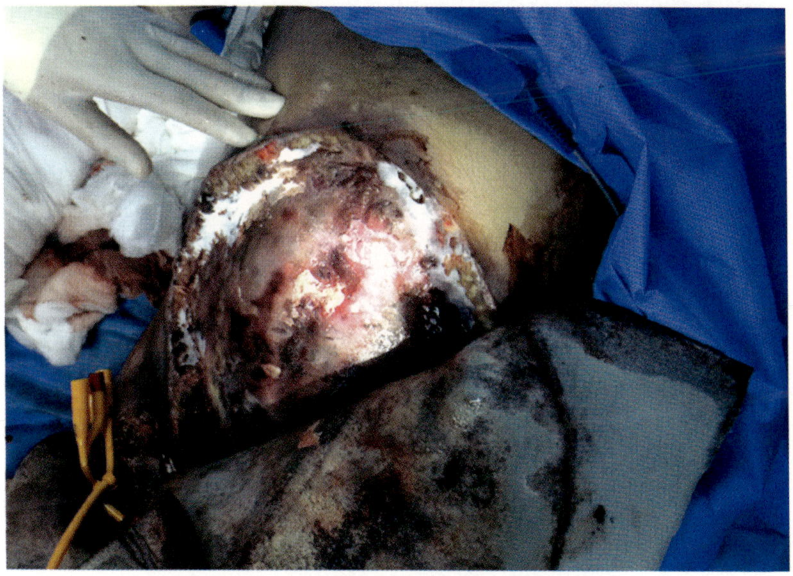

Fig. 17: Fungal infection of the surgical wound.

- The patient developed fungal infection evident as white patches on the amputated limb.
- Needed identification of fungus and appropriate antifungal.

CHEST INJURY (FIG. 18)

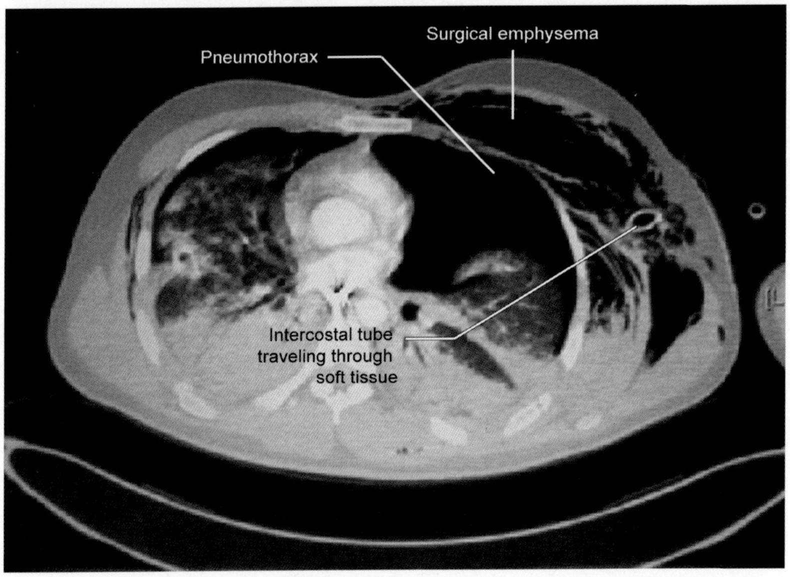

Fig. 18: Chest injury.

- Computed tomography (CT) scan of the patient who sustained thoracic injury.
- A large left pneumothorax and subcutaneous emphysema is visible.
- Patient needed ventilator support and thoracic epidural for effective pain control.

HEMOPERICARDIUM (FIG. 19)

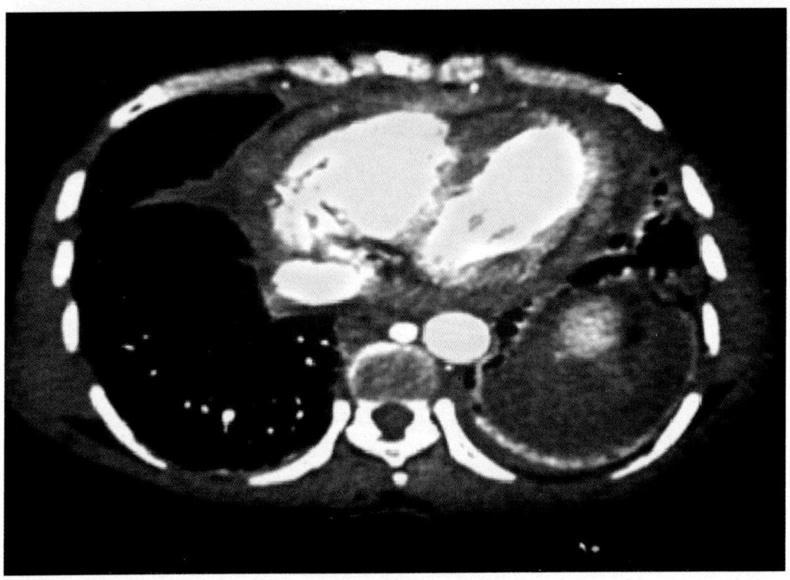

Fig. 19: Hemopericardium.

- The patient presented with stab wound chest and had muffled heart sounds on auscultation during primary survey. His initial vitals: blood pressure (BP) 80/50 mm Hg, heart rate 140 beats/min. Resuscitation was done and patient was stabilized. Computed tomography (CT) shows hemopericardium and left hemothorax. Patient had high likelihood of developing cardiac tamponade. High suspicion is warranted.

LIVER LACERATION (FIG. 20)

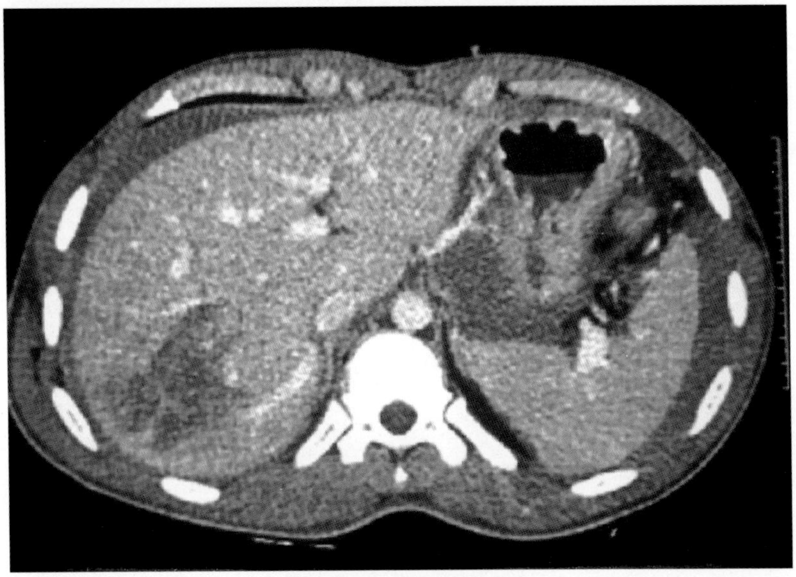

Fig. 20: Liver laceration.

- A patient with history of assault presented in shock. After primary survey and resuscitation, contrast-enhanced computed tomography (CECT) torso was ordered. The CT depicts liver laceration (grade 3) in segment 6 and 7 along with hemoperitoneum. Patient was managed nonoperatively with continuous monitoring.

PANCREAS LACERATION (FIG. 21)

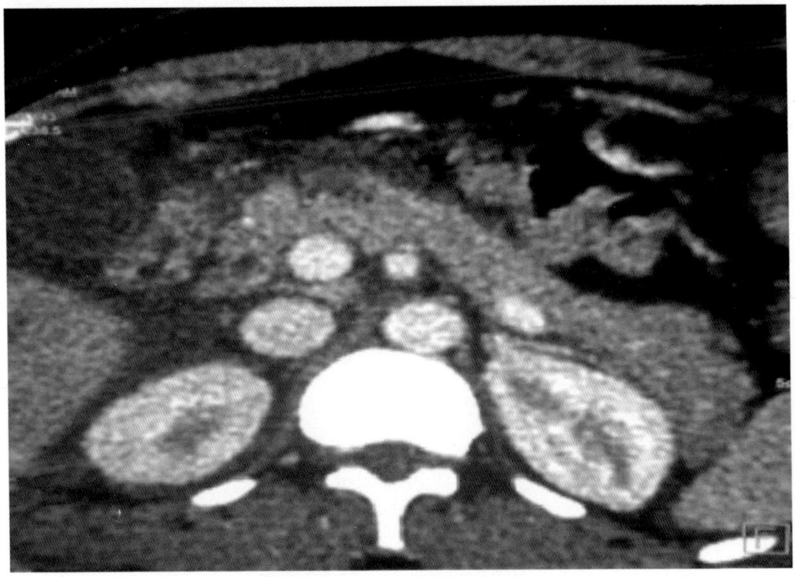

Fig. 21: Pancreatic laceration.

- The patient had history of steering wheel injury and presented with abdominal pain. On CECT torso, pancreatic injury is identified at junction of head and body. Patient underwent subsequent laparotomy.

SPLENIC INJURY (FIG. 22)

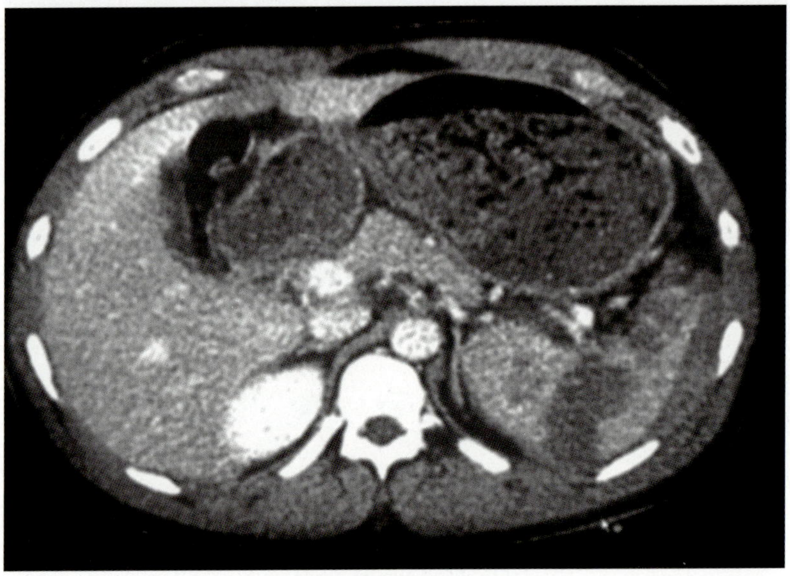

Fig. 22: Splenic injury.

- The earlier CECT illustrates grade 4 splenic laceration. Patient presented in shock and was stabilized during primary survey and admitted in intensive care unit (ICU) for close observation.

PNEUMOTHORAX (FIG. 23)

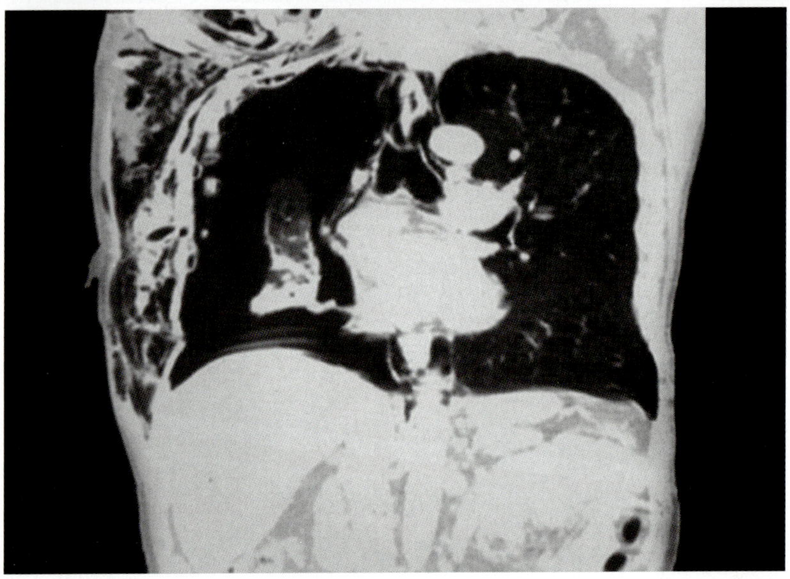

Fig. 23: Pneumothorax.

- The patient had history of RTI and sustained severe chest trauma. On presentation, his oxygen saturation was 80% and was breathing at the rate of 40 breaths/min. Air entry was absent on right side. Immediate chest tube was inserted. CT scan shows large pneumothorax with collapsed lung and massive subcutaneous emphysema. Most thoracic injuries are managed with chest tube insertion. Thoracotomy is required for few indications only.

RIB FRACTURES (FIG. 24)

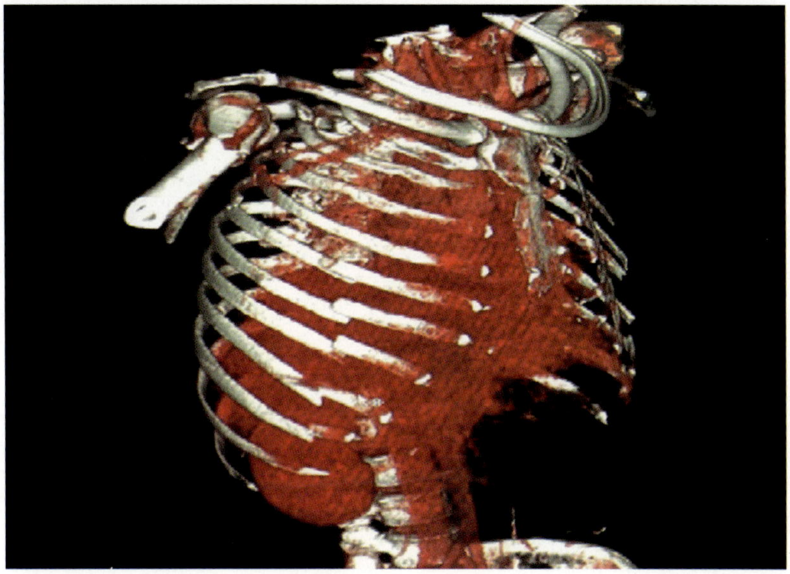

Fig. 24: Rib fractures.

- Volume rendered reconstructed CT image of a patient's chest who suffered direct chest injury and complained of difficulty in breathing and intense pain. The image shows multiple rib fractures. Epidural analgesia is preferred modality for pain relief in such patients.

PELVIC FRACTURES (FIG. 25)

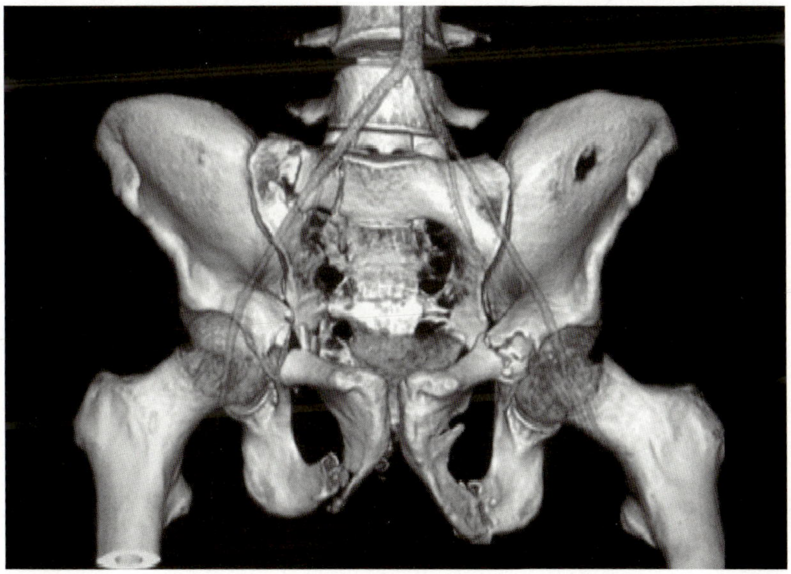

Fig. 25: Pelvic fractures.

- Computed tomography of pelvis illustrating bilateral superior and inferior pubic rami fractures. Such patient, if presents in shock require application of pelvic binder along with standard resuscitation.

EXTRADURAL HEMATOMA (FIG. 26)

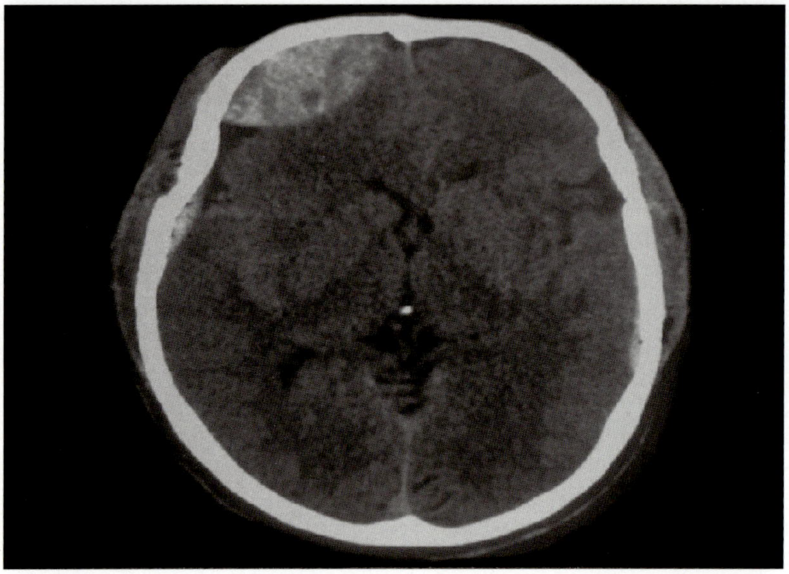

Fig. 26: Extradural hematoma.

- The patient presented with history of brief loss of consciousness following RTI. On noncontrast computed tomography (NCCT) head, an extradural hematoma (EDH) is identified on the right frontal region. Such patient may present in lucid interval but they have potential to deteriorate quickly. An urgent evacuation is often warranted.

SUBDURAL HEMATOMA (FIG. 27)

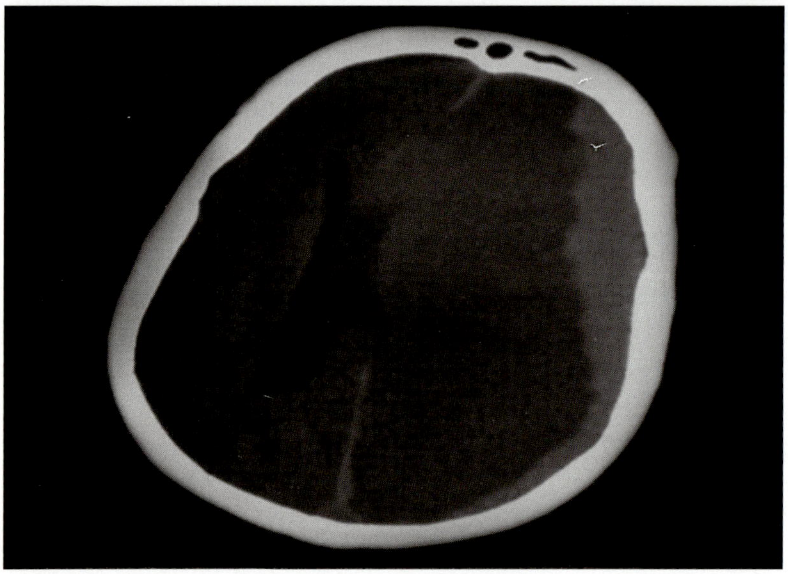

Fig. 27: Subdural hematoma.

- The NCCT head demonstrates subdural hematoma (SDH) crossing suture lines and mass effect (midline shift). Patient underwent urgent decompressive craniectomy to prevent herniation and permanent brain damage.

PARENCHYMAL CONTUSION (FIG. 28)

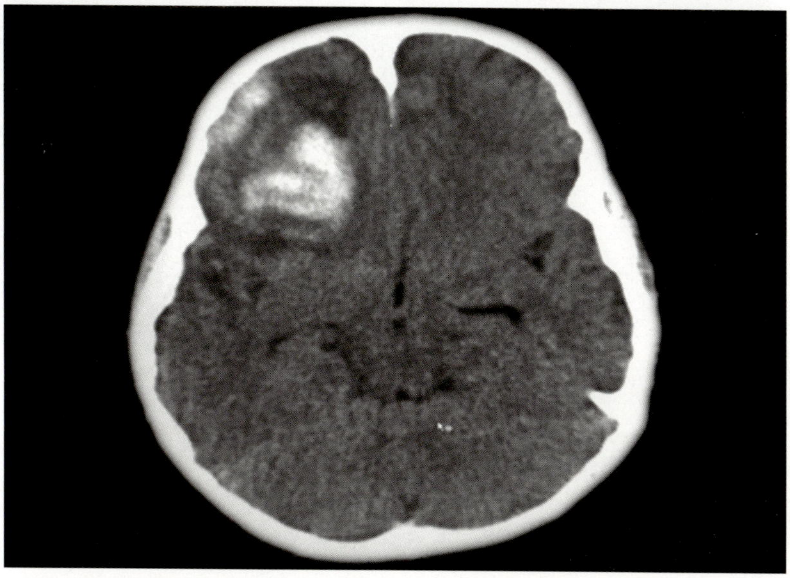

Fig. 28: Parenchymal contusion.

- The NCCT head shows right frontal contusion. Patient requires continuous monitoring for deterioration in Glasgow coma scale (GCS). Intracranial pressure (ICP) monitoring should be instituted and kept within normal levels.

ODONTOID FRACTURE (FIG. 29)

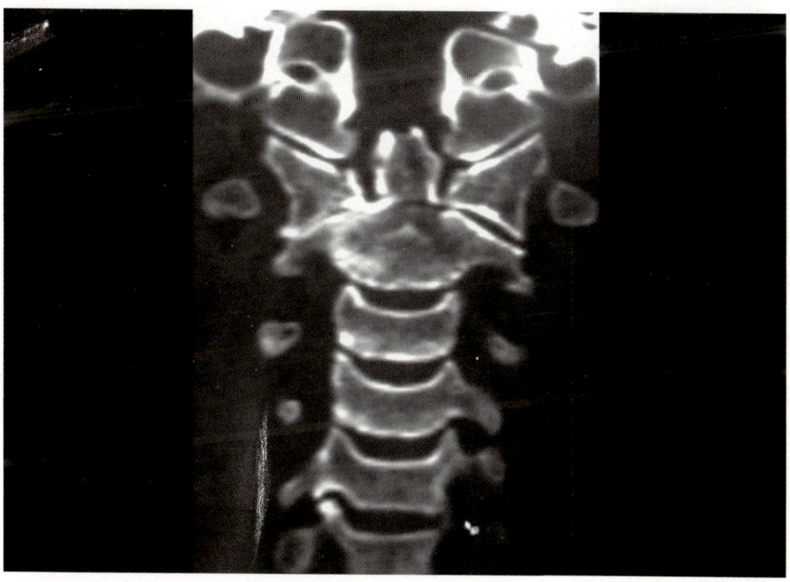

Fig. 29: Odontoid fracture.

- The patient presented with weakness in all the four limbs and pain in neck. NCCT spine shows type 2 fracture of odontoid process of C2 vertebra.

TRACHEAL INJURY (FIG. 30)

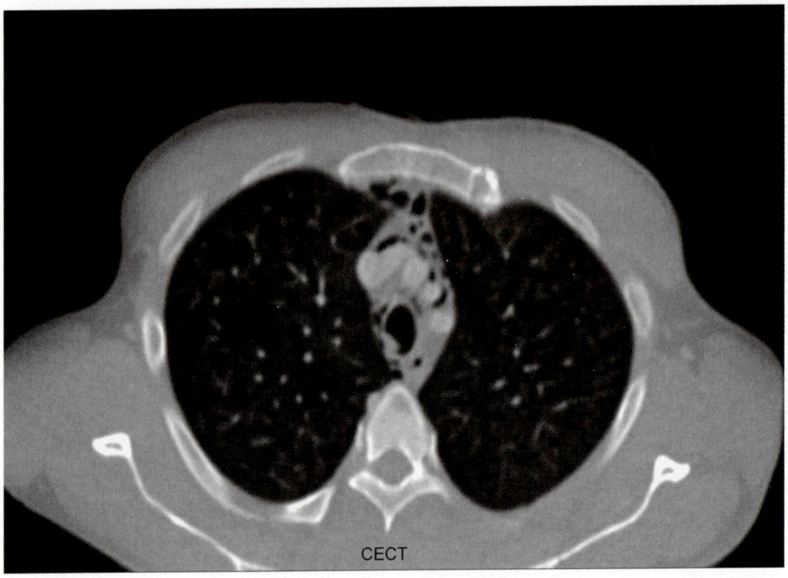

Fig. 30: Tracheal injury. (CECT: Contrast-enhanced computed tomography)

- The patient presented with history of injury to the neck and chest. Contrast-enhanced computed tomography (CECT) chest demonstrates tracheal injury at the right posterolateral aspect and air around the trachea and mediastinum. Close monitoring is needed. If there is excessive leak causing respiratory failure, surgery is warranted.

ASPIRATION PNEUMONITIS (FIG. 31)

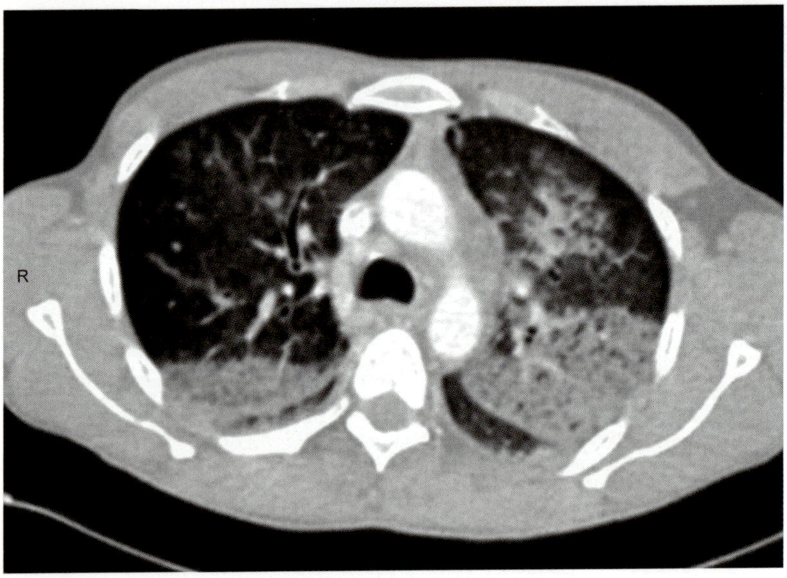

Fig. 31: Aspiration pneumonitis.

- The CECT shows bilateral aspiration changes as air space opacities. Patient presented with history of loss of consciousness and vomiting. Antibiotic may be needed if patient develops infection and new infiltrates.

PNEUMOPERITONEUM DUE TO BOWEL PERFORATION (FIG. 32)

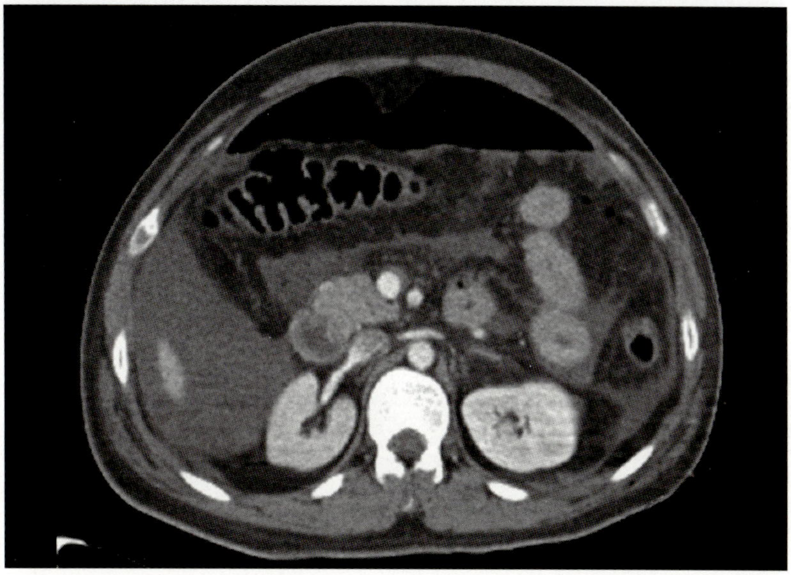

Fig. 32: Pneumoperitoneum due to bowel perforation.

- The CECT shows pneumoperitoneum secondary to bowel perforation. Immediate surgical exploration is indicated.

HEPATIC ARTERY DIGITAL SUBTRACTION ANGIOGRAPHY WITH EMBOLIZATION (FIG. 33)

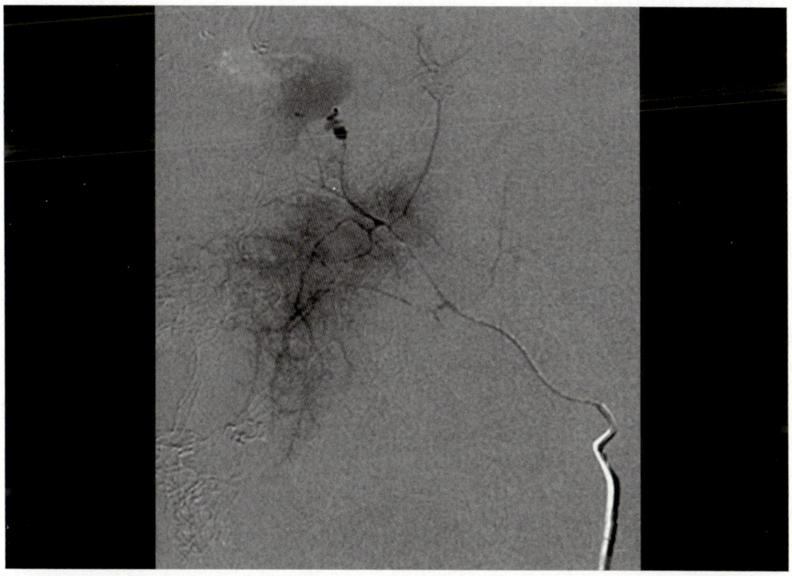

Fig. 33: Hepatic artery digital subtraction angiography with embolization.

- The patient presented with blunt trauma abdomen and shock due to hemoperitoneum identified on focused assessment with sonography for trauma (FAST). Immediate resuscitation along with digital subtraction angiography (DSA) was done. It showed active bleed from the branch of hepatic artery. Angioembolization was carried out to stop the bleeding. Patient was monitored further in ICU.

CERVICAL SPINE FRACTURE DISLOCATION (FIGS. 34A AND B)

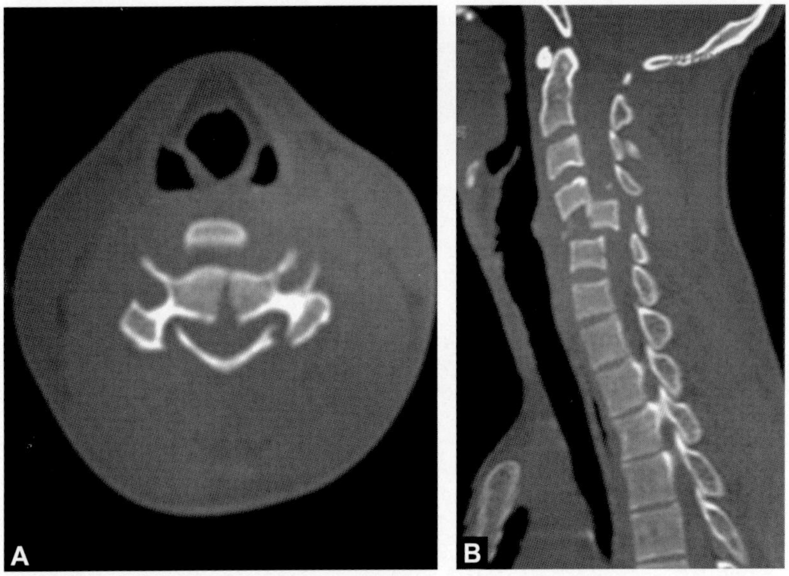

Figs. 34A and B: Cervical spine fracture dislocation.

- Patient presented with history of fall from height and complained of inability to move all the limbs. CT spine demonstrated cervical spine fracture dislocation at C5 level and spinal cord compression. He was managed with neck collar initially to prevent further deterioration and spinal surgery performed next day.

DISTAL SUPERFICIAL FEMORAL ARTERY TRANSECTION (FIG. 35)

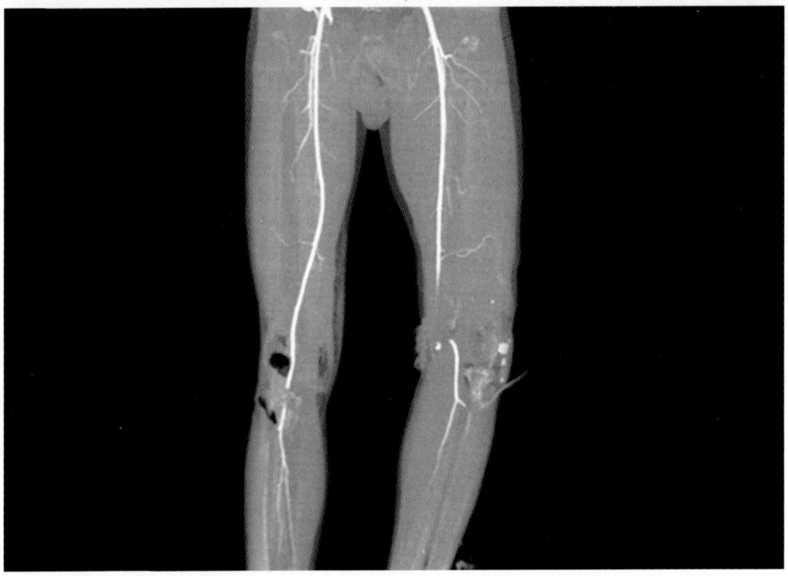

Fig. 35: Distal superficial femoral artery transection.

- The CT angiogram demonstrates distal left superficial femoral artery (SFA) transection just above the knee joint with reformation of the popliteal artery after around 4 cm. Patient underwent surgical exploration and repair.

SECTION 7

Microbiology

CHAPTER

16

Infection and Microbiology

Anand Shah, Camilla Rodrigues

SAMPLE COLLECTION (FIGS. 1 AND 2)

Blood Culture Collection (Fig. 1)

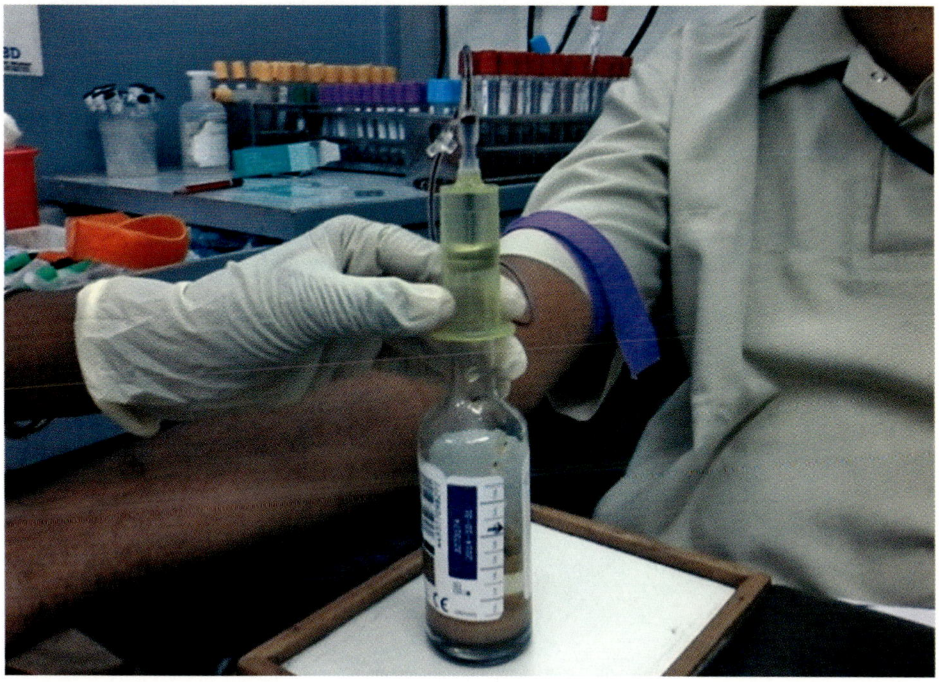

Fig. 1: Blood collection.

Skin disinfectants for blood culture collection:

- Most blood cultures are drawn by venipuncture. In order to minimize the risk of contamination with skin flora, the venipuncture site requires disinfection.
- Iodine-containing preparations require sufficient time to disinfect surfaces (30 seconds for tincture of iodine and 1.5–2 minutes for iodophors).
- Chlorhexidine gluconate [2% weight volume (w/v) that is equivalent to 10% volume/volume (v/v) in 70% isopropyl alcohol] requires the same amount of time as tincture of iodine (30 seconds), but is not associated with allergic reactions and does not need to be cleaned off the skin after the venipuncture is completed.
- Chlorhexidine is the recommended skin disinfectant for older infants, children, and adults, however, it is not indicated for use in infants less than 2 months.

Source: Adopted from CLSI 2007 guidelines for blood culture.

Blood collection procedure:

- Select a prominent vein, cleanse the area with 2% w/v chlorhexidine in 70% isopropyl alcohol and allow it to dry for 30 seconds.
- Without palpating the vein again, puncture the vein to draw the blood (if not confident of the vein, apply 2% chlorhexidine w/v in 70% isopropyl alcohol to the tip of the gloved finger for palpation.
- Disinfect the culture bottle rubber top with the same solution used earlier, and transfer into the required blood culture bottle.
- A blood culture set is advised for all blood culture requests and includes collection of both aerobic and anaerobic vial for each venepuncture.
- Volume of blood is 8–10 mL for each aerobic and anaerobic vial, 1–3 mL for pediatric culture bottle.

Urine Sample through Urinary Catheter Port (Figs. 2A and B)

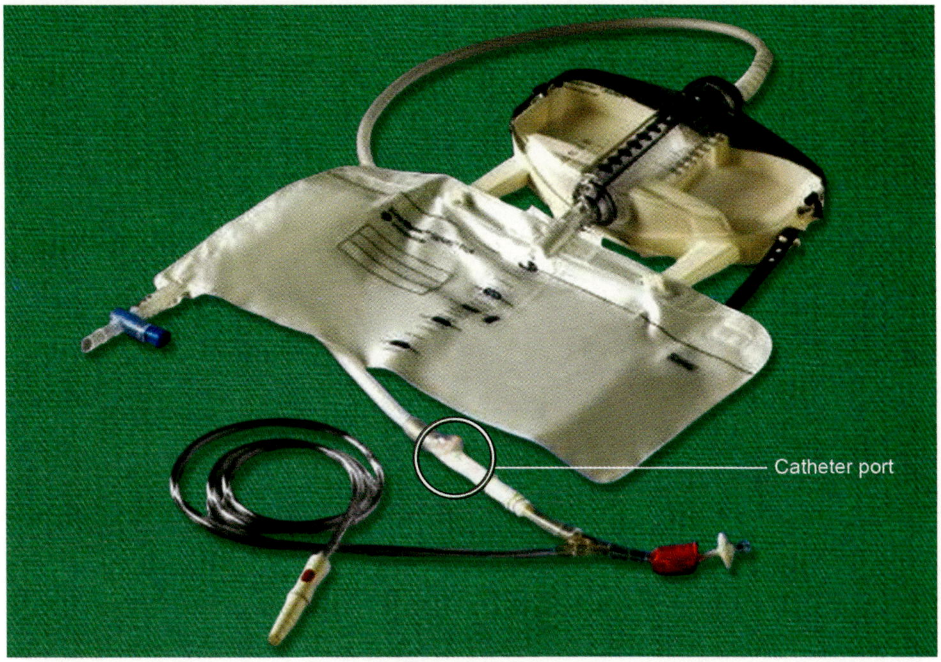

Fig. 2A: Urobag.

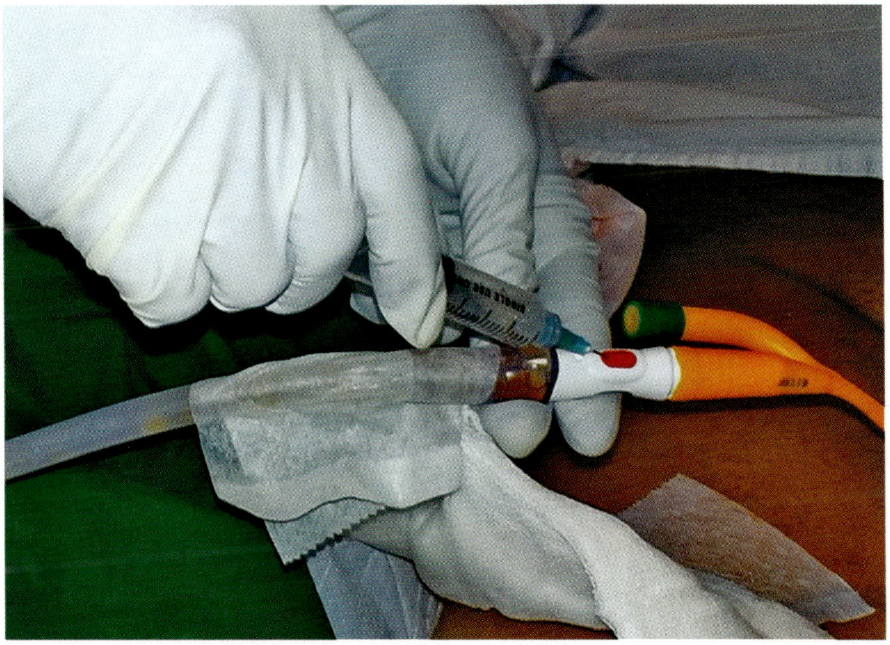

Fig. 2B: Urine collection through catheter port.

- Empty the drainage tube of urine.
- Clamp the drainage tube below the level of the specimen port for 15–30 minutes to allow a fresh sample to collect 20–30 mL urine aseptically.
- Transfer the sample into a sterile container and cap it tightly.

SKIN LESIONS (FIGS. 3 TO 6)

Herpes Simplex Skin Lesions (Fig. 3)

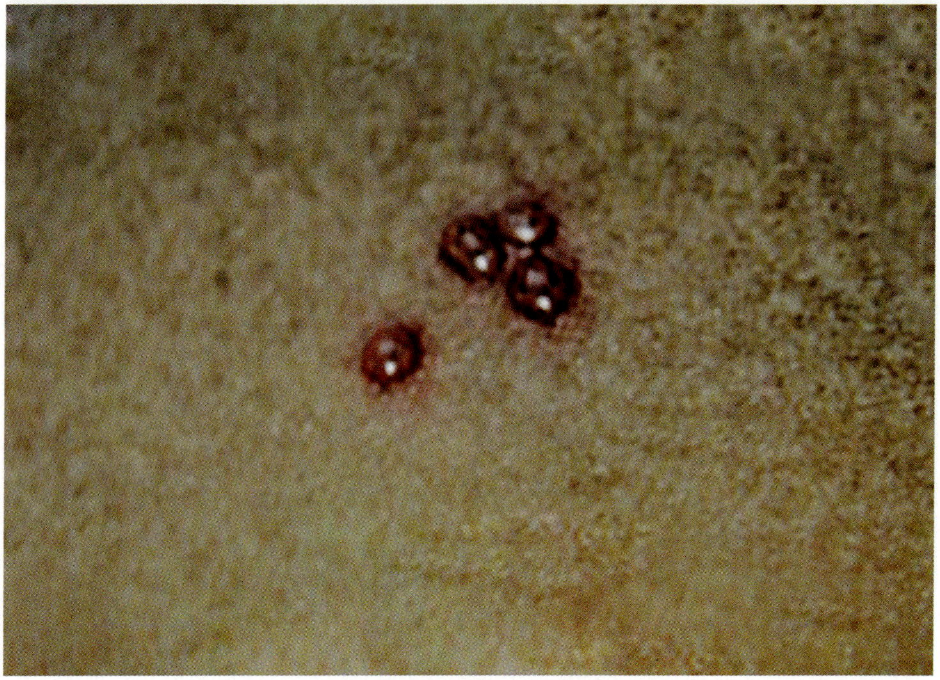

Fig. 3: Herpes simplex.

- Two types:
  1. *Herpes simplex virus (HSV) 1*: Isolated from lesions in and around mouth.
     - Transmitted by direct contact or droplet spread from cases or carriers.
  2. *HSV 2*: Majority of genital herpes infections.
     - Commonly transmitted venereally.
- Typical lesion is the "fever blisters" caused by reactivation in febrile patients. Most common site is the face—on the cheeks, chin, around the mouth, or on the forehead.
- Buccal mucosa is the most commonly affected. Gingivostomatitis and pharyngitis are the most frequent conditions in primary infection and recurrent herpes labialis in recurrent infection.
- Tzanck smear is a rapid, sensitive, and inexpensive diagnostic method. Polymerase chain reaction (PCR) based deoxyribonucleic acid (DNA) detection has replaced all the diagnostic modalities.

Chickenpox (Varicella) (Fig. 4)

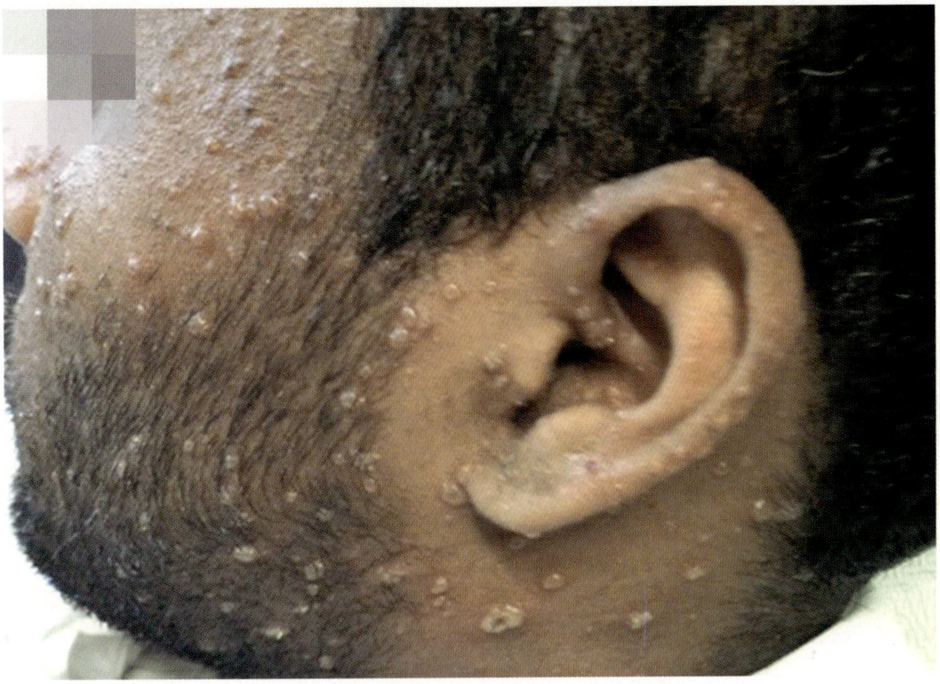

Fig. 4: Chickenpox skin lesions (varicella).

- Incubation period of about 2 weeks (7–23 days). Patient is considered to be infectious during the 2 days before and 5 days after the onset of the lesions.
- The rash is centripetal in distribution, affecting mainly the trunk and sparing the distal part of the limbs, very superficial without deeper layers of skin resembling a dewdrop lying on the skin.
- Evolution of rash is so rapid that various stages—macule, papule, vesicle, pustule, and scab—cannot be readily followed in individual lesions. The rash appears in crops during the first 3 or 4 days of the disease, so lesions of varying age can be noticed on the same patient. It matures very quickly, beginning to crust within 48 hours.
- When varicella occurs in adult, systemic symptoms may be severe, the rash very profuse and the entire disease much more intense. The rash may become hemorrhagic and occasionally bullous lesions appear.

Herpes Zoster (Figs. 5A and B)

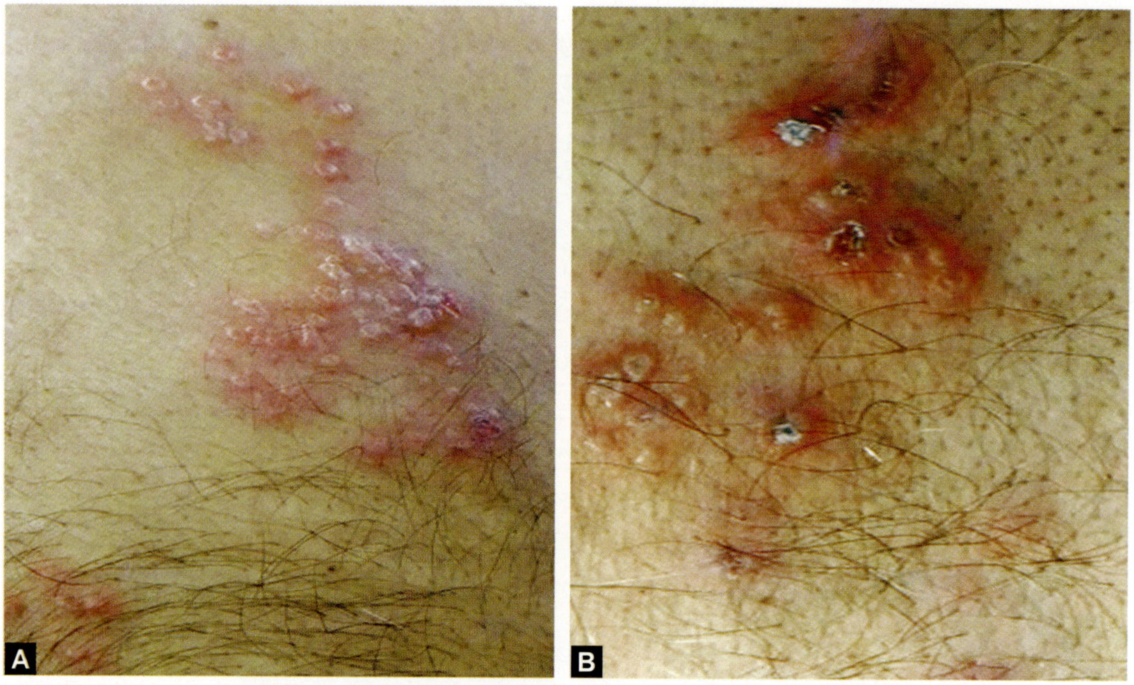

Figs. 5A and B: Herpes zoster skin lesions.

- Common after age of 50 years. Usually occurs in persons who had chickenpox several years earlier. The virus remaining latent in sensory ganglia, may be reactivated and triggered when immunity wanes or by some precipitating stimuli. This reactivation is associated with inflammation of the nerve and, accounts for neuritic pain that often precedes the skin lesions.
- The rash is typically unilateral and confined to the area supplied by a single sensory ganglion. Most common sites are the areas innervated by spinal cord segments D3 to L2 and the trigeminal nerve, particularly its ophthalmic branch. The rash heals in about 2 weeks but pain and paresthesia at the affected area may persist for weeks or months.
- Herpes zoster ophthalmicus is a common and troublesome complication. Other complications are lower motor neuron paralysis, meningoencephalitis, and generalized zoster.

Scrub Typhus (Figs. 6A and B)

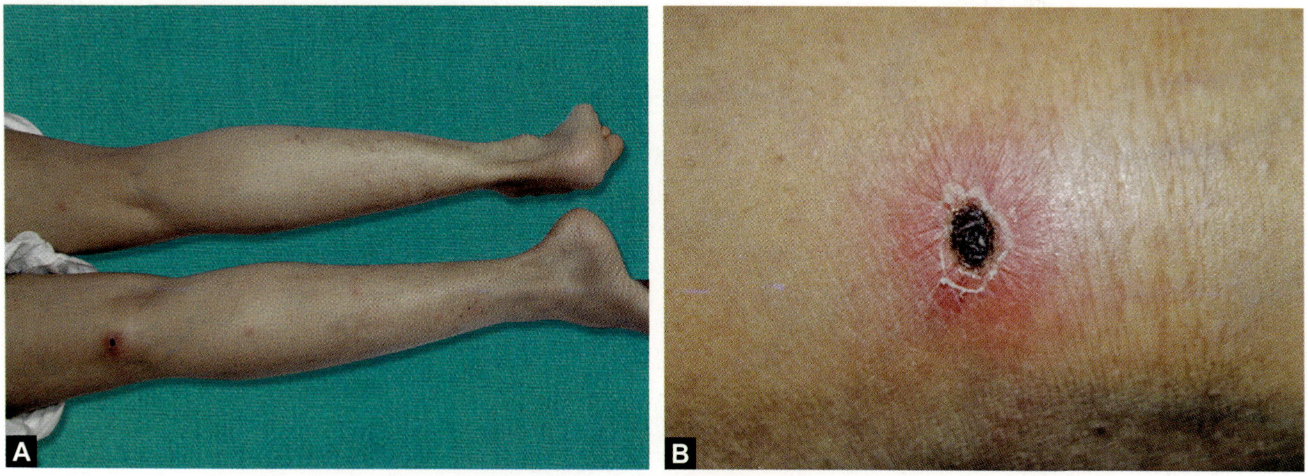

Figs. 6A and B: Scrub typhus eschar.

- It is caused by *Orientia tsutsugamushi* (formerly *R. tsutsugamushi, R. orientalis*). Transmitted by mite. Also known as chigger borne typhus.
- The incubation period is 1–3 weeks. Patient typically develops a characteristic eschar at the site of the mite bite, with regional lymphadenitis and a maculopapular rash. The disease sets in with fever, headache, and conjunctival injection. Encephalitis and pneumonia may be seen in severe cases.
- The Weil–Felix test, which detects cross-reacting antibodies against *Proteus vulgaris* antigens (OX 2 and OX 19) and *Proteus mirabilis* antigen (OX K). OX K agglutinins are found only in scrub typhus. However, some Indian data shows that this test is highly specific at 1:80 but not sensitive for scrub typhus. Anti-scrub typhus immunoglobulin M (IgM) on enzyme-linked immunosorbent assay (ELISA) has sensitivity of 86.5% but false-positive results occur with malaria, typhoid, and tuberculosis (TB).

STAIN AND CULTURE (FIGS. 7 TO 20)

Gram-positive Cocci (Fig. 7)

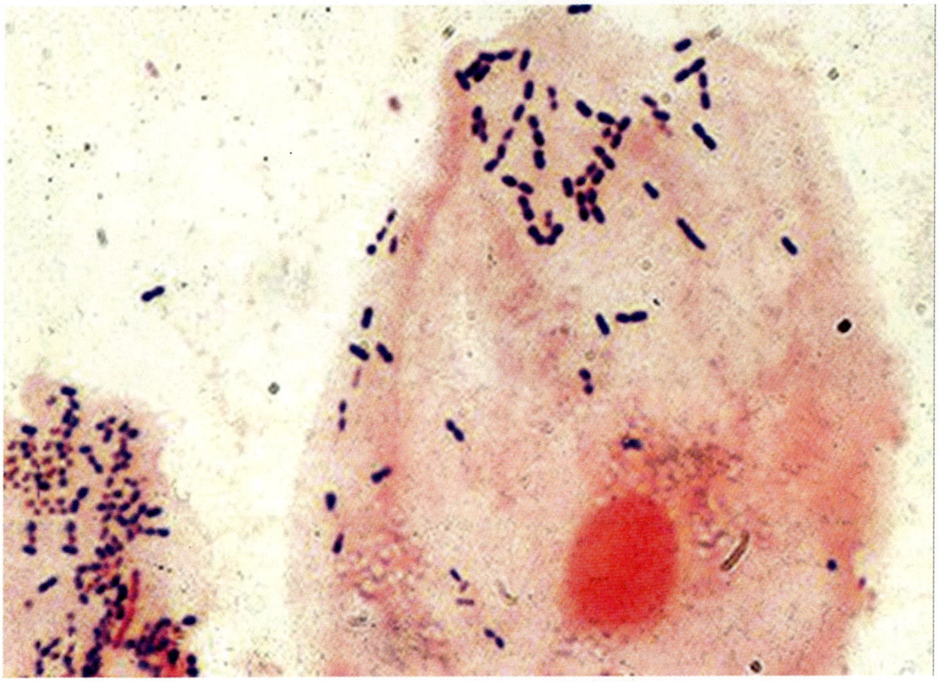

Fig. 7: Gram smear shows Gram-positive lanceolate-shaped diplococci.

- Appears violet-colored cocci against pink background. The Gram-positive cells have a more acidic protoplasm, which may account for their retaining the basic primary dye such as methyl violet, crystal violet, or gentian violet more strongly.
- Cocci may be arranged in pairs (diplococci), chains (streptococci), groups of four (tetrads) or eight (sarcina) or as grape-like clusters (staphylococci).

Gram-negative Bacilli (Fig. 8)

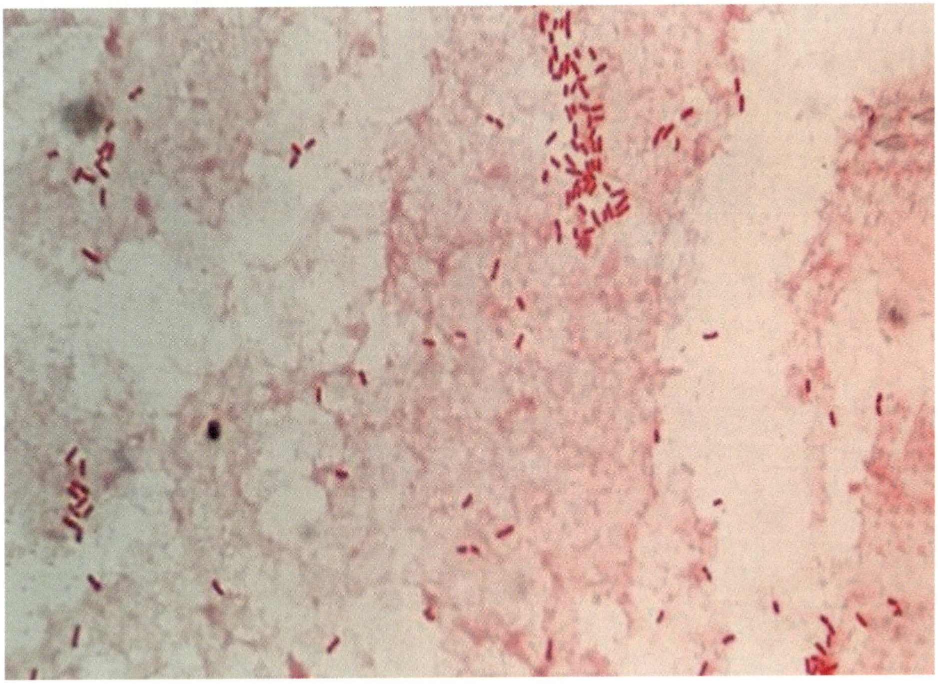

Fig. 8: Gram-negative bacilli.

- Appears pink- or orange-colored rods against pink or orange background. Presence of lipopolysaccharide in the cell wall does not allow the primary dye to retain and hence they take the color of counterstain such as carbol fuchsin, safranin, or neutral red.

Staphylococci (Fig. 9)

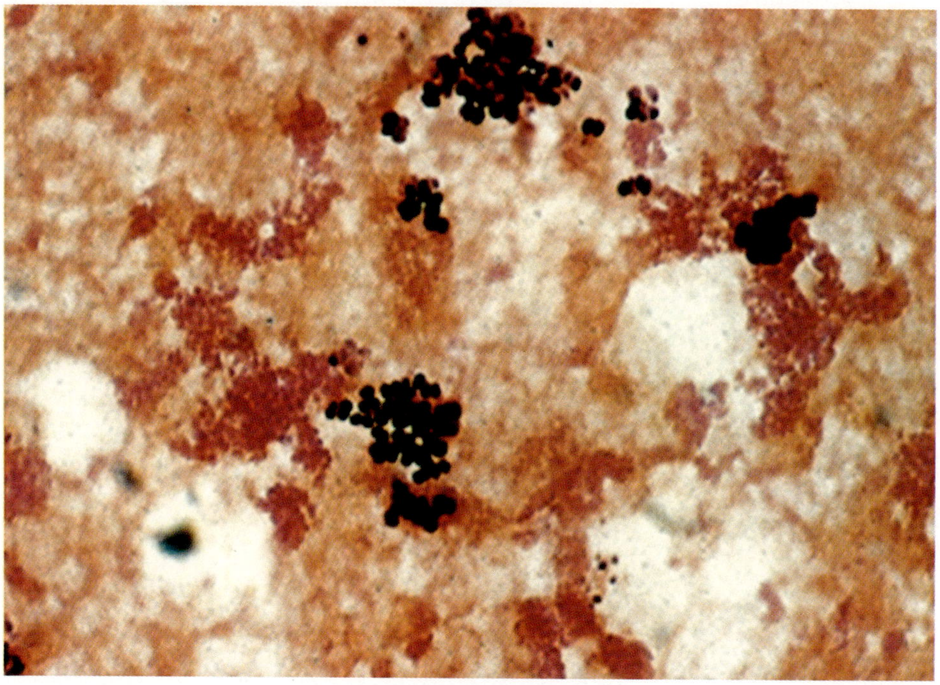

Fig. 9: Staphylococci.

- Gram-positive cocci arranged in grape-like clusters. Based on coagulase test, further divided into *Staphylococcus aureus* and coagulase-negative staphylococci (CoNS).
- *Staphylococcus aureus* causes various lesions based on its ability to invade breaks in body's defenses including skin lesions such as carbuncles and abscesses, and other infections such as osteomyelitis, pyoderma, pneumonia, endocarditis, and septicemia. It can also secrete various toxins that produce different manifestations such as food poisoning, toxic shock syndrome, and staphylococcal-scalded skin syndrome.
- Cons constitute a major component of the normal flora of the human body. Some species can produce human infections—*Staphylococcus epidermidis*, *Staphylococcus haemolyticus*, and *Staphylococcus saprophyticus*. *S. epidermidis* has a polysaccharide outer layer, which binds strongly to plastics, formation of biofilm, thus causes infections associated with central venous catheters (CVCs), cerebrospinal fluid (CSF) shunts, intraocular lenses, as well as prosthetic heart valves.
- Staphylococci are usually susceptible to penicillinase-resistant penicillins, such as methicillin and cloxacillin, and to aminoglycosides and macrolides. Methicillin-resistant *Staphylococcus aureus* (MRSA) stains are a dreaded cause of nosocomial infections.

Streptococci (Fig. 10)

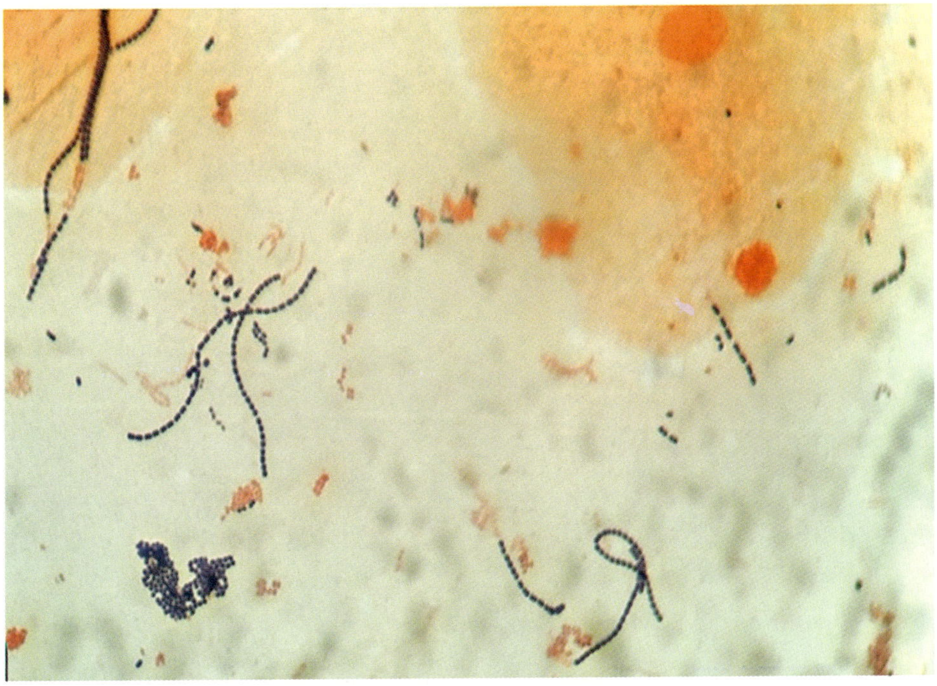

Fig. 10: Streptococci.

- Gram-positive cocci arrange in pairs or short and long chains. Hemolytic activity has been used as a preliminary criterion for classifying some streptococci thus:
  - *Alpha hemolysis*—incomplete lysis causing "greening" around colonies on blood agar; viridans group
  - *Beta hemolysis*—complete lysis; contains most of the major human pathogens
  - Gamma hemolysis—complete nonhemolytic.
- Streptococci are responsible for many human diseases, which are partly attributable to actual infection by the organisms (pharyngitis, impetigo, and pyogenic infection), from the release of bacterial toxins (scarlet fever) and from immunological cross-reactions associated with streptococcal antigens (glomerulonephritis and rheumatic fever).

Acid-fast Bacilli Stain (Fig. 11)

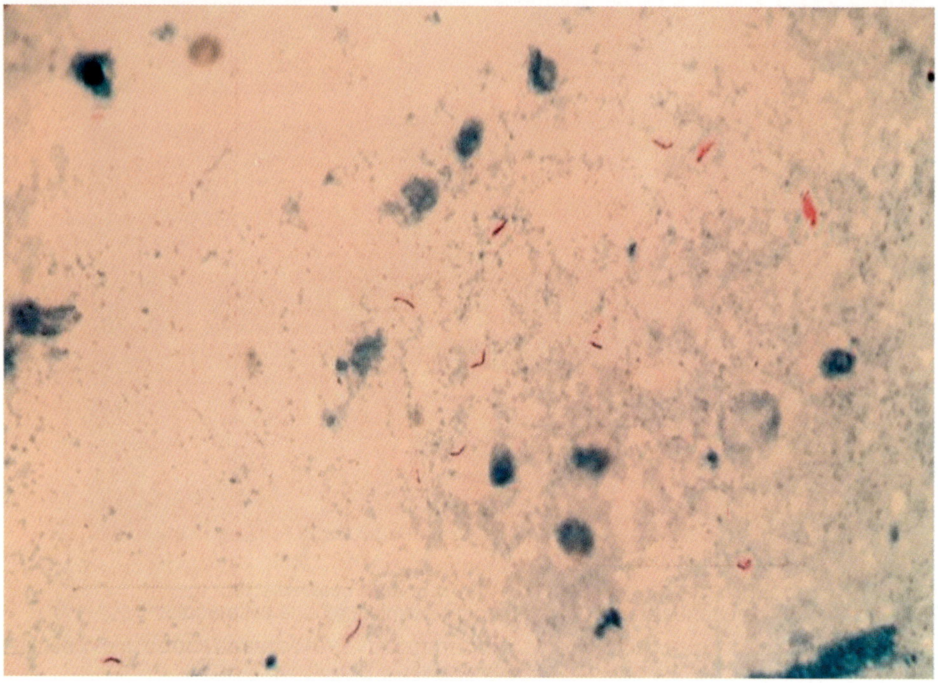

Fig. 11: Acid-fast bacilli stain.

- Acid fastness has been ascribed to high content and variety of lipids, fatty acids, and higher alcohols found in tubercle bacilli. It is related to the integrity of the cell and appears to be the property of lipid-rich waxy cell wall. Presence of mycolic acid in the cell wall of tubercle bacilli resists decolorization by 20% sulfuric acid and absolute alcohol for 10 minutes.
- These acid-fast bacilli (AFB) are seen as single, in pairs, or in clumps as beaded or barred forms.

India Ink Stain (Figs. 12 and 13)

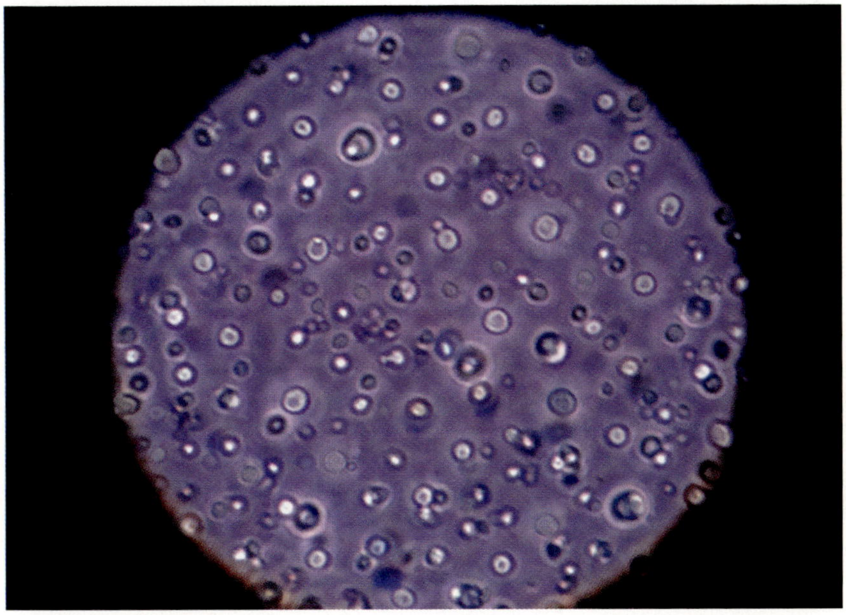

Fig. 12: India ink showing round, budding yeast cells suggestive of *Cryptococcus*.

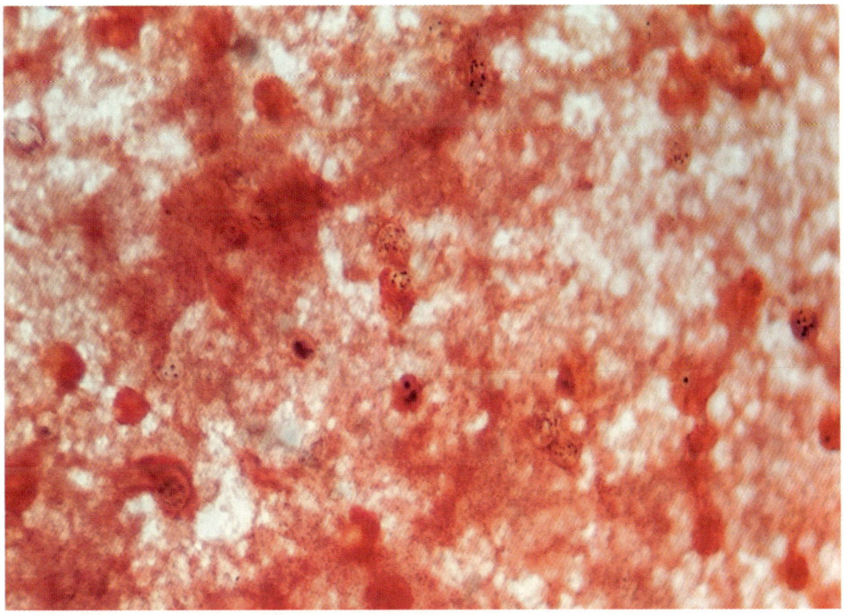

Fig. 13: Gram smear with round, budding yeast cells.

- The India ink stain is a negative stain. Here, the organism is mixed with India ink dye that provides a uniformly black-colored background against which unstained organism stand out in contrast. This is particularly helpful in the demonstration of capsule.

Fungal Stain

Septate Fungal Filaments (Fig. 14)

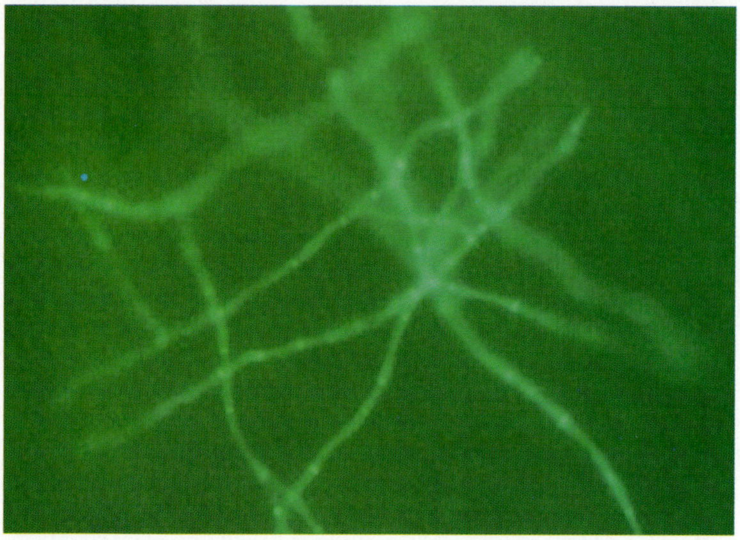

Fig. 14: Septate fungal filaments.

- *Septate fungal filaments*: 2–5 µm wide hyphae, even in diameter with narrow-angled branching and frequently septations are seen. Common examples are—*Aspergillus* species, *Fusarium* species, *Scedosporium* species, etc.

Aseptate Fungal Filaments (Fig. 15)

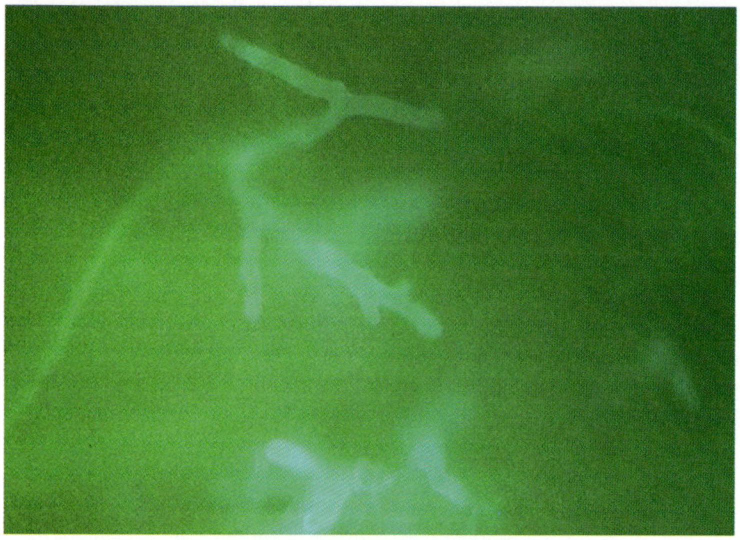

Fig. 15: Aseptate fungal filaments.

- *Aseptate fungal filaments*: 3–25 µm wide hyphae, uneven diameter with broad-angled branching, folded, or twisted on itself forming ribbon-like appearance and very sparse or no septa. Common examples are—*Mucor* species, *Rhizomucor* species, *Rhizopus* species, etc.

MALARIA PARASITE (FIGS. 16 TO 19)

Ring-form Trophozoites of *Plasmodium Falciparum* in a Thin Blood Smear (Fig. 16)

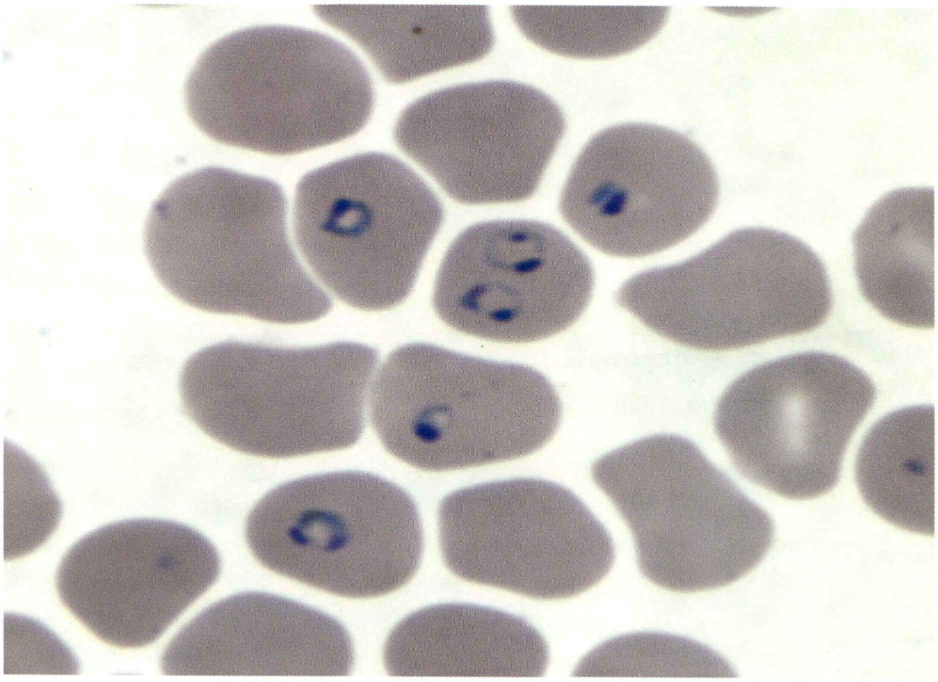

Fig. 16: Ring-form trophozoites of *Plasmodium falciparum*.

- Ring-form trophozoites (rings) of *Plasmodium falciparum* are often thin and delicate, measuring on average 1/5 the diameter of the red blood cell. Rings may possess two chromatin dots resembling the shape of "headphone". They may be found on the periphery of the red blood cell (RBC) (accolé, appliqué) and multiply. There is usually no enlargement of infected RBCs.

Gametocytes of *Plasmodium Falciparum* in a Thin Blood Smear (Fig. 17)

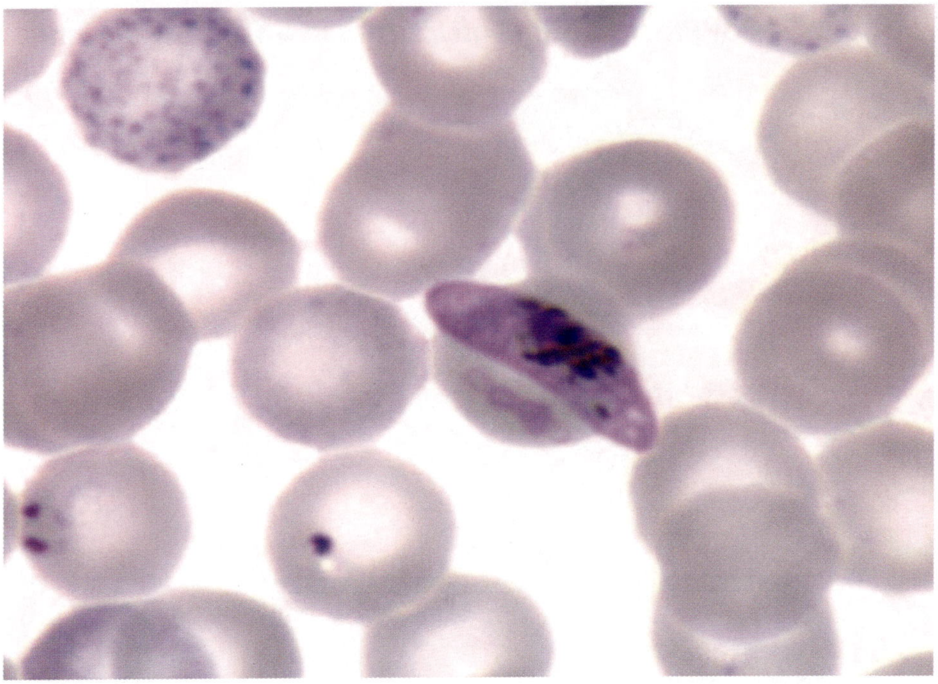

Fig. 17: Gametocytes of *Plasmodium falciparum.*

- Gametocytes of *Plasmodium falciparum* are crescent- or sausage-shaped, and are usually about 1.5 times the diameter of an RBC in length. The cytoplasm of the macrogametocytes (female) is usually a darker, deeper blue; the cytoplasm of the microgametocytes (male) is usually more pale. The red chromatin and pigment are more coarse and concentrated in the macrogametocytes than the microgametocytes.

Ring-form Trophozoites of *Plasmodium Vivax* in Thin Blood Smears (Fig. 18)

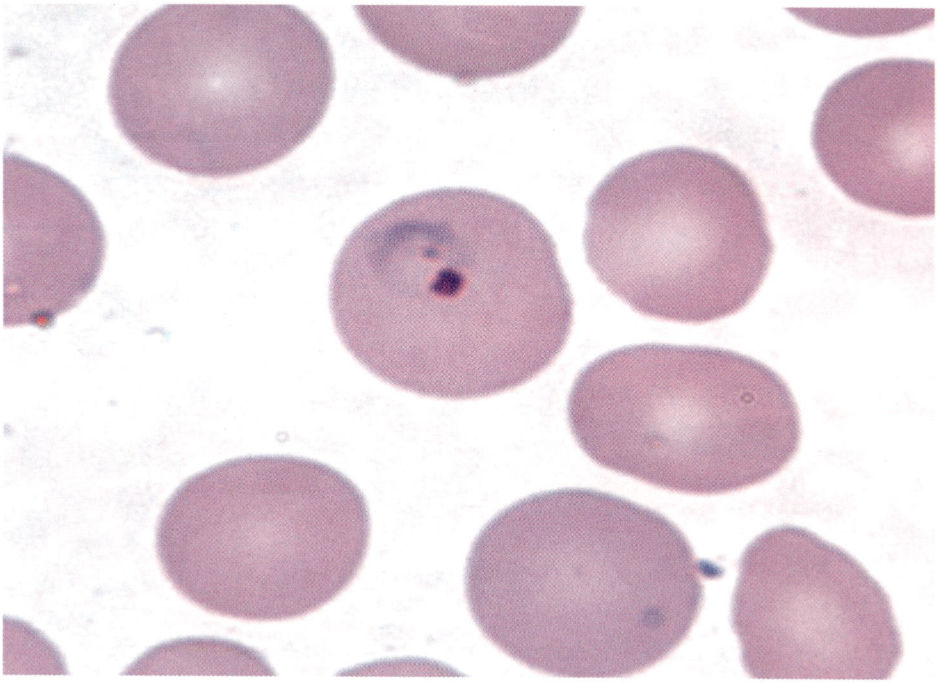

Fig. 18: Ring-form trophozoites of *Plasmodium vivax*.

- Ring-form trophozoites of *P. vivax* usually have a thick cytoplasm with a single, large chromatin dot. The cytoplasm becomes ameboid and Schüffner's dots may appear as the trophozoites mature. Infected RBCs are often larger than uninfected RBCs. Multiple-infected RBCs are not uncommon.

Schizonts of *Plasmodium Vivax* in Thick and Thin Blood Smears (Fig. 19)

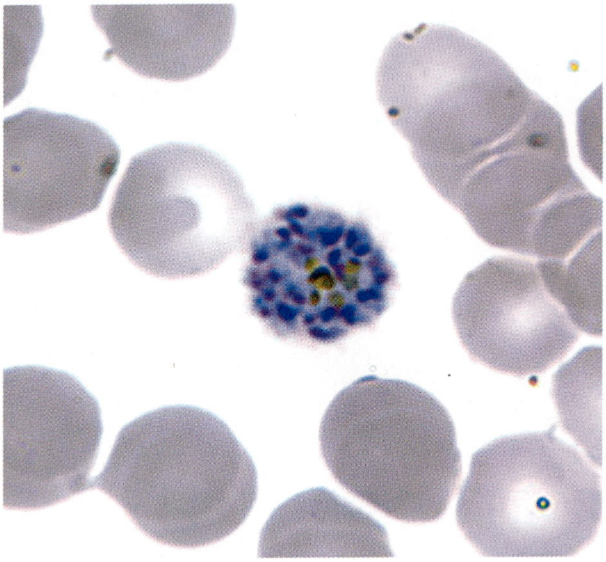

Fig. 19: Developing schizonts of *Plasmodium vivax.*

- Developing schizonts of *P. vivax* are large and ameboid. Chromatin is arranged in two or more masses; pigment is also usually arranged in more than one mass. Mature schizonts contain 12–24 merozoites, each of which contains a dot of chromatin and a mass of cytoplasm. Pigment is usually organized in one or two clumps. Like other stages, infected RBCs are usually larger than uninfected RBCs.

Hanging Drop Preparation (Figs. 20A and B)

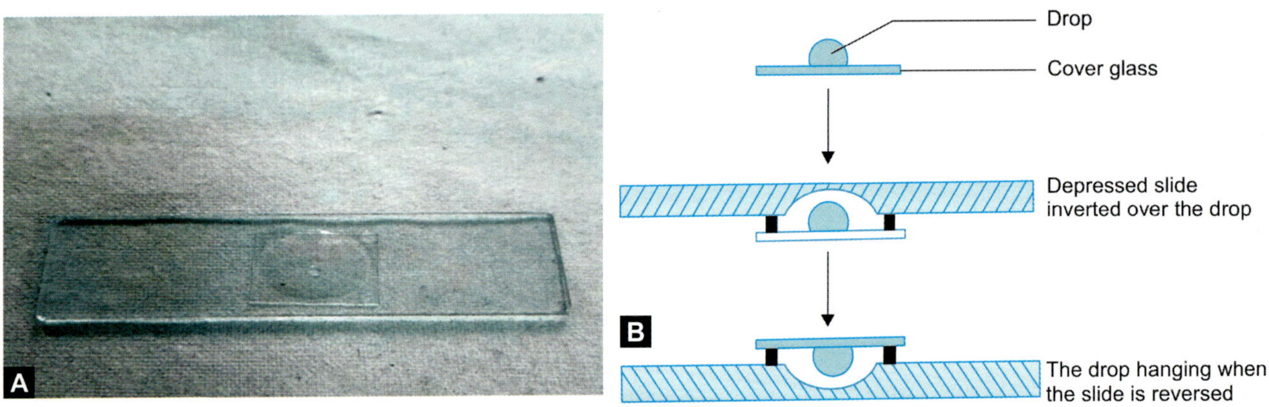

Figs. 20A and B: (A) Hanging drop slide; and (B) Hanging drop preparation.

- Hanging drop preparation is a special type of wet mount (in which a drop of medium containing the organisms is placed on a microscope slide), to observe the motility of bacteria.
- In this method, a drop of culture is placed on a coverslip that is encircled with petroleum jelly (or any other sticky material). The coverslip and drop are then inverted over the well of a depression slide. The drop hangs from the coverslip, and the petroleum jelly forms a seal that prevents evaporation. This preparation gives good views of microbial motility.
- This preparation is very useful to diagnose a suspected case of *Vibrio cholera. Vibrio cholera* is very rapidly motile organism and under hanging drop preparation, made directly from the stool sample, it shows the darting type of motility.

CHAPTER

17

Fungal Infections in Critical Care

Arunaloke Chakrabarti, MR Shivaprakash, Ashim Das

DIAGNOSIS

- The gold standards of diagnosis of invasive fungal infection are histopathological, cytopathological, or direct microscopic evidence or culture of yeasts or molds in a specimen derived from a sterile site.
- Diagnosis of invasive fungal infection often requires a biopsy or aspirates from sterile body sites and blood.
- Around 10% potassium hydroxide with calcofluor mount help in quick identification of fungi; Gram stain helps in yeast infection.
- Hematoxylin and eosin staining helps to evaluate tissue reaction, whereas fungus-specific stains such as Gomori's or Grocott's methenamine silver (GMS), periodic acid-Schiff (PAS), or Giemsa are useful for morphological diagnosis of infecting fungi.
- Slide culture mount helps in morphological identification, as mode of conidiation.

DIRECT MICROSCOPY (FIGS. 1 TO 5)

Gram Stain (Fig. 1)

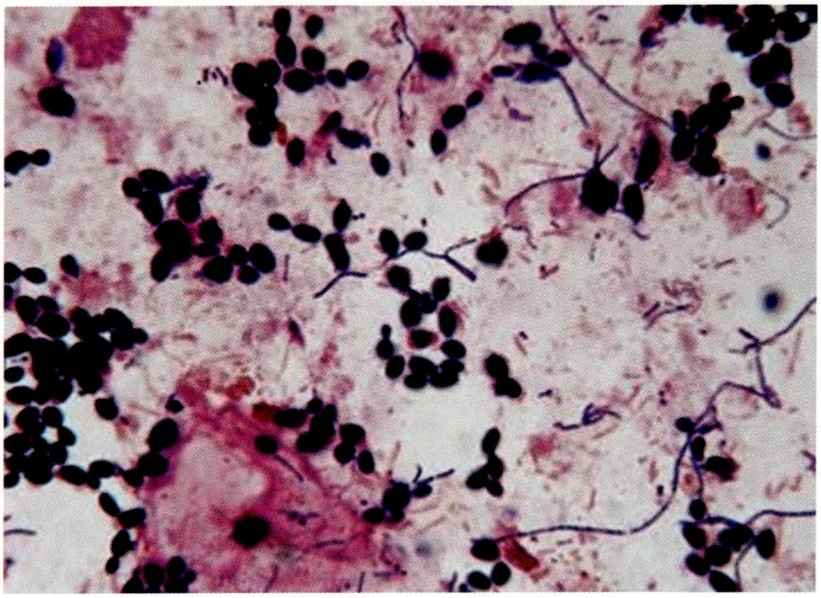

Fig. 1: Oval yeast cells suggesting *Candida* on Gram stain.

- Gram smear preparation from percutaneous nephrostomy pus sample showing budding yeast cells suggestive of *Candida* pyelonephritis.

10% Potassium Hydroxide Wet Mount (Fig. 2)

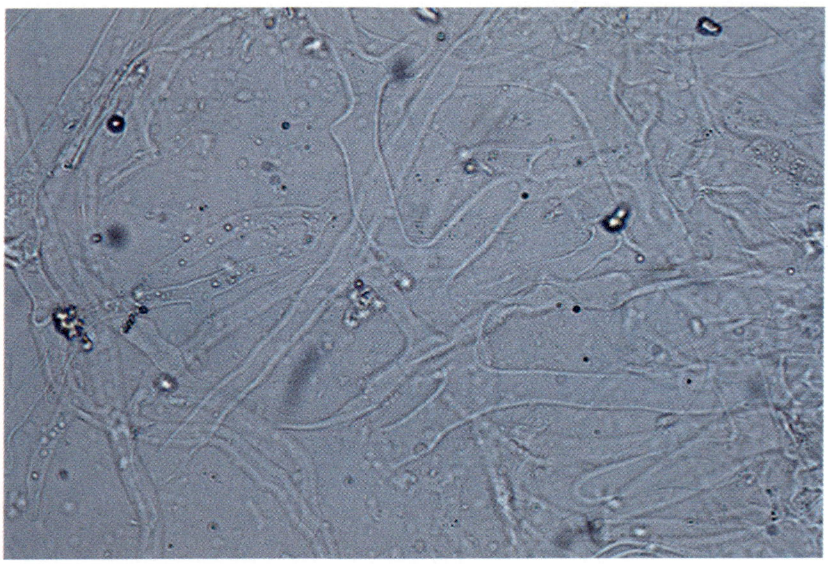

Fig. 2: Potassium hydroxide (10% KOH) wet-mount preparation of lung biopsy.

- Potassium hydroxide (10% KOH) wet-mount preparation of lung biopsy showing hyaline aseptate hyphae with right angle branching *Mucorales* on examination using bright field microscope.

Calcofluor Mount (Fig. 3)

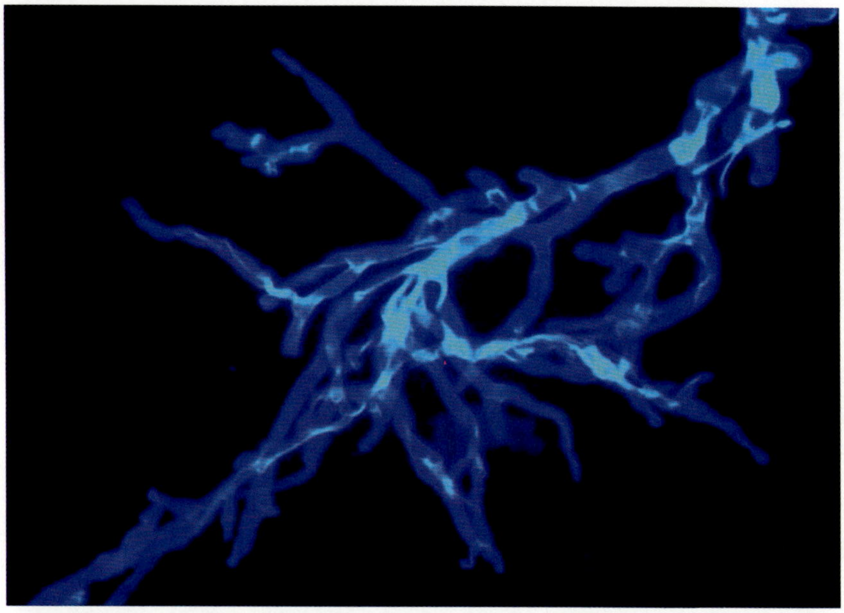

Fig. 3: Calcofluor–potassium hydroxide (KOH) mount preparation of lung biopsy.

- Calcofluor-KOH mount preparation of lung biopsy showing aseptate hyphae with acute angle suggesting that the agent is Mucorales on examination using fluorescent microscope.

India Ink Mount (Fig. 4)

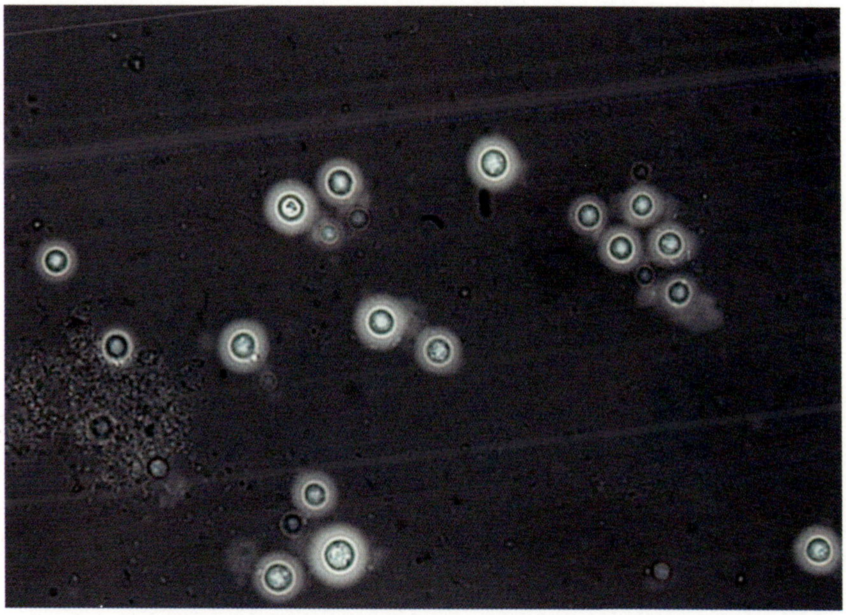

Fig. 4: *Cryptococcus* yeast cells stained with India ink.

- India ink preparation of cerebrospinal fluid (CSF) showing varying sizes of round yeast cells with clear unstained area around suggesting capsule production as in *Cryptococcus*.

Modified Acid-fast Stain (Fig. 5)

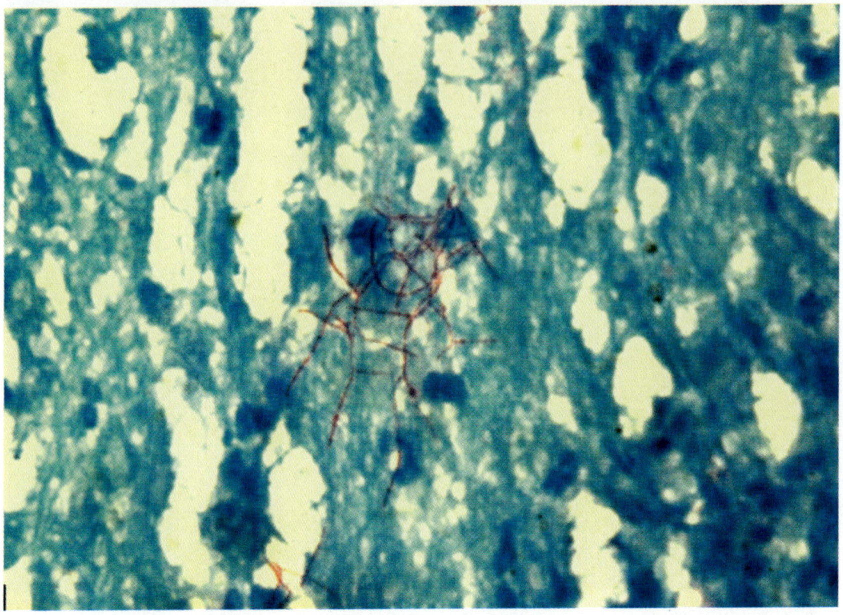

Fig. 5: Modified Ziehl–Neelsen stain (modified acid-fast stain).

- Modified Ziehl-Neelsen stain (modified acid-fast stain) of the pus sample showing acid fast, thin, and branching filaments of Nocardia.

INVASIVE CANDIDIASIS (FIGS. 6 TO 12)

Candida Meningoencephalitis (Figs. 6A to C)

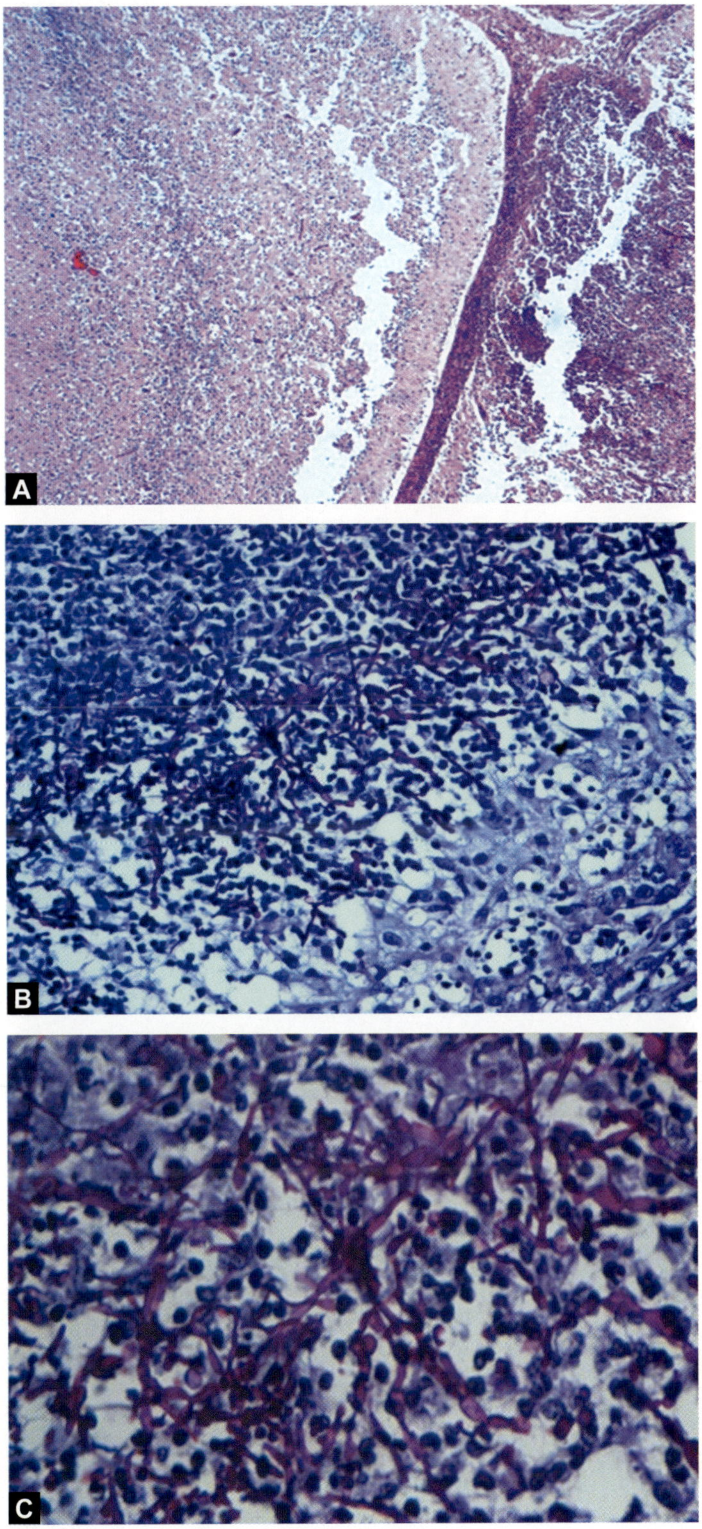

Figs. 6A to C: (A) Inflammation of meninges, involving cortical area; (B and C) Yeast cell and pseudohyphae of *Candida*.

Candida Albicans (Fig. 7)

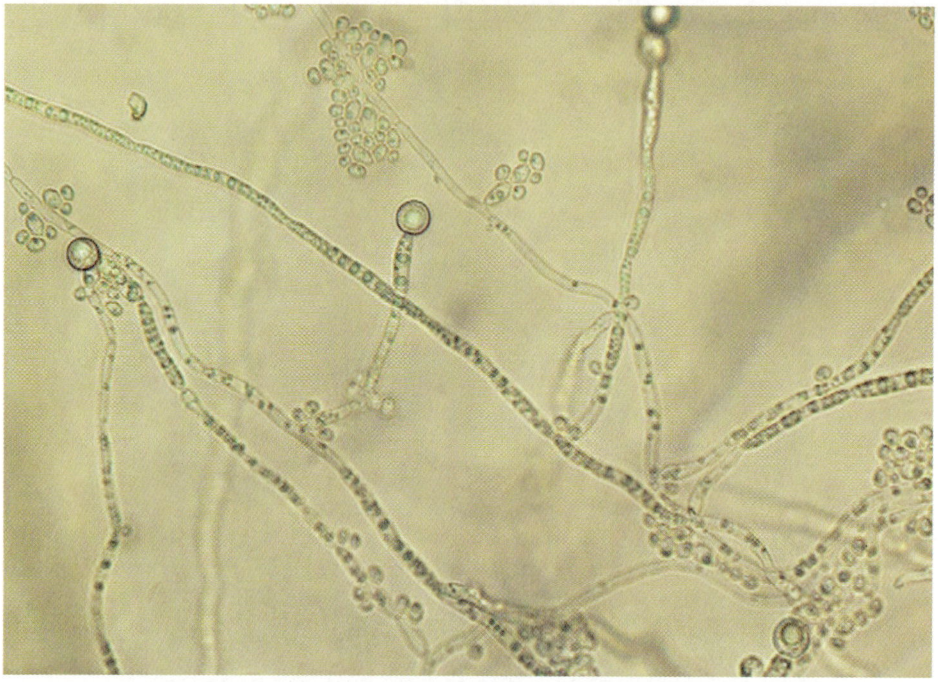

Fig. 7: *Candida albicans* showing the characteristic terminal chlamydoconidia on the Corn Meal Agar with Tween 80.

Candida Auris (Fig. 8)

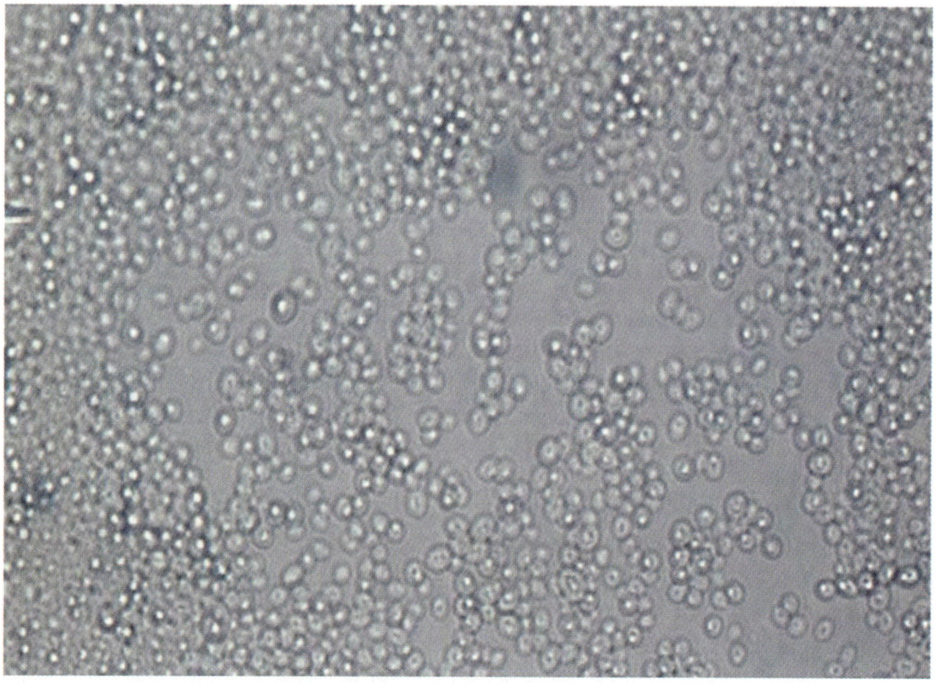

Fig. 8: *Candida auris* on Corn Meal Agar with Tween 80 showing only blastoconidia forms (no hyphal or pseudohyphal forms).

Candida Tropicalis (Fig. 9)

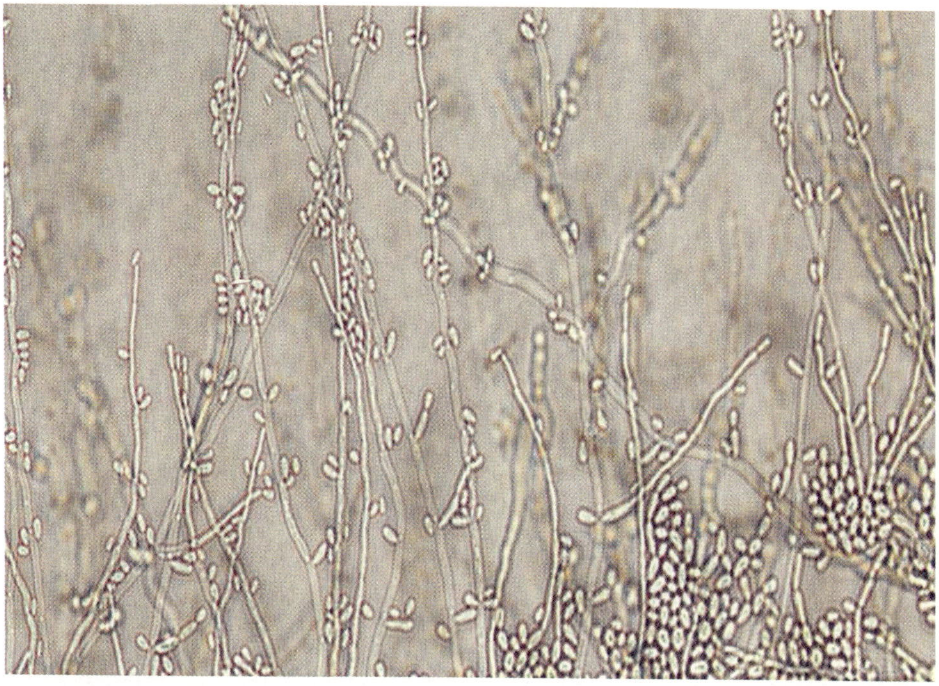

Fig. 9: Morphology of *Candida tropicalis* on Corn Meal Agar with Tween 80 showing abundant long pseudohyphae appears in the pattern of pine forest. Typically, blastoconidia are formed at or in-between septa.

Candida Glabrata (Fig. 10)

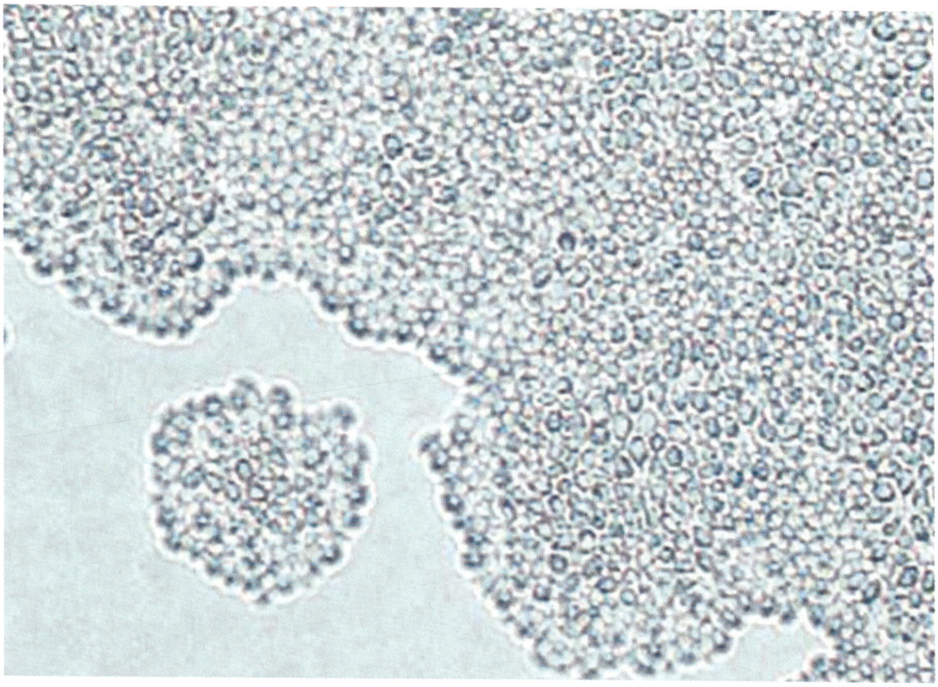

Fig. 10: *Candida glabrata* on Corn Meal Agar with Tween 80 showing only blastoconidia forms (the size of blastoconidia is smaller than *Candida auris*).

Candida Krusei (Fig. 11)

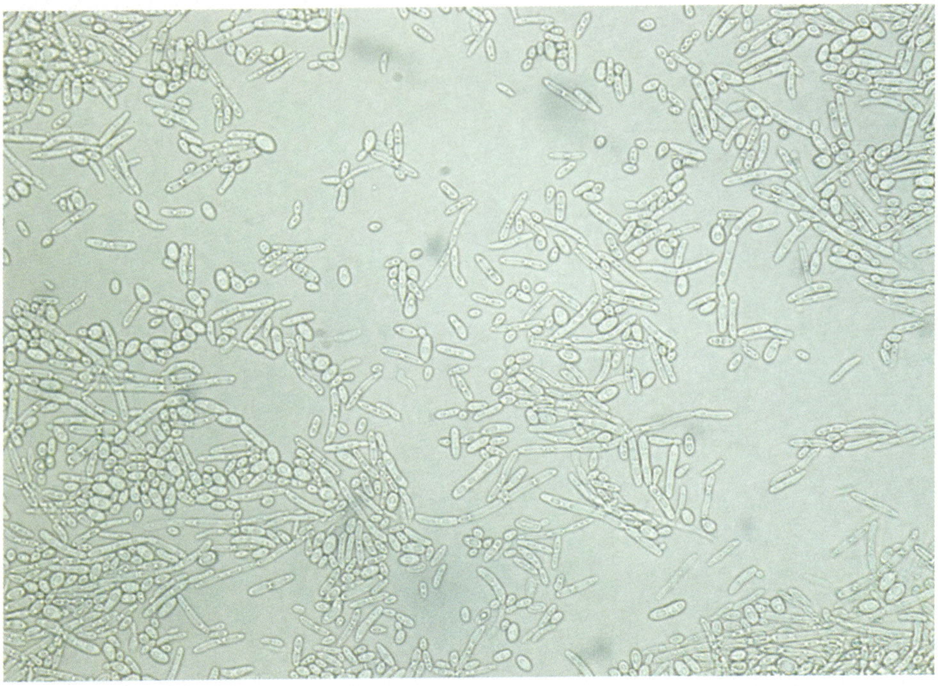

Fig. 11: *Candida krusei* on Corn Meal Agar with Tween 80 shows elongated budding yeasts with abundant pseudohyphae.

Candida Parapsilosis (Fig. 12)

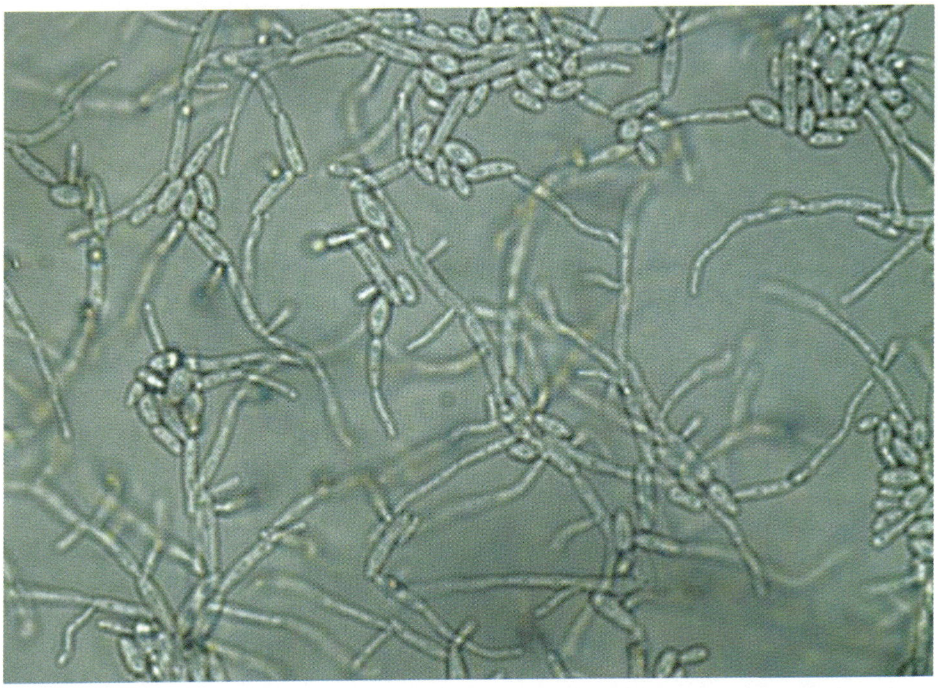

Fig. 12: *Candida parapsilosis* on Corn Meal Agar with Tween 80 showing oval to elliptical budding yeasts with pseudohyphae. Few hyphae broader than the others are also seen in the picture.

ACUTE INVASIVE TRICHOSPOROSIS (FIGS. 13 TO 15)

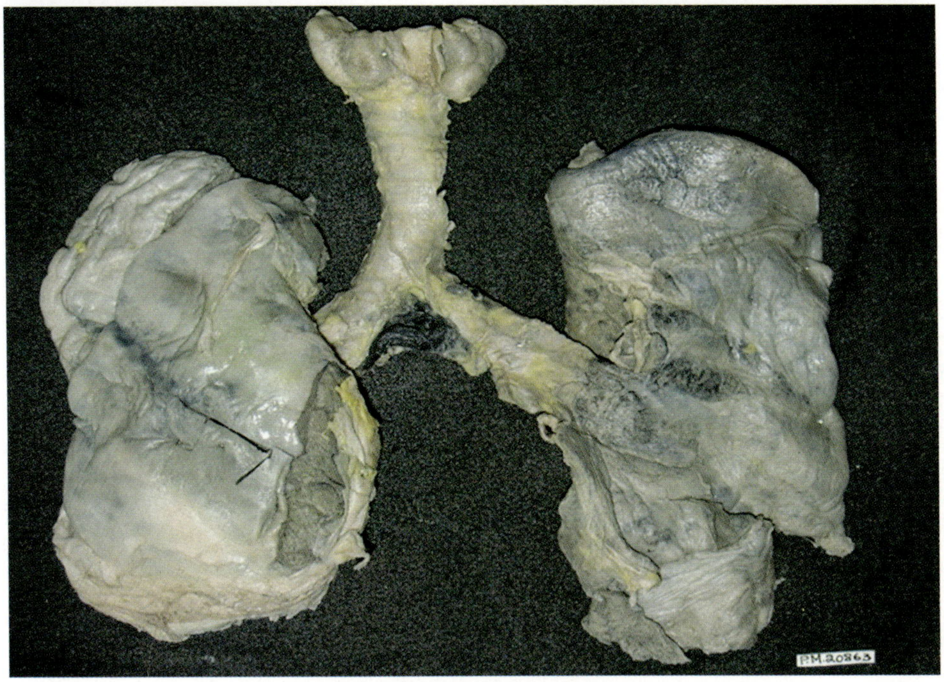

Fig. 13: Both lungs were consolidated with extensive pleuritis.

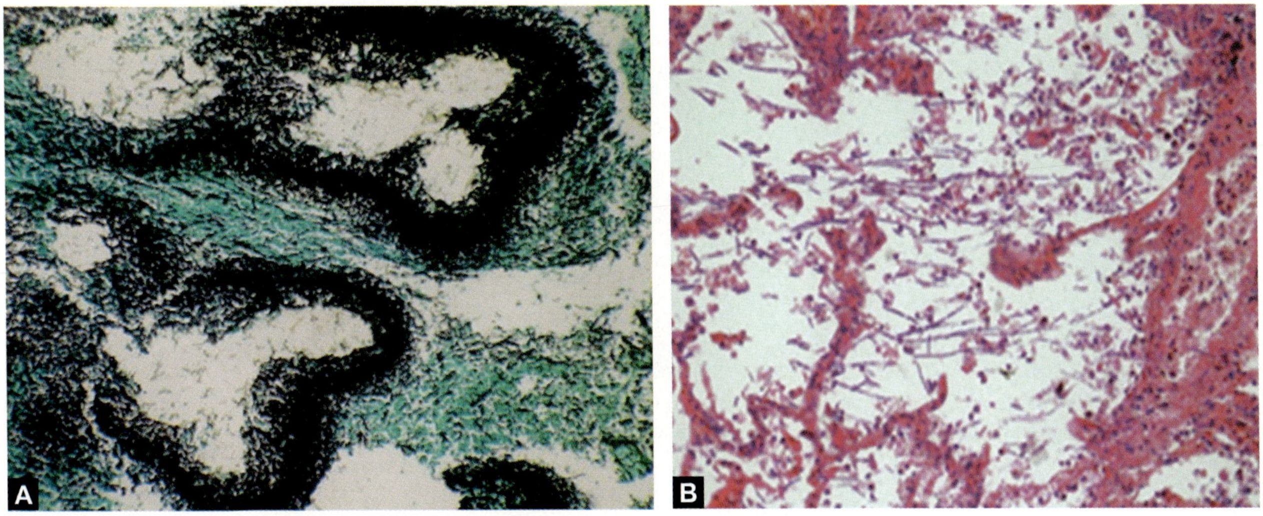

Numerous septate hyphae of *Trichosporon* in Grocott's and H & E stain

Figs. 14A and B: Numerous colonies of thin fungal septae in Grocott's stain and hematoxylin and eosin (H and E) stain.

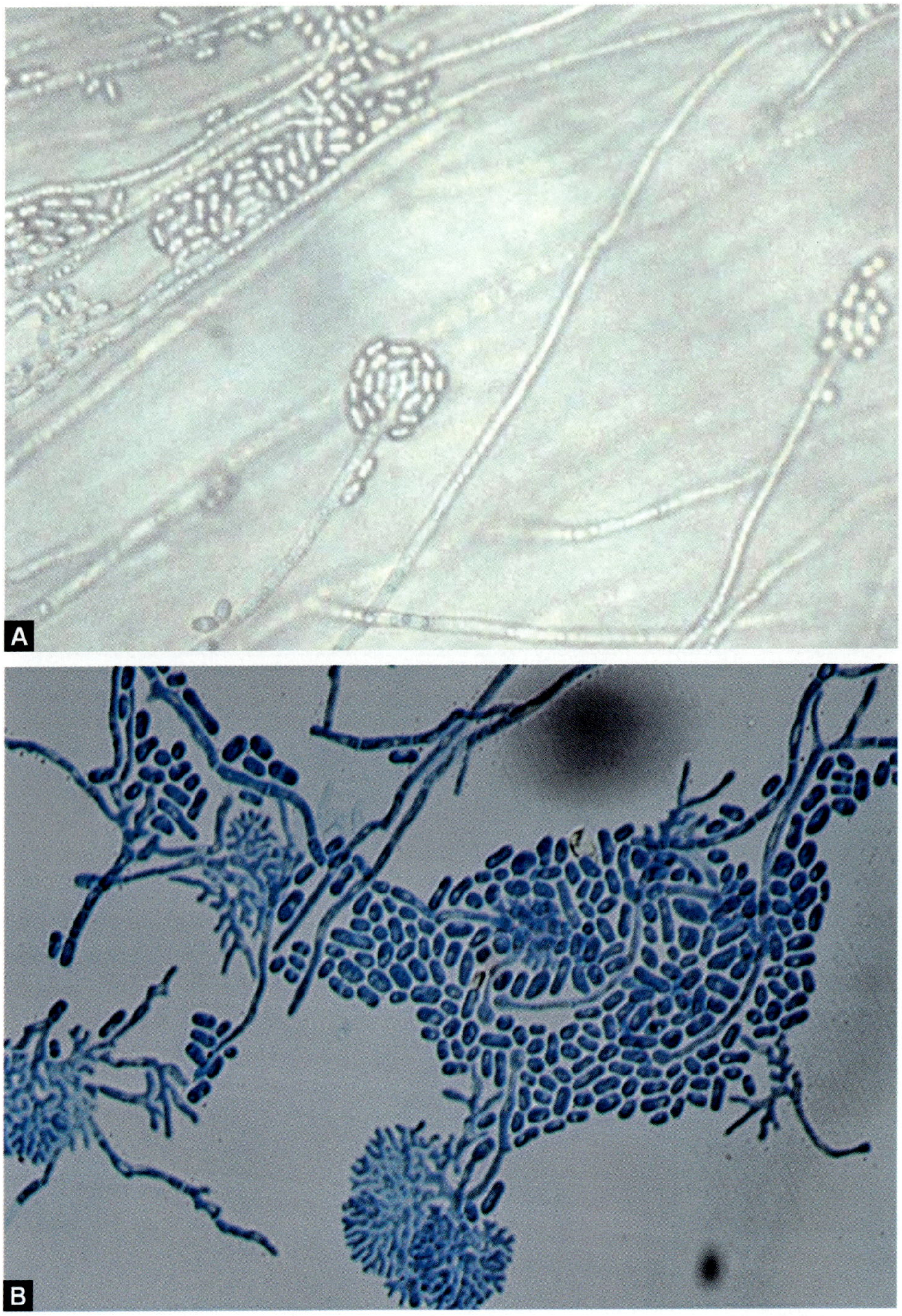

Figs. 15A and B: Slide culture of *Trichosporon* on the lactophenol cotton blue mount showing barrel-shaped arthroconidia. Appressoria (finger like projections) seen in this picture may be produced by few species of *Trichosporon*.

INVASIVE ASPERGILLOSIS (FIGS. 16 TO 25)

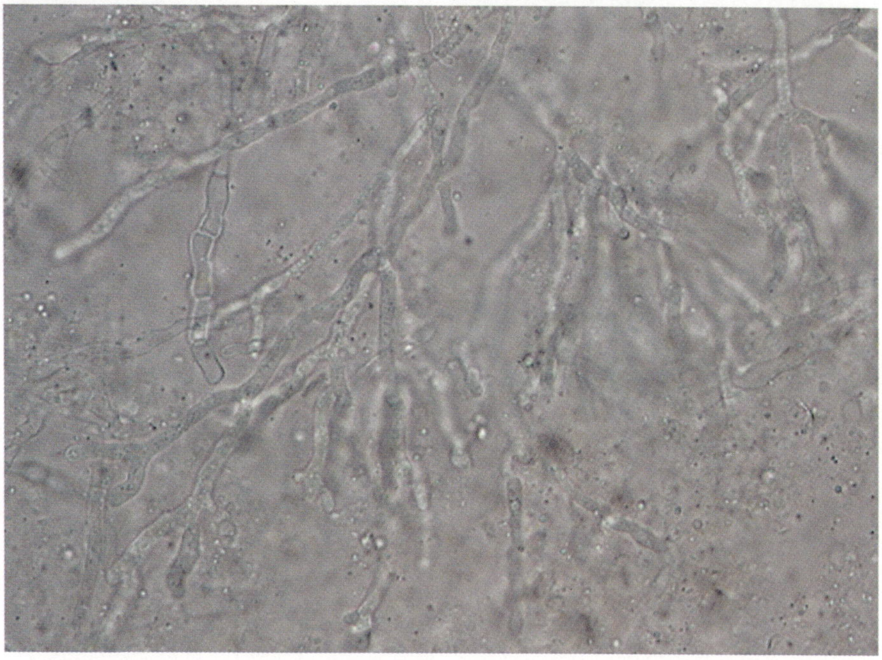

Fig. 16: Potassium hydroxide (10% KOH) wet-mount preparation of lung biopsy showing hyaline septate hyphae with acute angle branching suggesting *Aspergillus* on examination using bright-field microscope.

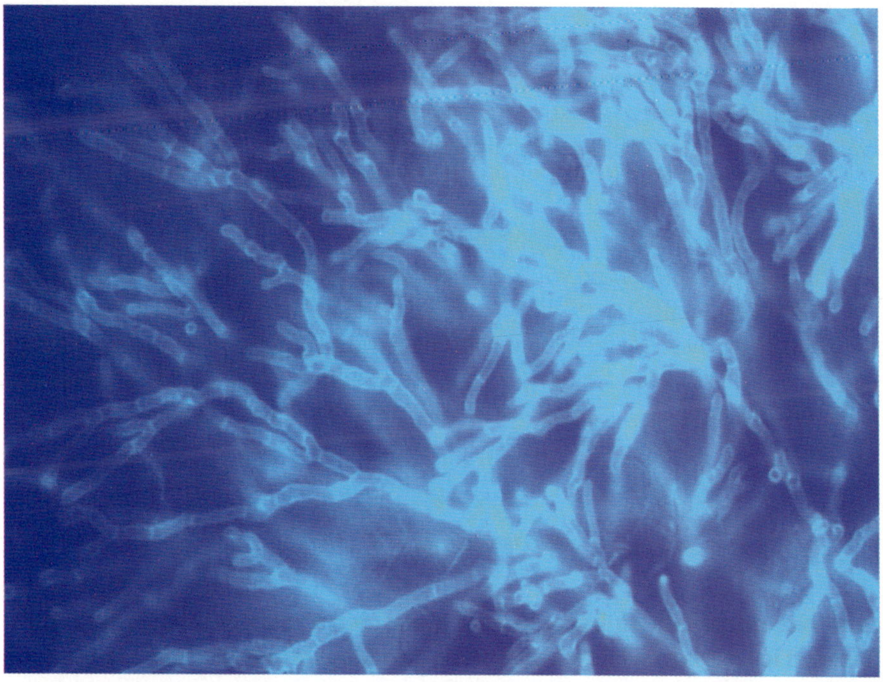

Fig. 17: Calcofluor–potassium hydroxide (KOH) wet-mount preparation of lung biopsy showing septate hyphae with acute angle branching suggesting *Aspergillus* on examination under fluorescent microscope.

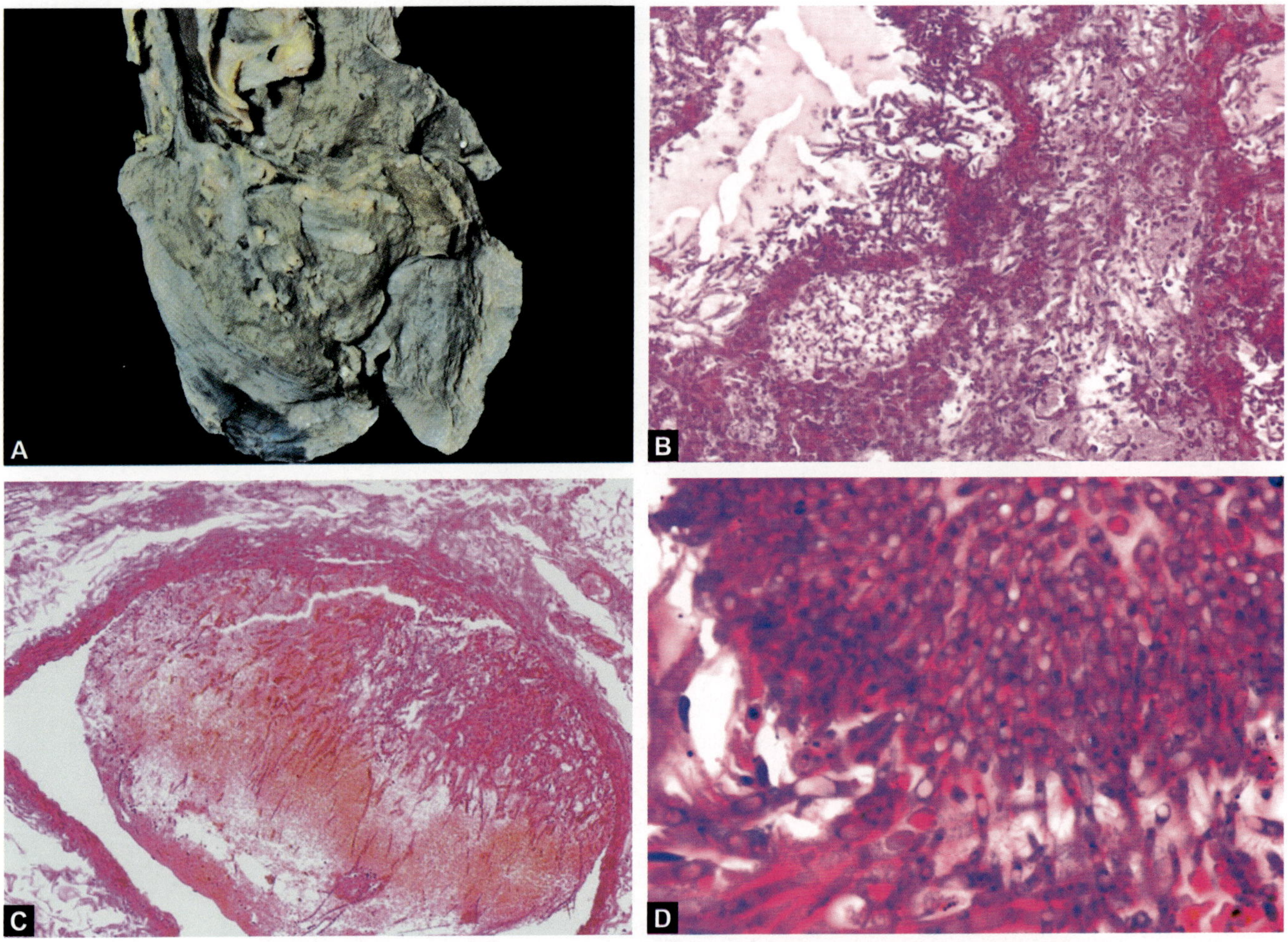

Figs. 18A to D: (A) Multiple nodular hemorrhagic areas in the lungs in a case of acute invasive pulmonary *Aspergillosis*; (B) Numerous hyphae of *Aspergillus*; (C and D) Vascular invasion by the fungi.

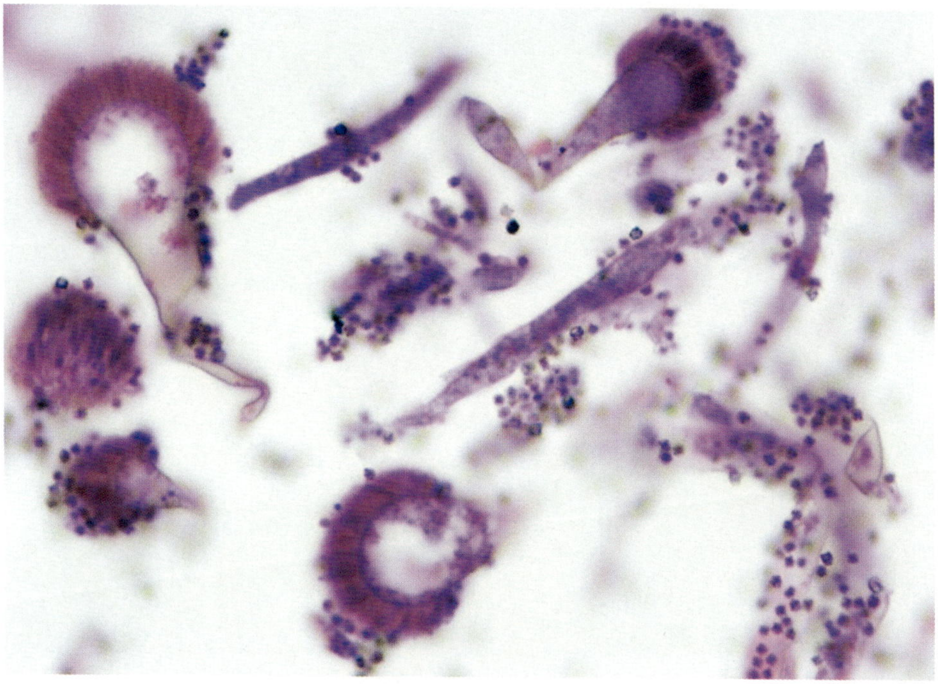

Fig. 19: Fungal ball.

- In the lung cavity, *Aspergillus*-producing fungal ball with vesicle formation and conidia (*Aspergillus* head).

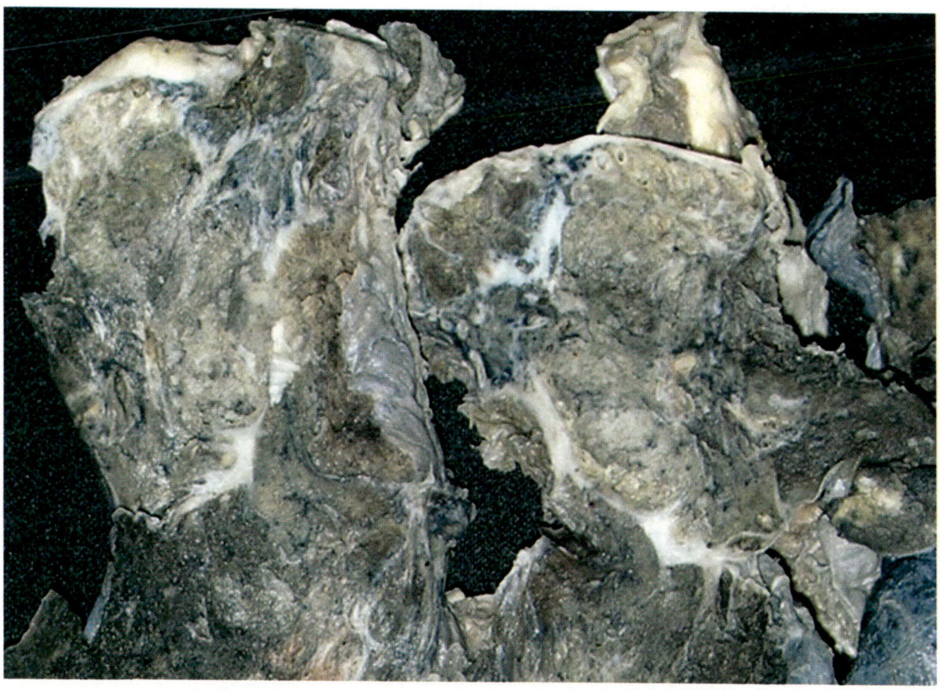

Fig. 20: Chronic pulmonary necrotizing *Aspergillosis*.

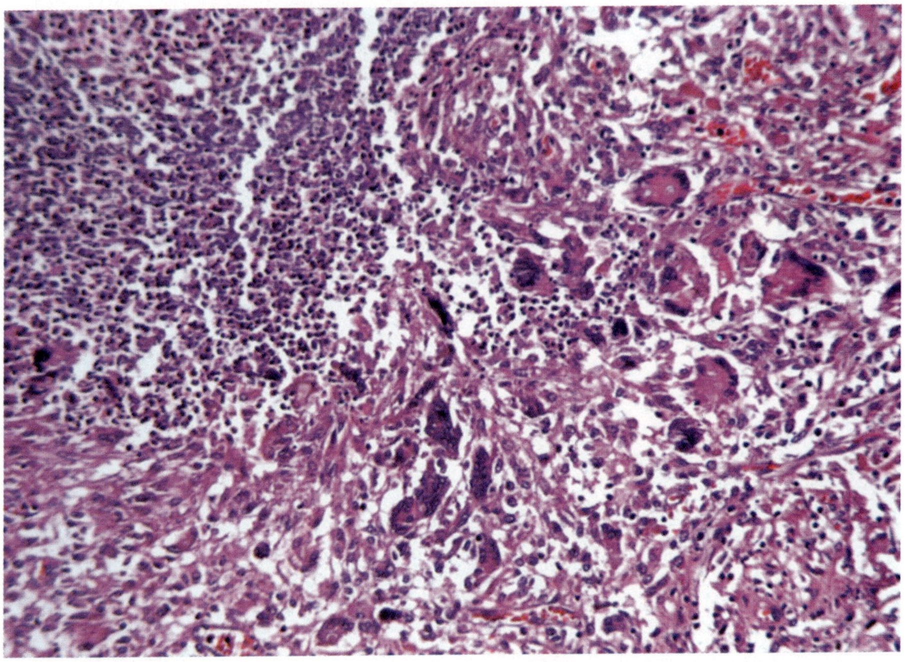

Fig. 21: The center of bronchi showed numerous neutrophils surrounded by eosinophils and giant cells in the surrounding lung parenchyma indicating invasion.

- Cut surface of lungs showing numerous gray areas involving the small dilated bronchi in a case of chronic pulmonary necrotizing *Aspergillosis*.

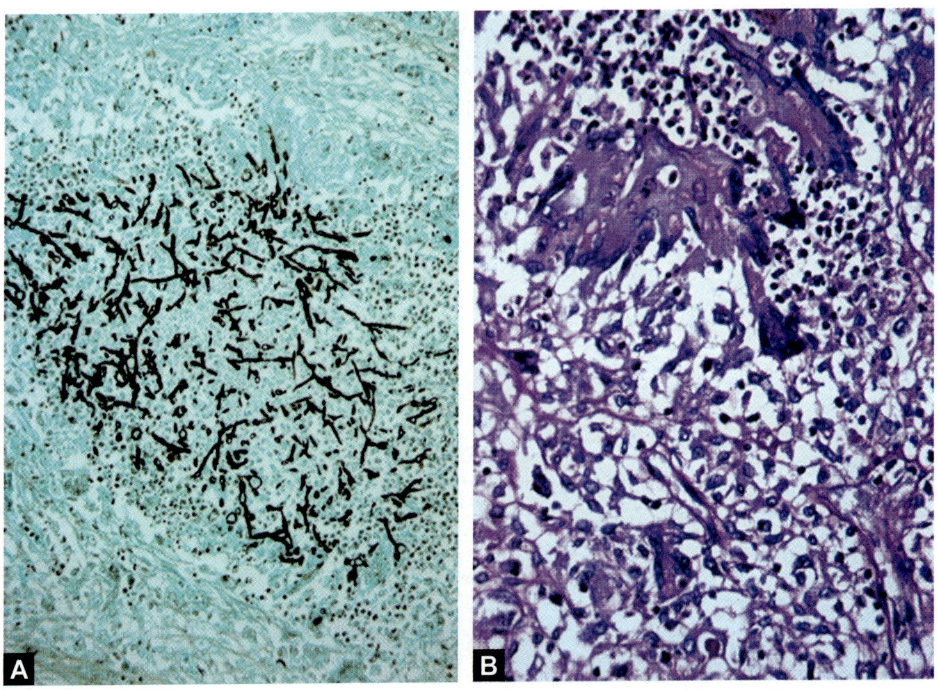

Figs. 22A and B: Numerous septate hyphae of *Aspergillus* in Grocott's stain and a few septate hyphae within the giant cells in periodic acid–Schiff (PAS) stain.

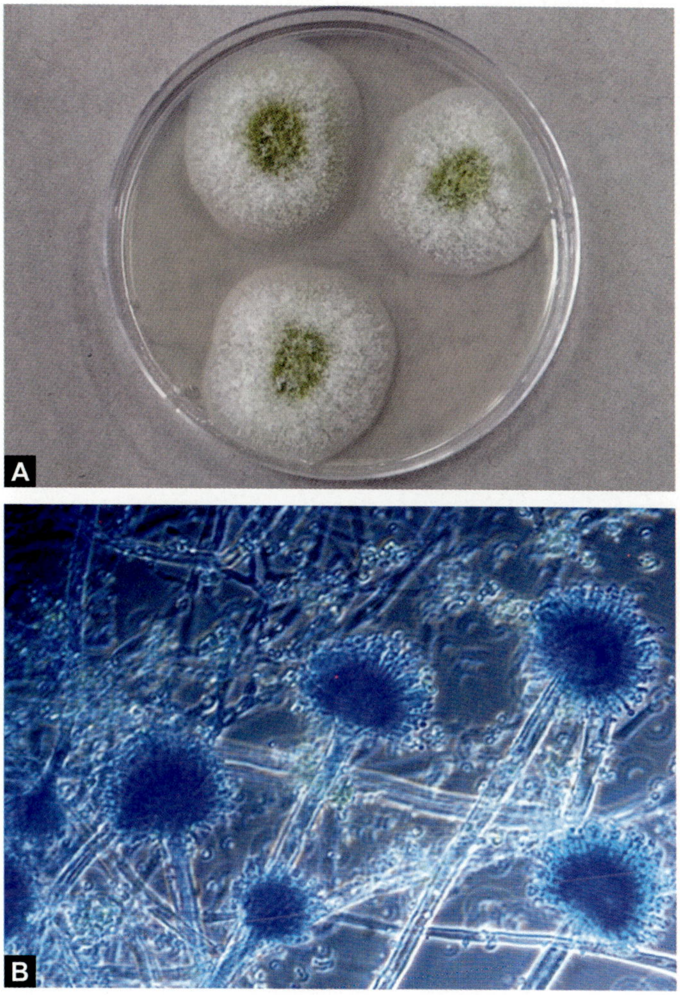

Figs. 23A and B: (A) Greenish yellow mycelial growth of *Aspergillus flavus* on Sabouraud's dextrose agar, a characteristic appearance of colonies; (B) *Aspergillus flavus* with rough conidiophore and globose to subglobose rough conidia (measuring 3–6 μm).

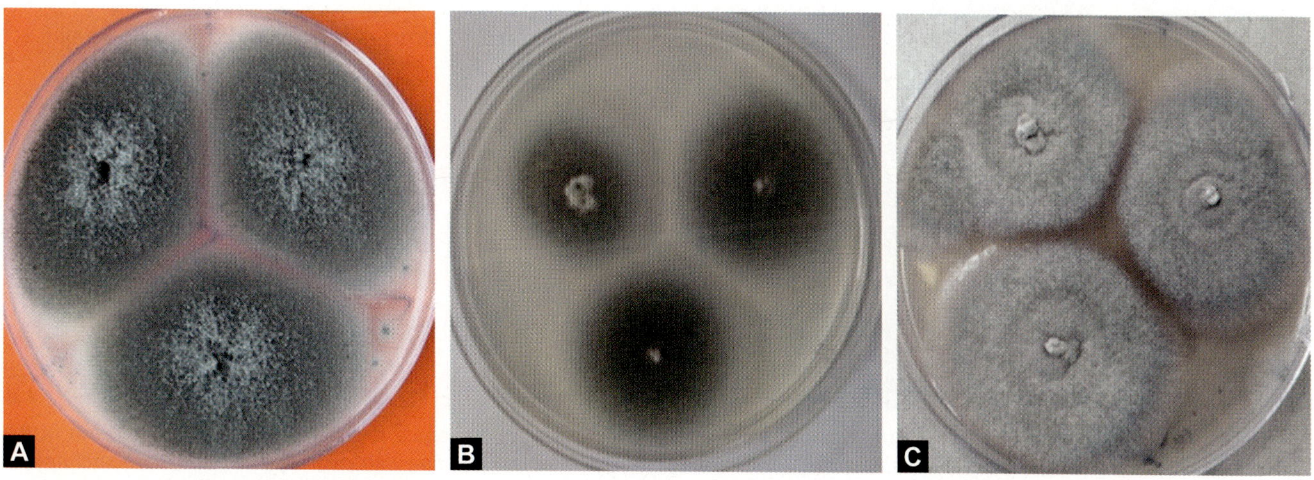

Figs. 24A to C: Colonies of *Aspergillus fumigatus* appearing dark green on—(A) Sabouraud's dextrose agar; (B) Malt Extract Agar; and (C) Grayish green on Czapek Dox Agar.

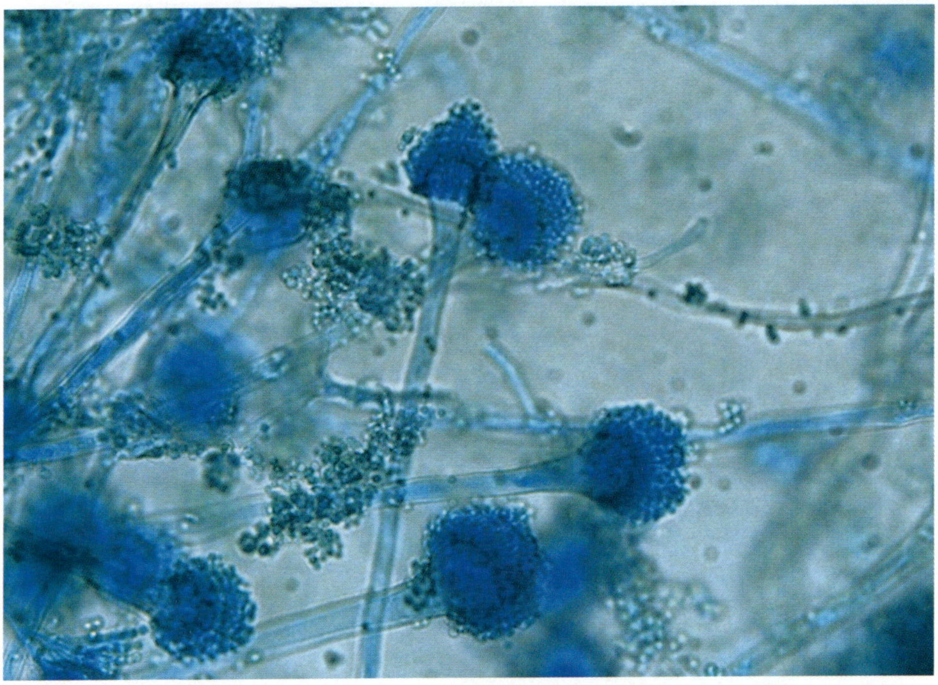

Fig. 25: Microscopic appearance of *Aspergillus fumigatus* on slide culture with small conidia (2.5–3 μm).

FIBROSING ASPERGILLUS MEDIASTINITIS (FIGS. 26A TO C)

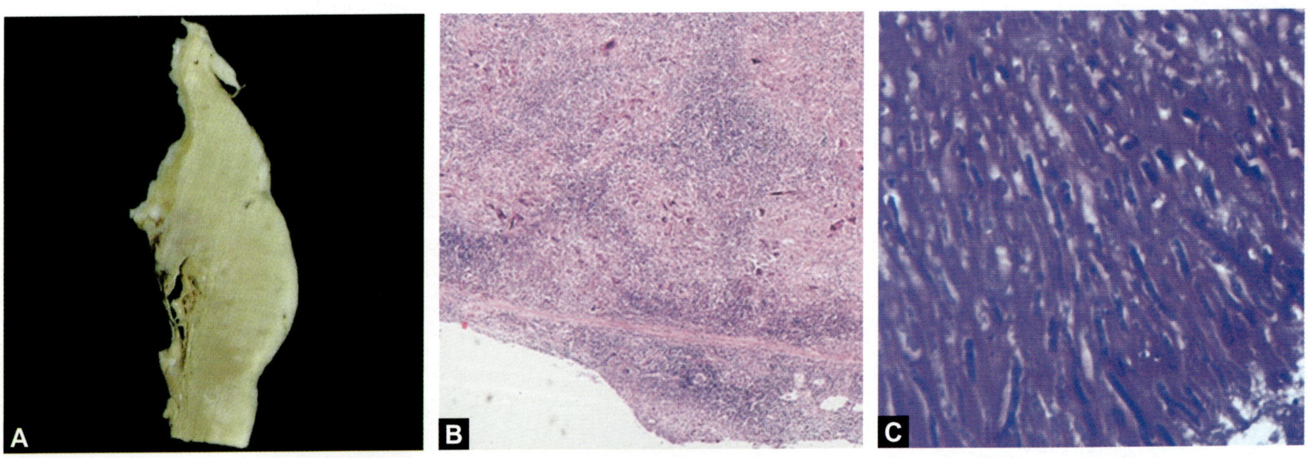

Figs. 26A to C: (A) Cut surface of the left ventricle showing the involvement of the entire wall thickness by the extension of the process of chronic fibrosing *Aspergillus mediastinitis*; (B) Extensive granulomatous response with involvement of the endocardium and myocardium in a background of fibrosis; (C) Periodic acid–Schiff (PAS) stain brings the hyphae much better as septate fungus with acute angle branching.

MUCORMYCOSIS (FIGS. 27 TO 32)

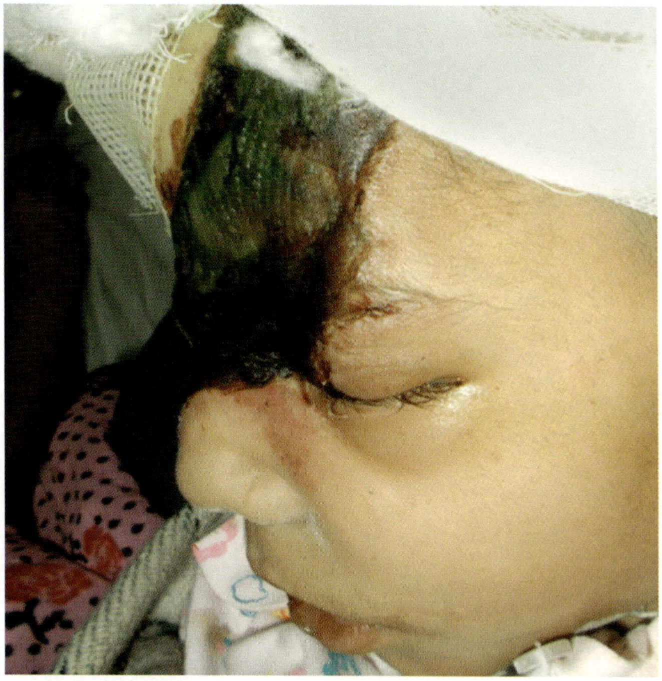

Fig. 27: Black necrotic patch on the nasal bridge, eyelid, and forehead of a child admitted to hospital suggesting mucormycosis.

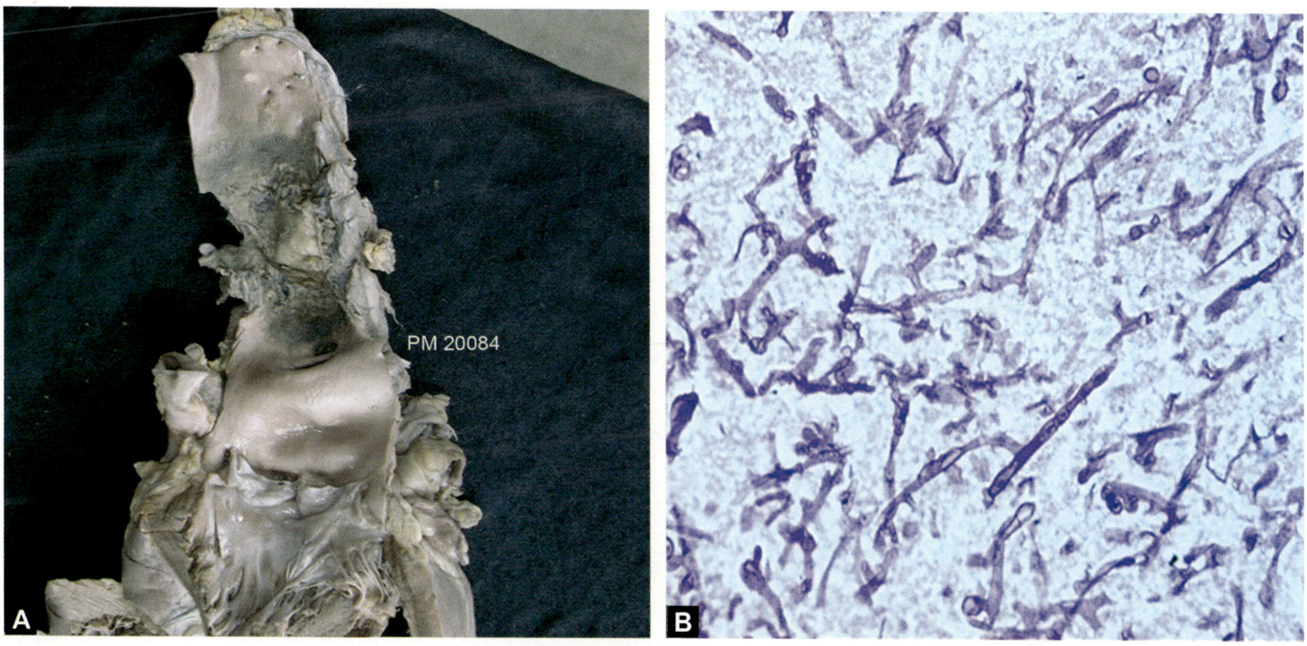

Figs. 28A and B: (A) Acute necrotizing mucormycosis of the arch of aorta and descending thoracic aorta in a thalassemia patient who received more than 100 units of blood transfusion; (B) Numerous hyphae of *Mucorales*, which are aseptate and with right-angle branching.

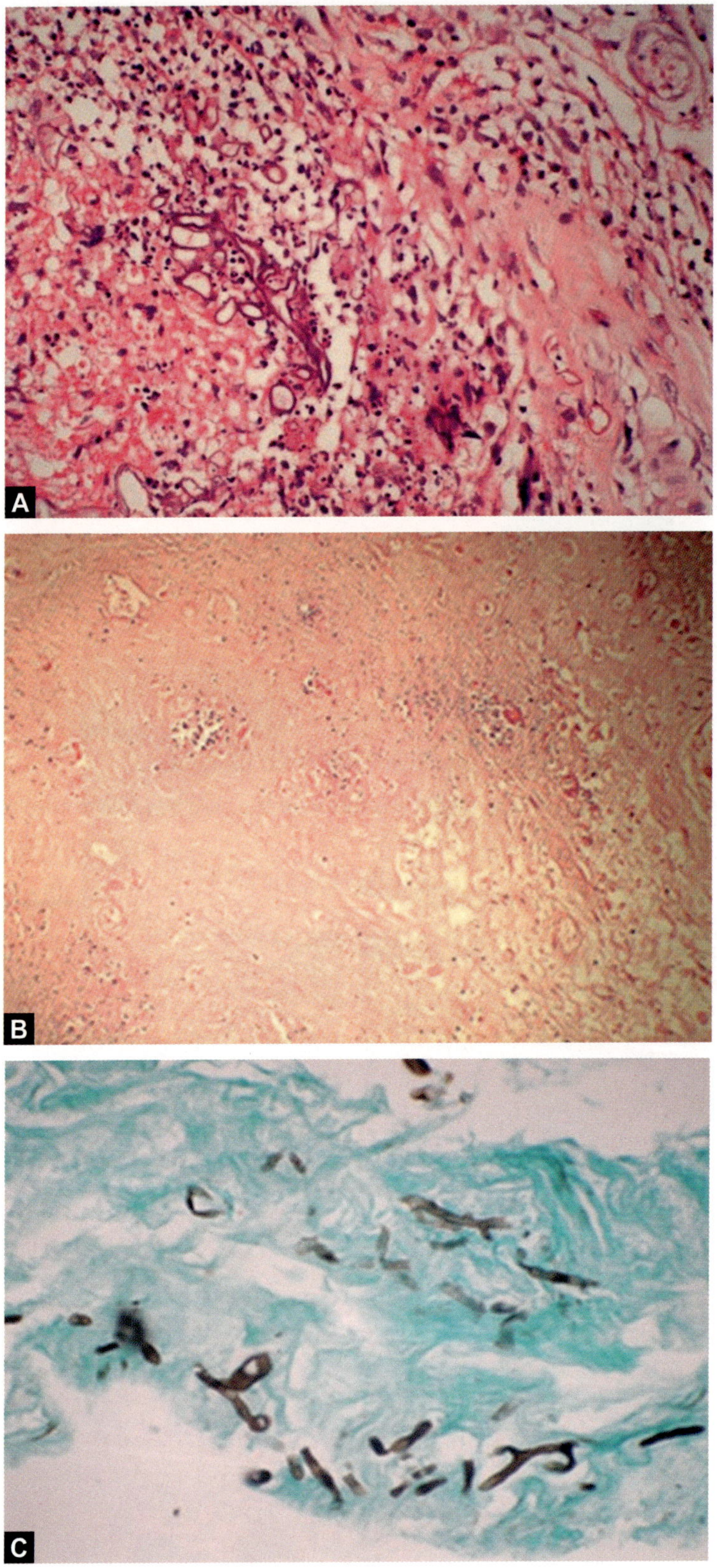

Figs. 29A to C: (A) Acute necrotizing fungal rhinosinusitis with many broad-aseptate hyphae suggesting mucormycosis in a background of necrotizing inflammation; (B) Extensive bland necrosis; and (C) Many broad-aseptate hyphae of mucormycosis in the background of bland necrosis.

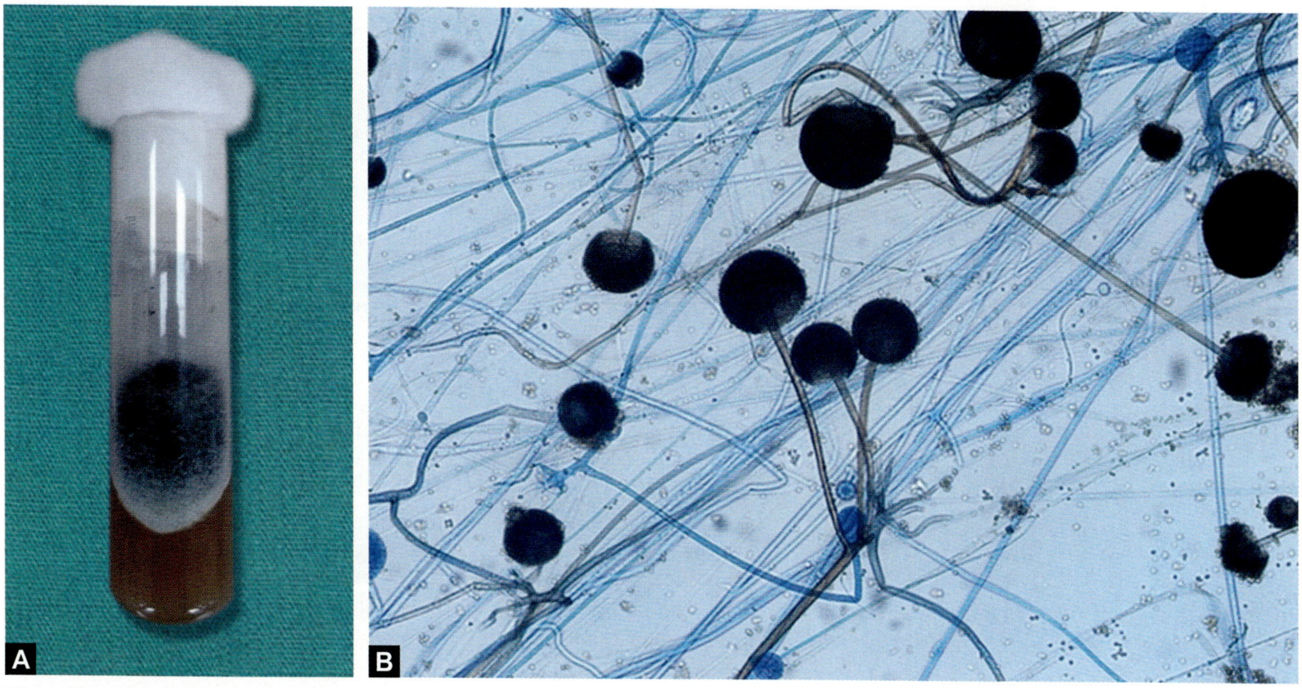

Figs. 30A and B: *Rhizopus arrhizus*: (A) Salt and pepper appearance of cottony growth with black gray to gray spores of *Rhizopus arrhizus* on Sabouraud's Dextrose Agar; and (B) *Rhizopus arrhizus* showing round sporangia at the end of the long sporangiophore that originate in groups opposite to the rhizoids.

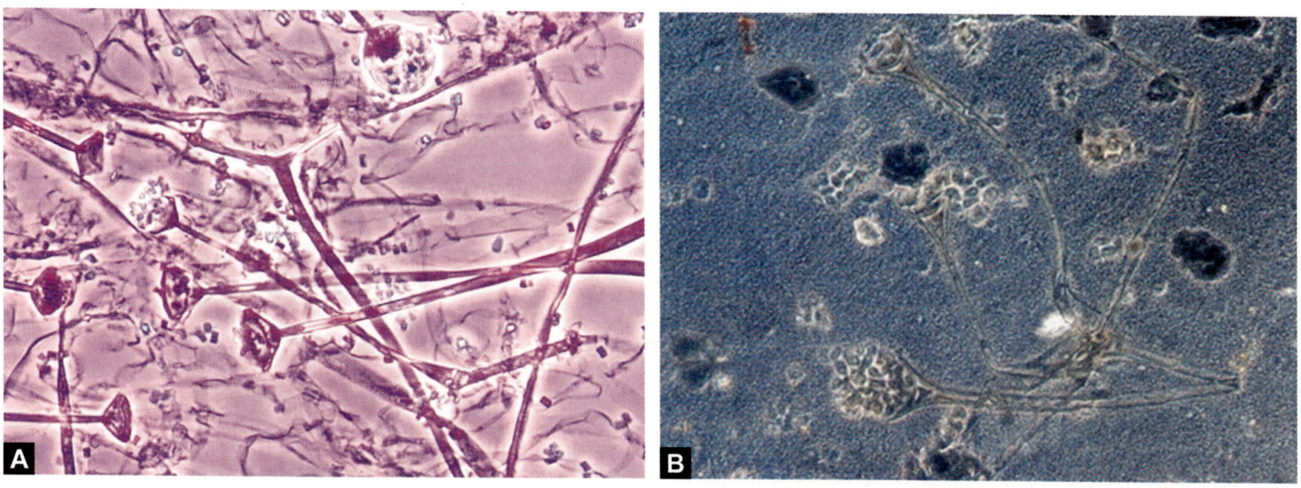

Figs. 31A and B: *Apophysomyces variabilis*: Scotch tape preparation of water agar culture stained with safranin (A) and lactophenol-cotton-blue stain (B) showing wine-glass appearance of apophysis filled with rectangular spores, the characteristic appearance of *Apophysomyces variabilis*.

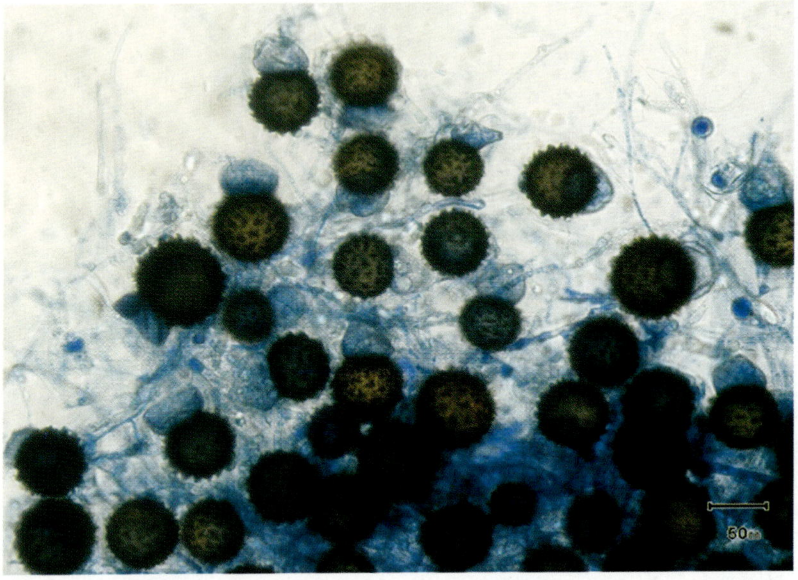

Fig. 32: *Rhizopus homothallicus*: Microscopic picture of *R. homothallicus* showing zygospores with varying length of suspensor cells. Absence or very few sporangia and sporangiospores are conspicuous with this species.

PHAEOHYPHOMYCOSIS (FIGS. 33A TO C)

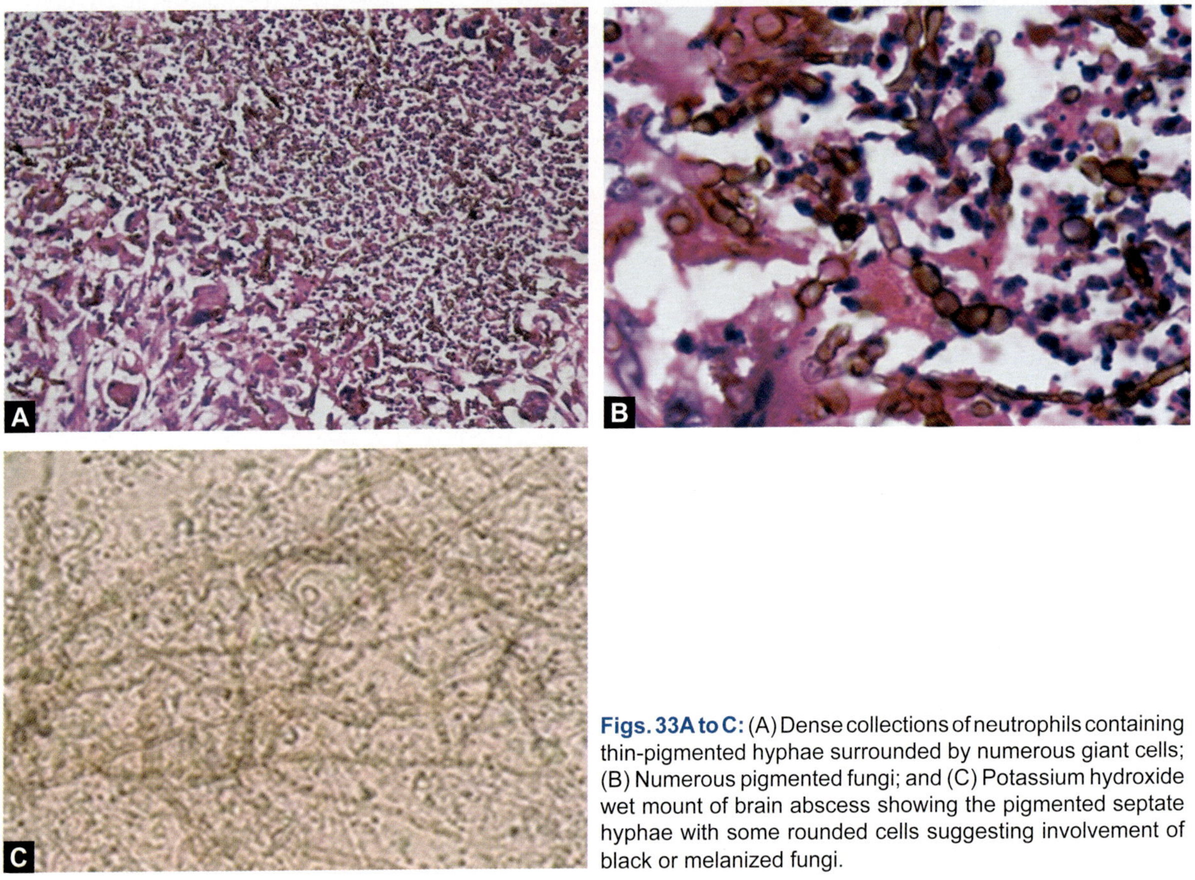

Figs. 33A to C: (A) Dense collections of neutrophils containing thin-pigmented hyphae surrounded by numerous giant cells; (B) Numerous pigmented fungi; and (C) Potassium hydroxide wet mount of brain abscess showing the pigmented septate hyphae with some rounded cells suggesting involvement of black or melanized fungi.

- The infections are usually caused by melanized fungi involving subcutaneous tissue or systemic infection. High frequency of *Cladophialophora bantiana* brain abscess is reported from India even in immunocompetent hosts.

CRYPTOCOCCOSIS LUNG INFECTION (FIGS. 34A TO C)

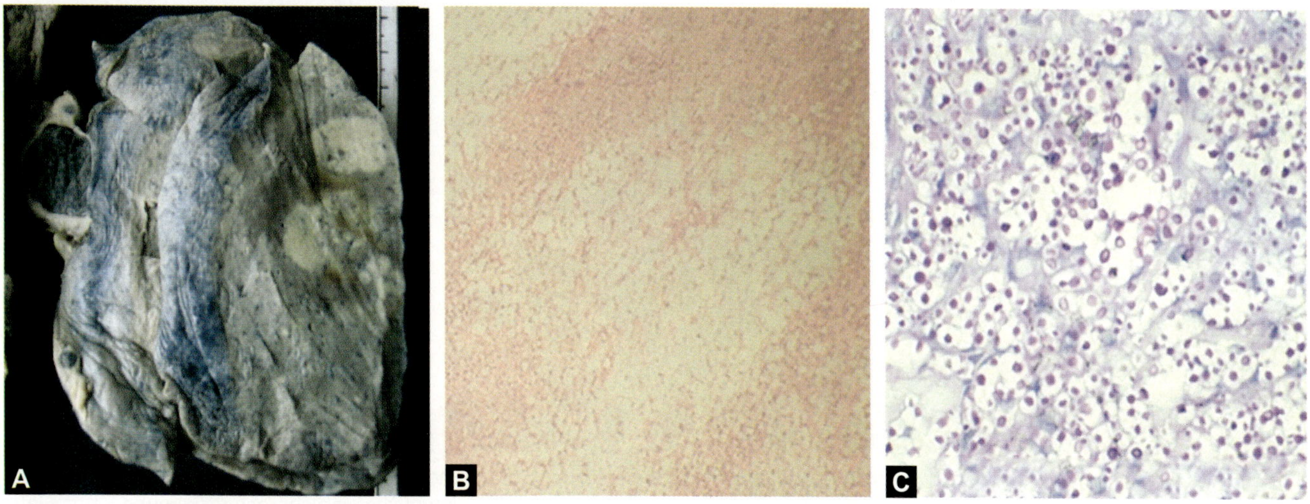

Figs. 34A to C: (A) Numerous gray nodules in both lungs in a case of bronchial asthma on steroid therapy; (B) Collections of yeast cells of *Cryptococcus* the gray areas; and (C) Periodic acid–Schiff (PAS) stain shows numerous *Cryptococcus* yeast cells.

CRYPTOCOCCOSIS CNS INFECTION (FIGS. 35A TO C)

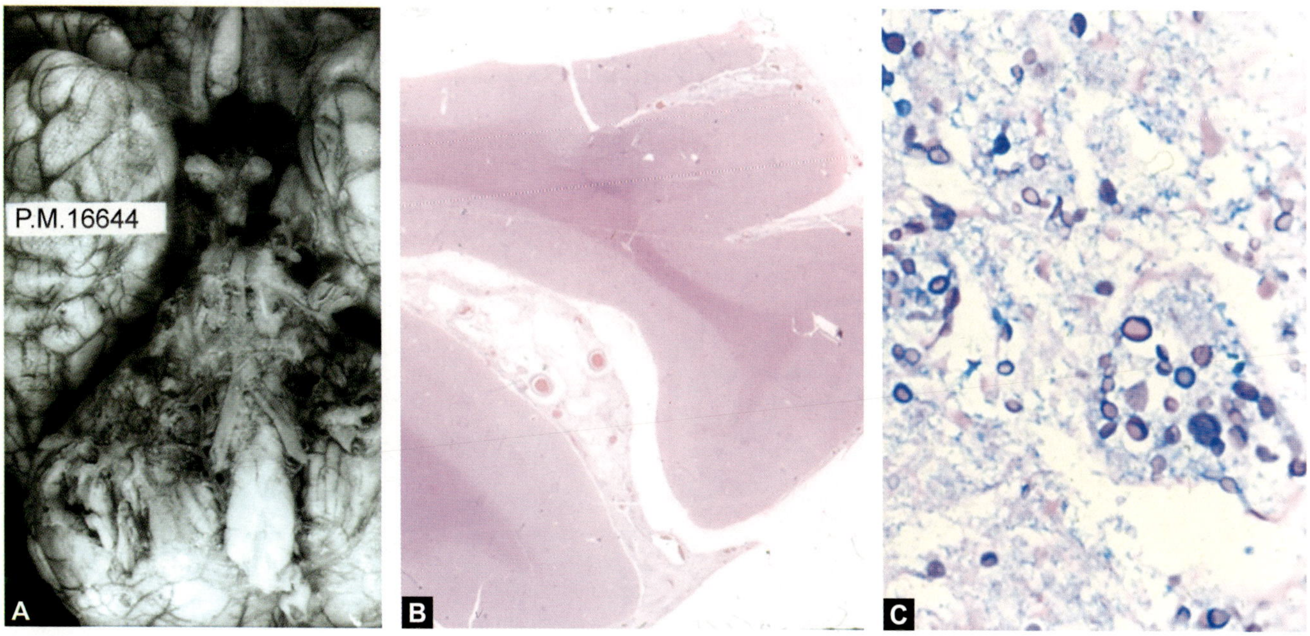

Figs. 35A to C: (A) Gross photograph of the brain shows exudate at the base of the brain and superolateral aspect; (B) Subarachnoid space showing *Cryptococcus*; (C) Periodic acid–Schiff (PAS) Alcian blue shows numerous *Cryptococcus*.

HISTOPLASMOSIS (FIGS. 36A TO C)

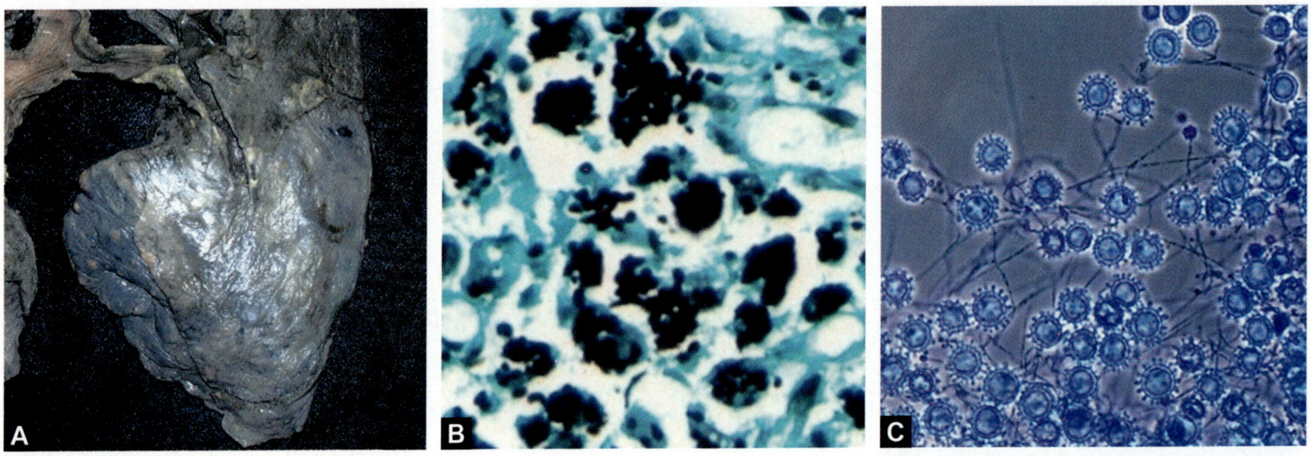

Figs. 36A to C: (A) Numerous gray nodules in lung of a renal transplant recipient; (B) Numerous yeast cells of *Histoplasma capsulatum* in Grocott stain; (C) Lactophenol-cotton blue mount of slide culture of *Histoplasma capsulatum* showing characteristic round tuberculate macroconidia on the short hyaline conidiophores. Few round microconidia are also visible.

- Histoplasmosis in critical care is a rare disease. In recent years, case numbers have increased in certain endemic areas.

PENICILLIOSIS (FIGS. 37A AND B)

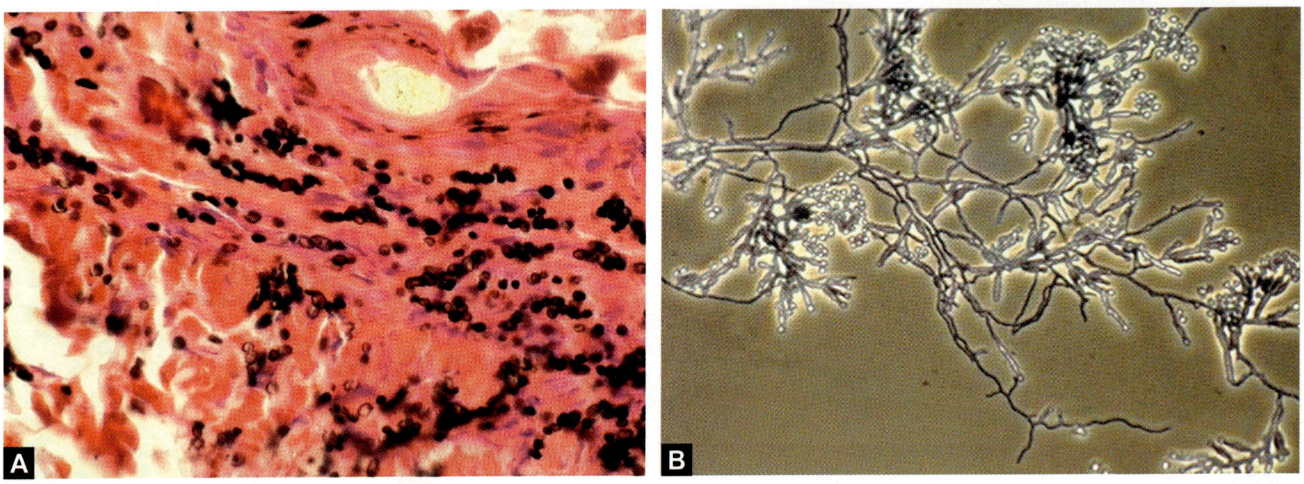

Figs. 37A and B: (A) *Talaromyces marneffei* seen as oval to elliptical yeast cells with few sausage-shaped cells with prominent septa in the tissue sections; (B) Slide culture of *Talaromyces marneffei* having biverticillate conidiophore containing three to five metulae bearing 3–6 phialides. Small smooth-walled globose conidia arise from phialides.

- Penicilliosis due to *Talaromyces marneffei* is common in endemic area (Southeast Asian countries). The disease is seen in critical patients of Northeast India especially in AIDS.

SCEDOSPORIOSIS AND FUSARIOSIS (FIGS. 38A AND B)

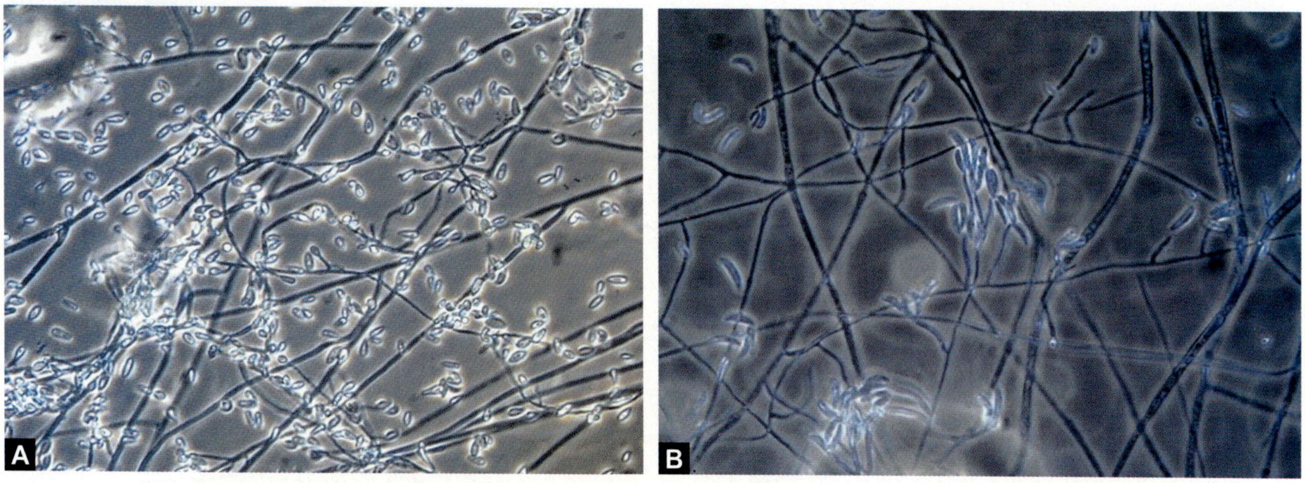

Figs. 38A and B: (A) Slide culture of *Scedosporium apiospermum* showing numerous single-celled clavate conidia borne on the short conidiophores laterally on the hyphae; (B) Slide culture of *Fusarium solani* showing clavate-shaped macroconidia with three to five septa along with few microconidia.

- These infections are increasingly reported in immunosuppressed patients, but may also be seen in immunocompetent patients in critical care. Histopathologically, the fungus is difficult to distinguish from *Aspergillosis*. Culture isolation helps to identify. These fungi may also be isolated from blood in disseminated infection.

PNEUMOCYSTOSIS (FIGS. 39A TO C)

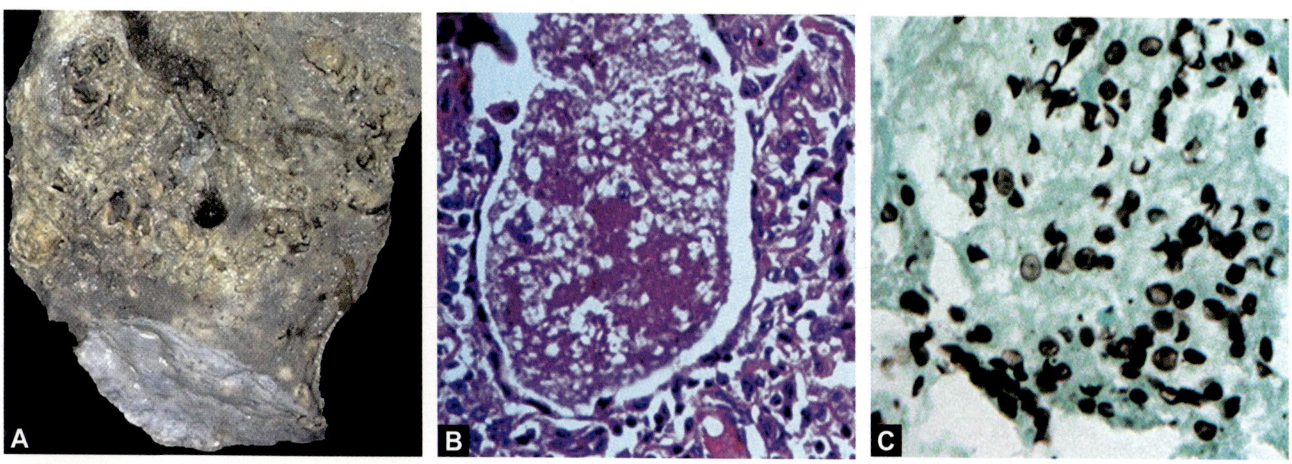

Figs. 39A to C: (A) Numerous cysts in the lower lobes of both lungs; (B) The alveoli are filled with frothy material; and (C) Cysts in Grocott stain.

- *Pneumocystis jiroveci* infections are increasingly recognized in critical care patients. Recent evidence shows that the infection may spread from one person to another.

CHAPTER

18

Equipment in Microbiology

Navin Kumar

SPECIMEN CONTAINERS (FIG. 1)

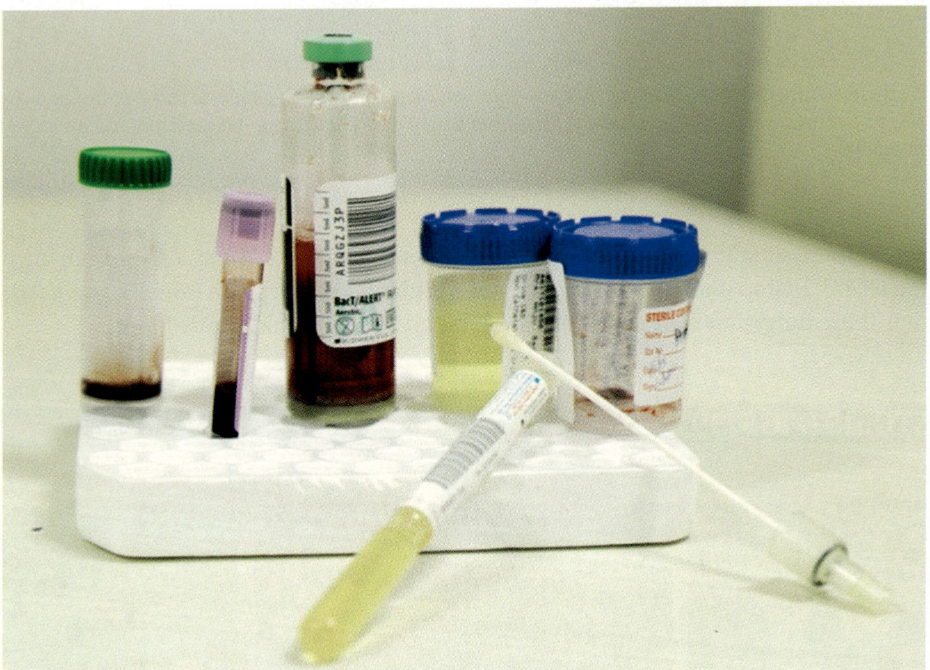

Fig. 1: Specimen containers used in microbiology.

- Selection of appropriate specimen is important for specific diagnostic test. The interpretation of microbiology test results depends upon quality of specimens received for analysis.

MICROSCOPY (FIG. 2)

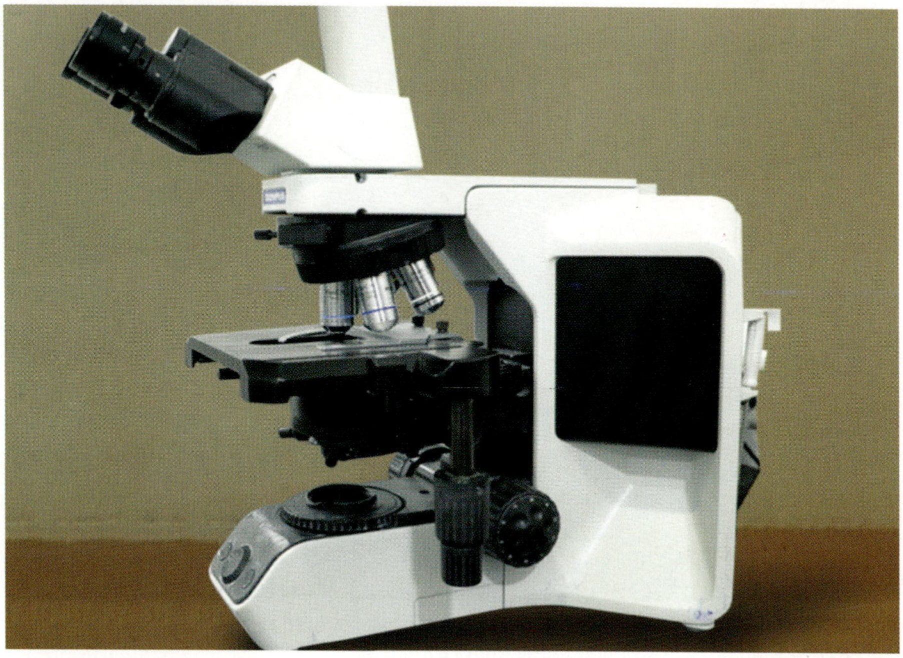

Fig. 2: Microscopy is the most common method used for detection of microorganisms in different clinical specimens. Bright-field microscopy (also known as light microscopy) and fluorescence microscopy have the widest use in clinical microbiology laboratory.

USE OF PERSONAL PROTECTIVE EQUIPMENT (FIG. 3)

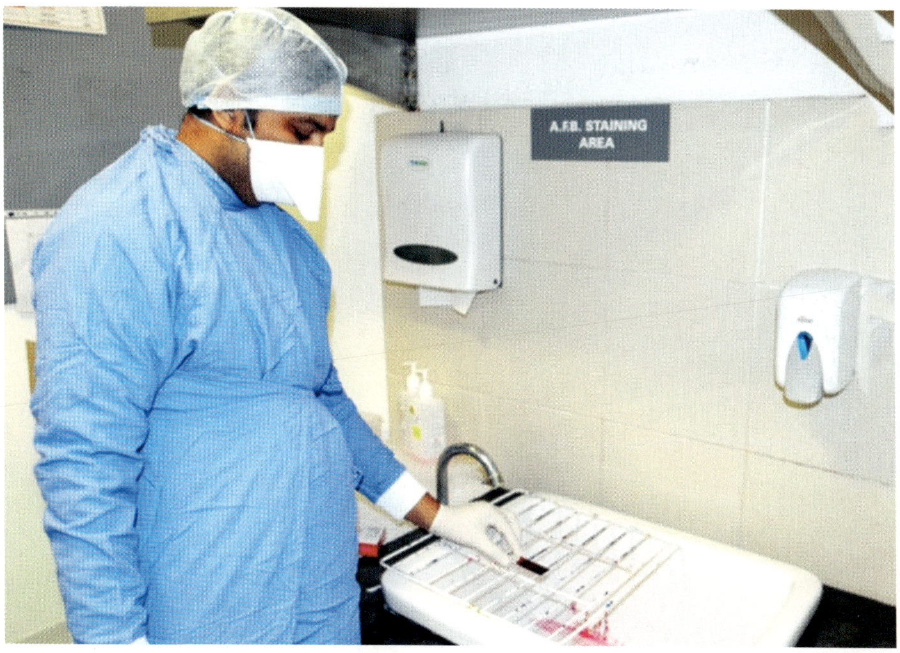

Fig. 3: Acid-fast staining is commonly used for detection of *Mycobacteria* in clinical specimens. It also provides preliminary identification information for bacteria grown in *Mycobacteria* culture. Appropriate personal protective equipment (PPE) are required for safety of healthcare workers working in tuberculosis laboratory.

VITEK®2 AUTOMATED MICROBIOLOGY SYSTEM (FIG. 4)

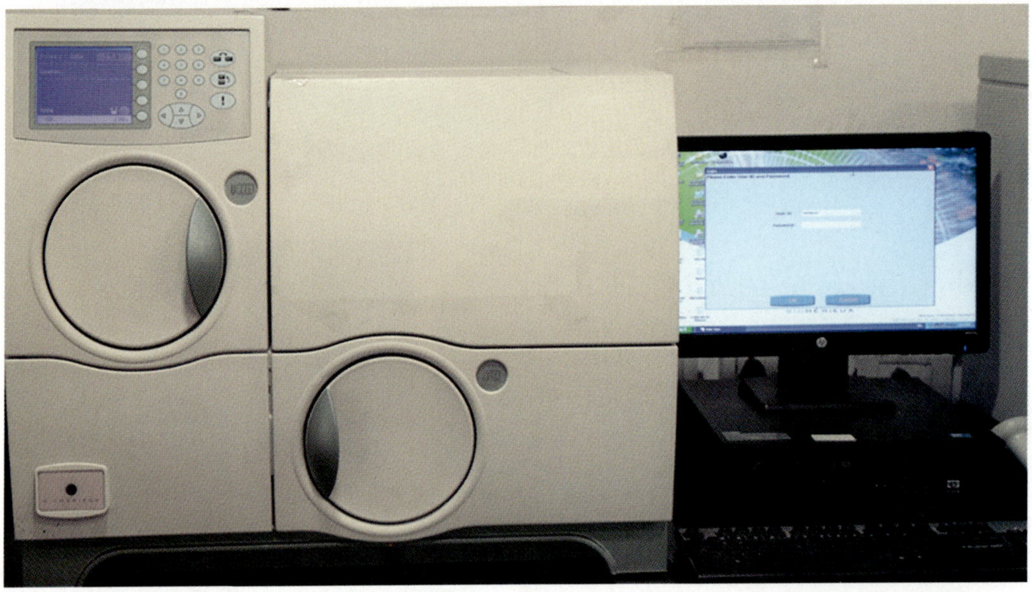

Fig. 4: VITEK®2 automated microbiology system for early identification of microorganisms and antimicrobial susceptibility testing. It also rapidly identifies resistance markers like extended-spectrum beta-lactamases (ESBL), vancomycin-resistant enterococci (VRE), and methicillin-resistant *Staphylococcus aureus* (MRSA). The early identification by automated system helps in optimizing antimicrobial therapy and improving patient care.

Table 1: Antibiotic sensitivity report showing minimum inhibitory concentration (MIC) values for different antibiotics.

Specimen type: Catheterized urine			
Category numb: / /		**Received** : 18/07/2017 17:13	
Clinical comment:		**Registered :** 18/07/2017 17:13	
Investigation	**Result**	**Biological reference interval**	
Aerobic C and S urine Organism	Comment		
0268 *Escherichia coli*			
Antibiotic	*Sensitivity*		*MIC value*
Ceftriaxone	R	≥	64
Gentamicin	S	≤	1
Nalidixic acid	R	≥	32
Nitrofurantoin	S	≤	16
Piperacillin/Tazobactam	S	≤	4
Trimethoprim/Sulfamethoxazole	S	≤	20
Ticarcillin	R		
Ertapenem	S	≤	0.5
Ciprofloxacin	R	≥	4
Ceftazidime	R		16
Amikacin	S	≤	2
Ampicillin	R	≥	32
Amoxicillin/Clavulanic acid	S		8

S: Sensitive; R: Resistant; I: Intermediate; Colony count 10^5 CFU/mL.

- Automated blood culture system has improved the detection of blood stream infections. The rapid detection of clinically significant bacteria and yeast in positive blood culture bottle helps in timely initiation of appropriate antibiotics.
- Ideally antibiotic sensitivity report should include minimal inhibitory concentrations (MICs) in order to determine the most effective antibiotic (Table 1).
- The MIC number is the lowest concentration of an antimicrobial agent that inhibits the growth of particular microorganism.
- The MIC is a quantitative method of susceptibility testing and provides the ability to precisely determine the concentration of antimicrobial agent required to inhibit growth of a pathogen.
- An MIC number for one antimicrobial agent cannot be compared to the MIC number for another agent.
- The choice of antibiotic should be based on the MIC number, the site of infection, and an antibiotic's breakpoint.

DISC DIFFUSION METHOD (FIG. 5)

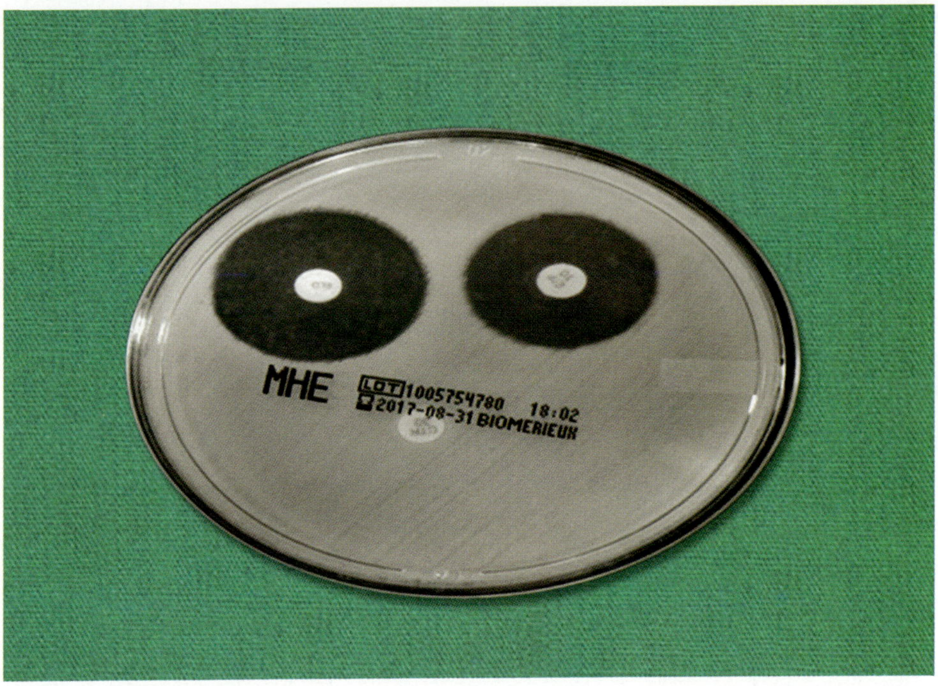

Fig. 5: *Escherichia coli* isolate sensitive to ertapenem (ETP) and resistant to ceftriaxone (CTR).

- Disc diffusion method is also used for detection of antibiotic sensitivity/resistance of micro-organisms grown in routine clinical specimens (Fig. 5).

MOLECULAR DIAGNOSTIC TECHNIQUE (FIGS. 6A AND B)

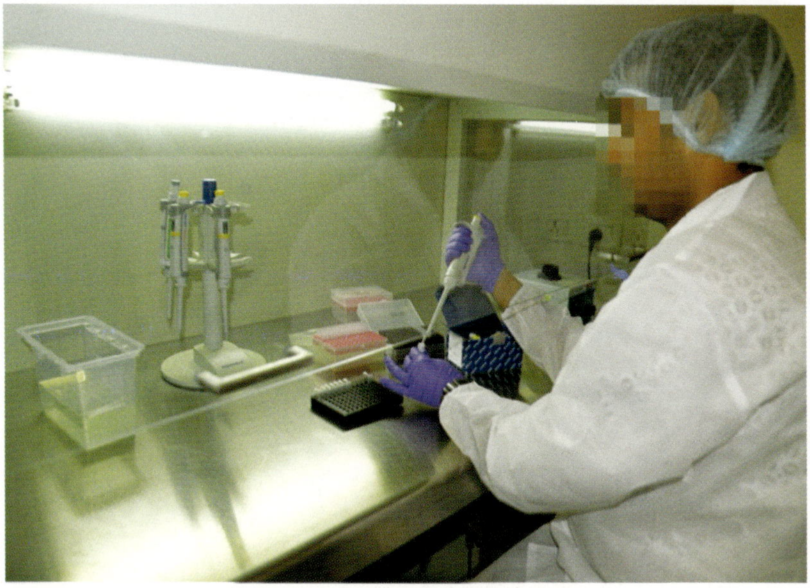

Fig. 6A: Real-time polymerase chain reaction (PCR) assay setup in laminar flow cabinet.

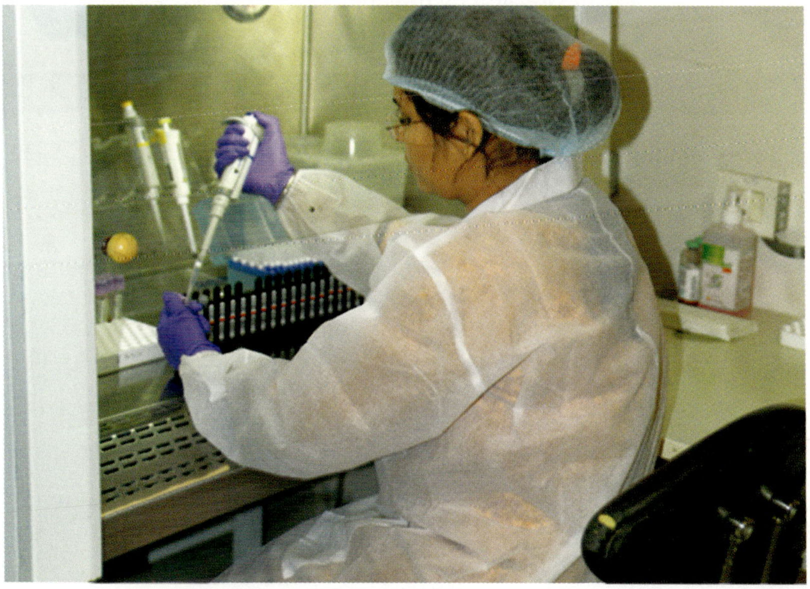

Fig. 6B: Sample processing for real-time polymerase chain reaction (PCR) in biosafety cabinet.

- Molecular methods have significantly improved the field of infectious disease diagnostics. The molecular infectious disease testing provides timely therapeutic clinical decisions and early infection control intervention.
- Extra care needs to be taken to avoid reagent contamination on PCR workstation. This workstation should be free of any biological material (DNA/RNA extracts, samples, and PCR products).
- Good laboratory practice should be followed all the time in PCR laboratory. Dedicated laboratory coats, gloves, and other personal protective equipment should be supplied in each work area of PCR laboratory to avoid cross-contamination.

ANAEROBIC JAR (FIG. 7)

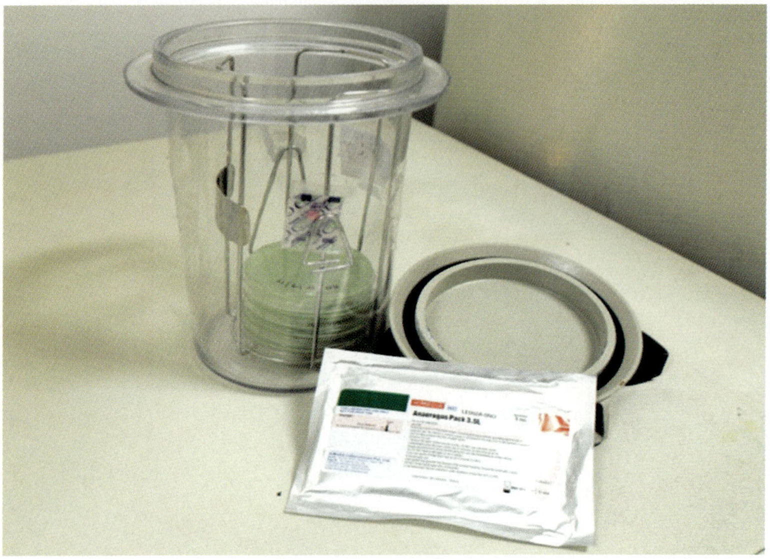

Fig. 7: Anaerobic jar.

- Anaerobic jar is used to produce anaerobic environment during the incubation of anaerobic culture in microbiology laboratory. It is assembled and incubated at 35–37°C. The atmosphere within the jar is free of oxygen, and consists mainly of nitrogen, with some carbon dioxide and hydrogen.

LIQUID CULTURE OF TUBERCULOSIS (FIG. 8)

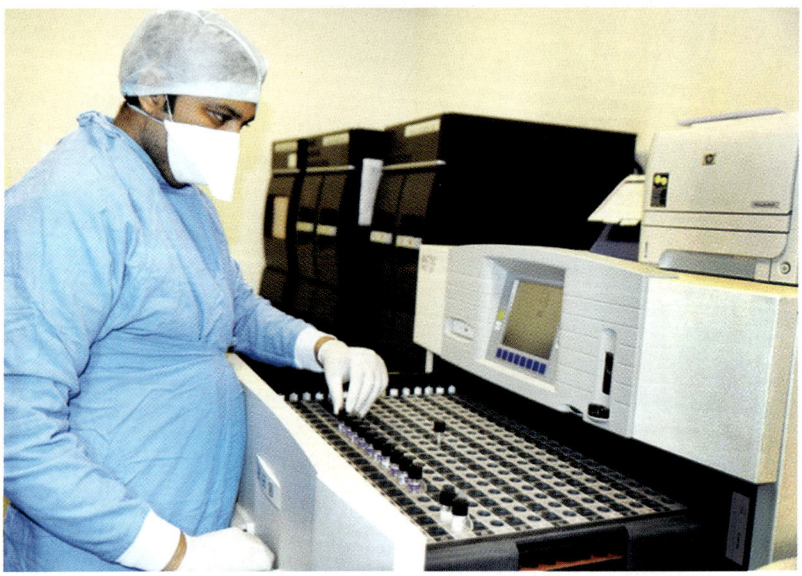

Fig. 8: Liquid culture of tuberculosis.

- Liquid culture medium is used for detection of *Mycobacterium tuberculosis* and *Mycobacterium* other than Tuberculosis (MOTT). It has increased sensitivity and detection rate from specimens with low-bacilli count along with reduced detection time in comparison to solid TB culture medium.

INCUBATOR (FIGS. 9A AND B)

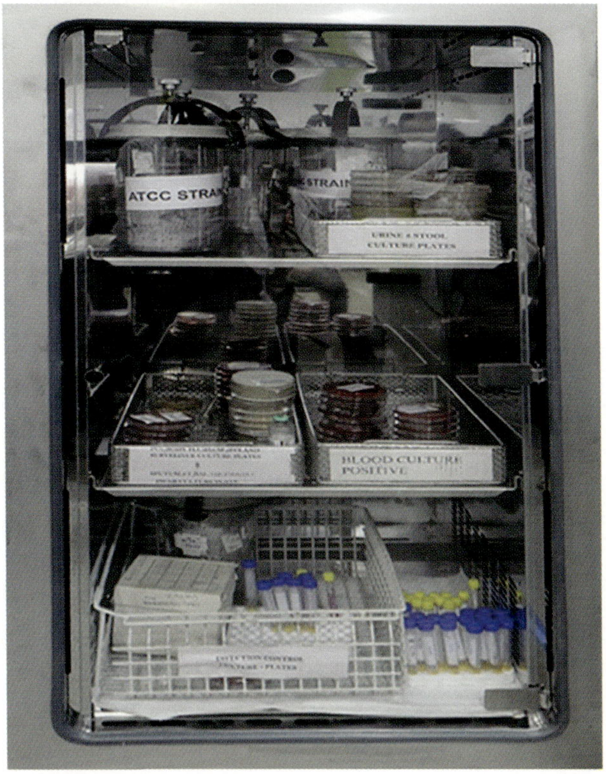

Fig. 9A: Incubator holding culture plates and liquid culture medium.

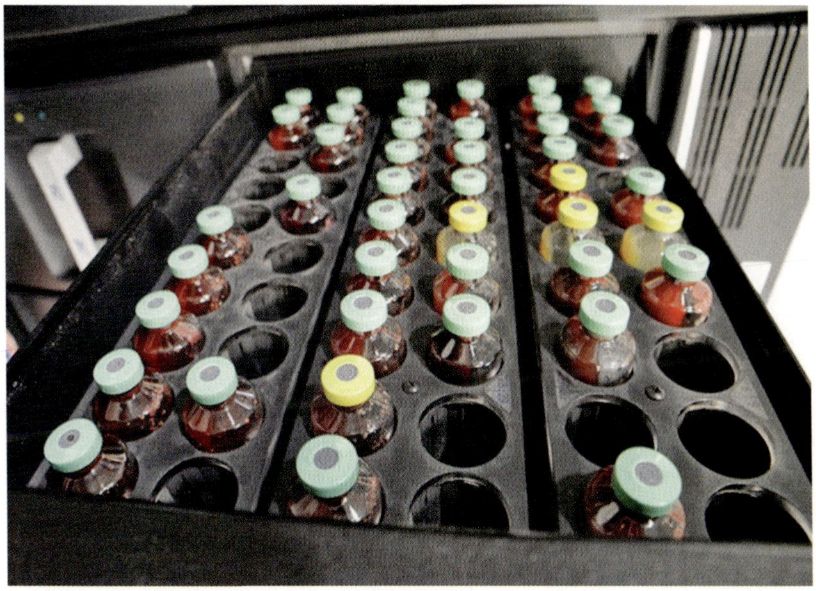

Fig. 9B: Automated blood culture system holding blood culture bottles for continuous incubation.

- In microbiology laboratory, incubators are used to maintain progressive growth of organisms by regulating temperature, humidity and ventilation.

SECTION 8

Miscellaneous

CHAPTER 19

Nephrology

Manju Aggarwal, Vijay Joshi

CT SCAN IMAGE OF THE ABDOMEN OF AN ADOLESCENT SHOWING NEPHROCALCINOSIS IN THE NATIVE AND TRANSPLANT KIDNEY (FIGS. 1A TO E)

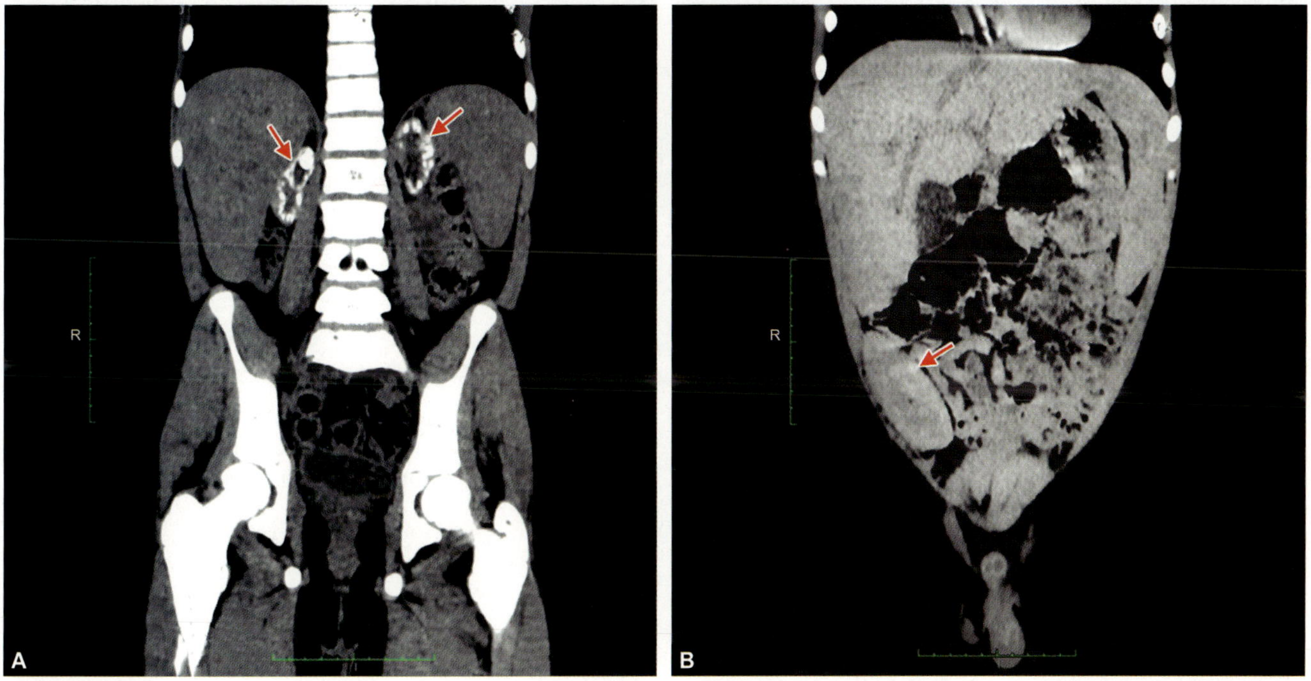

Figs. 1A and B: (A) Nephrocalcinosis in native kidneys primary hyperoxaluria; (B) Nephrocalcinosis in transplant kidney primary hyperoxaluria.

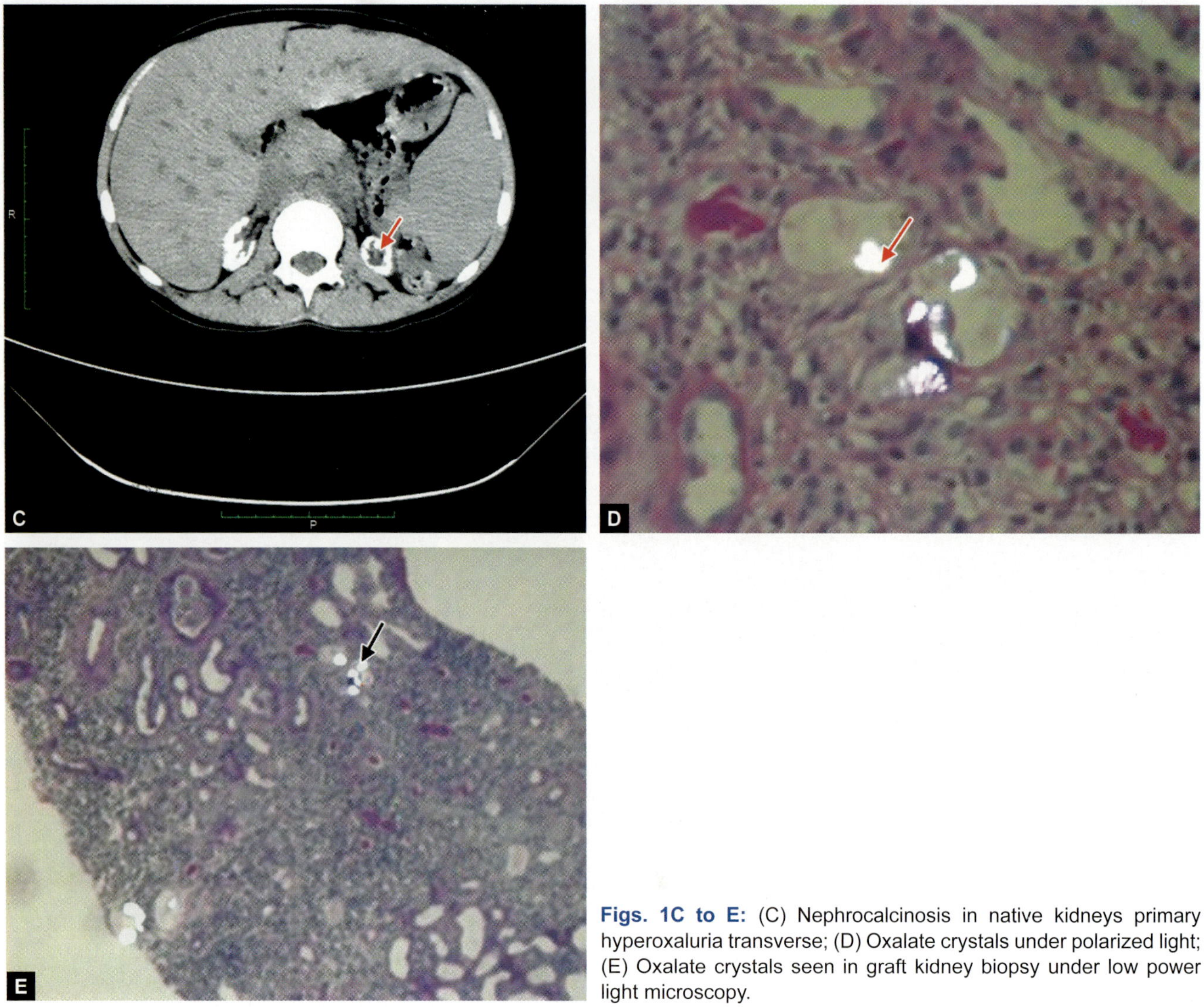

Figs. 1C to E: (C) Nephrocalcinosis in native kidneys primary hyperoxaluria transverse; (D) Oxalate crystals under polarized light; (E) Oxalate crystals seen in graft kidney biopsy under low power light microscopy.

- CT scan image of the abdomen of an adolescent showing nephrocalcinosis in the native and in the transplant kidney.
- Patient under went first renal transplant for advanced renal failure few years back.
- He lost his graft kidney within 2 years and was re-evaluated for second transplant.
- Graft kidney biopsy was done showing oxalate crystals in graft kidney tissue on polarized light microscopy and a CT image of the abdomen revealed both native kidneys and graft kidney nephrocalcinosis, establishing a diagnosis of primary hyperoxaluria.
- Patient later underwent simultaneous liver and kidney transplant and is on long-term chelation of urinary oxalate with potassium citrate.
- Primary hyperoxaluria is a autosomal recessive disorder.
- Glyoxylate converts to poorly soluble oxalate because of AGXT/GRHPR enzyme deficiencies.
- Cause nephrocalcinosis and nephrolithiasis and systemic oxalate deposits later on.

MRI OF RENAL VIEN THROMBOSIS (FIGS. 2A TO C)

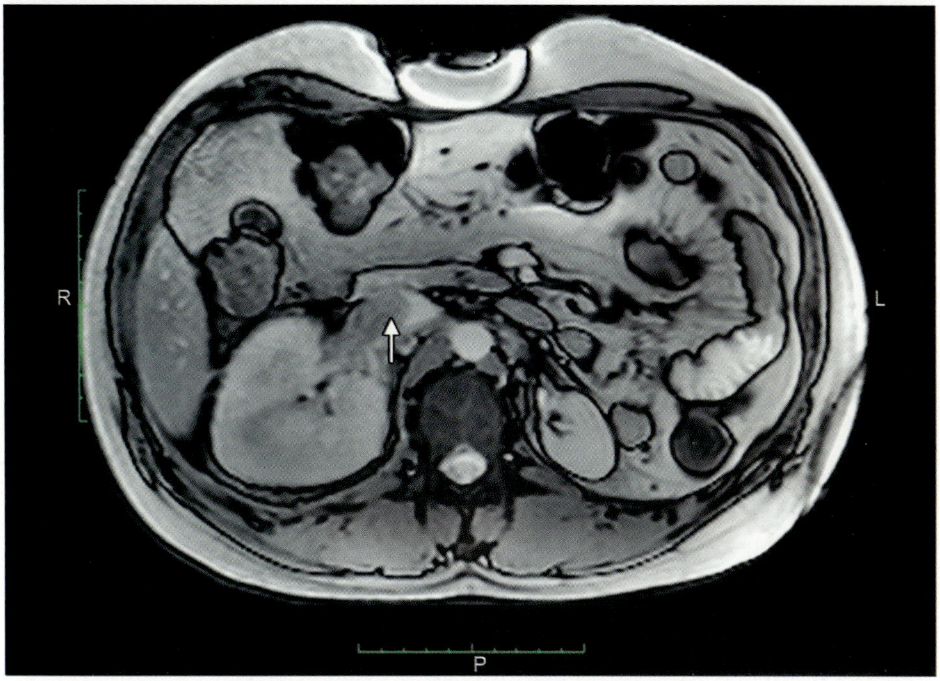

Fig. 2A: Right renal vein thrombosis transverse.

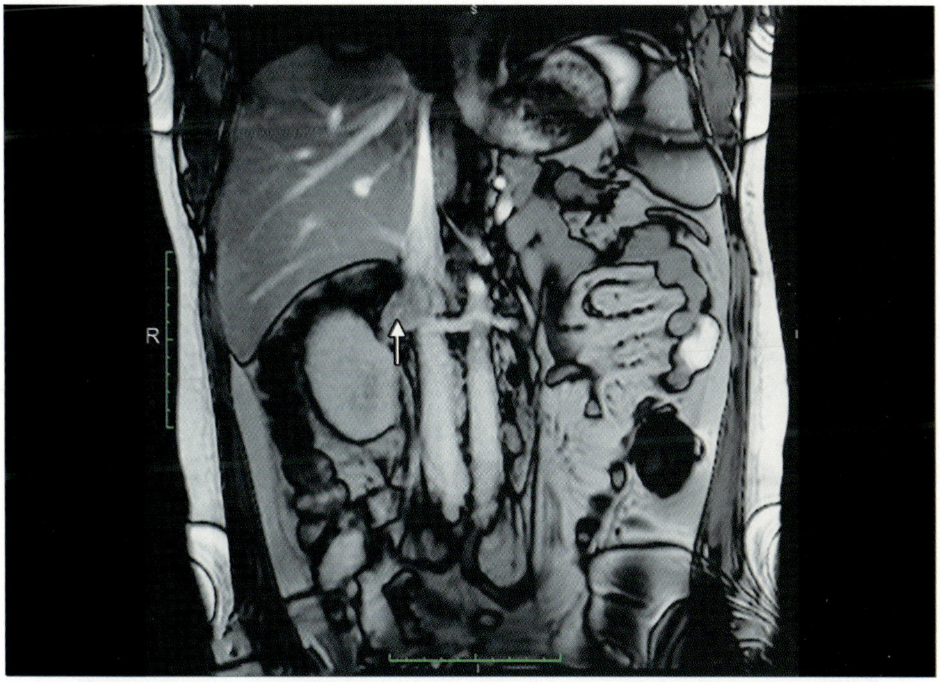

Fig. 2B: Right renal vein thrombosis coronal.

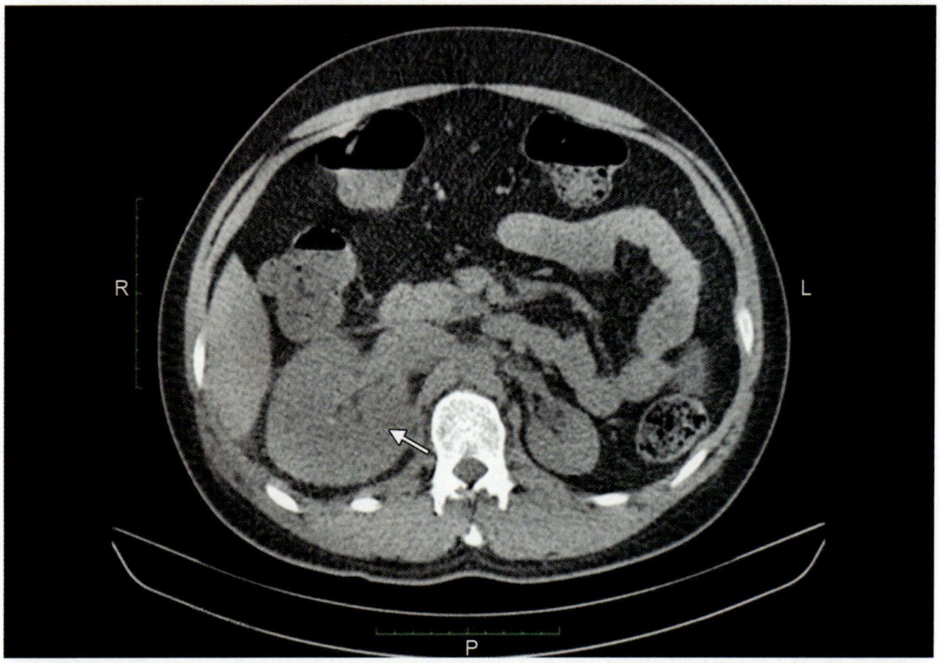

Fig. 2C: Right renal vein thrombosis with enlarged right kidney and a small left kidney.

- An MRI of a patient with acute kidney injury secondary to renal vein thrombosis.
- Patient was a young adult who presented to casualty with gross hematuria, flank pain and renal dysfunction.
- The patient had an underlying procoagulant state secondary to presence of beta-2-GP1 antibody.
- Renal vein thrombosis is seen as a complication of nephrotic syndrome (particularly membranous nephropathy) with severe hypoalbuminemia (Sr. albumin <2.5 mg/dL).
- It can also be seen in patients with renal cell carcinoma and in deceleration injury to the abdominal and renal vessels.

CT SCAN OF ACUTE CORTICAL NECROSIS (FIGS. 3A AND B)

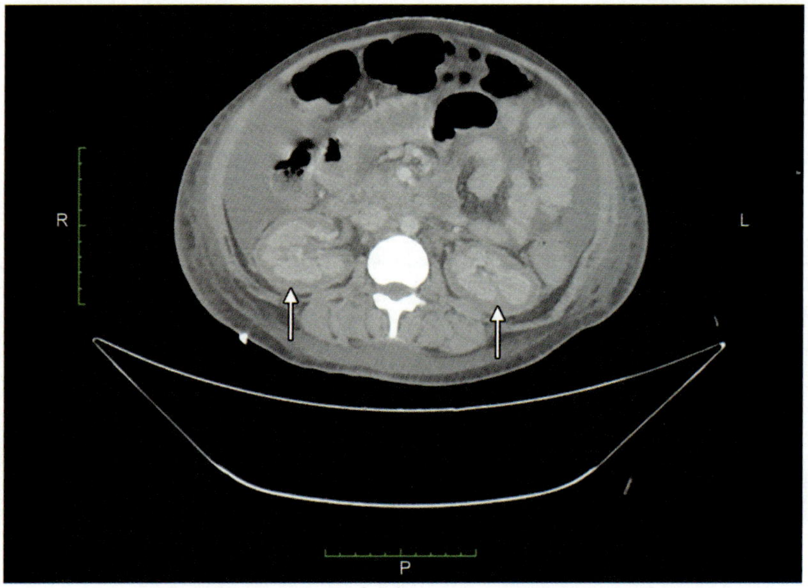

Fig. 3A: Diffuse acute cortical necrosis after in transfer.

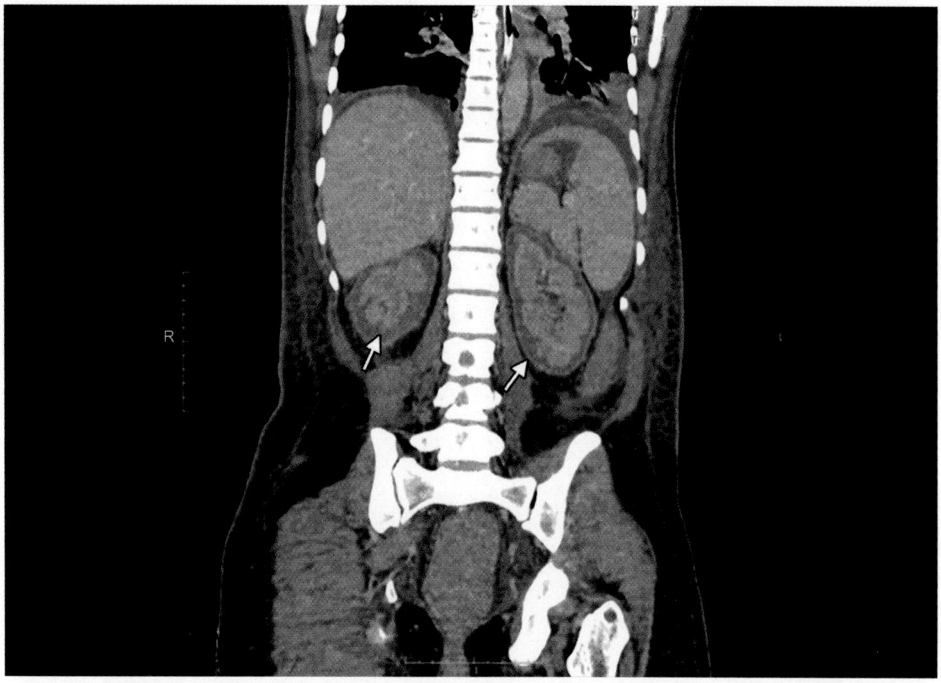

Fig. 3B: Diffuse acute cortical necrosis after postpartum hemorrhage (PPH) in coronal section contrast-enhanced CT scan of the abdomen.

- Contrast enhanced CT scan of the abdomen of a young lady with acute kidney injury (AKI) secondary to postpartum hemorrhage (PPH) causing acute cortical necrosis.
- This patient is a young-lady with AKI secondary to PPH causing acute cortical necrosis.
- Patient was admitted with dialysis dependent AKI and anuria after an episode of massive PPH.
- In view of persistent anuria contrast, CT image of the kidneys was done that showed absent perfusion in the cortices of both kidneys with small area of juxta capsular viable tissue producing 'cortical rim sign.'
- Common causes of acute cortical necrosis include snake bite poisoning AKI, PPH, septic abortions, severe sepsis and severe thrombotic microangiopathy (TMA).
- Diffuse cortical necrosis portends poor prognostic outcome in terms of kidney recovery.
- It can definitively be confirmed on a kidney biopsy.
- Late follow-up of cortical necrosis can show cortical calcification on X-ray/ultrasound imaging.

X-RAY WRIST AND PELVIS SHOWING VASCULAR CALCIFICATION (FIGS. 4A AND B)

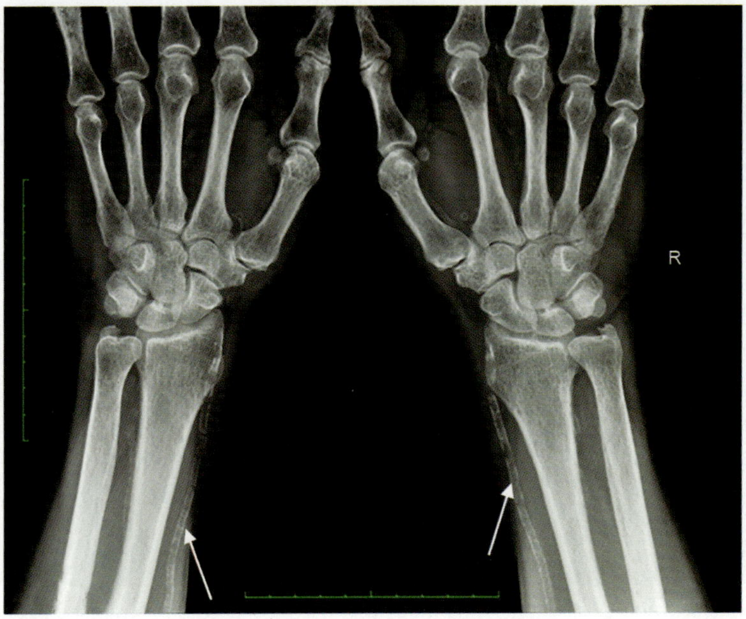

Fig. 4A: X-ray wrist vascular calcification of radial arteries.

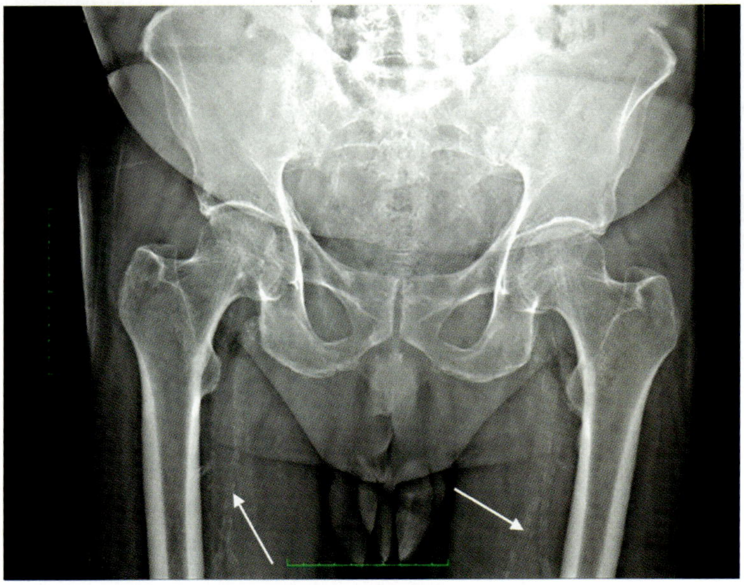

Fig. 4B: X-ray pelvis vascular calcification of femoral arteries.

- X-ray pelvis and wrist of a patient with chronic kidney disease (CKD) on maintenance hemodialysis showing vascular calcification in the femoral and radial arteries.
- Linear vascular calcification represents medial calcification (Monckeberg's medial sclerosis) as against intimal calcification seen in non-CKD patients.
- Vascular calcification has a high prevalence in predialytic and dialytic CKD patients.
- Its prevalence is higher in diabetic patients and increases with age and dialysis vintage.
- It is associated with higher risk of cardiovascular events and all-cause mortality in CKD.

CT OF ACUTE EMPHYSEMATOUS PYELONEPHRITIS (FIG. 5)

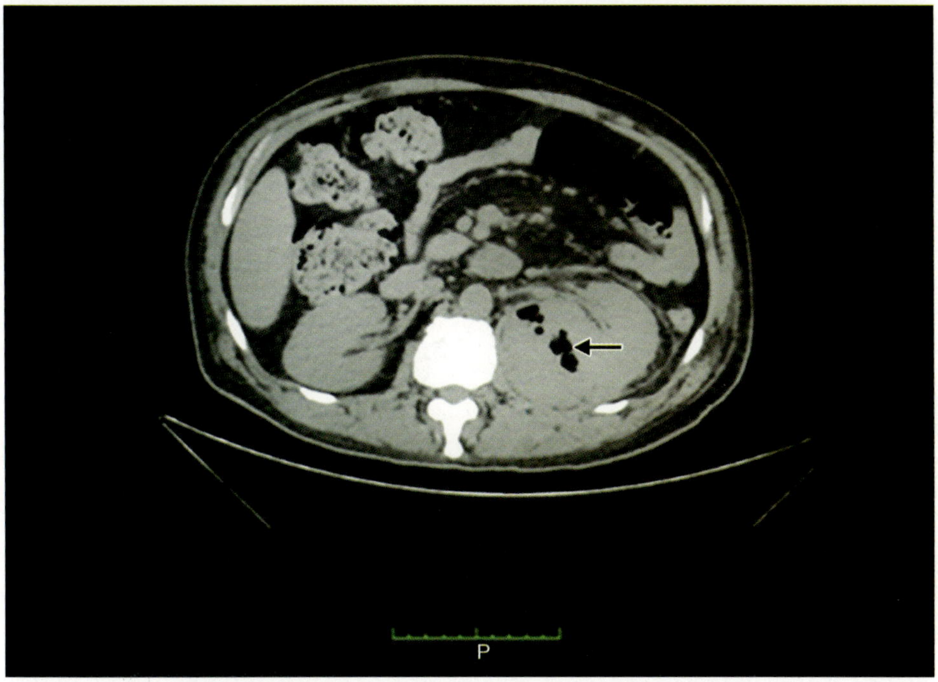

Fig. 5: Emphysematous pyelonephritis with renal abscess.

- Contrast-enhanced CT images of a patient with acute emphysematous pyelonephritis and acute kidney injury.
- Image shows gas shadow in the left kidney with collection in the subcapsular space suggestive of abscess.
- Patient was treated with antibiotics and percutaneous drainage of abscess.
- Emphysematous pyelonephritis is a serious disease with high mortality.
- It is commonly associated with diabetic patients and *E. coli* is the most common cause.
- Ipsilateral nephrectomy is indicated in most cases with higher grades and deteriorating renal function and general condition of the patient.

ULTRASOUND IMAGE OF GRAFT HYDRONEPHROSIS (FIG. 6)

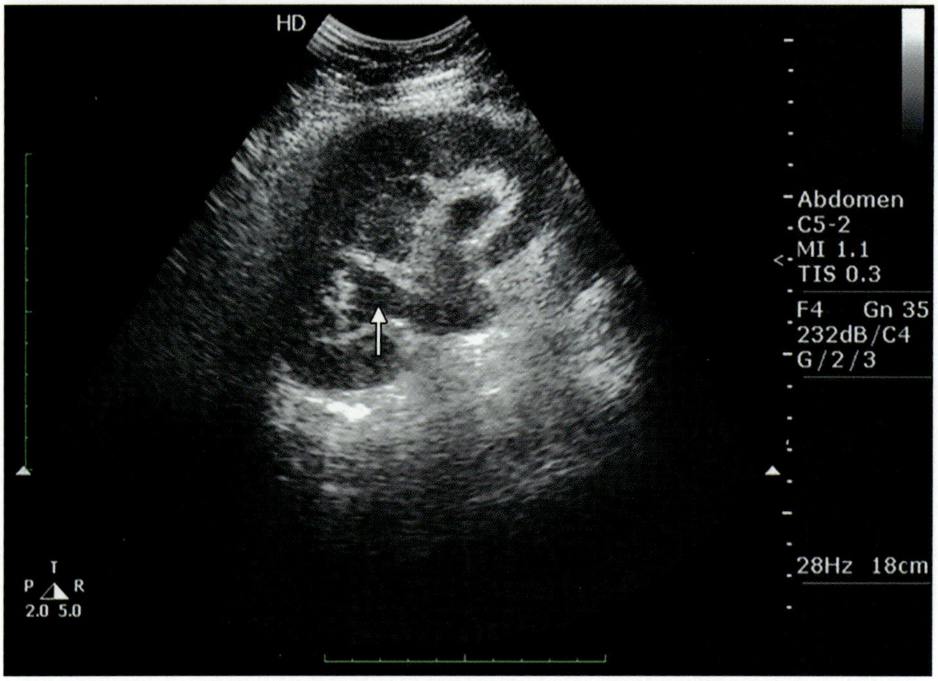

Fig. 6: USG image hydronephrosis in transplant kidney.

- Hydronephrosis of graft kidney is secondary to external compression of the ureter from a lymphocele or an urinoma in the early post-transplant period (<1 month).
- Later in the course, ureteric strictures are a common cause of graft hydronephrosis.
- The index patient presented with decreased urine output and graft dysfunction 8 months post-transplant.
- Ultrasound imaging of graft kidney revealed hydronephrosis.
- Patient underwent percutaneous nephrostomy followed by retrograde stenting of graft ureter.
- Her renal functions improved following relief of obstruction.

TRANSPLANTED KIDNEY WITH ACUTE ANTIBODY-MEDIATED REJECTION (FIG. 7)

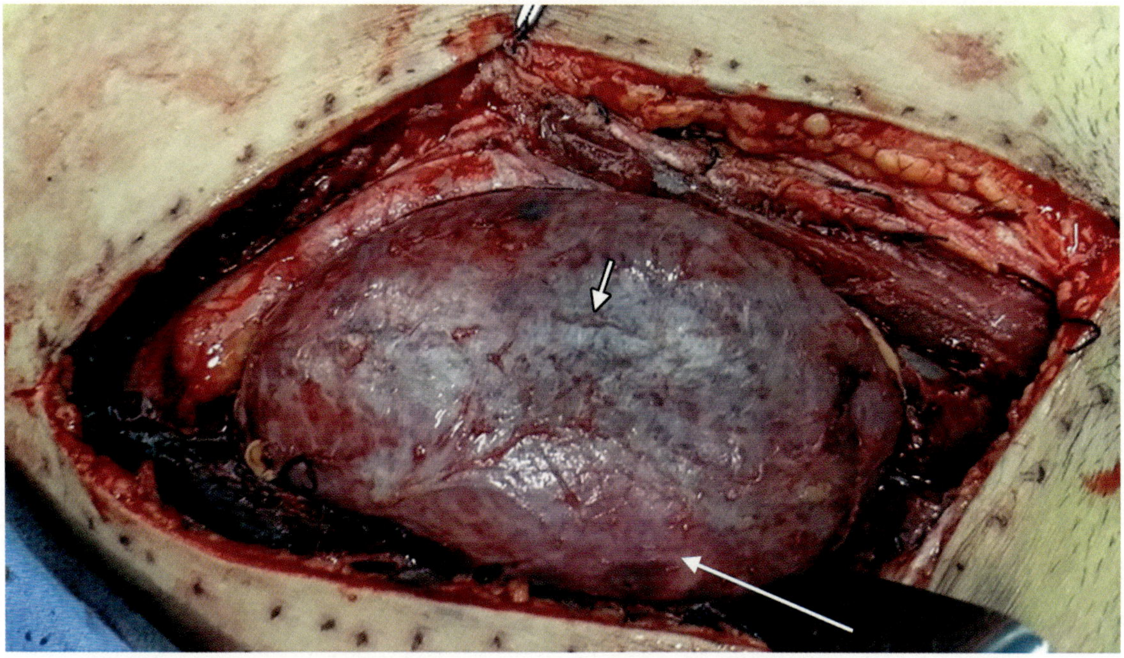

Fig. 7: Graft nephrectomy after severe antibody-mediated rejection.

- Transplant kidney showing bluish black kidney with oozing in a patient with acute antibody-mediated rejection; the kidney is in the process of graft nephrectomy.
- Early fulminant rejection results in severe thrombotic microangiopathy and cortical necrosis leading to a nonviable kidney.
- This patient underwent an ABO-incompatible renal transplant 10 days prior.
- Graft dysfunction occurred on 7th postoperative day.
- An USG-Doppler revealed patent main vessels with no parenchymal flow.
- Graft kidney biopsy revealed extensive cortical necrosis with thrombotic microangiopathy.
- It confirmed the diagnosis of severe antibody-mediated rejection in an ABO-incompatible transplant.
- Acute rejection rates in ABO-incompatible renal transplant.
- Indications for graft nephrectomy are (1) Allograft failure with ongoing symptomatic rejection causing fever, malaise, hematuria, and graft pain; (2) Infarction due to thrombosis; (3) Severe infection of the allograft such as emphysematous pyelonephritis; and (4) Allograft rupture.

HEMODIALYSIS PROCEDURE (FIGS. 8A TO C)

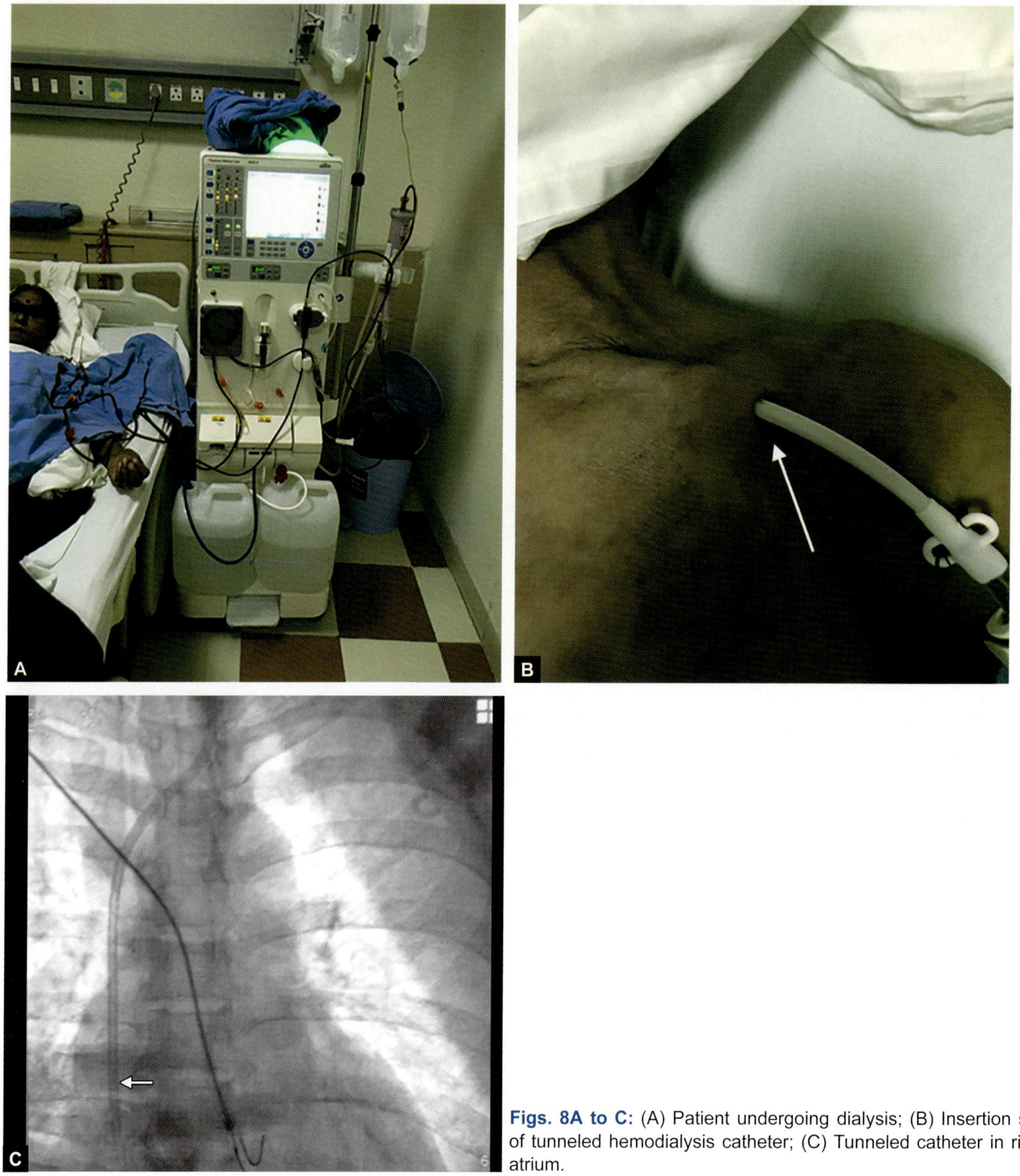

Figs. 8A to C: (A) Patient undergoing dialysis; (B) Insertion site of tunneled hemodialysis catheter; (C) Tunneled catheter in right atrium.

- The patient is undergoing dialysis through left internal jugular tunneled catheter.
- The cuff can be seen approximately 2 cm from the exit site.
- The tip of the catheter is seen in the right atrium in the fluoroscopy image.
- Tunneled catheters have a lower incidence of infections than nontunneled catheters, however, they are inferior to arteriovenous (AV) fistulas/AV grafts as a major vascular access for long-term hemodialysis.

CANNULATION OF ARTERIOVENOUS FISTULA FOR HEMODIALYSIS (FIGS. 9A AND B)

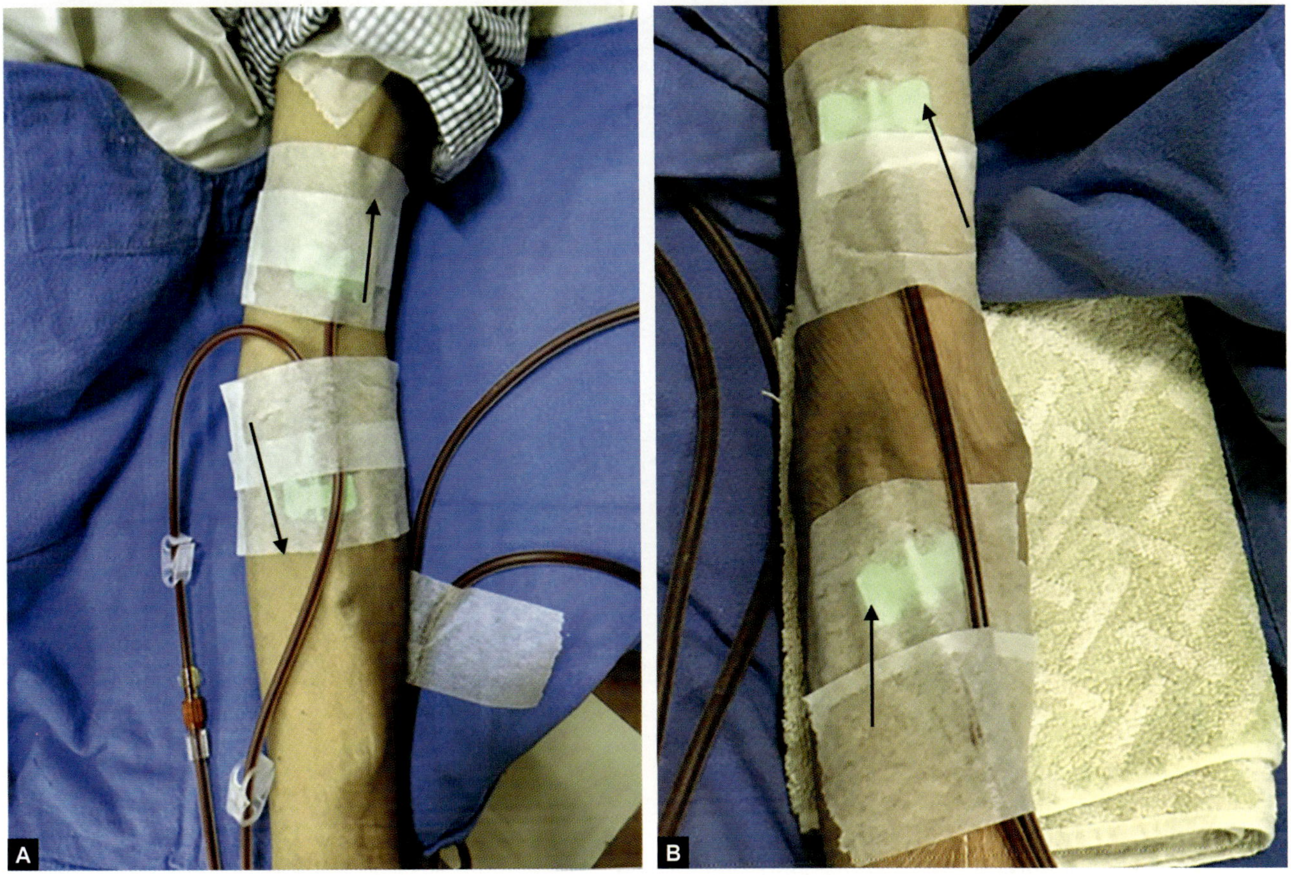

Figs. 9A and B: (A) Fistula cannulation—needles in opposite direction; (B) Fistula cannulation—needles in same direction.

- Cannulation of arteriovenous fistula for hemodialysis.
- Proximal end (downstream) is venous and distal end (upstream) is arterial, *cannulated in opposite directions* (Fig. 9A).
- Cannulation done in same direction (Fig. 9B).
- Cannulation of the AV fistula is generally done with two 16 g/17 g dialysis needles.
- The needles are placed into the dilated arterialized vein.
- The needle for dialyzer inlet is placed more upstream, at least 3 cm away from the anastomosis.
- The arterial needle may be used pointing upstream or downstream.
- The venous needle for return of blood to the heart, should point downstream approximately 5 cm away from the upstream needle.
- This recommended distance reduces the chances of access recirculation.
- Cannulation can be done using two methods, viz. buttonhole and rope ladder technique.
- The rope ladder technique uses entire length of dilated vein for repeated cannulation. This method avoids the risk of weakening the venous wall which happens in cases of repeated cannulations in the same areas.

PATIENT WITH SEVERE GOUT (FIGS. 10A AND B)

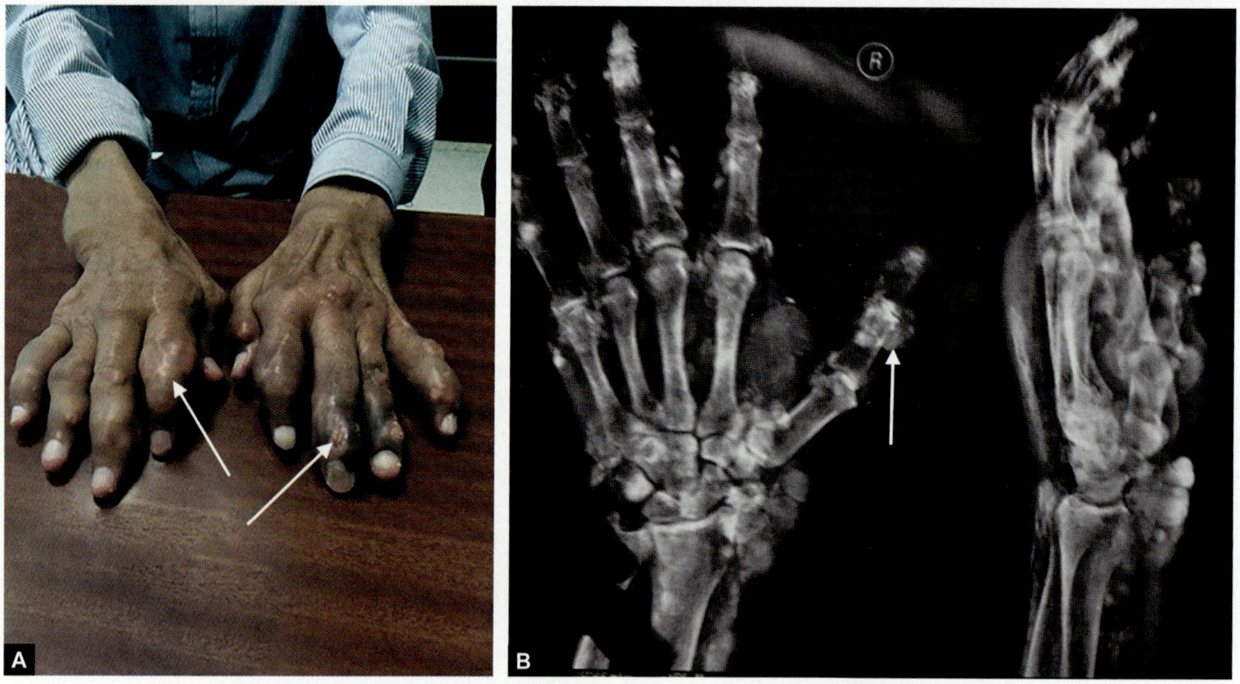

Figs. 10A and B: (A) Gout; (B) Gouty tophi wrist X-ray showing multiple gouty tophi in the fingers.

- A patient of severe gout with X-ray of wrist showing multiple gouty tophi in the fingers.
- This patient was from a middle-eastern country and had gouty pain for many years.
- He now presented with chronic kidney disease.
- Hyperuricemia and gout is associated with renal stones.
- Effective treatment with xanthine oxidase inhibitors can prevent tophaceous gout.

NONTUNNELED HEMODIALYSIS CATHETER (FIG. 11)

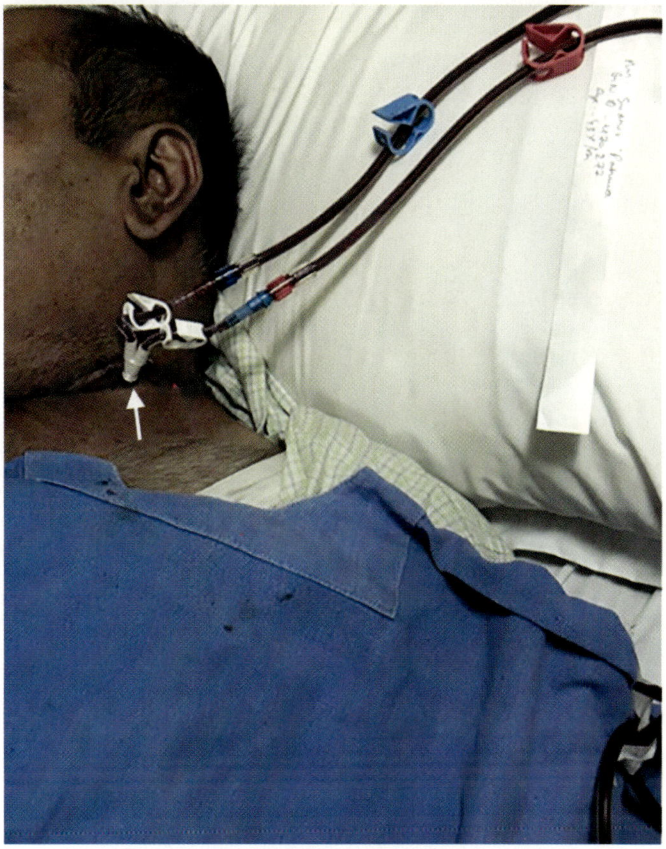

Fig. 11: Nontunneled hemodialysis catheter.

- Nontunneled catheter is the most common mode of venous access for urgent initiation of hemodialysis in acute kidney injury and CKD without pre-existing AV fistula.
- A large bore vein is required to attain blood flow rates of 250–350 mL/min for dialysis.
- Nontunneled catheter has two ports, viz. red port/arterial end for blood flow to dialysis machine and blue port/venous end for return of dialyzed blood to the heart.
- Most common site for venous access is right internal jugular vein, followed by left internal jugular and femoral vein.
- Subclavian vein access is associated with significant rates of venous stenosis.
- Nontunneled catheters are associated with increased risk of bacteremia as against AV fistula/tunneled catheters.

BRACHIOCEPHALIC ARTERIOVENOUS FISTULA SHOWING ANEURYSMAL DILATATION AND TORTUOSITY (FIG. 12)

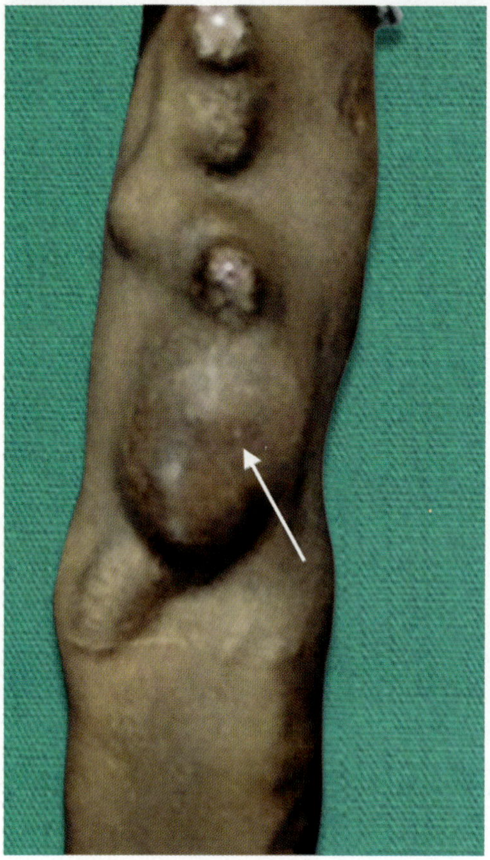

Fig. 12: Left brachiocephalic AV fistula showing aneurysmal dilatation and tortuosity in a patient on long-term hemodialysis.

- A picture of left brachiocephalic arteriovenous fistula showing aneurysmal dilatation and tortuosity in a patient on long-term hemodialysis.
- Aneurysmal dilatations of AV fistulas are at increased risk of rupture and life-threatening bleed.
- Repeated cannulation in the same areas leads to aneurysm formation due to weakened vessel wall.
- The preferred method of cannulation to reduce the chances of aneurysms is rope ladder technique.

AUTOLOGOUS LOWER EXTREMITY ARTERIOVENOUS FISTULA (FIGS. 13A AND B)

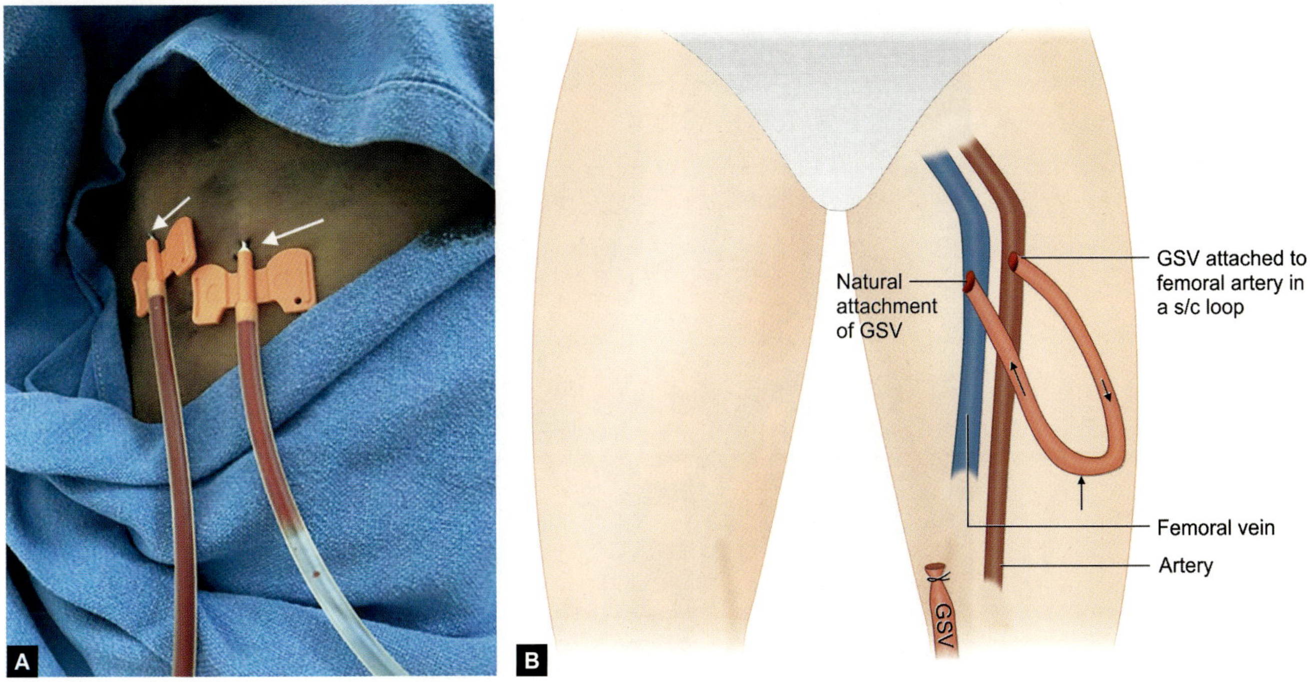

Figs. 13A and B: (A) Saphenofemoral vein loop arteriovenous fistula cannulation; (B) Saphenofemoral loop arteriovenous fistula cannulation schematic. (GSV: Great saphenous vein)

- A patient of CKD on maintenance dialysis through autologous lower extremity arteriovenous fistula.
- The patient had multiple access failure with no venous access in the upper limb.
- Left great saphenous vein was looped, transposed and anastomosed to left femoral (superficial femoral artery).
- Patient is presently on dialysis through the access.
- Lower limb venous access is an alternative to upper limb access in case of central venous stenosis/exhausted upper limb access.
- Various types of venous access include:
  1. Autologous lower extremity AV fistula (index case).
  2. Synthetic lower extremity AV graft.
  3. Lower extremity central venous catheter.

MUCORMYCOSIS OF KIDNEY (FIGS. 14A TO D)

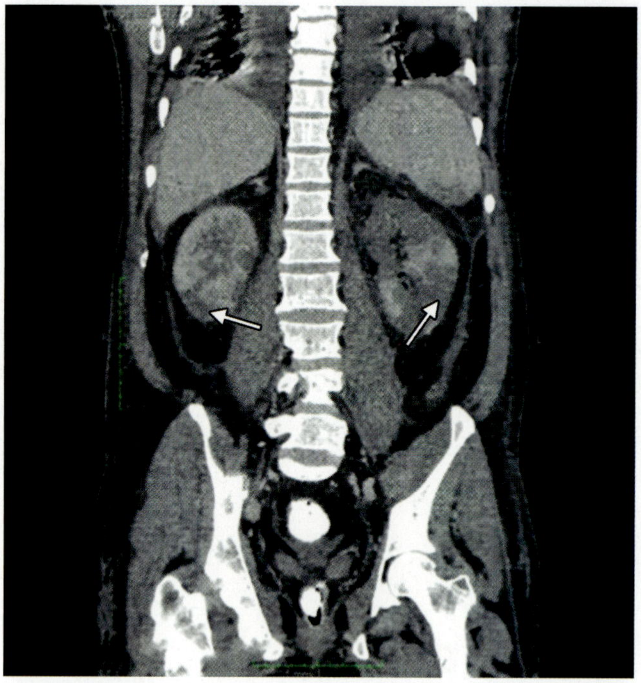

Fig. 14A: Renal infarction in a case with mucormycosis of kidney.

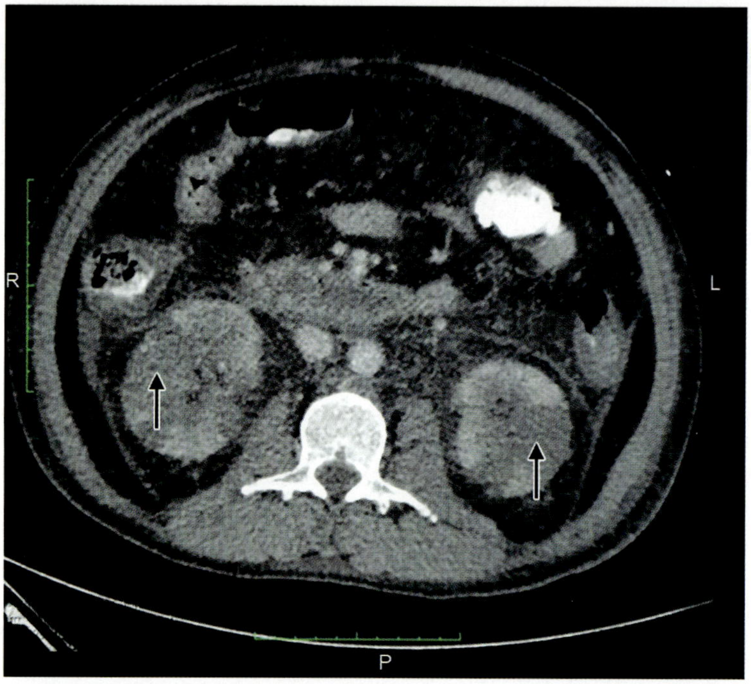

Fig. 14B: Renal infarction in a case with mucor of kidney transverse.

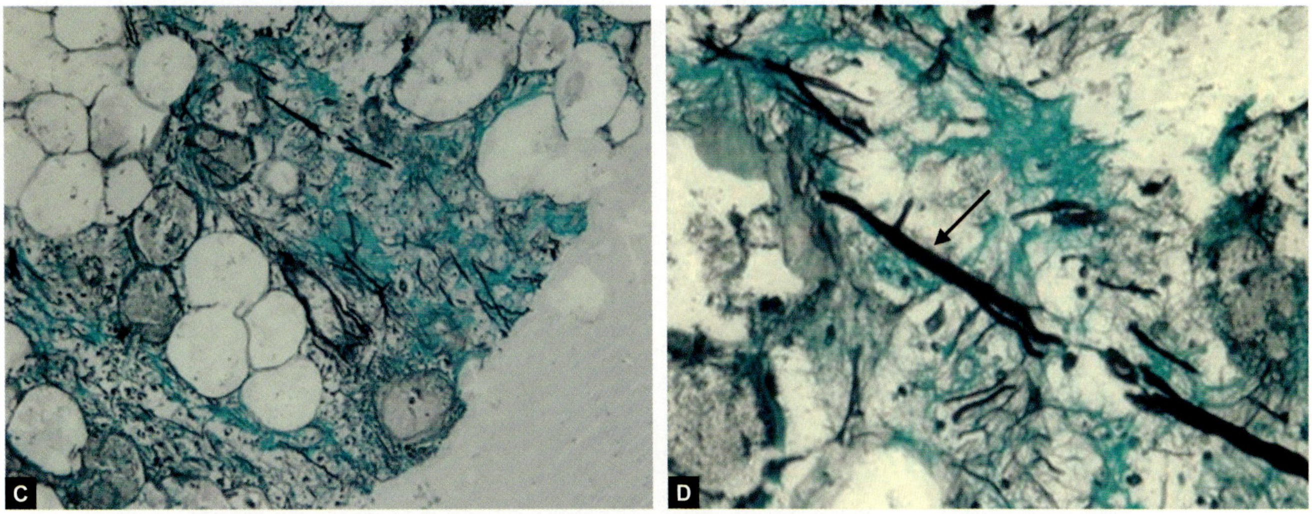

Figs. 14C and D: Renal biopsy showing mucor.

- CT and kidney biopsy images of a patient who presented with fever, oliguria of acute onset, and flank pain of 2 weeks duration.
- Initial features were suggestive of pyelonephritis.
- CT scan of abdomen revealed extensive bilateral renal infarction in an otherwise healthy individual.
- Patient underwent renal biopsy for further diagnosis which revealed acute diffuse cortical necrosis with presence of broad aseptate hyphae of mucormycosis in the necrotic debris of the perirenal fatty tissue.
- It was a rare case of isolated renal mucormycosis in a taxi driver from rural area who was immunocompetent.
- Antifungal treatment with amphotericin b was started and patient advised bilateral nephrectomy.
- He refused to consent for nephrectomy.
- He succumbed to his illness after 1 week.
- Mucormycosis is an opportunistic infection seen in immunocompromised individuals like those with acquired immunodeficiency syndrome (AIDS), solid organ transplant recipients, diabetes mellitus, intravenous (IV) catheter/ drug abuse, etc.
- It is a life-threatening infection which needs urgent treatment with antifungals and most of the times, nephrectomy in case of renal involvement.

DMSA SCAN WITH SPECT IMAGE (FIG. 15)

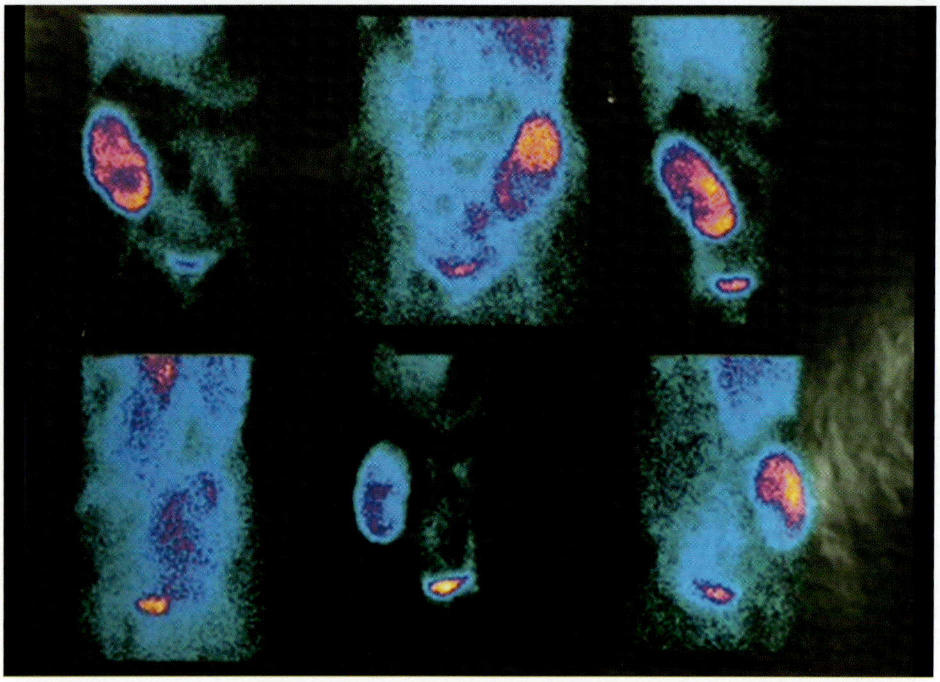

Fig. 15: SPECT image of a renal transplant recipient who underwent DMSA scan.

- Single-photon emission computed tomography (SPECT) image of a renal transplant recipient who underwent dimercaptosuccinic acid (DMSA) scan.
- Renal transplant recipient underwent a DMSA scan to evaluate for higher baseline creatinine.
- DMSA scan with SPECT image shows wedge-shaped infarction in the lower pole of the graft kidney.
- Donor kidney retrieved after donor nephrectomy had a small accessory artery which possibly was injured during the surgery leading to infarction of the portion of kidney being supplied.
- Presence of accessory artery in donor kidney is associated with occurrence of silent vascular infarcts in the graft kidney.
- Larger infarctions are associated with a baseline creatinine above the normal range.
- DMSA scan is established as a standard of care investigation modality for infarction and pyelonephritis in the native kidneys.
- The same principle was used to investigate vascular insults in the transplant recipients.

CONTINUOUS RENAL REPLACEMENT THERAPY (FIGS. 16A AND B)

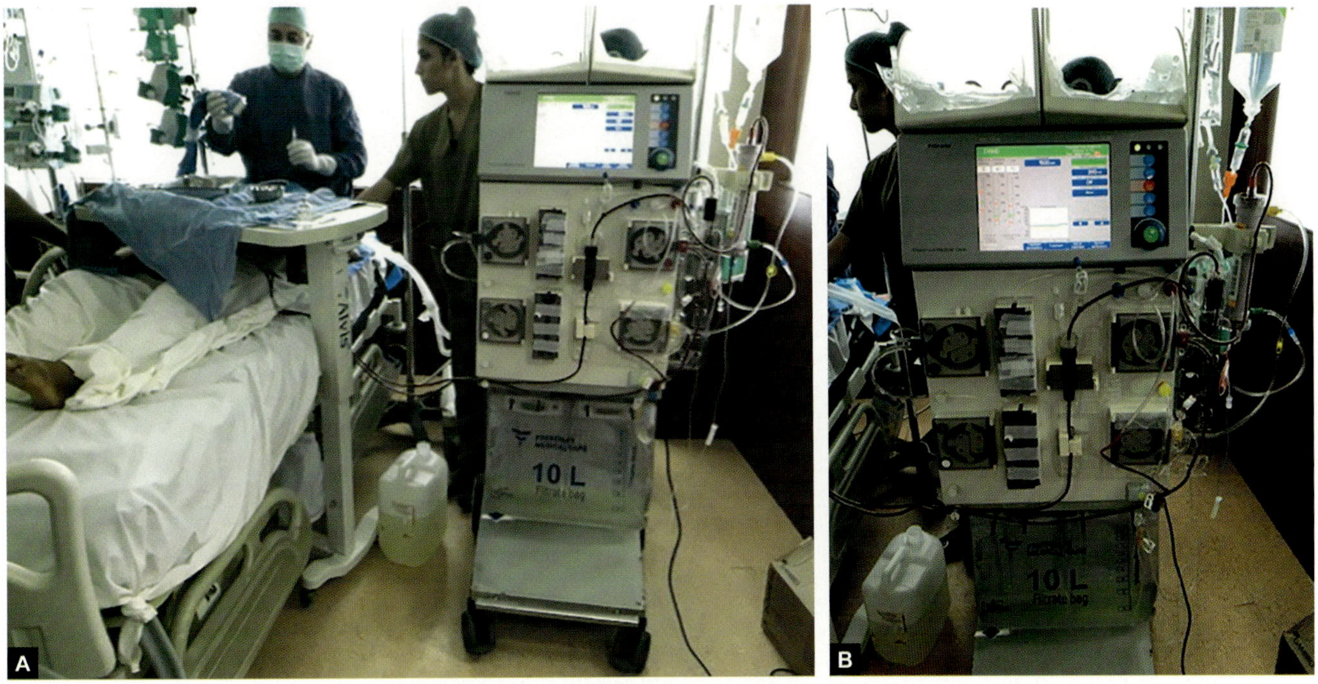

Figs. 16A and B: (A) A patient undergoing continuous renal replacement therapy (CRRT); (B) CRRT connections.

- Images showing a patient undergoing continuous renal replacement therapy (CRRT) and CRRT connections.
- CRRT is a modality of slow dialysis used in patients who are critically ill and have acute kidney injury (AKI).
- This patient was admitted with scrub typhus and AKI in anuric state, with severe metabolic acidosis and hypotension requiring multiple inotropic support.
- He was given CRRT support with which his acidosis improved and cumulative fluid load improved.
- CRRT is a modality used in hemodynamically unstable patients in the ICU.
- Modes of CRRT include:
    - CVVHD—continuous venovenous hemodialysis.
    - CVVH—continuous venovenous hemofiltration.
    - CVVHDF—continuous venovenous hemodiafiltration.
    - SCUF—slow continuous ultrafiltration.
- The image shows CRRT machine.
- It has a touch screen monitor for programming the desired functions for dialysis.
- Four pumps are also seen, viz. Pumps for dialysis fluid, blood, substitution fluid (HF/HDF mode) and effluent.
- An effluent bag with effluent is seen hanging on hooks which have weight sensors.
- There is a heparin pump, dialyzer connected to the dialyzer stand.
- Blood is flowing countercurrent to the dialysis fluid in the dialyzer as seen in the connection.
- Above the monitor are the weight sensing trays for dialysis fluid placement.

DIGITAL INFARCTION SECONDARY TO VASCULAR STEAL PHENOMENON (FIG. 17)

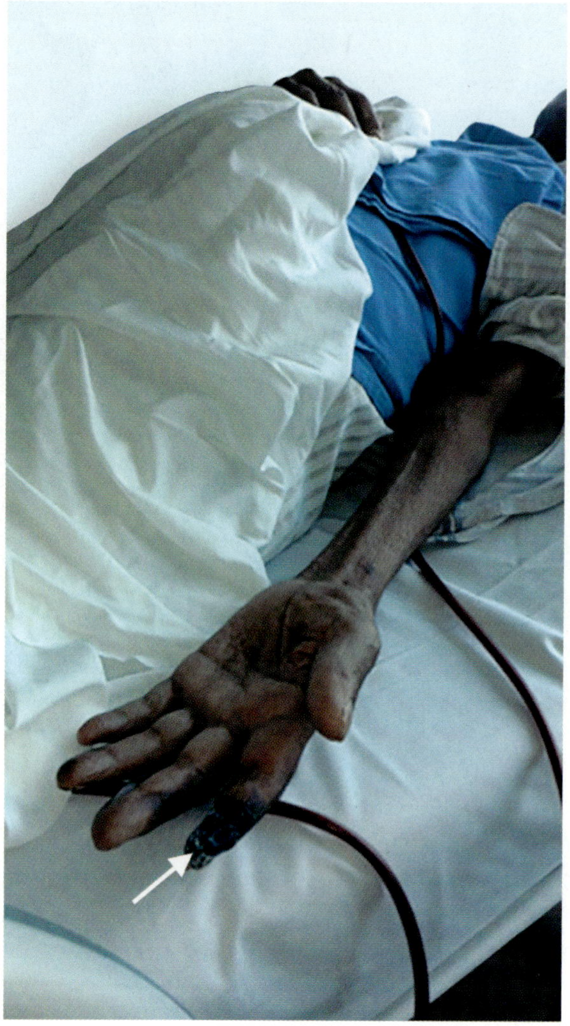

Fig. 17: A patient with digital infarction secondary to vascular steal phenomenon.

- Patient is a case of diabetic CKD on maintenance dialysis through AV fistula.
- He developed digital ischemic infarction secondary to vascular steal phenomenon.
- Vascular access-induced upper limb ischemia is a serious complication that without prompt intervention may lead to amputation.
- Elderly patients, diabetics, and patients with peripheral or coronary arterial occlusive disease are most at risk of ischemia.
- Access-induced ischemia occurs more often with proximally located fistulas.
- Pain during hemodialysis (HD) is a characteristic early symptom.
- Surgical management is indicated for flow reduction and other measures.

LEFT BRACHIOCEPHALIC TRUNK STENOSIS (FIG. 18)

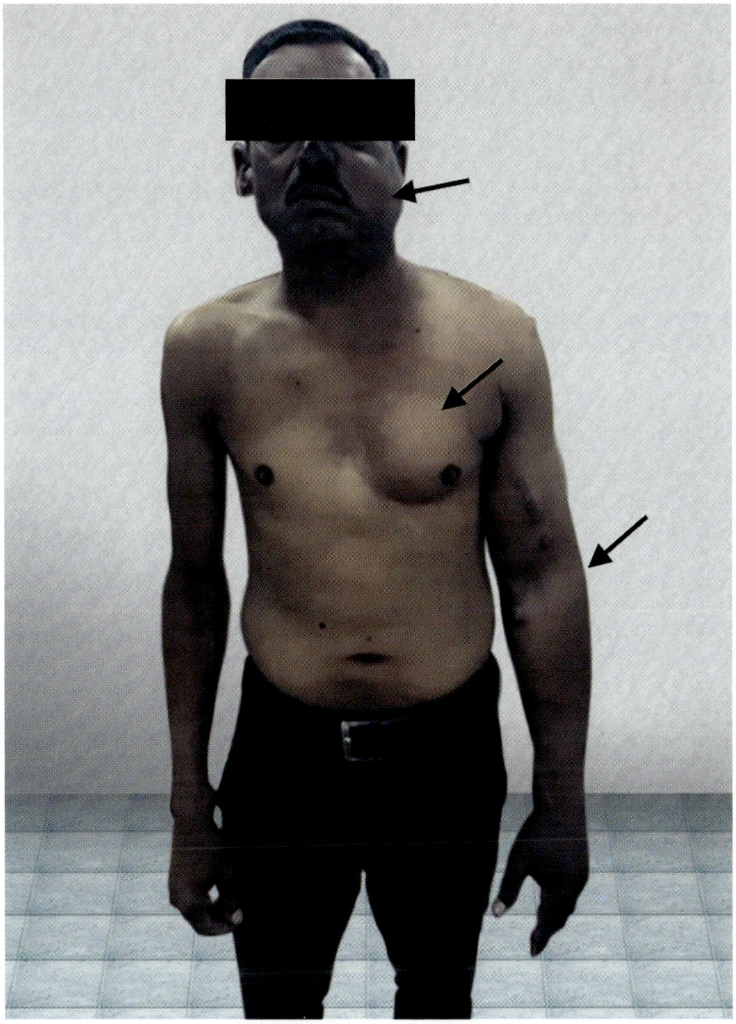

Fig. 18: A patient with left brachiocephalic trunk stenosis.

- Patient had gradually increasing edema of left upper limb, face and left side of chest.
- Doppler ultrasound and CT venogram of left upper limb and neck veins revealed stenosis of the left brachiocephalic trunk.
- Patient underwent fluoroscopic-guided percutaneous balloon angioplasty with opening up of the stenosis.
- Following balloon angioplasty, there was restoration of flow and reduction of edema.
- Central venous stenosis is a common problem in patients on maintenance dialysis secondary to venous catheters.
- Endovascular/surgical management is indicated in such cases to relieve symptoms and restore flows.

CHAPTER 20

Ocular Emergencies: Illustration and Management

Sonam Yangzes, Aniruddha Agarwal, Jagat Ram

INTRODUCTION

The eye is a very delicate and important organ of the body. Even though the eyelids play a protective role from direct injuries, many forms of trauma of conditions may make the eye susceptible to vision loss. Ocular emergencies are an important cause of preventable blindness and the key to it lies in early diagnosis and prompt management. This section highlights several such ocular conditions along with the clinical features and treatment. An ICU physician may recognize the signs and symptoms and make an early referral to his/her ophthalmology colleague and even initiate baseline therapy to avoid worsening of the condition.

OCULAR CHEMICAL BURNS (FIGS. 1A AND B)

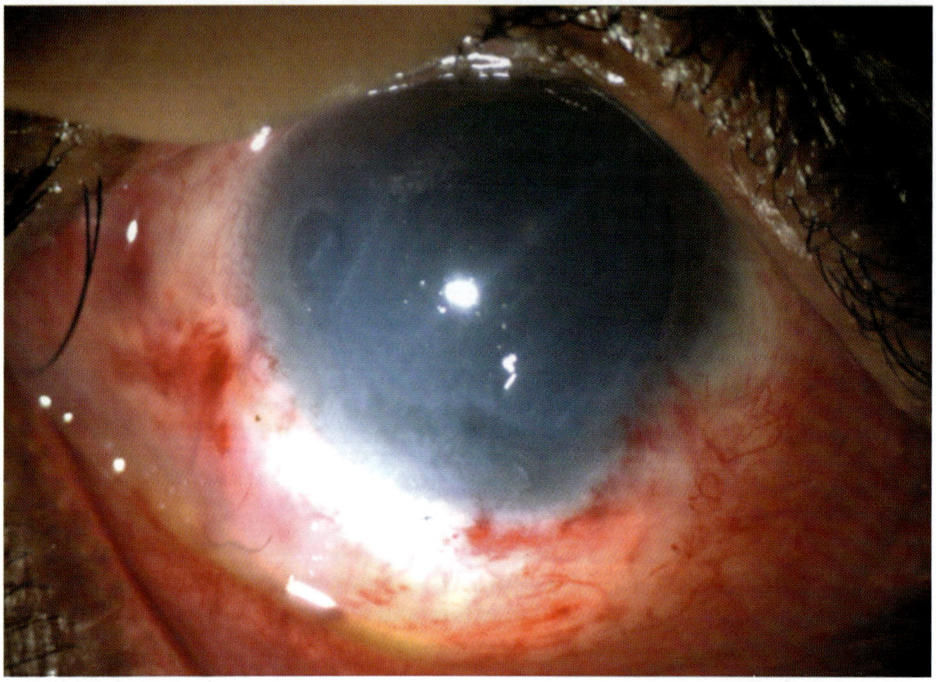

Fig. 1A: Alkali injury in right eye. Note the presence of inferior 180° limbal ischemia with associated corneal and conjunctival defect.

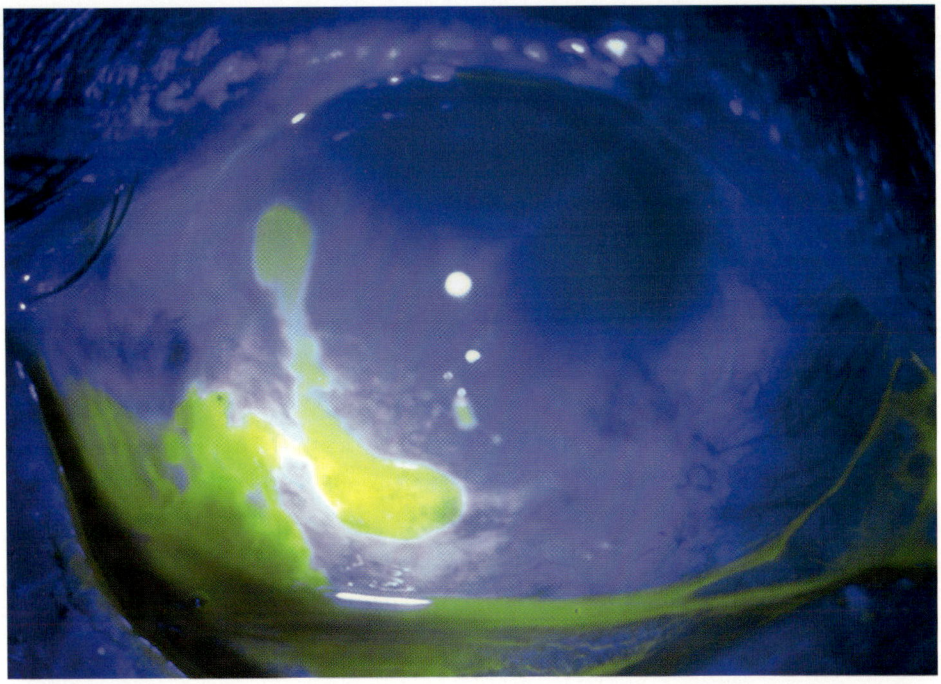

Fig. 1B: Fluorescein stain in blue light shows extent of corneal and conjunctival epithelial defect.

Chemical injury can occur due to either alkali or acidic material instilled in the eye. Alkali injury is more severe as the alkali penetrates deeper tissue while acid tends to undergo saponification and, hence, less severe injury. Nonetheless, all chemical injury cases need to be promptly managed in the form of copious irrigation with saline or Ringer lactate or even tap water.

Signs

- Corneal and conjunctival epithelial defects.
- Limbal ischemia.
- Chemosis and hemorrhage may be seen.

Treatment

After prompt and copious irrigation, slit lamp evaluation using fluorescein stain must be done to measure extent of epithelial defect. Topical cycloplegic agents along with antibiotic drops must be used. Oral as well as topical steroids in the first 7–10 days to control inflammation. Oral and topical steroids must be tapered soon during reparative phase. Frequent use of preservative-free tear substitutes in addition to gel formulation at night is advised. Oral tetracycline and vitamin C also reduce collagen lysis and stromal melting.

CORNEAL ULCER (FIG. 2)

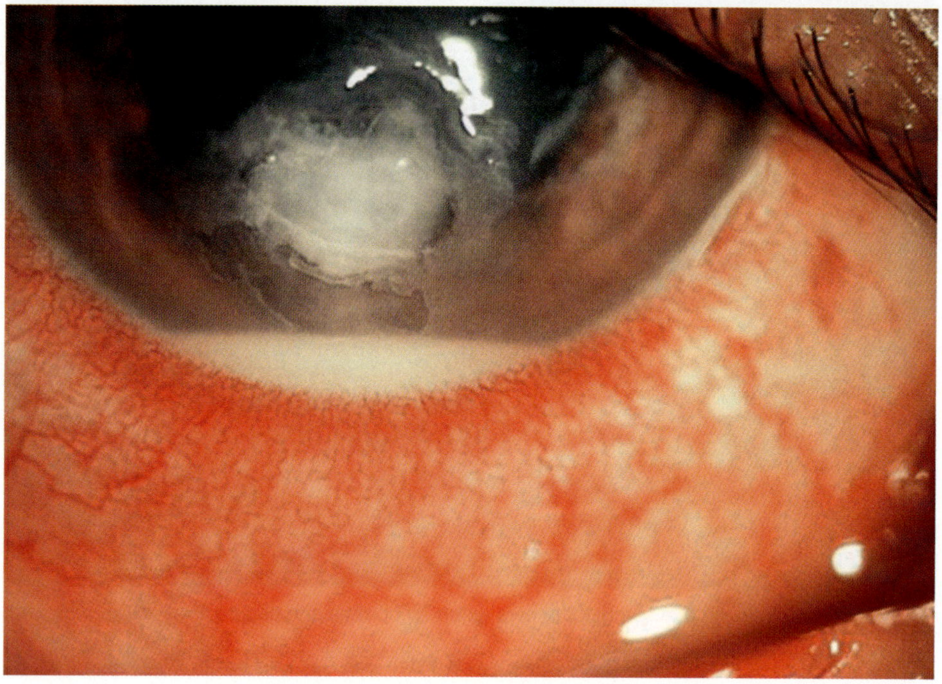

Fig. 2: Corneal ulceration with infiltrate and hypopyon.

An ulcer is defined as epithelial defect with underlying infiltrate. Cases with bacterial keratitis usually report with a sudden onset and rapid progression, while fungal ulcers have a more indolent course. In cases with sterile ulceration with peripheral location, one must rule out connective tissue disorders (Table 1).

Symptoms

Redness, photophobia, discharge, decreased vision, and moderate-to-severe pain associated with lid swelling.

Signs

Epithelial defect, mucopurulent discharge, stromal edema, anterior chamber reaction, with or without hypopyon. Fungal ulcers present with more symptoms than signs. Typical signs of fungal ulcer include dry-looking ulcer with convex hypopyon.

Table 1: The predisposing factors in case of corneal ulcer.

Ocular	*Systemic*	*Occupational*
Topical medications	Stevens–Johnson syndrome	Gardeners
Trauma	Diabetes mellitus	Farmers
Contact lens	Connective tissue disorders	Animal handlers
Ocular surgery/exposure keratitis in ICU	Extremes of age	
Allergic eye disease (shield ulcer)	AIDS	

(AIDS: Acquired immunodeficiency syndrome; ICU: Intensive care unit)

Management (Table 2)

We must collect corneal scrapings to find the causative organisms. Steps of sample collection include: (1) Topical anesthetic is applied. (2) Purulent material is removed by a sterile cotton swab and discarded. (3) Lid speculum may be used (to prevent eyelashes contaminating—the Kimura spatula/BP No. 15 blade) or assistant should hold the lids apart. (4) Tissue should be obtained from interface between normal and visibly involved stroma. (5) Multiple corneal scrapings under slit lamp magnification need to be collected. (6) Material is inoculated directly onto various media.

Table 2: Differential diagnosis of microbial keratitis.

Slowly progressive localized	*Rapidly progressive diffuse*

Bacteria:
Fungi:
• Filamentous fungi:
  - *Fusarium*
  - *Aspergillus*
  - *Dematiaceous*
• Yeast-like:
  - *Candida*
• Gram negative:
  - *Moraxella*
  - *Serratia*
• Gram positive:
  - *Staphylococcus epidermidis*
  - Alpha-hemolytic streptococci
  - Other than *Streptococcus pneumoniae*
  - Actinomycetales:
    ▪ *Actinomyces*
    ▪ *Nocardia*
	Bacteria:
	• Gram negative:
	  - *Pseudomonas*
	  - *Enterobacteriaceae*
	  - Mixed infection
	• Gram positive:
	  - *Staphylococcus aureus*
	  - *Streptococcus pneumoniae*
	  - Beta-hemolytic streptococci
	Protozoa:
	• *Acanthamoeba*
	• *Microsporidia*

Treatment

Ulcers are initially treated as bacterial until proved otherwise with culture or smear. In cases with very high index of suspicion of another form of infection, one may add antifungal or antimicrobial agent sensitive to organism.

Medical Therapy

Broad spectrum fortified antibiotics are used frequently along with cycloplegic agents, antiglaucoma medications and lubricating eye drops. Combined fortified cefazolin sodium (5%)/vancomycin (5%) and tobramycin (1.3%)/amikacin (5%) are given hourly for the initial 48 hours. Following initial response to therapy, dosage is reduced to 2 hourly or monotherapy in the form of broad spectrum antibiotic is given. Systemic therapy is given only in severe cases with scleral involvement, impending perforations or associated endophthalmitis. Natamycin (5%) and voriconazole (1%) are used in cases of filamentous fungal infections. In case of yeast-related ulceration, amphotericin B (0.15%) has a role. Topical antibiotics are routinely given even in proven fungal keratitis to prevent bacterial infection. In cases of stromal abscess or deeper ulcers, intracameral or intrastromal antibiotics or antifungals have a role.

Surgical Therapy

Therapeutic keratoplasty or patch graft is performed in cases with corneal perforation or melt. In cases with less than 2 mm of perforation, cyanoacrylate glue can be used to seal the perforation.

ACUTE ANGLE-CLOSURE GLAUCOMA (FIG. 3)

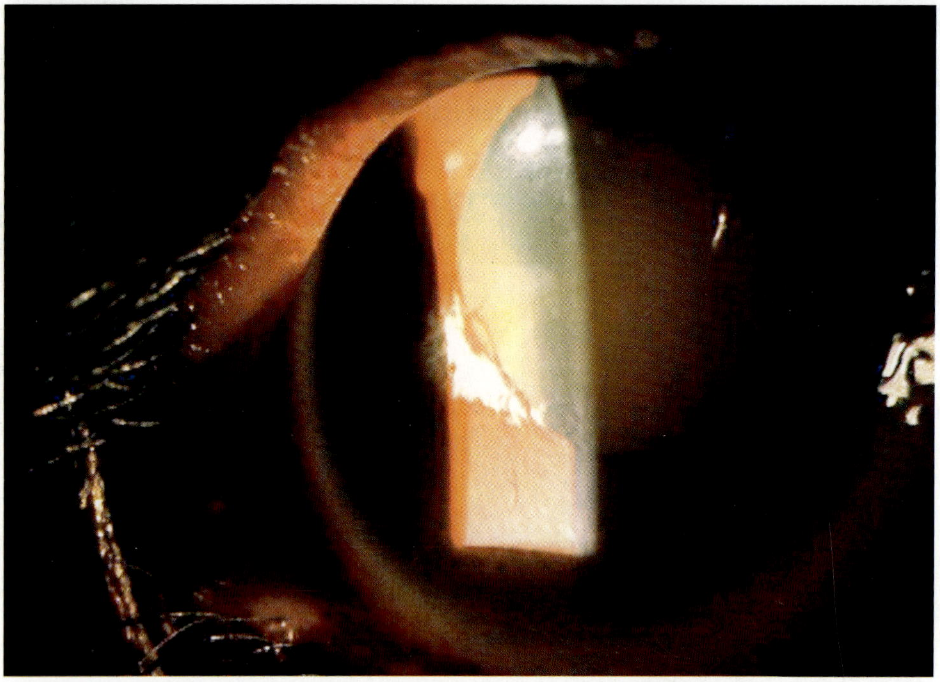

Fig. 3: Acute angle-closure glaucoma. Shallow anterior chamber with iris atrophy.

Symptoms

Ocular pain, colored halos, blurred vision, nausea, and vomiting.

Signs

Raised intraocular pressure (IOP), conjunctival injection, corneal edema, fixed and mid-dilated pupil, and closed angle.

Management

Urgent reduction in IOP with oral or intravenous (mannitol) antiglaucoma medications. Compression gonioscopy is done to determine trabecular blockage and to break acute attack. Topical antiglaucoma therapy such as beta-blockers (timolol—0.5%), alpha-2 agonists (brimonidine—0.15%), and carbonic anhydrase inhibitors (dorzolamide—2%) are used. Topical steroids are used to control the inflammation. Definitive treatment in pupillary block glaucoma after the anterior chamber becomes quiet and cornea clears is in the form of laser iridotomy or surgical iridectomy.

LENS-INDUCED GLAUCOMA (FIG. 4)

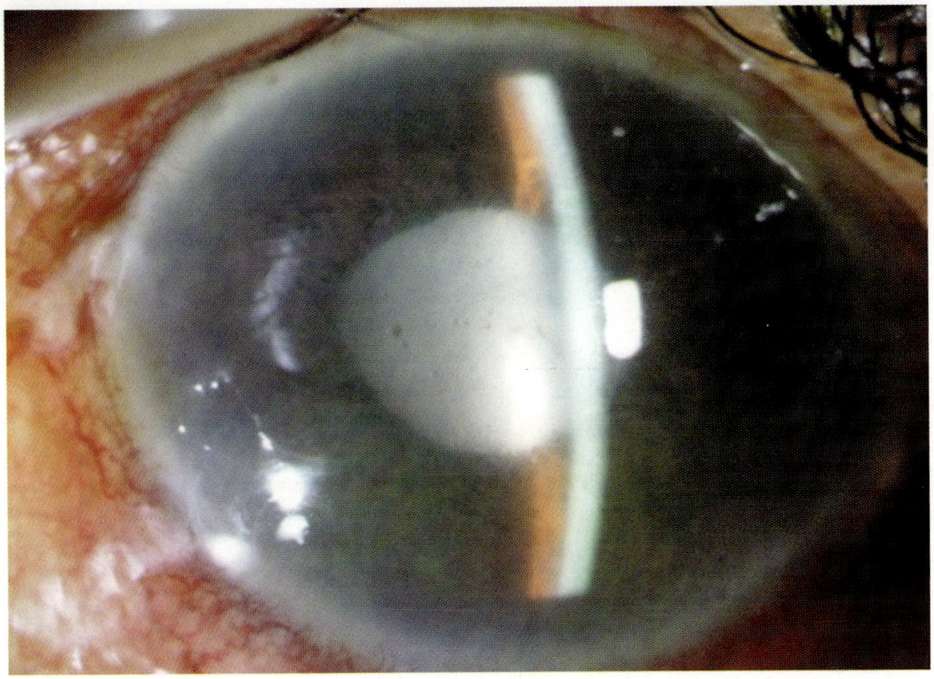

Fig. 4: Phacomorphic glaucoma. Shallow anterior chamber (AC) with intumescent white cataract.

Phacomorphic Glaucoma

Phacomorphic glaucoma is caused by closure of anterior due to intumescent lens. The mechanism of glaucoma is pupillary block.

Symptoms: Blurring of vision associated with pain and photophobia.

Signs: Corneal edema, mid-dilated pupil, shallow anterior chamber.

Management: The management of phacomorphic glaucoma includes control intraocular pressure with oral and topical carbonic anhydrase inhibitors and hyperosmotic agents. Laser iridotomy may help in breaking an attack though definitive treatment remains cataract extraction.

PHACOLYTIC GLAUCOMA (FIG. 5)

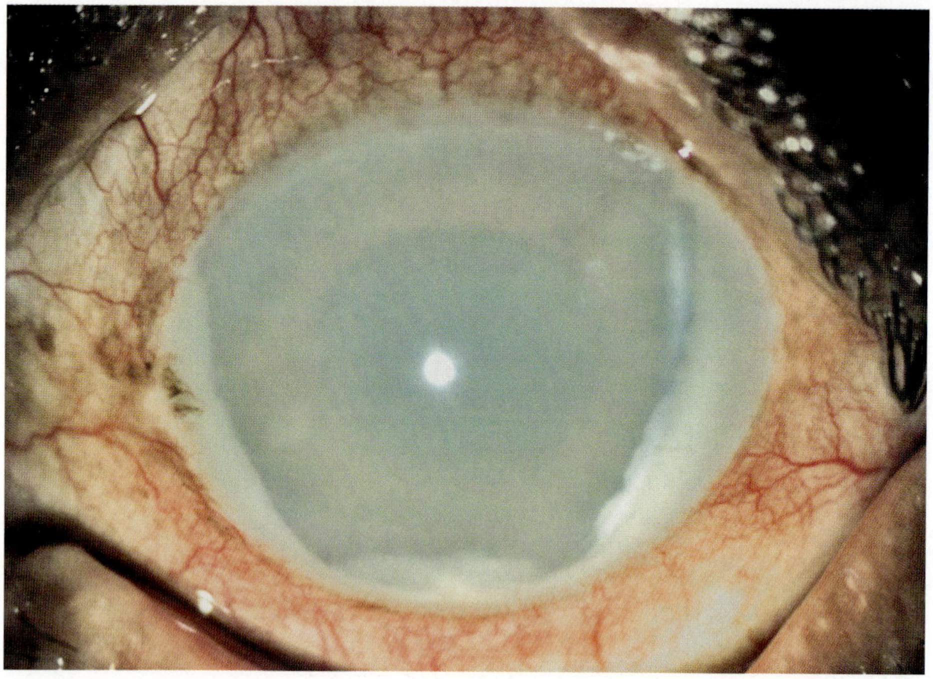

Fig. 5: Phacolytic glaucoma: corneal edema with presence of whitish lens matter deposit in the anterior chamber.

Mechanism

Leakage of lens matter through intact lens capsule with subsequent obstruction of trabecular meshwork.

Symptoms

Blurring of vision, pain and photophobia.

Signs

Marked increase in intraocular pressure, whitish material in anterior chamber with a hypermature cataract. Associated corneal edema, hypopyon may be present.

Management

The steps of management include immediate control of IOP and reduction of inflammation. Topical beta blockers (timolol 0.5% BD), alpha-2 agonists (brimonidine 0.1–0.2% TDS) and carbonic anhydrase inhibitors (CAIs) (dorzolamide 2% TDS) are used. Oral CAIs (acetazolamide 250 mg TDS), topical cycloplegic (atropine 1%) and topical steroids (prednisolone acetate 1%/betamethasone 0.5%) are added. Cataract removal is performed after control of IOP.

PENETRATING EYE INJURY (FIG. 6)

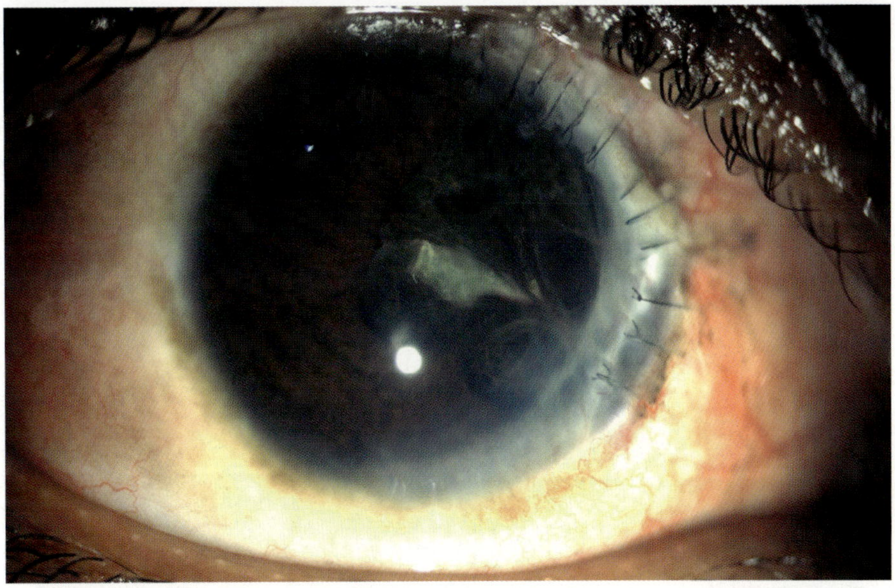

Fig. 6: Penetrating eye injury.

Every case of ocular trauma must be evaluated carefully for signs of penetrating injury. Presence of full thickness scleral or corneal laceration with uveal tissue prolapse, shallow anterior chamber, full chamber hyphema, subconjunctival hemorrhage, peaked or irregular pupil, iridodialysis, and vitreous or lens matter in anterior chamber. Presence of an intraocular foreign body.

Management

Promptly patch the affected eye and plan primary repair as soon as possible.

OPTIC NEURITIS (FIG. 7)

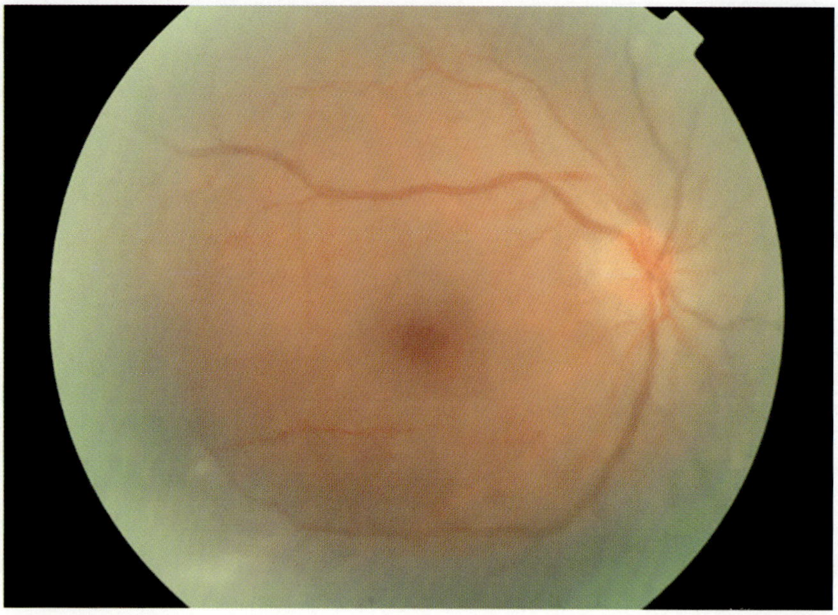

Fig. 7: Fundus photograph of a 25-year-old male diagnosed with optic neuritis. There is presence of disk hyperemia and blurring of the disk margins.

Symptoms

Painless loss of vision over hours to days occurs in patients with optic neuritis. Vision loss can be subtle or profound. Reduced visual acuity, color, and contrast vision are noted on examination. Optic neuritis is usually unilateral, but may rarely be bilateral. More often affecting females aged between 18 and 45. Orbital pain is usually associated with eye movement. There may be other focal neurological symptoms.

Signs

Signs of optic neuritis include—relative afferent pupillary defect (RAPD); decreased visual acuity; decreased color vision; patchy visual field defects; swollen optic disk; and other focal neurological signs.

Investigation and Management

Complete ophthalmic and neurological examination must be performed. Additional laboratory analysis includes—blood count/erythrocyte sedimentation rate (ESR); magnetic resonance imaging (MRI) brain and orbit; intravenous steroid (methylprednisolone). There are no indications for oral corticosteroids as initial treatment in cases of optic neuritis.

CENTRAL RETINAL ARTERY OCCLUSION (FIG. 8)

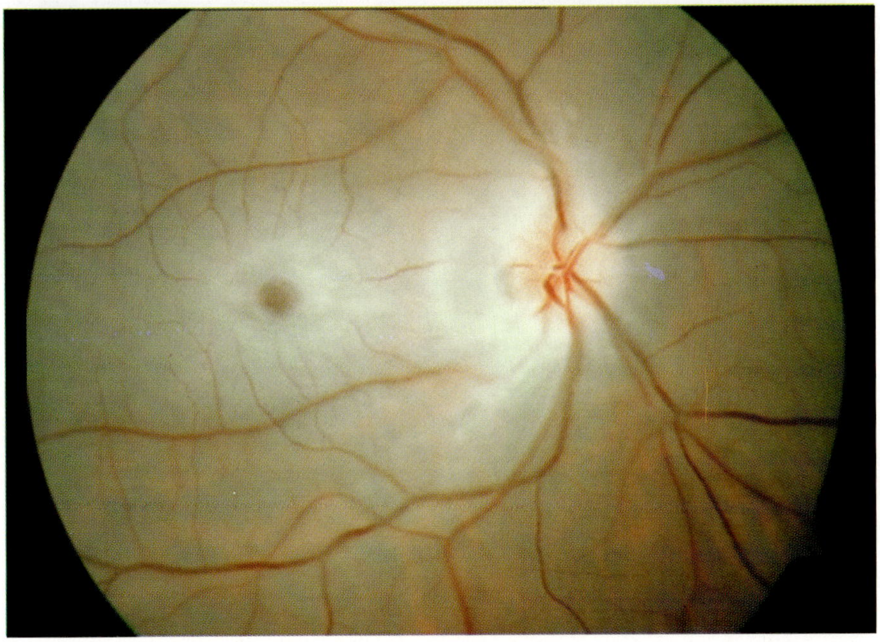

Fig. 8: Fundus picture showing ischemic pale retina with "cherry-red spot".

Central retinal artery occlusion (CRAO) presents with sudden, painless, and profound visual loss developing over seconds with RAPD. Fundus examination shows retinal opacification located in the posterior pole with normal-looking peripheral fundus. There may be a cherry-red spot in 90% of patients within 1 week of onset retinal arterial changes include—boxcar/cattle trucking; attenuation of arterioles; sheathing of arteries. Optic disk changes include—initial disk edema in 22% with development of disk pallor due to optic atrophy. Emboli may be seen in retinal arteries in 20–40% patients. Most common emboli are cholesterol emboli (Hollenhorst plaques).

Management

Initial conservative management for CRAO includes ocular massage, anterior chamber paracentesis, hyperbaric oxygen therapy, oral acetazolamide, and use of vasodilators such as sublingual isosorbide dinitrate. Invasive management options include selective ophthalmic artery catheterization through femoral artery and injection of thrombolytic agents.

ENDOPHTHALMITIS (FIGS. 9A AND B)

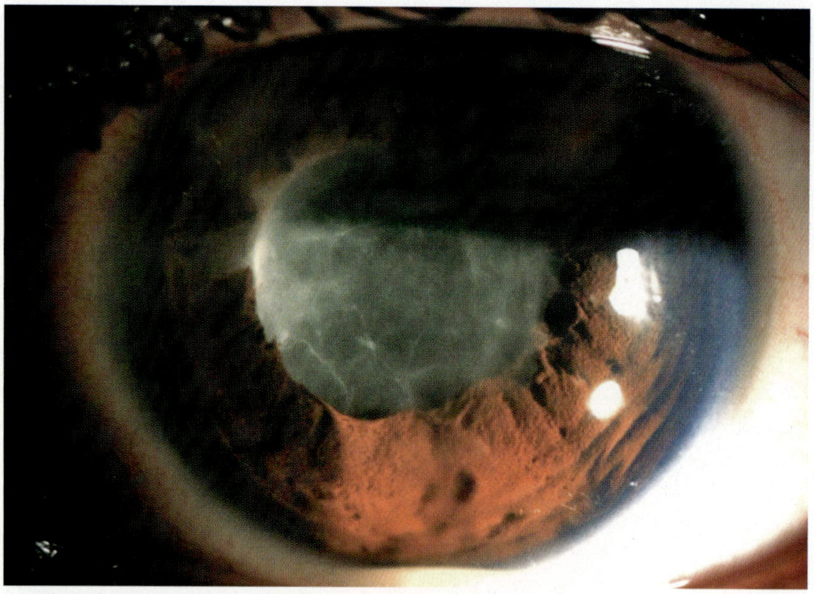

Fig. 9A: Postoperative endophthalmitis. Fibrin on anterior lens surface and hypopyon.

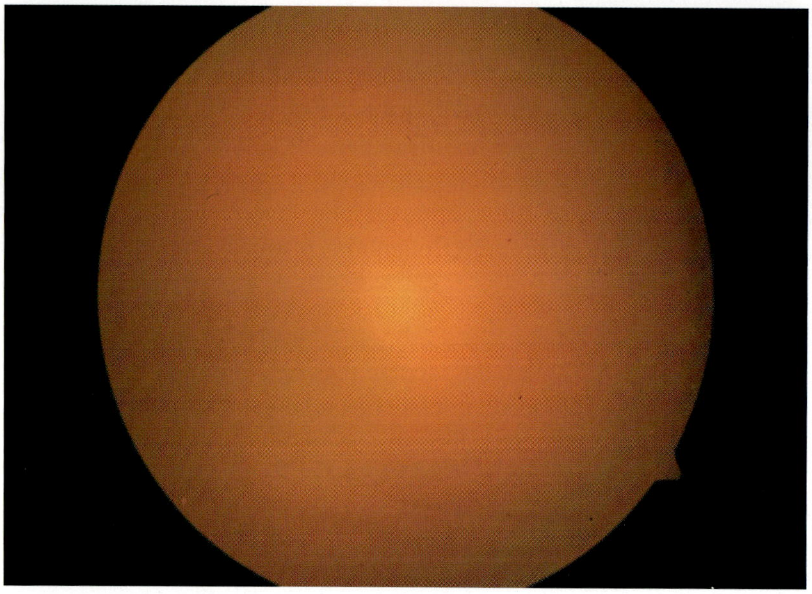

Fig. 9B: Fundus photograph shows presence of distinct yellow glow suggestive of vitreous exudates in a patient with endophthalmitis.

Endophthalmitis refers to purulent inflammation of vitreous and/or aqueous humor. It can follow trauma, ocular surgery, or after administration of intravenous fluids (endogenous endophthalmitis).

Symptoms

Sudden onset blurring of vision associated with redness following ocular surgery or trauma.

Signs

Hypopyon, fibrin, anterior chamber reaction, vitreous cells and membranes, and decreased red reflex.

Organisms

Coagulase-negative *Staphylococcus*: *Staphylococcus epidermidis* is the most common organism responsible for post-operative endophthalmitis. Others include *Staphylococcus aureus*, *Streptococcus* species, *Bacillus* species, and Gram-negative bacteria (*Pseudomonas*, *Aerobacter*, *Escherichia coli*, *Klebsiella*, *Proteus* species, etc.). Fungal endophthalmitis may be associated with history of trauma with vegetative matter.

Treatment

According to the endophthalmitis study (EVS), if visual acuity is light perception or worse, pars plana vitrectomy with intravitreal antibiotics is considered. In cases with better visual acuity, antibiotics can be given after taking a vitreous tap for culture and sensitivity.

The patient must be admitted and started on intravenous antibiotics along with topical antibiotics and cycloplegic agents. Intravenous antibiotics may be repeated after 48 hours of first injection. If inflammation does not decrease, the early vitrectomy may be considered.

BLOWOUT FRACTURE OF ORBIT (FIG. 10)

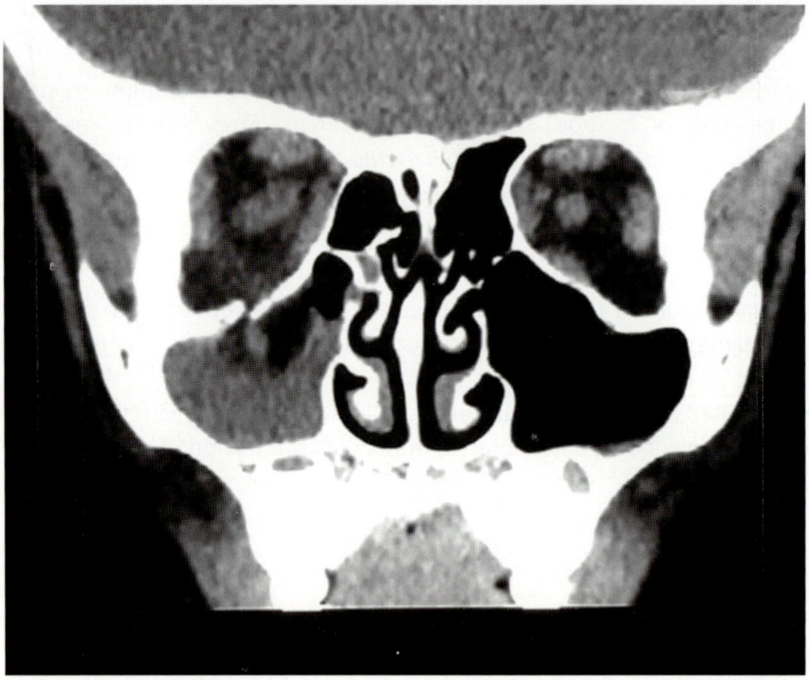

Fig. 10: Coronal CT image of blowout fracture.

Symptoms

Pain (especially on vertical movement), local tenderness, diplopia, eyelid swelling and crepitus after nose blowing. A "white" blow-out fracture occurs with orbital injury with the findings of minimal periorbital hemorrhage, sunken globe, restricted eye movement in an unwell child.

Signs

Nose bleed, ptosis and localized tenderness. The sensation of affected cheek may be decreased compared with that of the contralateral side. Infraorbital nerve involvement is demonstrated by anesthetized upper teeth and gums on the affected side.

Investigations

Computed tomography (CT) scan of the orbits and brain (axial and coronal scans) must be performed. There are two broad categories of blowout fractures: (1) open door—large, displaced, and comminuted; (2) trapdoor, which is linear, hinged, and minimally displaced.

Treatment

The steps of treatment include—broad-spectrum oral antibiotics; nasal decongestants; urgent neurological consultation; and surgical intervention. Immediate surgical repair (within 24–48 hours) is performed in cases with evidence of muscle entrapment or nonresolving bradycardia. Heart block, nausea, vomiting, or syncope. Other cases may be operated after 1–2 weeks, if patients have persistent diplopia along with evidence of muscle distortion or herniation.

ORBITAL CELLULITIS (FIG. 11)

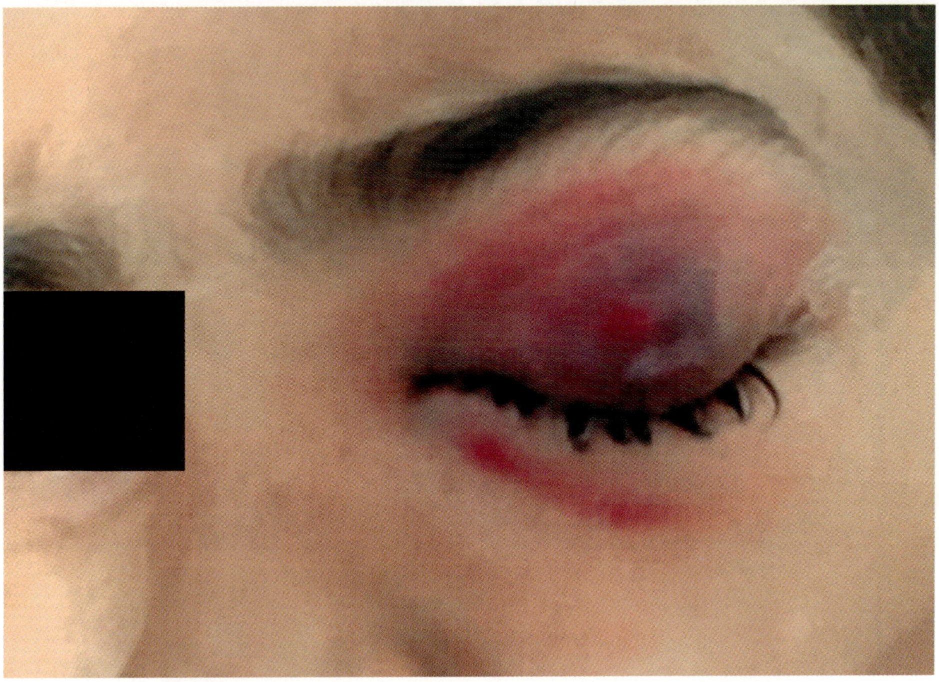

Fig. 11: Orbital cellulitis in a young boy with history of trauma 2 weeks ago.

Orbital cellulitis is the infection of soft tissues of the orbit behind the orbital septum. The main source is either from the adjacent sinuses or through blood. In some cases, eyelid trauma can lead to inflammation of the septum.

Signs

The most distinctive features are proptosis and limitation of ocular motility. Variable signs include—conjunctival chemosis, orbital pain, reduced visual acuity, and afferent pupillary defect. The onset of infection is usually acute and is characterized by headache, fever, eyelid edema, rhinorrhea, and increasing malaise. Intraorbital abscesses cannot possibly be detected on the basis of clinical examination alone.

Imaging

High-resolution CT scans (axial and coronal views) are essential in the initial assessment and management of all forms of orbital cellulitis.

Treatment

The mainstay of treatment remains parenteral antibiotics. These drugs should be continued for 10–14 days for bacteremia. The antibiotic coverage must be evaluated daily and changed, whenever necessary, according to the clinical course and the culture results. The best culture material will be obtained from direct sinus aspiration or by drainage of a subperiosteal or orbital abscess. In severe infections with typical clinical features, intravenous administration of amphotericin B may be appropriate before laboratory confirmation of the infection is obtained. In case of a diabetic patient especially in ketoacidosis, we must rule out a possibility of mucormycosis. One should employ a multifaceted and multidisciplinary approach with consultation between ophthalmologist, otorhinolaryngologist, and pediatric/adult physician where appropriate.

RETINAL HEMORRHAGES AND PAPILLOPATHY (FIGS. 12A TO C)

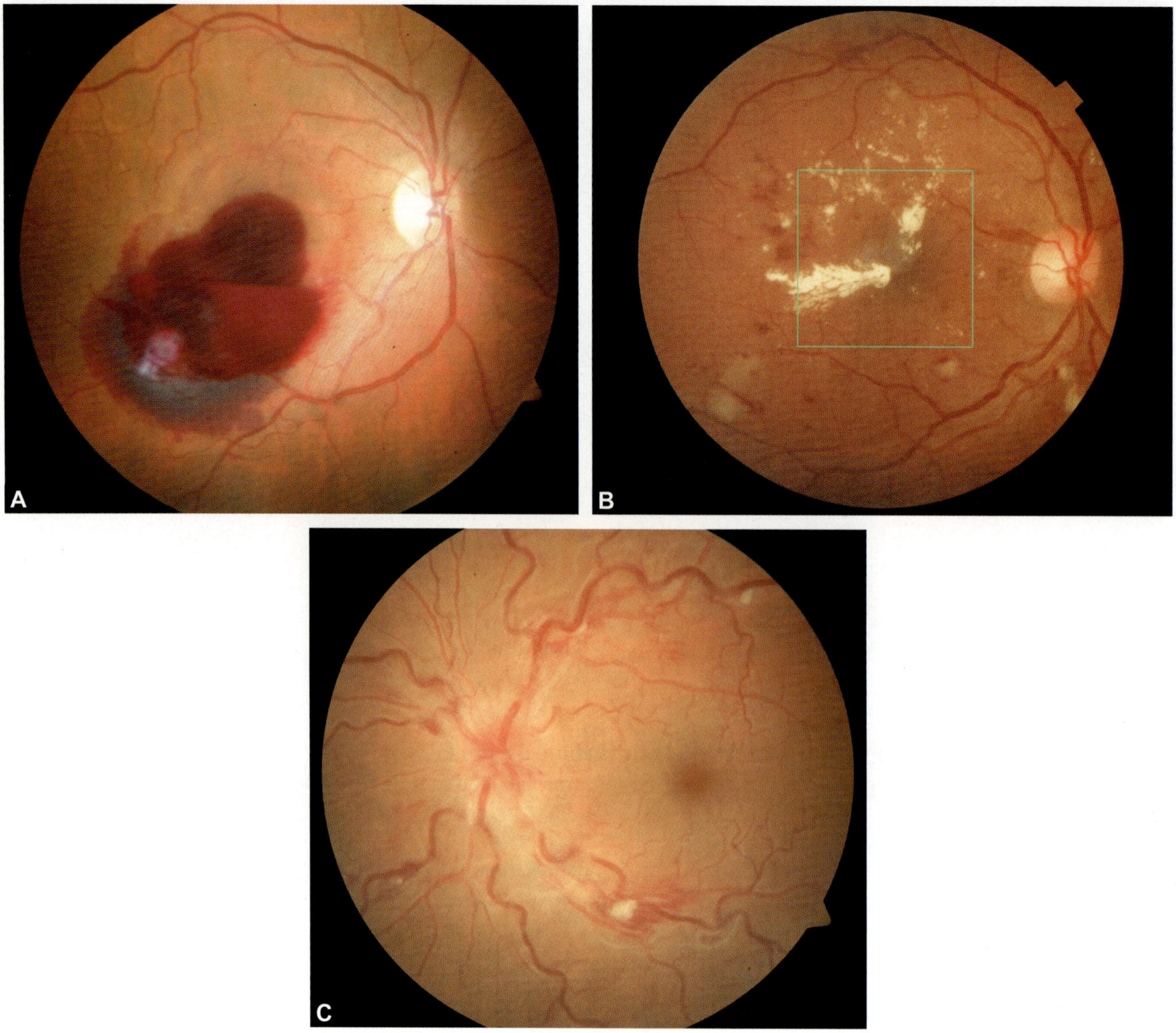

Figs. 12A to C: Retinal hemorrhages and papillopathy.

Sometimes, conditions such as retinal hemorrhages due to various conditions such as diabetic retinopathy may present with loss of vision which may be sudden in onset.

Signs

Retinal hemorrhages, cotton wool spots, microaneurysms, venous beading and tortuosity, optic disc edema and macular edema.

Treatment

The basic principle of treatment is to identify the underlying etiology. If the disease is caused due to diabetes mellitus, these patients require systemic metabolic control and assessment of laboratory parameters. In the presence of macular edema, treatment may be initiated with antivascular growth factor injections which are given intravitreally.

CHAPTER 21

Rheumatology

Sham Santhanam, Vinod Ravindran, Indrajit Agarwal

MALAR RASH AND ORAL ULCERS (FIGS. 1A AND B)

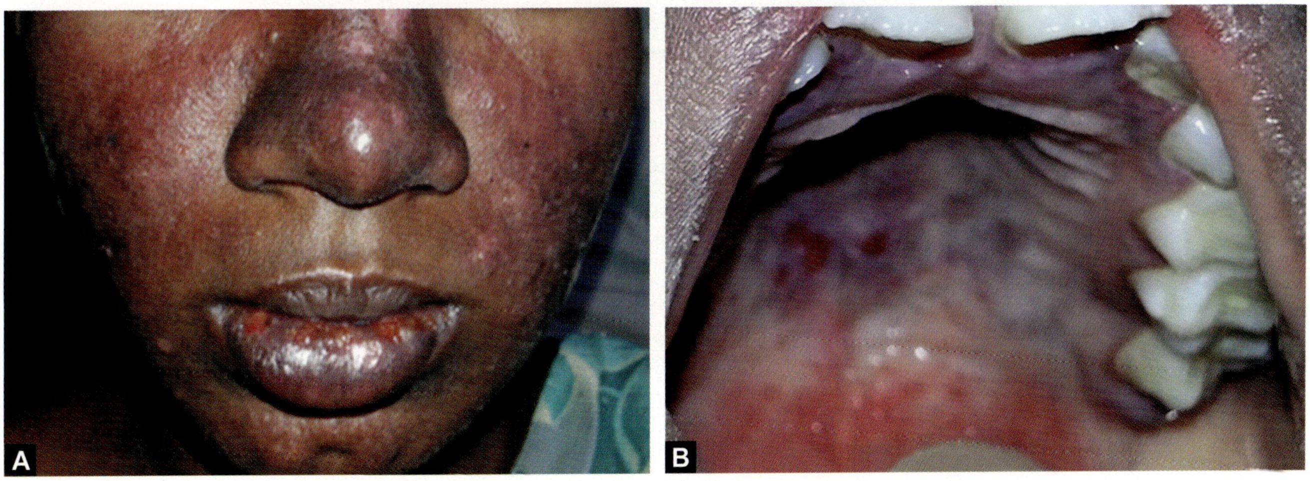

Figs. 1A and B: (A) Malar rash of systemic lupus erythematosus (SLE) with oral mucositis; (B) Palatal ulcer in SLE.

- "Malar rash" also known as butterfly rash is the typical lesion of acute cutaneous lupus. It is an acute, lupus erythematosus (LE) specific lesion.
- The malar rash in systemic lupus erythematosus (SLE) generally spares the nasolabial fold unlike the rash in dermatomyositis. It usually occurs in the setting of an active systemic disease and internal organ involvement need to be looked for.
- The lesion may be pruritic or painful and are accompanied by oral ulcerations.
- Oral ulcers can be painless or painful (discoid lesions). Palatal ulcers are more specific for SLE. Both malar rash and oral ulcers are part of the classification criteria for SLE.
- SLE can present with emergencies like lupus pneumonitis, diffuse alveolar bleed, neuropsychiatric complications, macrophage activation syndrome, etc.

DISCOID LUPUS ERYTHEMATOSUS (FIG. 2)

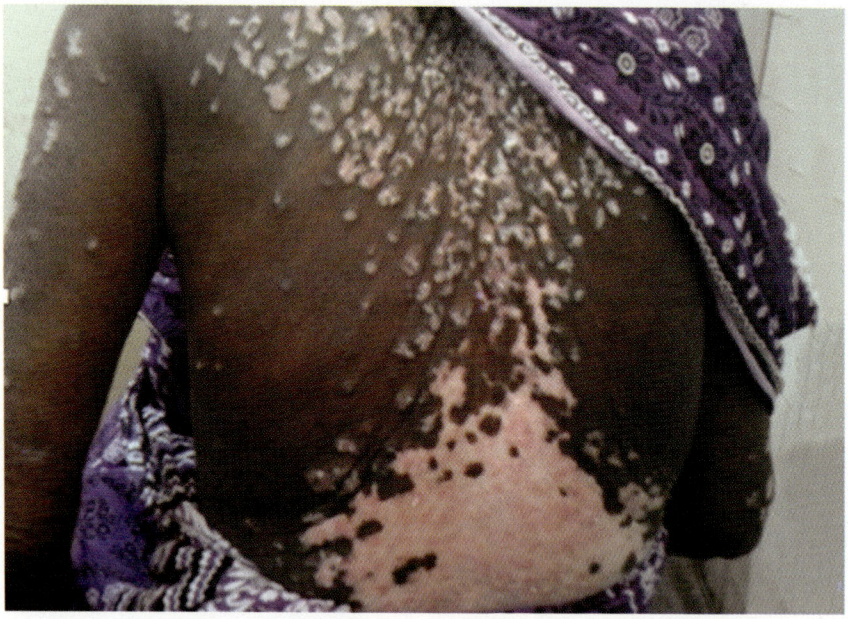

Fig. 2: Generalized discoid lupus erythematosus (DLE) seen over the trunk.

- Discoid lupus is a common form of chronic cutaneous lupus.
- It usually involves the face, scalp (common), and ears. In localized DLE, the lesions are found above the neck and, if present, both above and below, it is termed as "generalized DLE".
- It can also present as oral ulcer, malar rash, blepharitis, madarosis, and cicatrizing conjunctivitis.
- Squamous cell carcinoma can complicate a long-standing DLE lesion.
- Generalized DLE has a higher frequency of constitutional symptoms and systemic involvement.

RELAPSING POLYCHONDRITIS (FIG. 3)

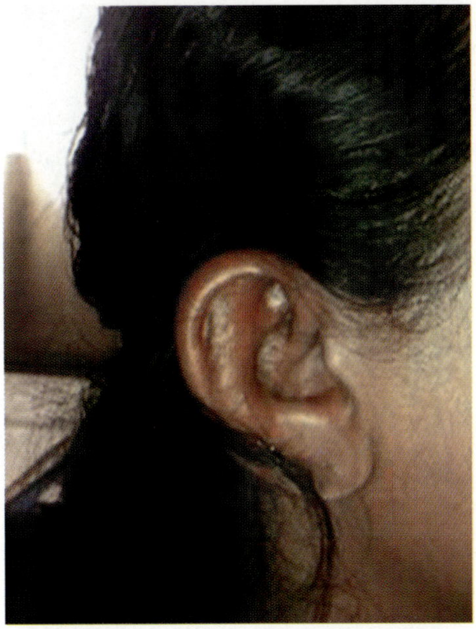

Fig. 3: Inflammation of the pinna in a case of relapsing polychondritis (RP).

- Relapsing polychondritis (RP) typically presents with recurrent episodes of inflammation of auricular cartilage with sparing of ear lobule.
- Recurrent episodes cause damage of cartilage and flopping over (cauliflower ear). It can also involve the nasal cartilage causing saddle nose deformity.
- The inflammation of tracheobronchial tree can lead to localized or diffuse obstruction leading to respiratory difficulty.
- RP may be associated with other inflammatory arthritis, connective tissue disorders, and even myelodysplastic syndrome.
- It can cause systemic vasculitis, eye involvement in the form of episcleritis/scleritis.

GRANULOMATOSIS WITH POLYANGIITIS (FIG. 4)

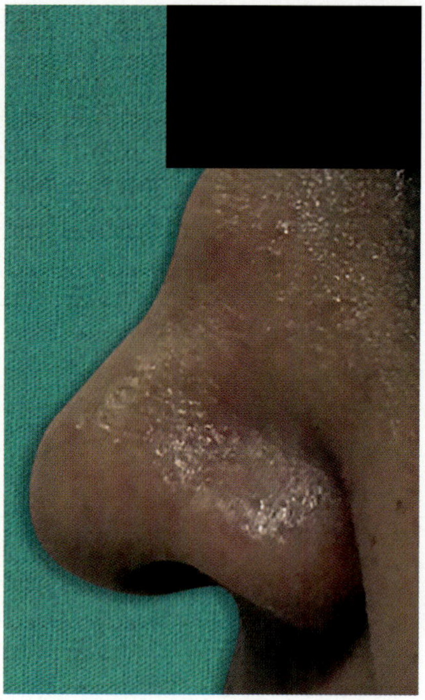

Fig. 4: Granulomatosis with polyangiitis (GPA) (also called as Wegener's granulomatosis) causing saddle nose deformity.

- Nasal inflammation is common in Wegener's granulomatosis (WG), causing mucosal erosions, septal perforation, and nasal bridge collapse leading to saddle nose deformity.
- Other causes of saddle nose deformity are RP, Hansen's disease, congenital syphilis, nasal trauma, and cocaine abuse.
- Alveolar hemorrhage, crescentic glomerulonephritis, subglottic stenosis, and scleritis are some of the serious manifestations in WG.
- Antineutrophil cytoplasmic antibody (c-ANCA) is positive in 80–90% of patients.
- Cyclophosphamide or rituximab can be used for induction therapy along with steroids.

SCLERODERMA (FIGS. 5A AND B)

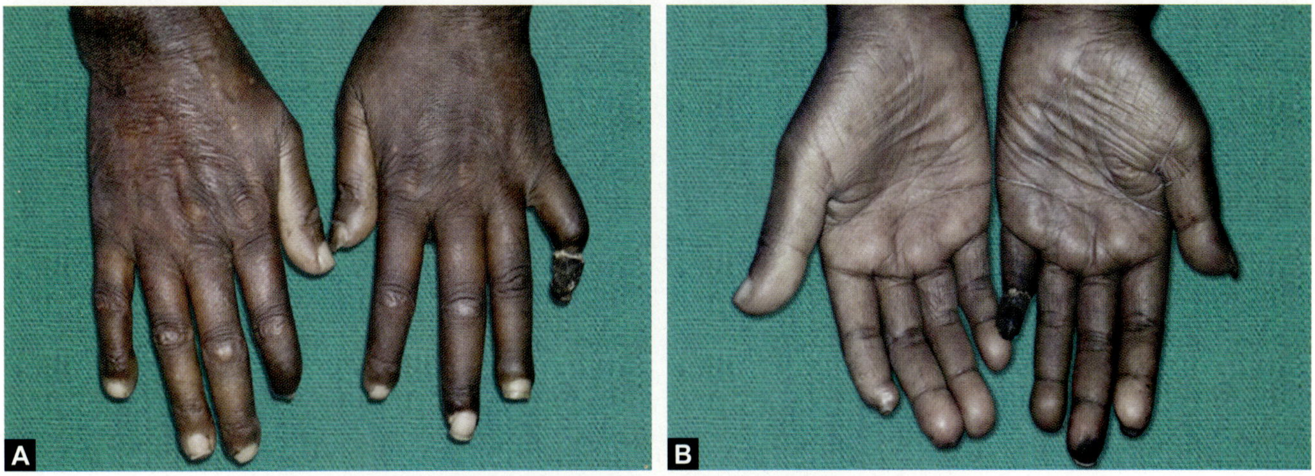

Figs. 5A and B: Digital gangrene in a patient with scleroderma.

- Dry gangrene can be one of the complications in scleroderma. It can occur due to severe Raynaud's phenomenon, coexisting macrovascular (common—ulnar artery) disease or thrombosis due to secondary antiphospholipid antibody syndrome.
- Calcium channel blockers are the initial therapy for Raynaud's phenomenon followed by phosphodiesterase (PDE) inhibitors and endothelin (ET) receptor antagonists.
- Intravenous prostaglandins are the drug of choice for critical ischemia.
- Scleroderma renal crisis, severe pulmonary hypertension, and exacerbation of interstitial lung disease (ILD) are some of the serious manifestations of scleroderma.

GOUTY ARTHRITIS (FIGS. 6A AND B)

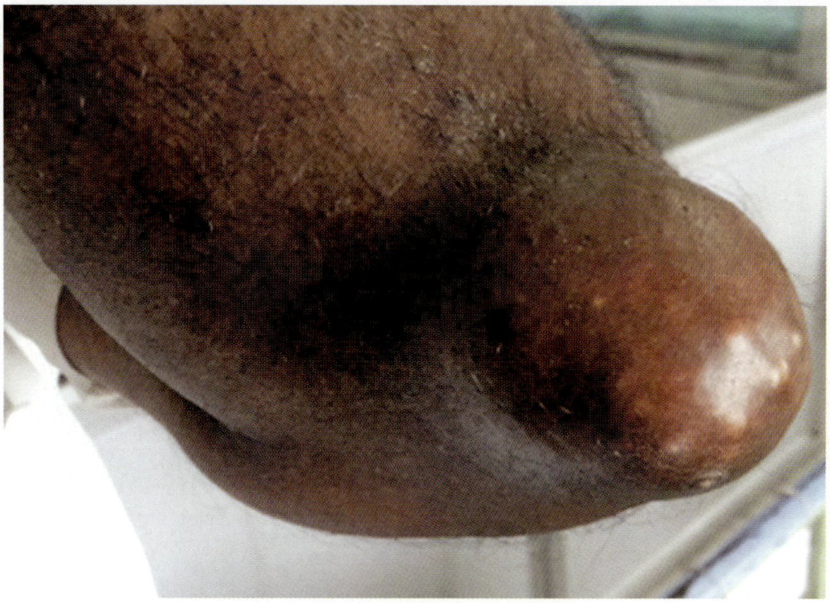

Fig. 6A: Gouty tophi at the olecranon bursa.

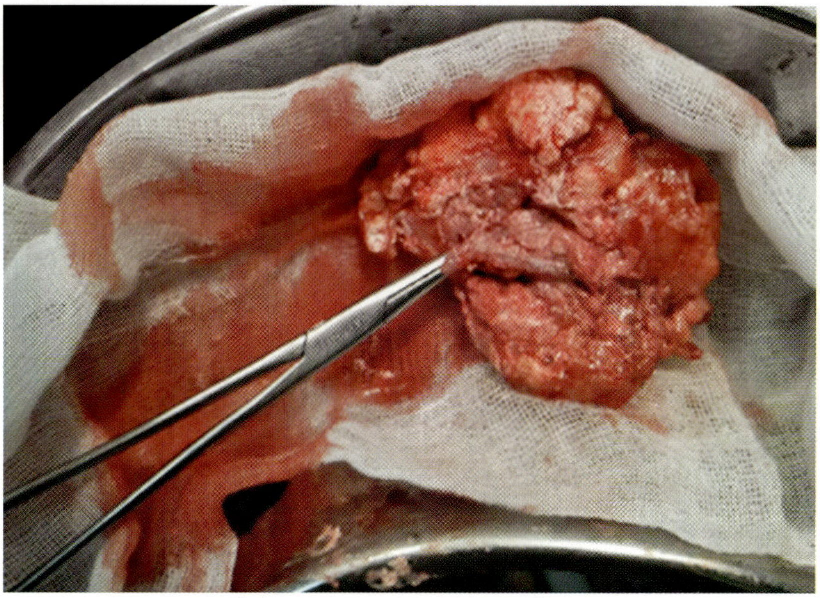

Fig. 6B: Surgically excised large tophi.

- Acute gouty arthritis is considered as a medical emergency due to the severity of pain.
- It can be commonly seen in critical care setting. Surgery, acute coronary syndrome, and cerebrovascular accident are some of the precipitating factors.
- Patients present with excruciating pain and swelling of first metatarsophalangeal (MTP) joint, followed by involvement of instep, ankle joint, etc.
- They can have fever, local erythema, and swelling and can be mistaken for cellulitis. Even the leukocyte counts can be elevated during an acute attack.
- Colchicine, nonsteroidal anti-inflammatory drugs (NSAIDs), and steroids are the drugs used to terminate an acute attack.

JUVENILE DERMATOMYOSITIS (FIG. 7)

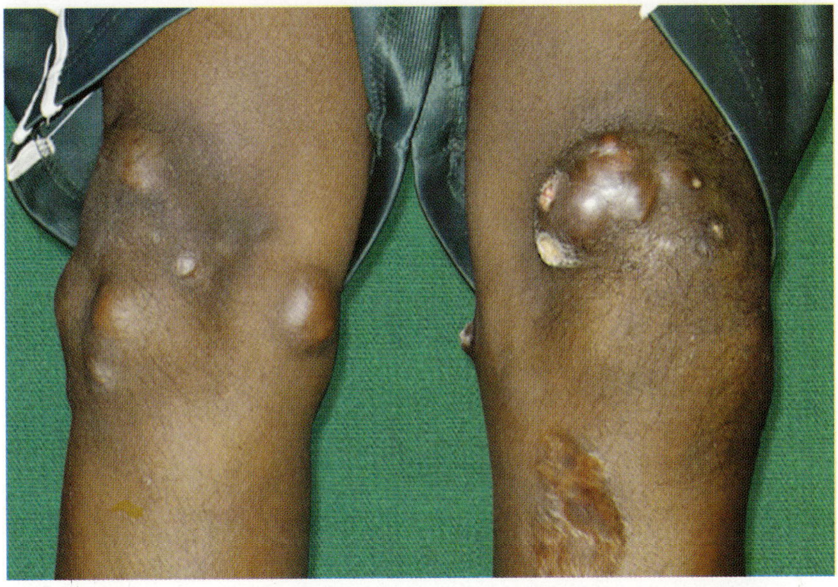

Fig. 7: Calcinosis cutis in a patient with juvenile dermatomyositis (JDM).

- Dystrophic calcification can occur in juvenile dermatomyositis (JDM) when the disease is active and when not adequately treated.
- It can cause ulceration, secondary infection and cellulitis, nerve entrapment, and joint contractures.
- JDM patients can present with severe muscle weakness, respiratory failure, aspiration pneumonia, and rarely vasculitis of gastrointestinal system (poor prognostic factor).
- Common cutaneous signs are heliotrope rash, Gottron papules, malar rash, and "V" and "shawl" sign rashes.
- Steroids, hydroxychloroquine, methotrexate, intravenous immunoglobulin, and rituximab are used in management, depending on the disease severity.

CUTANEOUS POLYARTERITIS NODOSA (FIGS. 8A AND B)

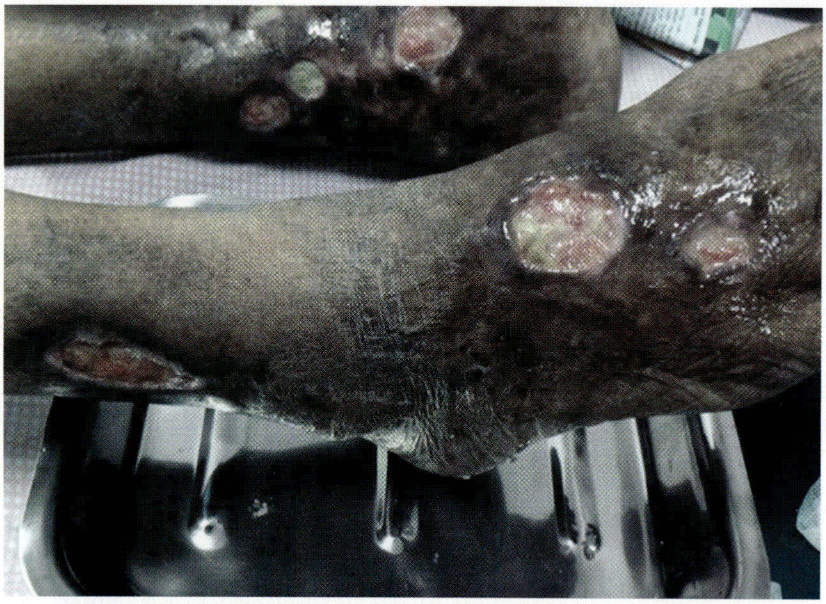

Fig. 8A: Nonhealing ulcers in cutaneous polyarteritis nodosa (PAN/c-PAN).

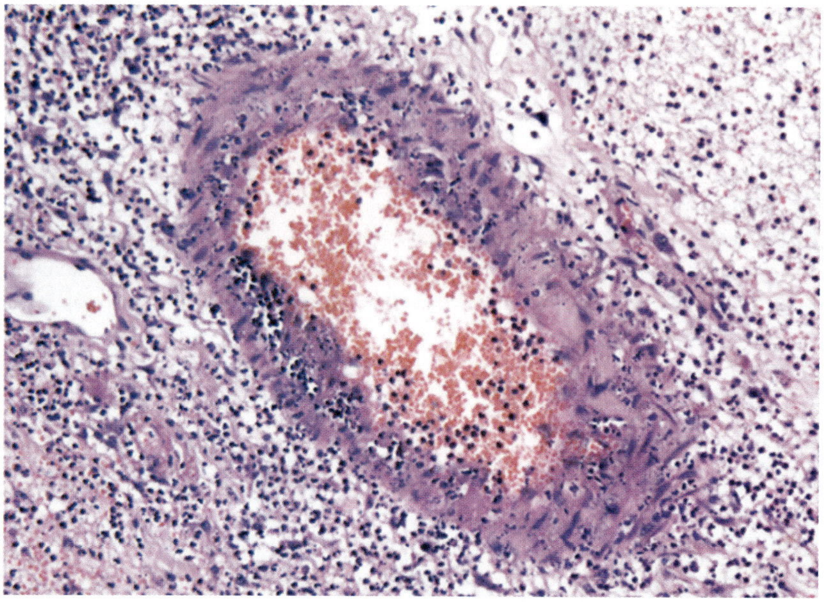

Fig. 8B: Histopathology hematoxylin and eosin (H and E) stain showing leukocytoclastic vasculitis.

- Cutaneous polyarteritis nodosa (c-PAN) is a rare form of cutaneous vasculitis without systemic involvement. It is a benign form of vasculitis with relapsing and remitting course.
- It presents as painful nodules, cutaneous ulceration, and livedo reticularis localized to the lower extremity.
- Diagnosis is confirmed by skin biopsy revealing leukocytoclastic vasculitis of small- and medium-sized vessels.
- Drugs used for treatment of c-PAN are steroids, azathioprine, cyclophosphamide, and other immunosuppressives.
- Any patient with leukocytoclastic vasculitis needs to be worked for various etiologies like ANCA-associated vasculitis, cryoglobulinemic vasculitis, etc. and also the degree of systemic involvement.

HENOCH-SCHONLEIN PURPURA (FIG. 9)

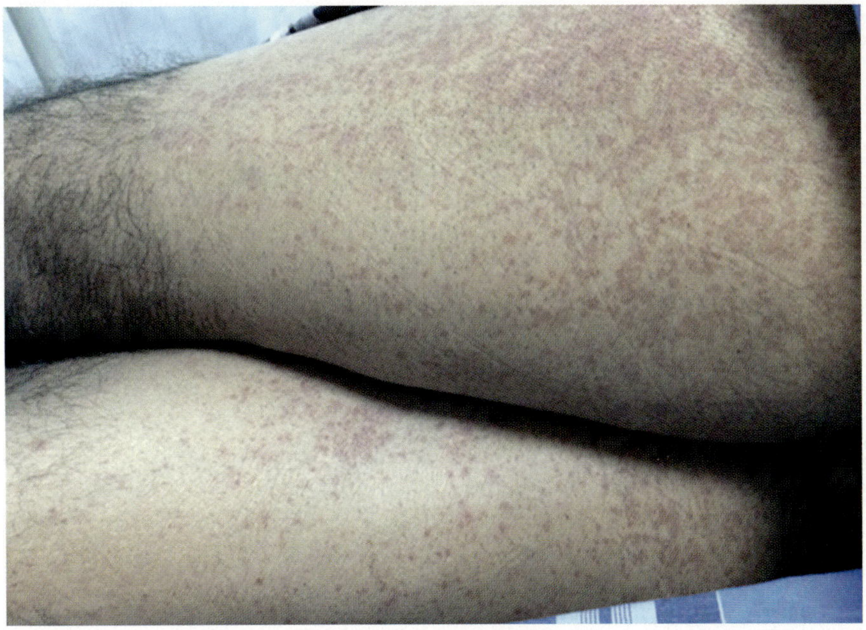

Fig. 9: Adult onset Henoch-Schonlein purpura (HSP) with purpuric lesions on extensor aspect of both thighs.

- Henoch-Schonlein purpura (HSP) is a common form of childhood vasculitis. Purpuric rash is usually present over dependent areas of buttocks and lower extremities.
- It consists of a tetrad of large joint arthritis, hematuria/proteinuria, diffuse abdominal pain, and predominant immunoglobulin A (IgA) deposits on skin biopsy.
- Gastrointestinal involvement, renal disease, and arthralgias are more common in adults and rarely associated with even malignancy.
- Usually, it is a benign and self-limiting illness but may develop severe nephritis, gastrointestinal vasculitis, alveolar hemorrhage (rarely), and may need high dose of steroids.

GIANT CELL ARTERITIS (FIG. 10)

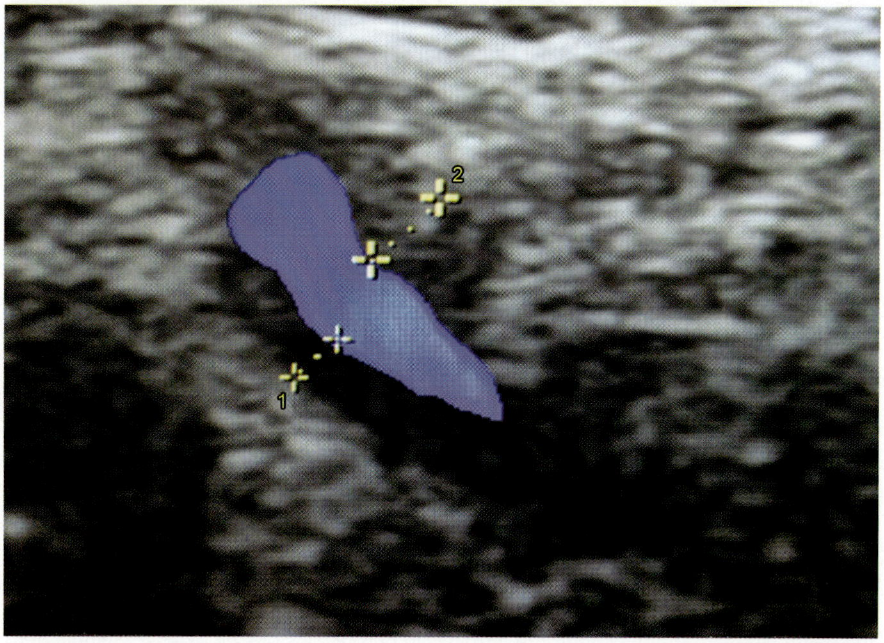

Fig. 10: 'Halo sign' (Circumferential wall thickening due to vessel wall edema) seen in color Doppler ultrasonography (CDUS) of a patient with giant cell arteritis (GCA).

- A diagnosis of giant cell arteritis (GCA) should be considered in any elderly patient more than 50 years with a new onset headache, jaw claudication, visual symptoms, and an elevated erythrocyte sedimentation rate (ESR).
- Diagnosis is generally confirmed by temporal artery biopsy or to look for a halo sign on temporal artery Doppler.
- Visual symptoms like visual loss and diplopia are common in GCA. Vision loss (due to anterior ischemic optic neuropathy) lasting more than few hours is not usually reversible.
- Early recognition and treatment with steroids can prevent blindness.
- About 40% of patients present with atypical manifestations like pyrexia of unknown origin, large-vessel disease, otolaryngeal/neurological manifestations, myocardial infarction, and tumor-like lesions.[11]

DIFFUSE ALVEOLAR HEMORRHAGE (FIG. 11)

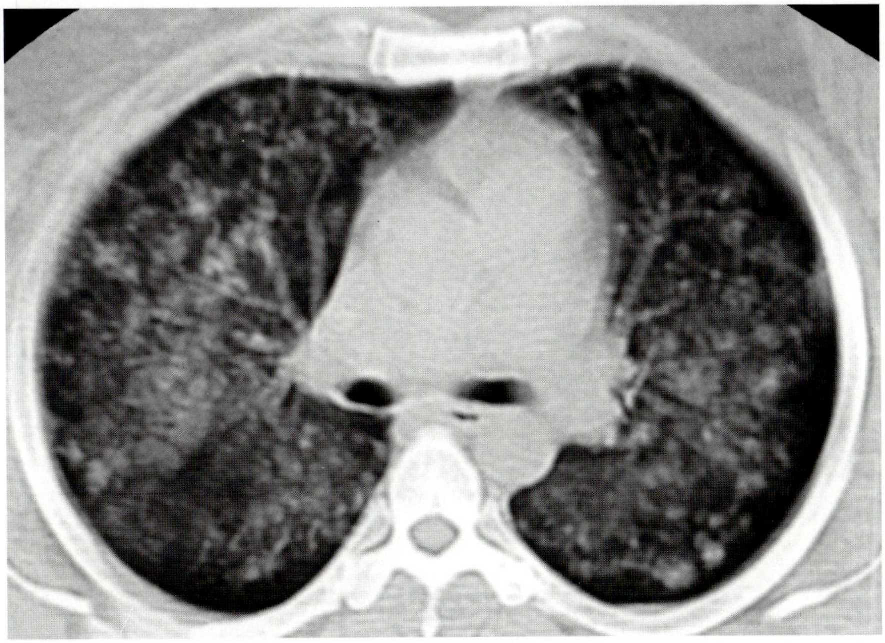

Fig. 11: Computed tomography (CT) chest showing diffuse alveolar hemorrhage (DAH) in a patient with antineutrophil cytoplasmic antibody (ANCA)-associated vasculitis.

- Diffuse alveolar hemorrhage (DAH) is a medical emergency and has to be recognized promptly. Patient presents with dyspnea, hemoptysis (not always), and breathlessness.
- Common causes of DAH are ANCA-associated vasculitis, systemic lupus erythematosus (SLE), antiphospholipid antibody syndrome (APS), Goodpasture's syndrome, and rarely cryoglobulinemic vasculitis.
- Fall in hemoglobin, raised DL_{CO} values, and diffuse alveolar shadowing on imaging are indicators of DAH.
- Coexisting renal involvement in the form of rapidly progressive glomerulonephritis may be present.
- Pulse steroids, cyclophosphamide, rituximab, and plasma exchange are the various treatment modalities depending on the etiology.

AVASCULAR NECROSIS (FIG. 12)

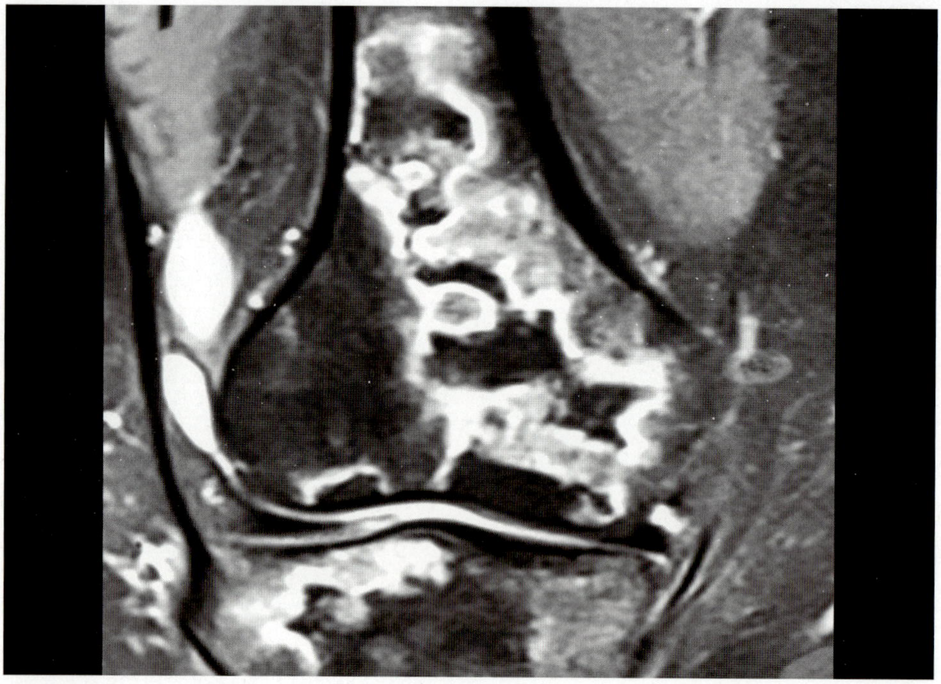

Fig. 12: Magnetic resonance imaging (MRI) knee joint: Multifocal avascular necrosis (AVN) of both femur and tibia in a patient with systemic lupus erythematosus (SLE) and secondary antiphospholipid antibody syndrome (APS).

- Avascular necrosis (AVN) is the end result of interruption of blood supply and is often seen in patients with SLE and APS.
- Commonly affected sites are femoral heads, tibial plateau, and femoral condyles.
- AVN should be suspected in patients with groin pain, which worsens on weight-bearing.
- Use of high-dose steroids and coexisting APS are well-known risk factors in SLE patients.
- Magnetic resonance imaging (MRI) is currently considered the gold standard imaging. Treatment is usually surgical and depends on the stage of disease.

VERRUCOUS ENDOCARDITIS (FIG. 13)

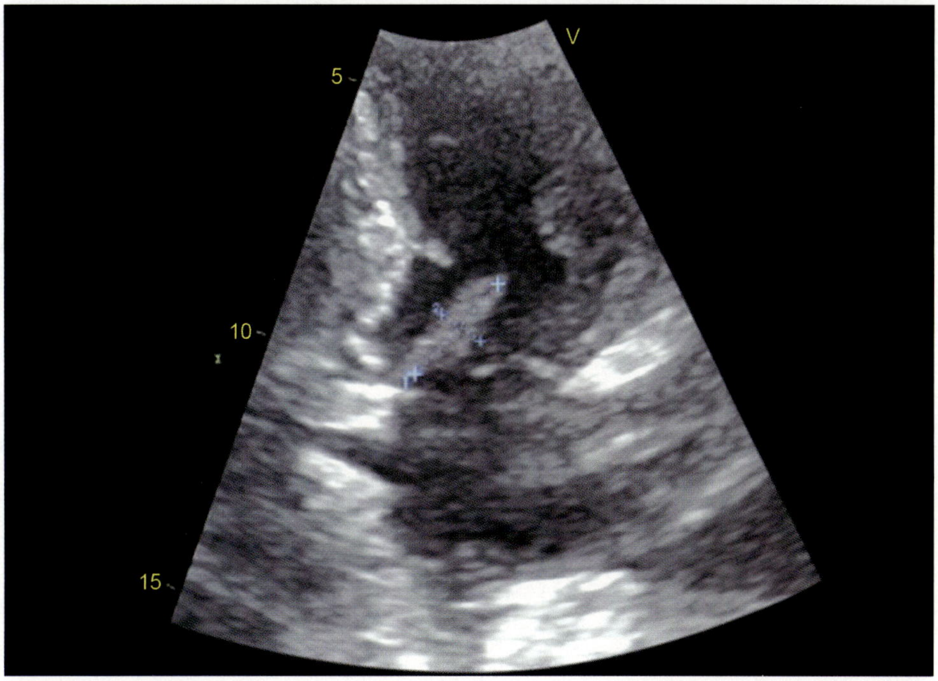

Fig. 13: Echocardiography showing mitral valve vegetation in a SLE patient with secondary APS.

- Verrucous endocarditis (Libman-Sacks) affects the mitral valve more frequently followed by aortic valve.
- It can predispose to infective endocarditis and embolic manifestations rarely.
- Antiphospholipid antibodies may play a role in the development of vegetations in Libman-Sacks endocarditis.
- Anticoagulation should be started to prevent embolic complications and the role of steroids is controversial.

EPISCLERITIS (FIG. 14)

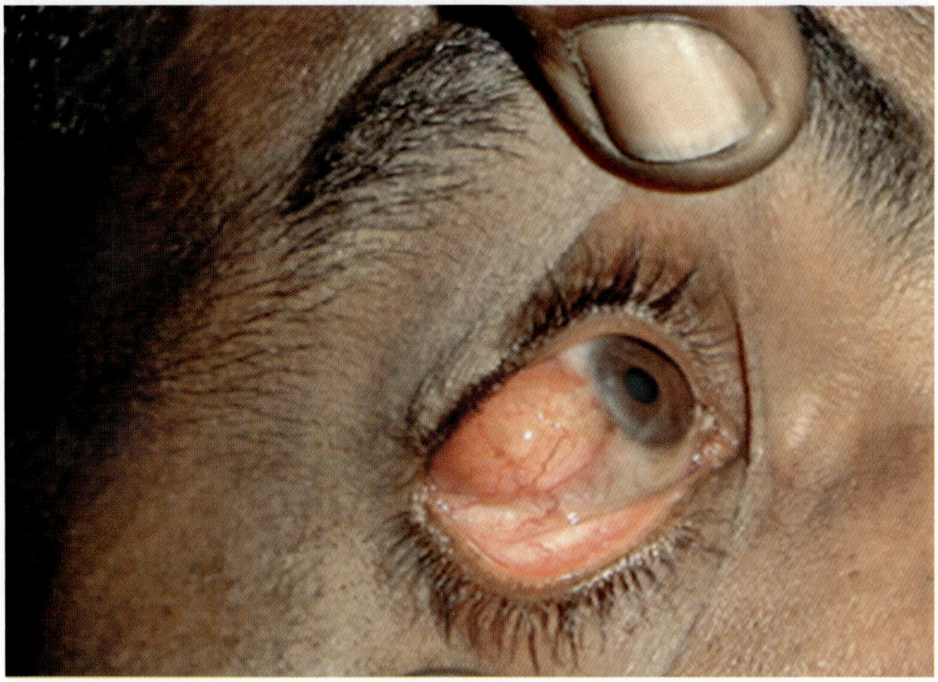

Fig. 14: Nodular episcleritis of eye in a patient with rheumatoid arthritis.

- Episcleritis usually causes painless red eye. The engorged blood vessels stop at the limbic border and move with light pressure. In contrast, scleritis presents with pain and can be vision threatening.
- Rheumatoid arthritis and Sjögren's syndrome are some of the rheumatological causes for episcleritis and ANCA associated vasculitis, SLE, rheumatoid arthritis, and relapsing polychondritis (RP) for scleritis.
- Episcleritis can be managed with topical anti-inflammatory agents but scleritis usually requires systemic or intraocular immunomodulating therapy.

INTERSTITIAL LUNG DISEASE (FIG. 15)

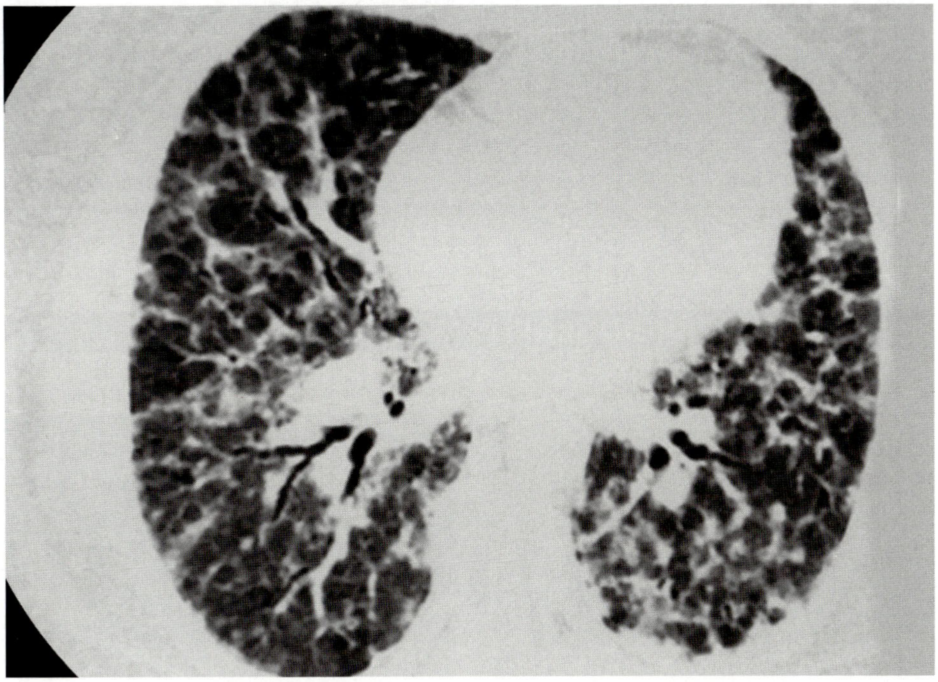

Fig. 15: High-resolution computed tomography (HRCT) chest shows ILD—usual interstitial pneumonia (UIP) pattern.

- Rheumatic diseases commonly associated with interstitial lung disease (ILD), are scleroderma, rheumatoid arthritis, dermatomyositis/polymyositis, and Sjögren's syndrome.
- Nonspecific interstitial pneumonia (NSIP) and usual interstitial pneumonia (UIP) are the common ILD types. UIP has patchy heterogeneous involvement with fibrosis and honeycombing and predominantly subpleural in location.
- Patients with ILD can have infective exacerbations and certain subsets (e.g. myositis-associated ILD) can have a rapidly progressing type.
- HRCT chest is the imaging modality of choice and during acute exacerbations bronchoscopy and bronchoalveolar lavage (BAL) may help in ruling out concomitant infection.
- Management is with steroids, cyclophosphamide, rituximab, mycophenolate mofetil, and azathioprine.
- It is a progressive disease, requiring repeated ICU admission and domiciliary oxygen therapy.

CHAPTER

22

Hemodynamic Monitoring and Equipment in Cardiac ICU

Prajeesh M Nambiar, Yatin Mehta

TRANSESOPHAGEAL ECHOCARDIOGRAPHY (FIGS. 1A TO C)

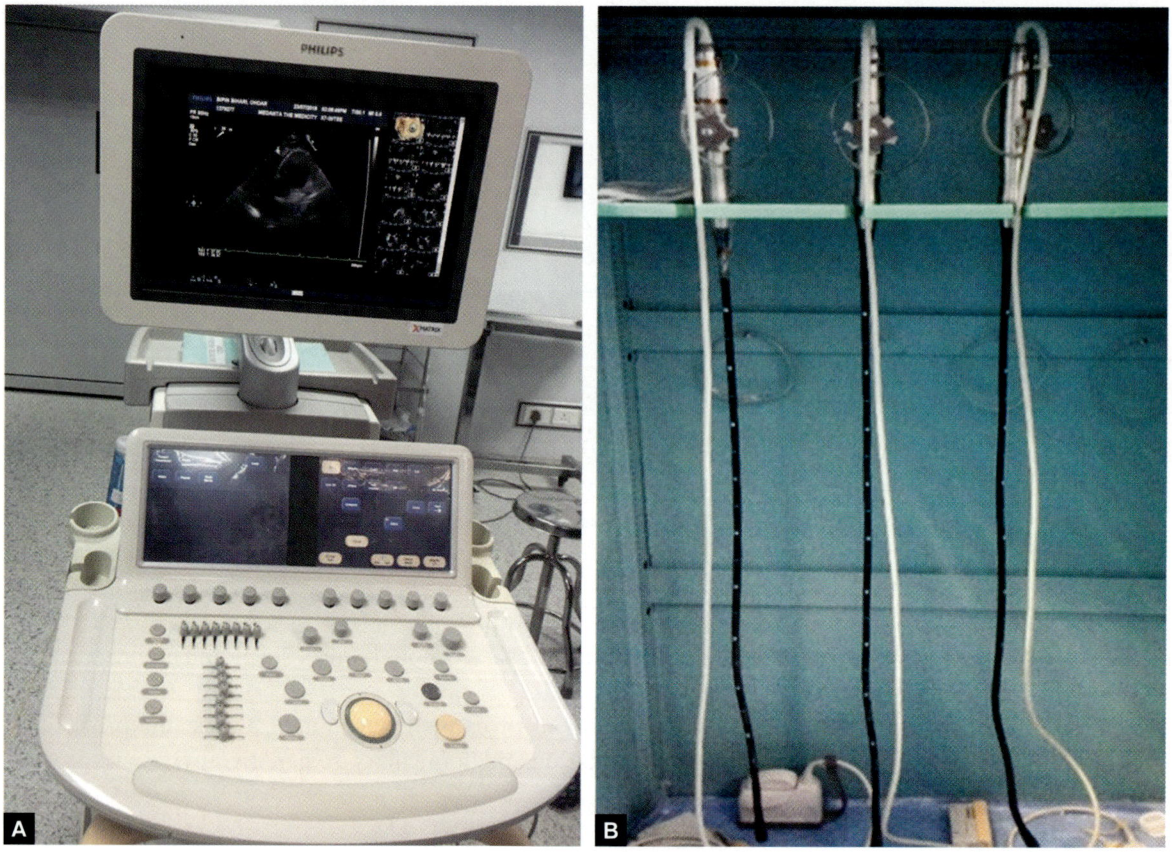

Figs. 1A and B: (A) Echocardiography (ECHO) machine with a four-chamber view of the heart; (B) Storage of transesophageal echocardiography (TEE) probes.

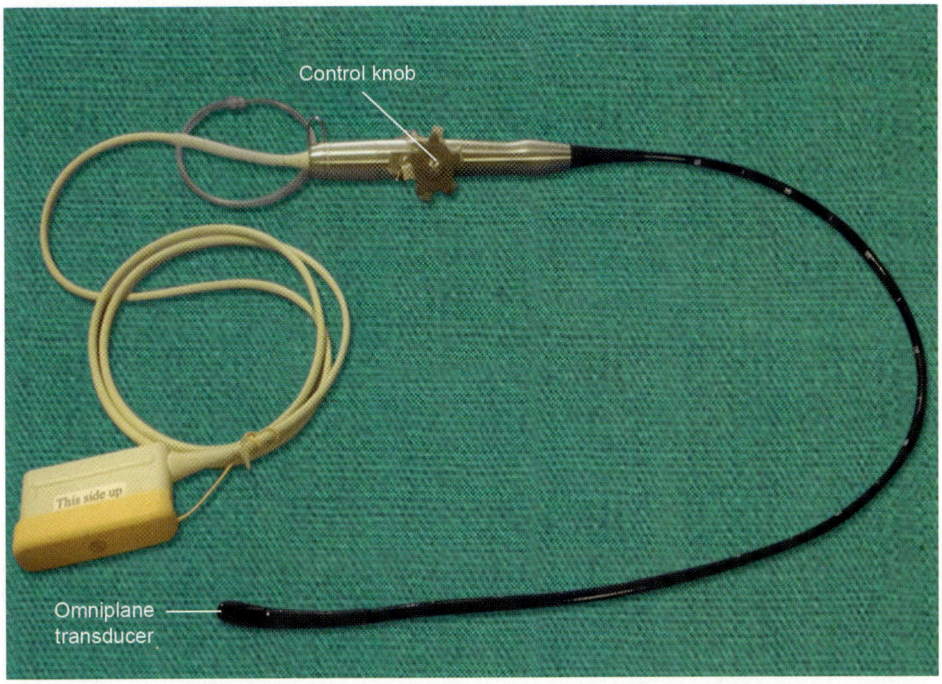

Fig. 1C: Transesophageal echocardiography (TEE) probe.

- A semi-invasive procedure used intraoperatively during surgeries and for percutaneous interventional procedural guidance in hybrid operating rooms, cardiac catheterization laboratory, and intensive care unit (ICU).
- Modern era of transesophageal echocardiography (TEE) began in 1982 with the introduction of flexible probes, which could be manipulated and phased array transducers.
- Pulse wave Doppler (PWD) and continuous wave Doppler (CWD) principles are used in quantification of valvular pathologies.
- The TEE probes with systems capable of producing real time 3D images are widely used.

PULMONARY ARTERY CATHETER (FIGS. 2A TO F)

- Pulmonary artery (PA) catheterization was first performed by Lewis Dexter in 1945.
- The idea of a flow-directed PA catheter was developed by Swan and Ganz in 1970.
- Addition of a thermistor allowed the monitoring of cardiac output.
- Based on the principle of thermodilution.

Pulmonary Artery Catheter (Swan-Ganz) (Figs. 2A and B)

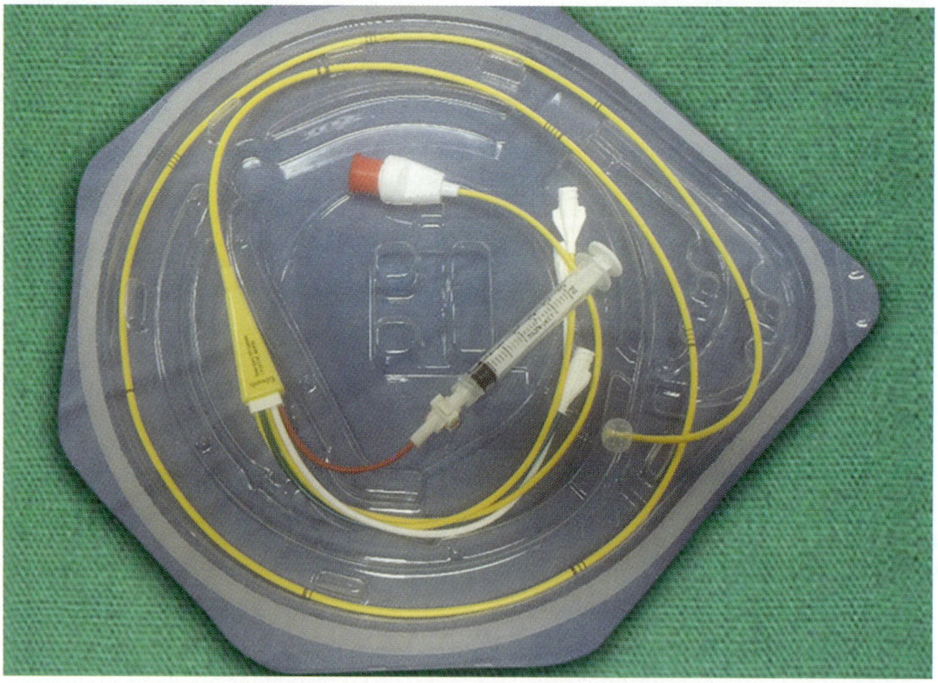

Fig. 2A: Swan-Ganz catheter in packing.

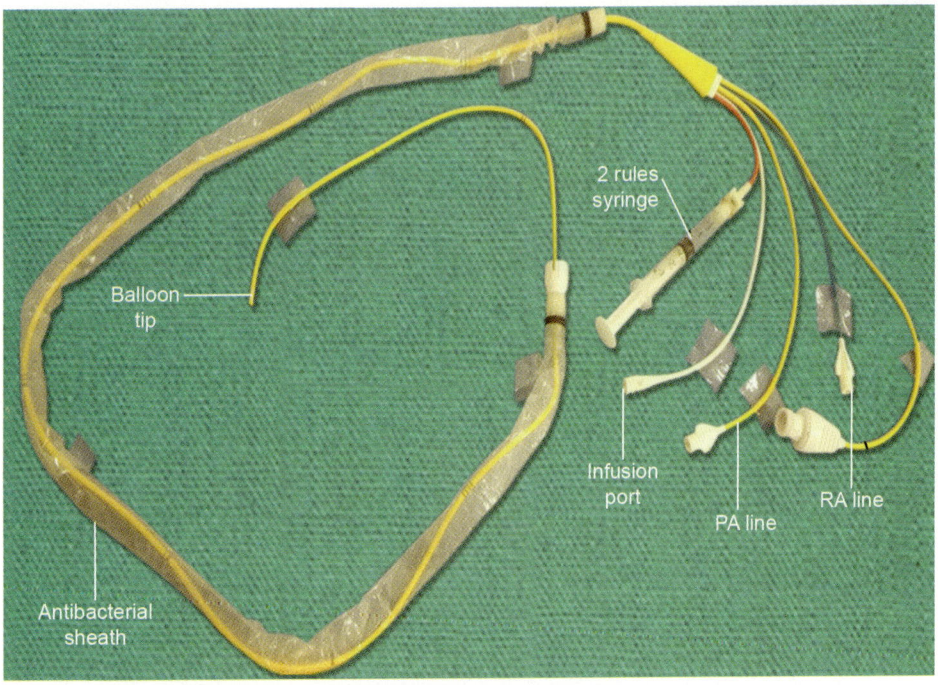

Fig. 2B: Swan-Ganz catheter.

- Swan-Ganz pulmonary artery catheter comes in sizes ranging from:
  - 5 Fr—75 cm length
  - 7.5 Fr—110 cm (5-lumen catheter)
  - 6 Fr—110 cm length
  - 7 Fr—110 cm length (4-lumen catheter).
- Parameters measured—right atrial pressure (RAP), pulmonary artery pressure (PAP), pulmonary artery occlusion pressure (PAOP), cardiac output (CO), blood temperature, mixed venous oxygen saturation.
- Derived parameters—cardiac index (CI), systemic vascular resistance (SVR), pulmonary vascular resistance (PVR), systemic vascular resistance index (SVRI), pulmonary vascular resistance index (PVRI), left ventricular stroke work index (LVSWI), and right ventricular stroke work (RVSW).

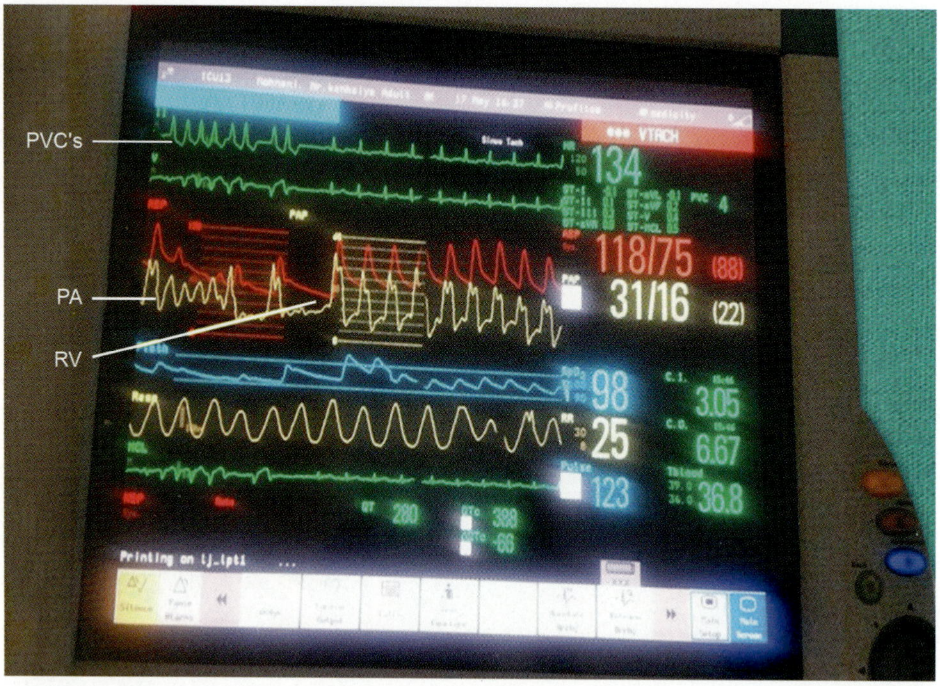

Fig. 2C: Pulmonary artery (PA) and right ventricle (RV) traces in premature ventricular contraction (PVC). Happens as the catheter migrates to RV.

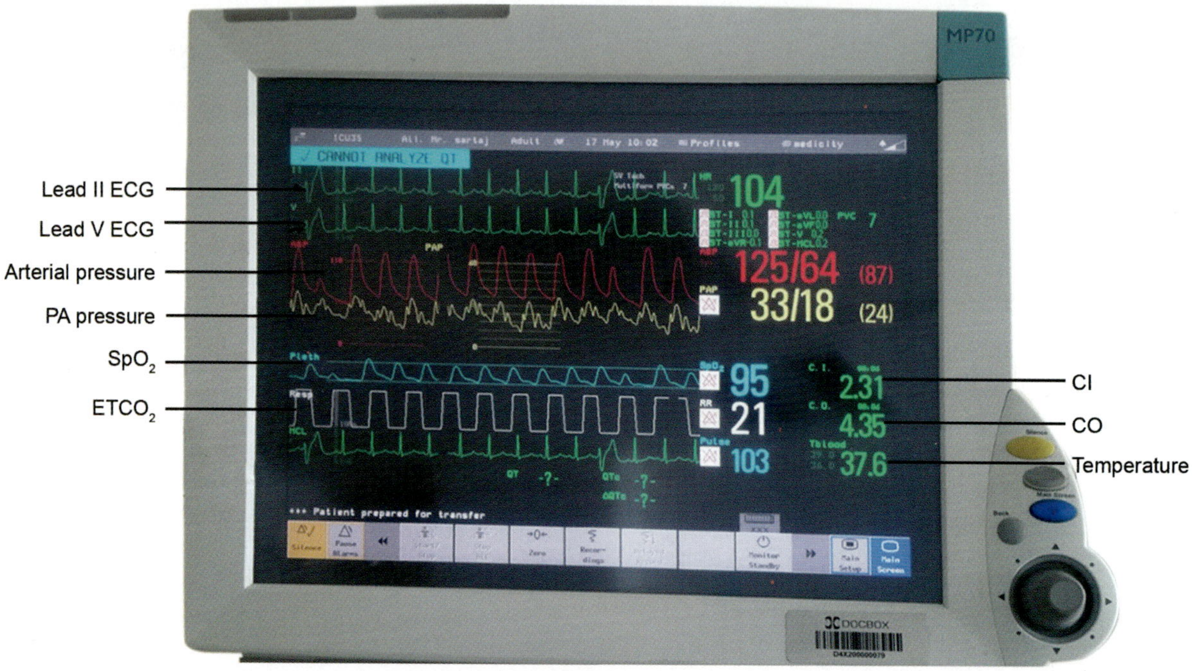

Fig. 2D: Multiparameter hemodynamic or cardiac monitor. (ECG: Electrocardiogram; PA: Pulmonary artery; SpO_2: Peripheral capillary oxygen saturation; $ETCO_2$: Partial pressure or maximal concentration of carbon dioxide; CI: Cardiac index; CO: Cardiac output)

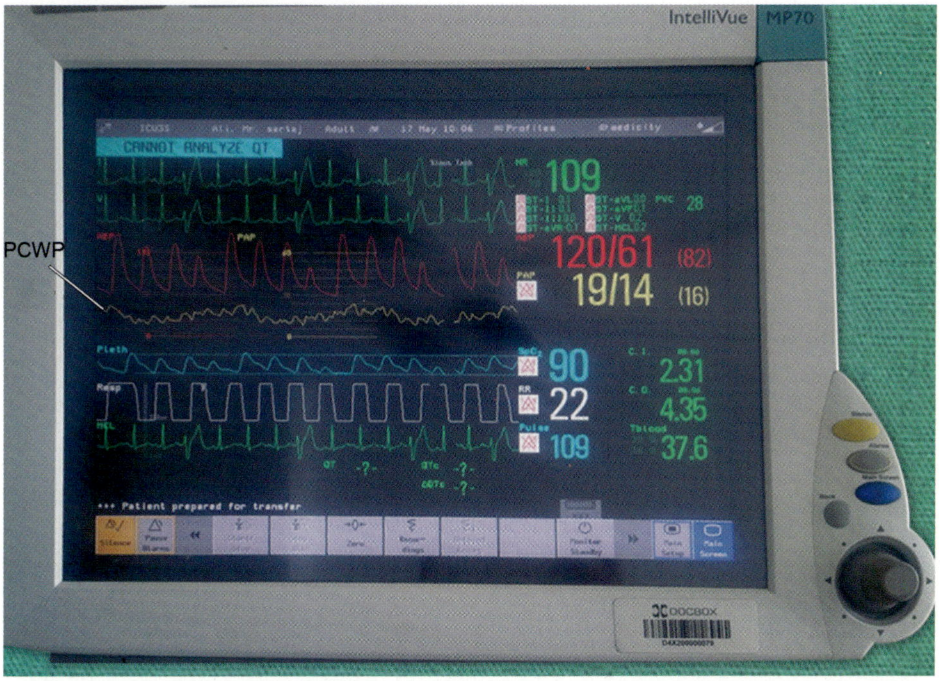

Fig. 2E: Wedge tracing. Pulmonary capillary wedge pressure (PCWP) measured end expiration.

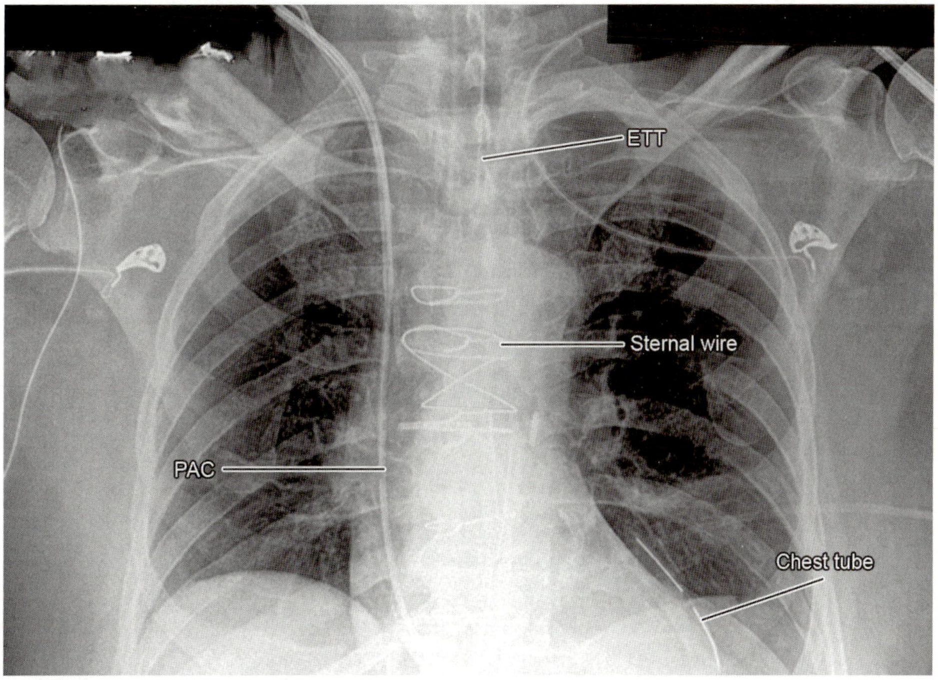

Fig. 2F: Swan-Ganz X-ray position. (ETT: Endotracheal tube; PAC: Pulmonary artery catheter).

Continuous Cardiac Output Pulmonary Artery Catheter (Figs. 3A and B)

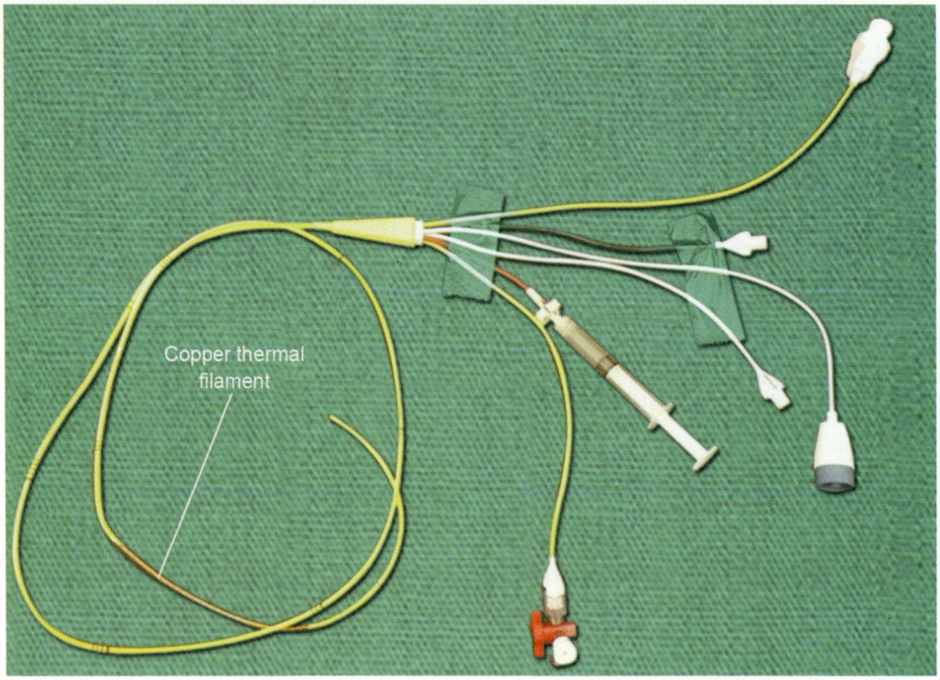

Fig. 3A: Continuous cardiac output pulmonary artery catheter (PAC).

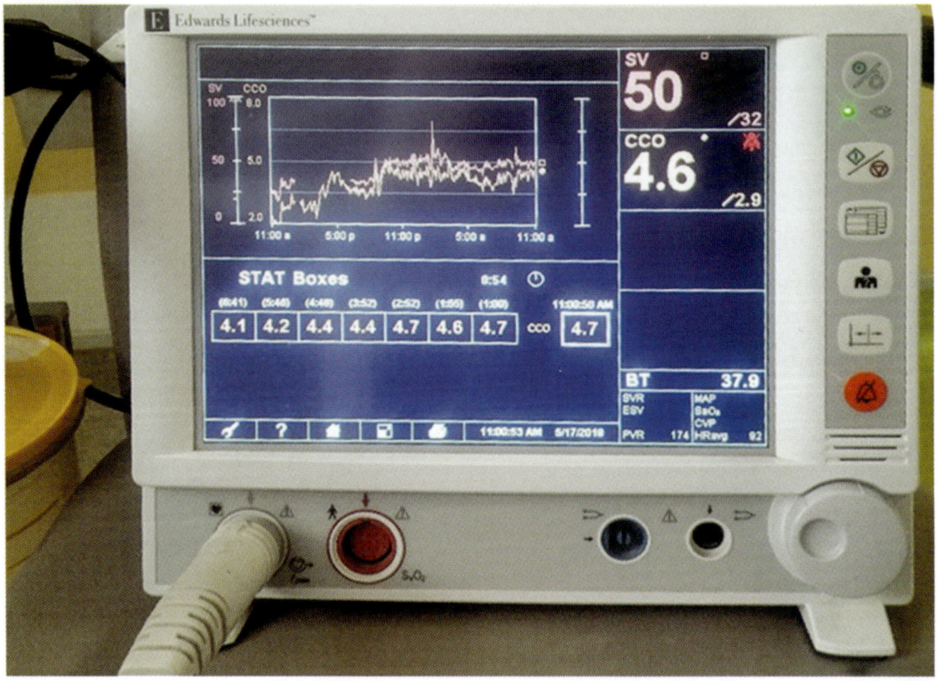

Fig. 3B: Continuous cardiac output (CCO) monitor.

- A thermal filament on the pulmonary artery (PA) catheter emits intermittent bursts of thermal energy.
- A compatible Vigilance II monitor uses the thermal energy to calculate CO based on the principle of thermodilution.

Pulse Contour-based Hemodynamic Monitoring Systems FloTrac (Figs. 4A to C)

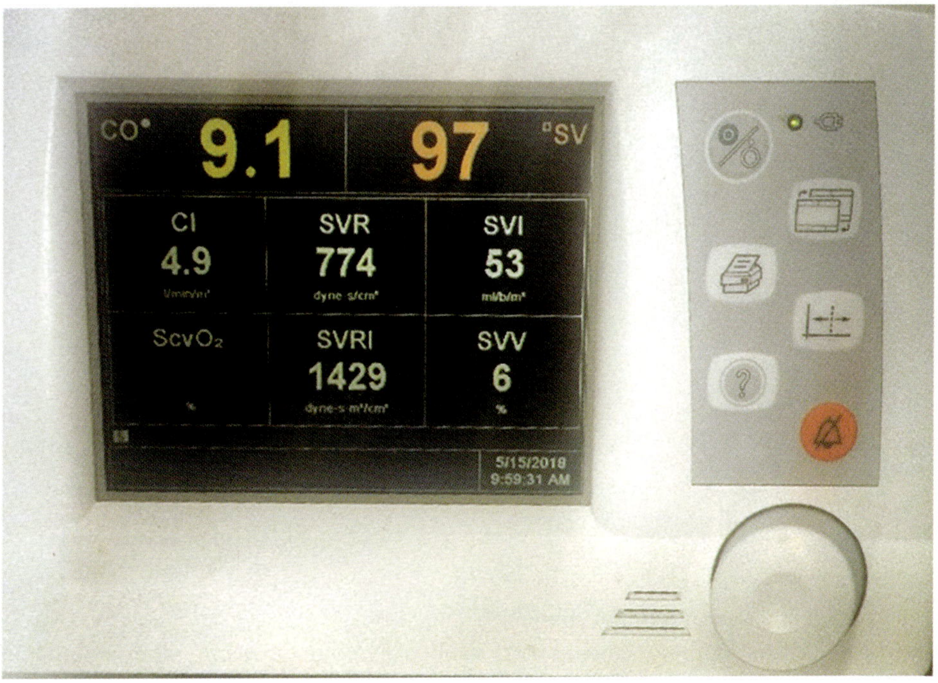

Fig. 4A: Parameters from FloTrac. SVV—Sensitive indicators of preload and volume responsiveness in patients on mechanical ventilation with a tidal ventilation of at least 8 mL/kg. (CI: Cardiac index; SVR: Systemic vascular resistance; SVI: Stroke volume index; SVV: Stroke volume variation).

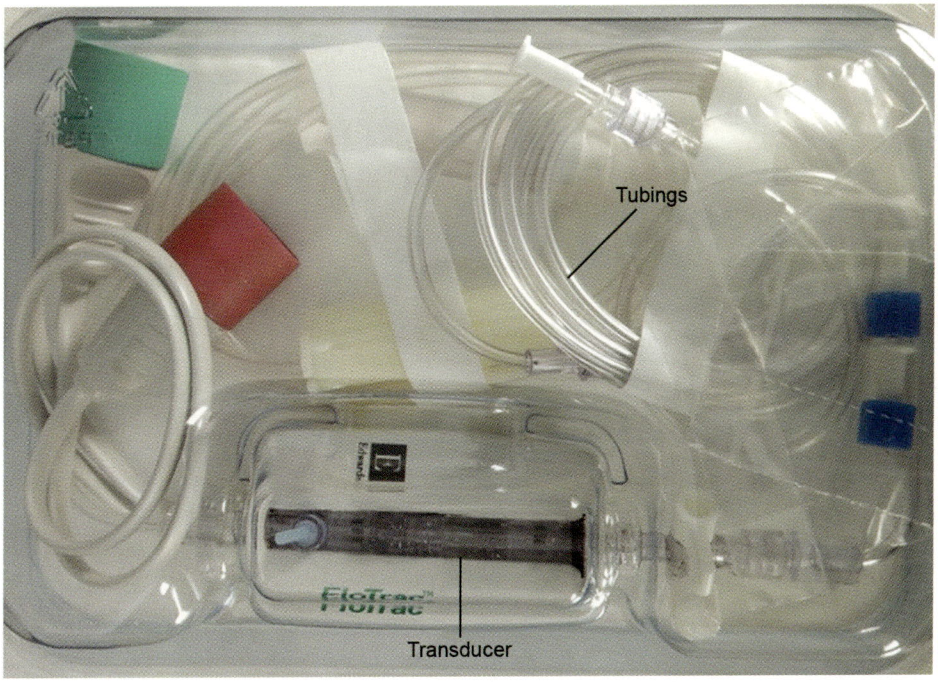

Fig. 4B: FloTrac transducer.

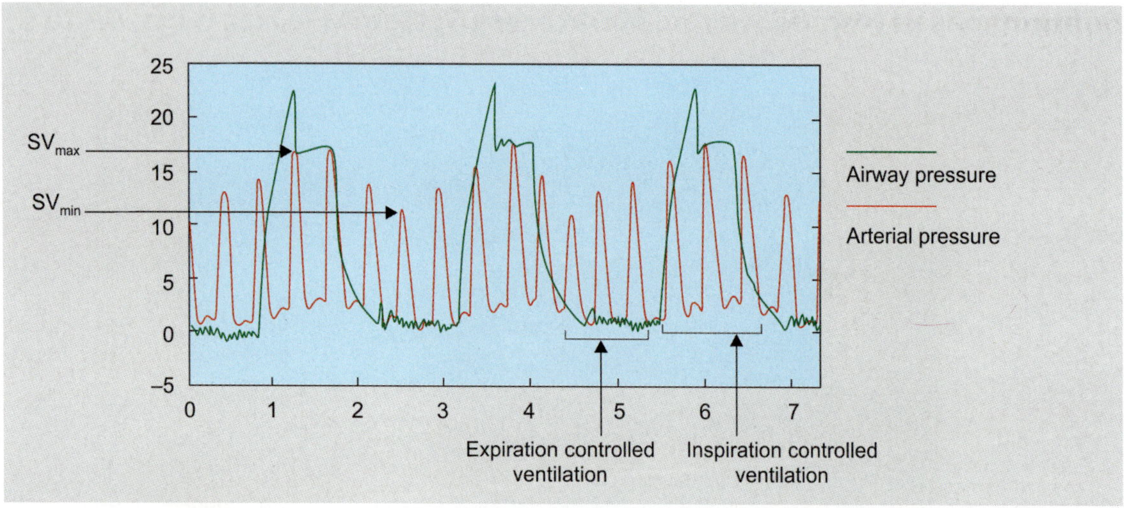

Fig. 4C: Stroke volume variation (SVV), SVV >20% hypovolemia (SV_{max}: Stroke volume maximum; SV_{min}: Stroke volume minimum; SV_{mean}: Stroke volume mean).

- Consists of FloTrac sensor and Vigileo monitor (EV 1,000).
- Requires a peripheral arterial catheter and central venous catheter operator independent, needs no external calibration.
- Requires patient demographics and physical characteristics.
- Arterial pressure waveform is analyzed each 20 seconds at 100 Hz resulting in 2,000 data points.
- Inaccurate in vasoplegic patients, aortic regurgitation, intra-aortic balloon pump (IABP), aortic pathology, and atrial fibrillation (AF).
- $\% \text{ SVV} = \dfrac{SV_{max} - SV_{min}}{SV_{mean}}$

Transpulmonary Thermodilution—PiCCO System (Fig. 5)

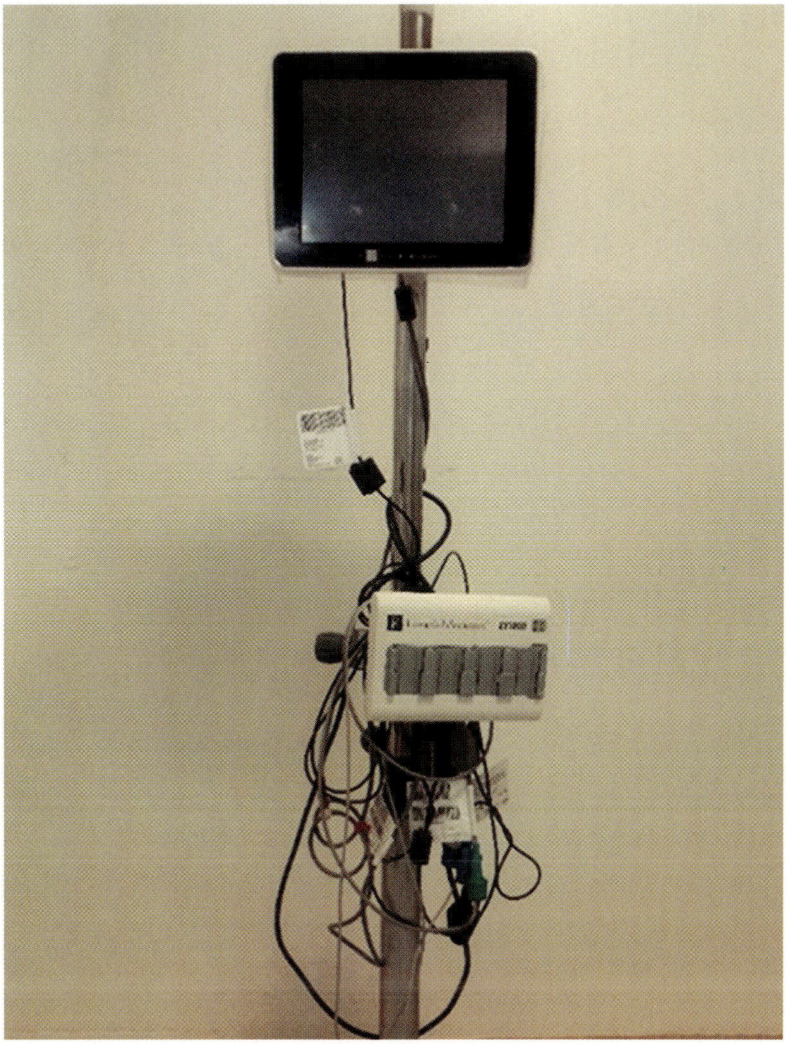

Fig. 5: Pulse contour cardiac output (PiCCO) monitor.

- Requires both central venous (internal jugular or subclavian) and central arterial (femoral artery) catheterization, Vigilance II monitor.
- The area under the systolic portion of the arterial waveform is analyzed to calculate the stroke volume (SV).
- Arterial compliance is derived from the systemic vascular resistance and the diastolic portion of the arterial waveform.
- Uses transpulmonary thermodilution for calibration.
- Gives an estimate of SVV, global end-diastolic volume (GEDV), and extravascular lung water (EVLW).
- Not accurate in arrhythmias or aortic pathology.

LITHIUM DILUTION CARDIAC OUTPUT (LiDCO) (FIGS. 6A AND B)

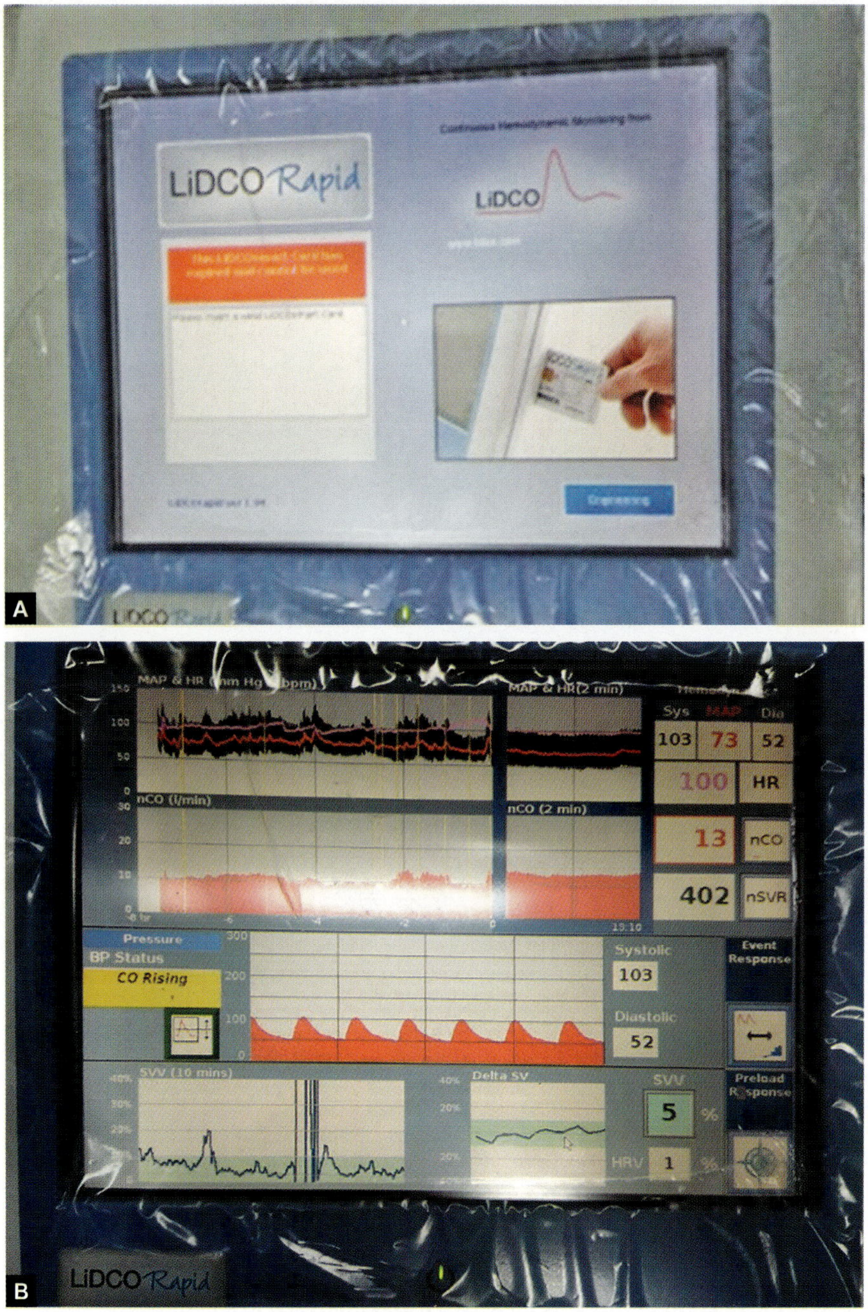

Figs. 6A and B: (A) LiDCO monitor; (B) LiDCO view monitor.

- LiDCO combines the principle of pulse contour analysis with lithium indicator dilution for the evaluation of SV and SVV.
- Manual recalibration is required after any acute hemodynamic changes or any interventions which alter the vascular tone.
- Needs a peripheral or central arterial catheter.
- Contraindicated in patients on lithium therapy.

NEAR-INFRARED SPECTROSCOPY (FIGS. 7A AND B)

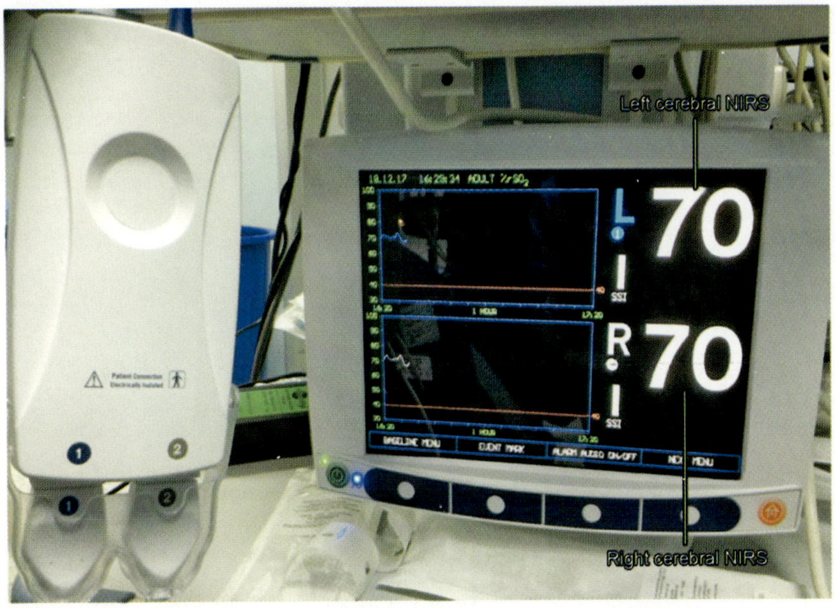

Fig. 7A: Near-infrared spectroscopy (NIRS) monitor.

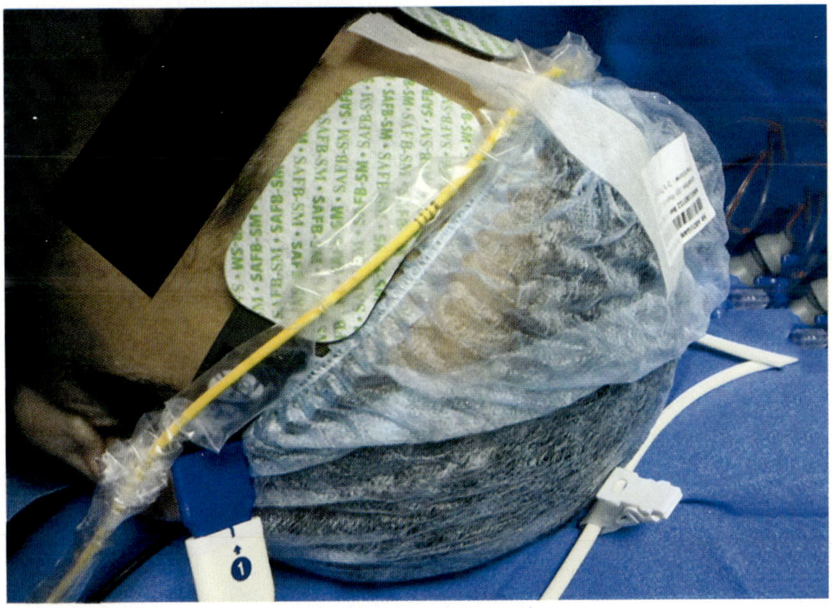

Fig. 7B: NIRS electrodes on forehead.

- First described in 1977 by Franz Jobsis.
- Monitors regional cerebral oxygen saturation ($rScO_2$).
- Noninvasive self-adhesive optode pads having integrated receptors and transmitter are applied on to the forehead skin.
- Uses light in the near-infrared spectrum (NIRS): 700–950 nm.
- *Principle*: Modification of Beer–Lambert's law, measures the concentration of oxygenated hemoglobin in relation to the total hemoglobin concentration.

TEMPORARY EXTERNAL PACEMAKERS (FIG. 8)

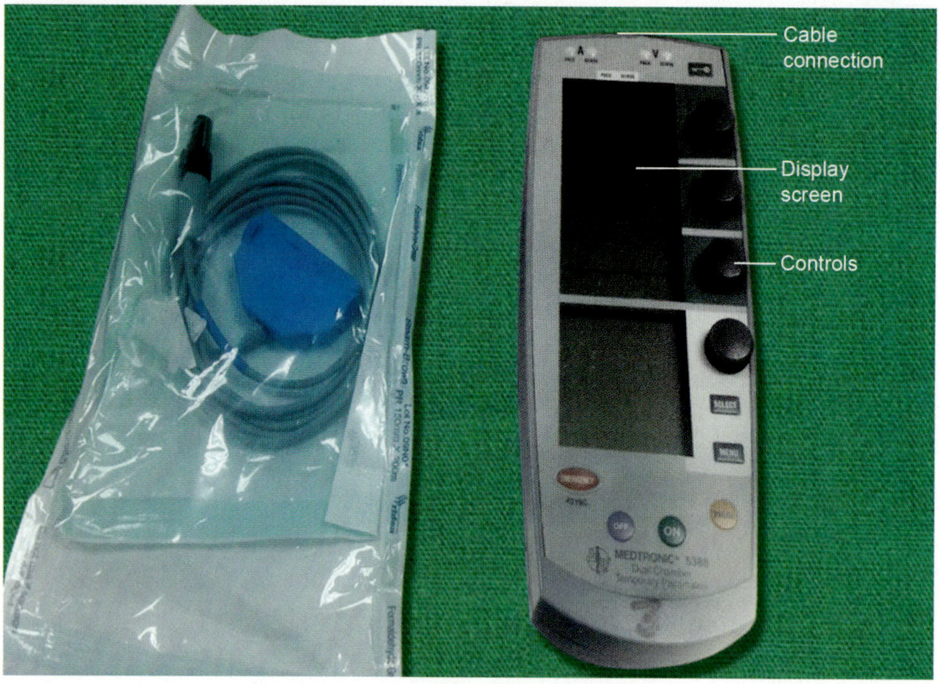

Fig. 8: External pacemaker with cable.

- Indicated in symptomatic bradycardia, bridge to permanent pacing in advanced second- or third-degree atrioventricular (AV) heart block.
- Used along with a cardiac pacing lead system (epicardial and transvenous).
- Needs continuous monitoring of the patient in ICU.
- *Modes used*: DDD, DOO, DDI, AAI, AOO, VVI, and VOO.
- *Pacing rate*: 30–200 ppm.
- *Amplitude*: Atrial—0.1–20 mA, ventricular—0.1–25 mA.
- *Sensitivity*: Atrial—0.4–10 mv, ventricular—0.8–20 mv.
- Transvenous pacing is required in ER or ICU.

EXTRACORPOREAL MEMBRANE OXYGENATOR (FIG. 9)

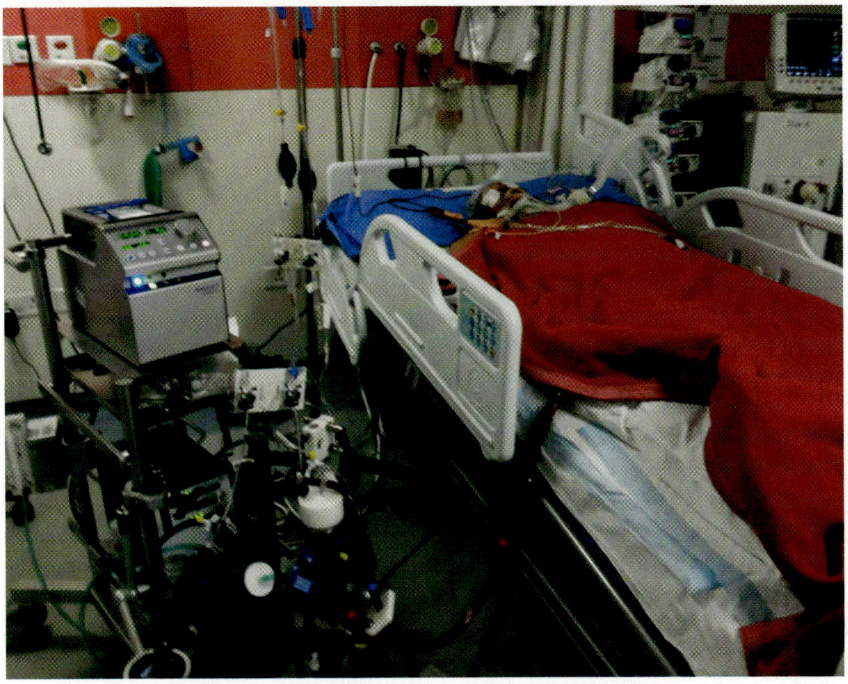

Fig. 9: Patient on extracorporeal membrane oxygenator (ECMO).

Bartlett et al. 1975–1976, successfully applied bedside cardiopulmonary bypass (CPB) to treat a newborn with meconium aspiration, marking the beginning of ECMO in critical care.

- Types:
  - Venoarterial (VA) ECMO
  - Venovenous (VV) ECMO
- *VV ECMO* involves venous blood from the patient being accessed from the large central veins (via the "access line") and returned to the venous system near the right atrium (via the "return line") after it has passed through an oxygenator. It provides support for severe respiratory failure, e.g. acute respiratory distress syndrome (ARDS) when no major cardiac dysfunction exists.
- *VA ECMO* involves venous blood from the patient being accessed from a large central veins and returned to a major artery after it has passed through the oxygenator. It provides support for severe cardiac failure (usually with associated respiratory failure) most commonly after cardiac surgery, cardiogenic shock after acute coronary syndrome (ACS), aluminum phosphide poisoning, myocarditis, etc.

THROMBOELASTOGRAPHY (FIGS. 10A TO C)

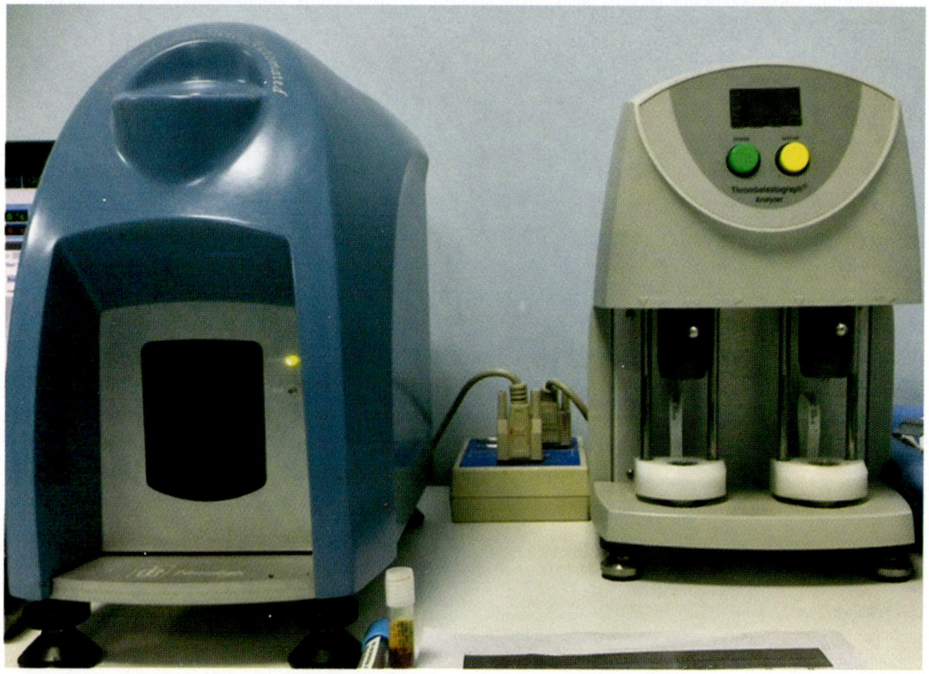

Fig. 10A: Thromboelastography (TEG) machine.

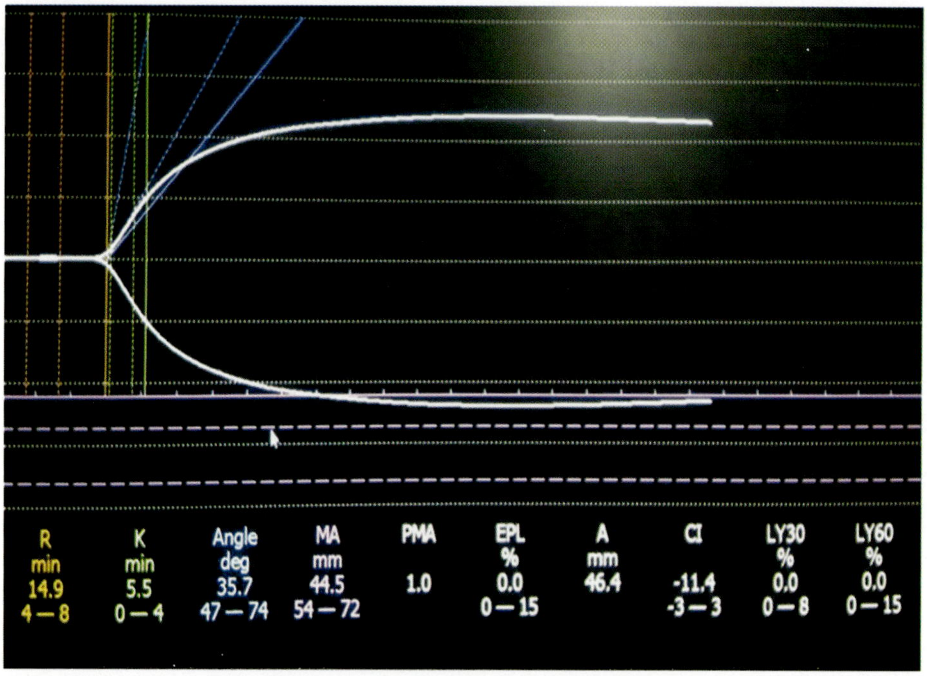

Fig. 10B: Normal thromboelastography (TEG) graph.

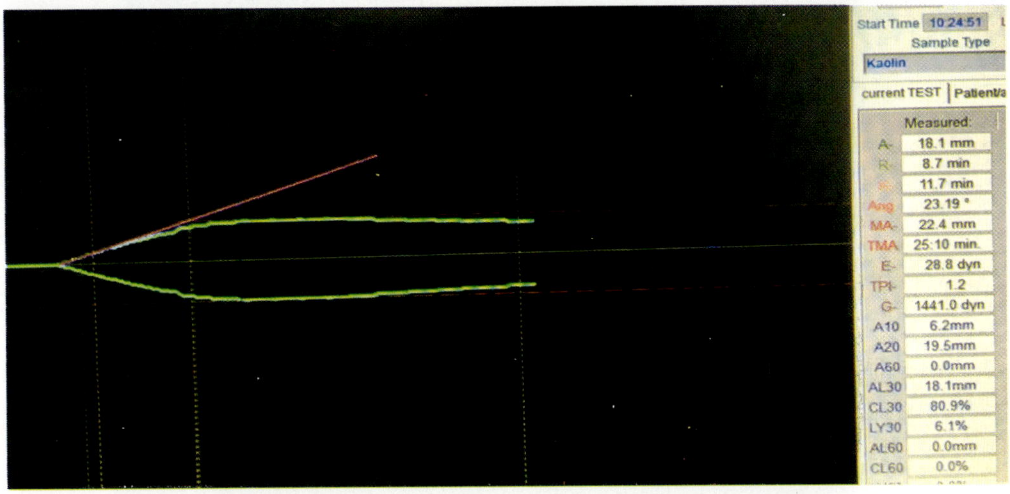

Fig. 10C: Reduced alpha angle and maximal amplitude (MA).

- Developed by Hartert in 1948, used to diagnose coagulation abnormalities.
- Can be performed onsite in operating room or in the laboratory, gives an information of the integrity of coagulation cascade, platelet function, platelet fibrin interaction, and fibrinolysis.
- Used for point-of-care testing (POCT) of coagulation cascade, by viscoelastic properties of the clot.
- *Parameters measured*:
  - *R value*: Reaction time—time for initial fibrin formation—coagulation factors
  - K value: Speed of clot formation
  - *Alpha angle*: Index of speed of clot formation
  - *MA (maximum amplitude)*: Clot strength, platelet function, and interaction with fibrin
  - *A60*: Amplitude 60 minutes after MA
  - *LY30:* Clot lysis 30 minutes after MA—fibrinolysis
  - *LY60*: Clot lysis 60 minutes after MA—fibrinolysis.

ACTIVATED CLOTTING TIME (FIGS. 11A AND B)

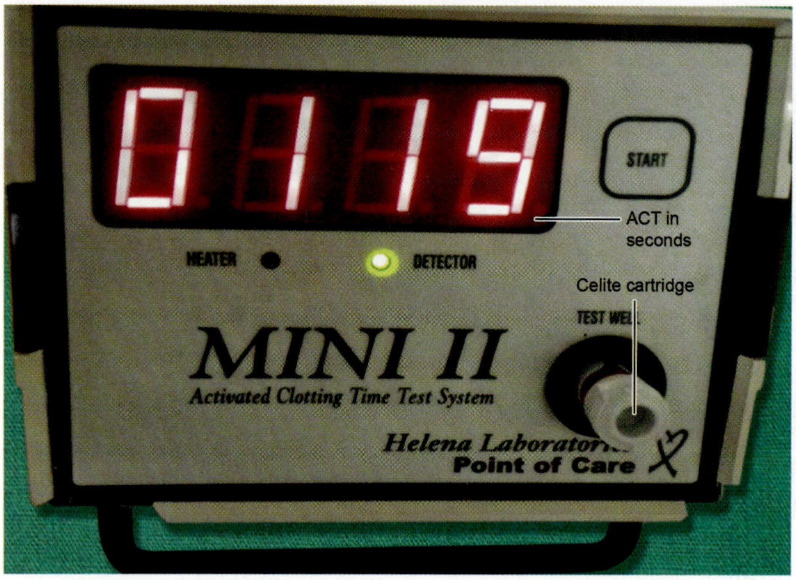

Fig. 11A: Activated clotting time (ACT) machine with cartridge.

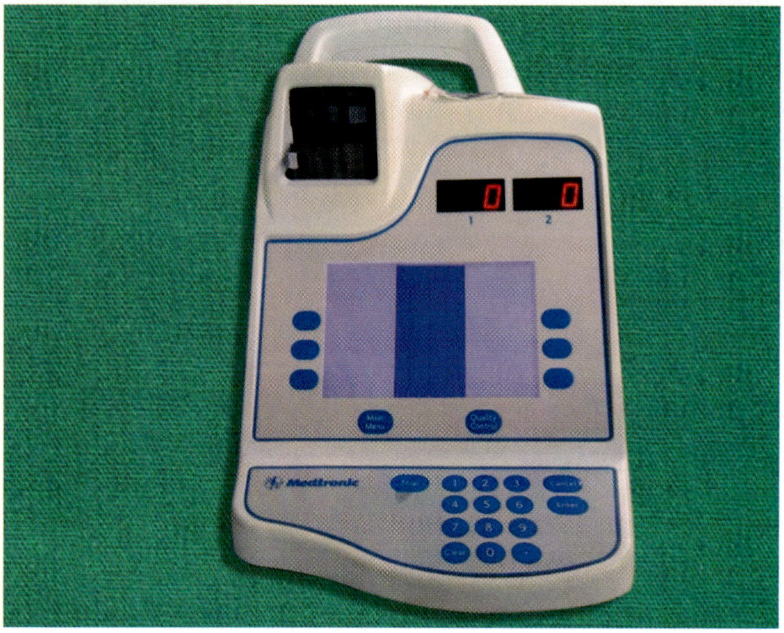

Fig. 11B: Activated clotting time (ACT) machine.

- First introduced by Hattersley in 1966.
- Whole blood is added to a test tube containing an activator—diatomaceous earth (Celite) or kaolin—activates the intrinsic coagulation pathway.
- Hemochron-activated clotting time (ACT) device (International Technidyne, Edison, NJ)—Celite activator.
  - Hemotec ACT device (Medtronic Hemotec) kaolin activator
- Most widely used to monitor heparin effect during cardiac surgeries and catheterization laboratory procedures and extracorporeal membrane oxygenation (ECMO).

NONINVASIVE CARDIOMETRY (FIGS. 12A TO C)

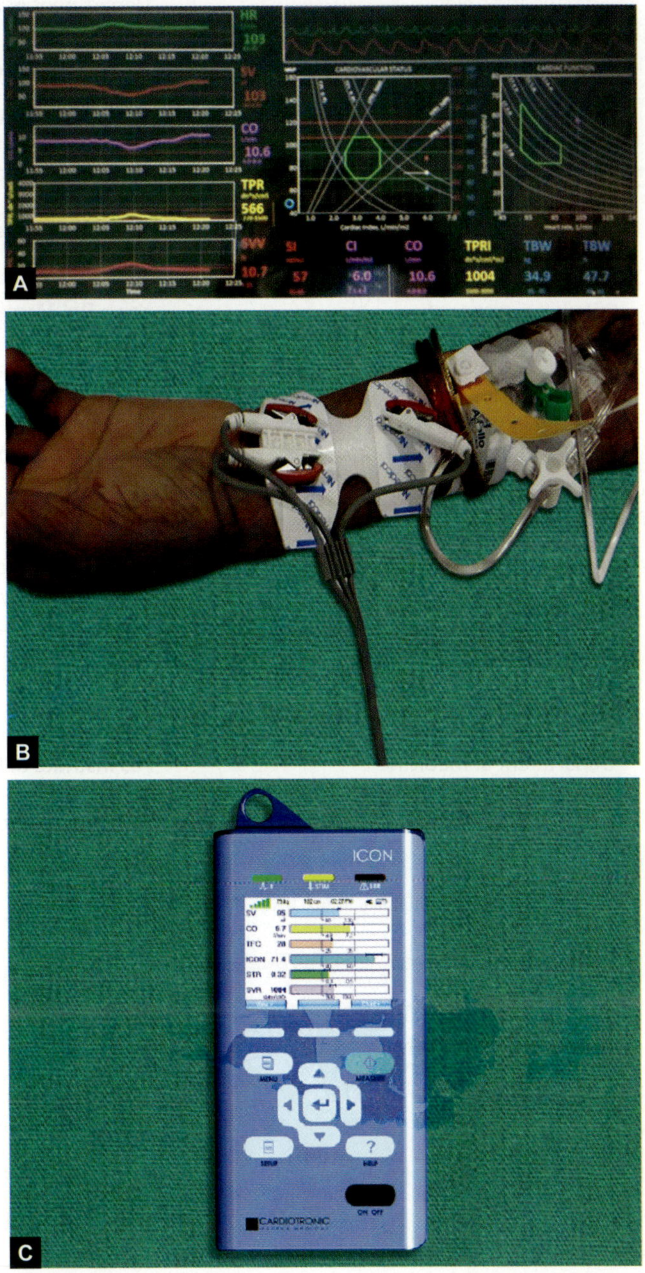

Figs. 12A to C: (A) NICaS noninvasive monitor; (B) NICaS noninvasive peripheral leads; (C) ICON—electrical cardiometry.

- Easy to use and noninvasive technology.
- Helps in continuous monitoring of hemodynamic variables—stroke volume, cardiac output, total peripheral resistance, total body water, etc.
- Clinically validated against pulse contour analysis and thermodilution techniques.
- *Principle*: Bioimpedance (impedance cardiography):
  - *Thoracic bioimpedance*: ICON (electrical cardiometry), OSYPKA medical
  - *Regional (whole body) impedance cardiography*: Noninvasive cardiac system (NICaS), NIMedical
  - *Bioreactance*: NICOM, Cheetah medical.
- *Limitations*: Aortic valve stenosis, aortic regurgitation, aortic dissection, and peripheral vascular diseases.

INTRA-AORTIC BALLOON PUMP (FIGS. 13A TO E)

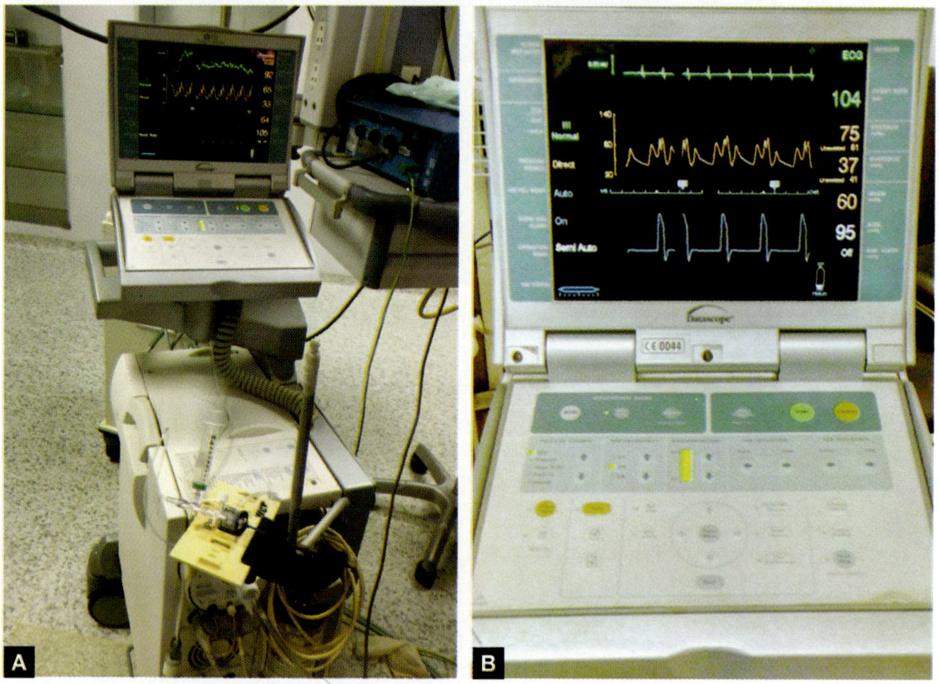

Figs. 13A and B: (A) Intra-aortic balloon pump (IABP) console; (B) IABP monitor and control.

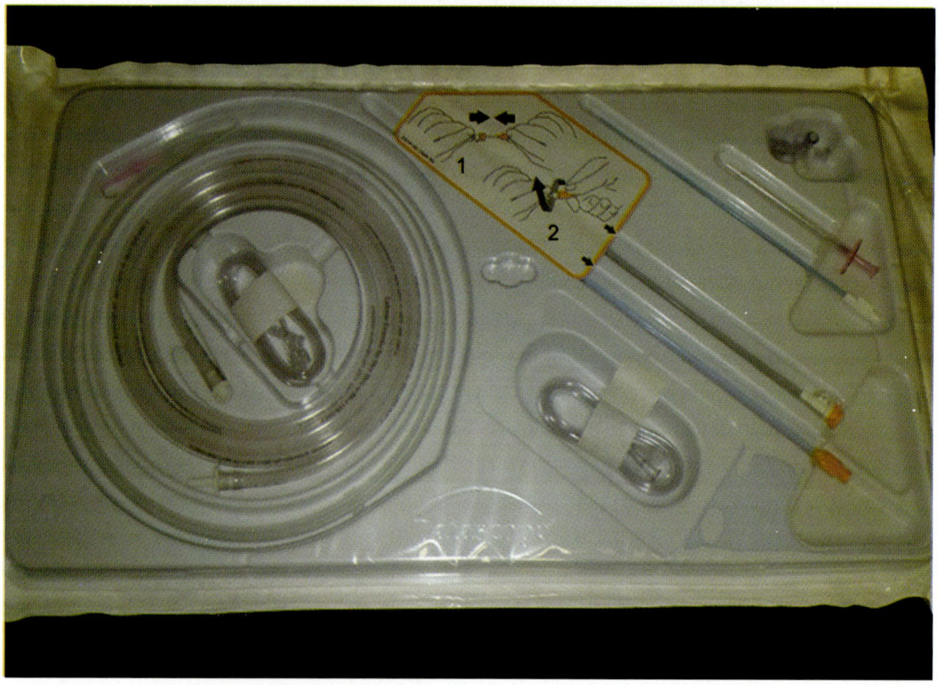

Fig. 13C: Insertion kit for use with intra-aortic balloon catheters.

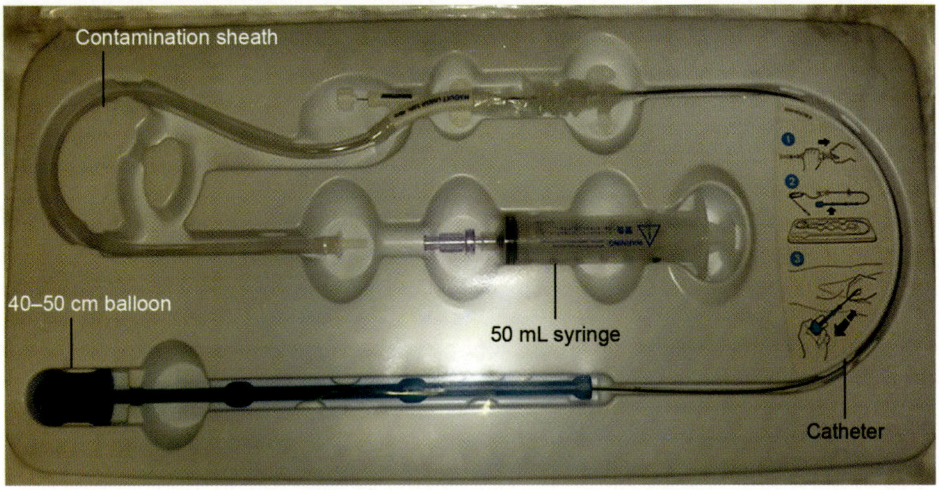

Fig. 13D: Intra-aortic balloon (IAB) catheter.

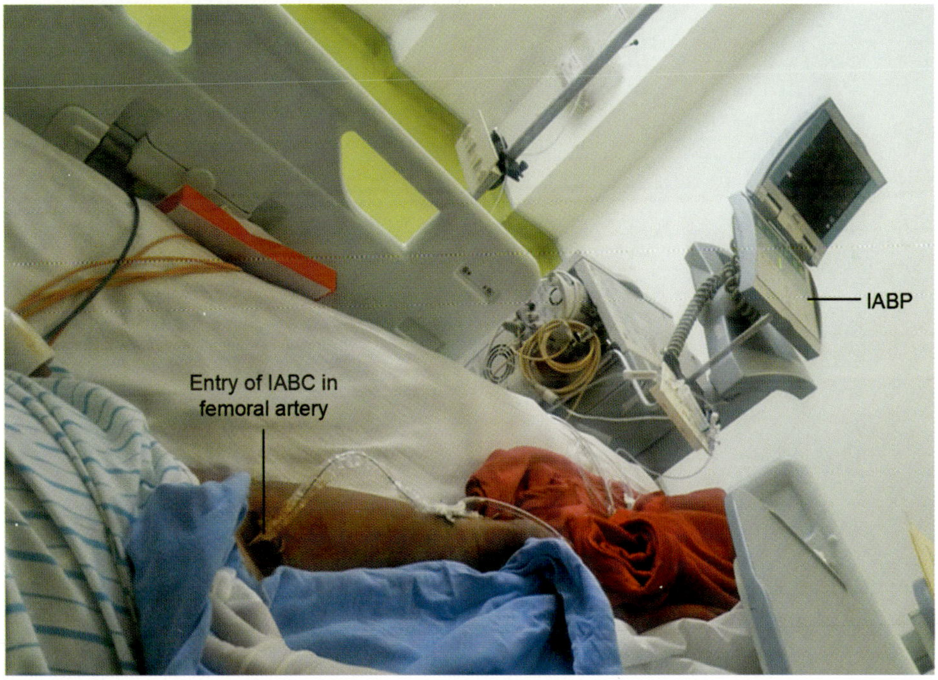

Fig. 13E: Entry of intra-aortic balloon catheter (IABC) and intra-aortic balloon pump (IABP).

- Invented by Adrian Kantrowitz in late 1960s.
- Most common mechanical support for the failing heart improving the myocardial supply/demand ratio.
- Augments the myocardial perfusion by increasing the coronary blood flow during diastole and unloading the left ventricle during systole.
- Alternately inflating and deflating balloon in the proximal descending aorta with helium or carbon dioxide gas.
- Synchronized to the cardiac cycle by the electronics of the balloon console.

CHAPTER

23

Hematology

Rahul Bhargava, Amrita Ramaswamy, Nitin Sood, Shalini Goel, Ritesh Sachdev

MALARIAL PARASITE (FIGS. 1 AND 2)

Plasmodium Falciparum (Figs. 1A and B)

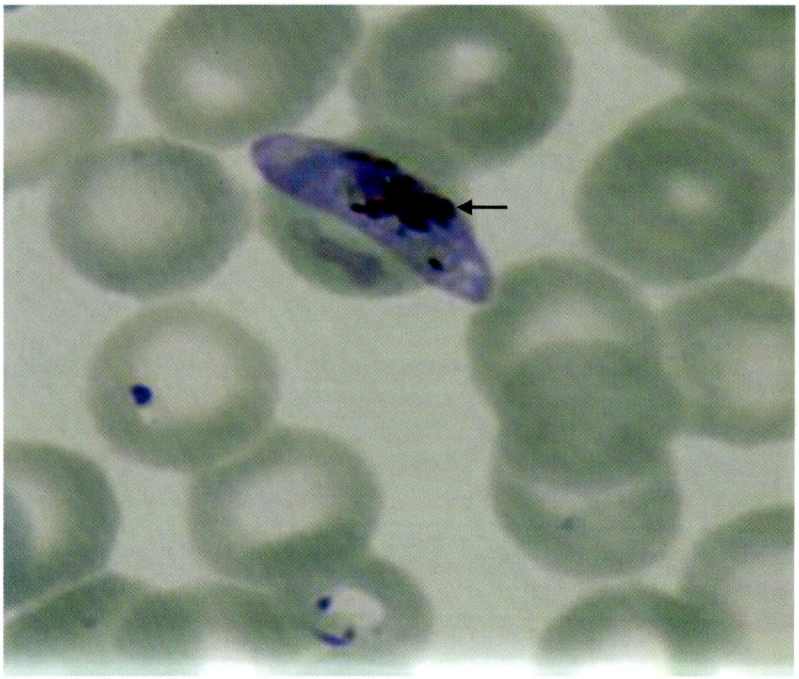

Fig. 1A: Gametocyte of *P. falciparum* in a thin blood smear. Also seen in this image are ring-form trophozoites.

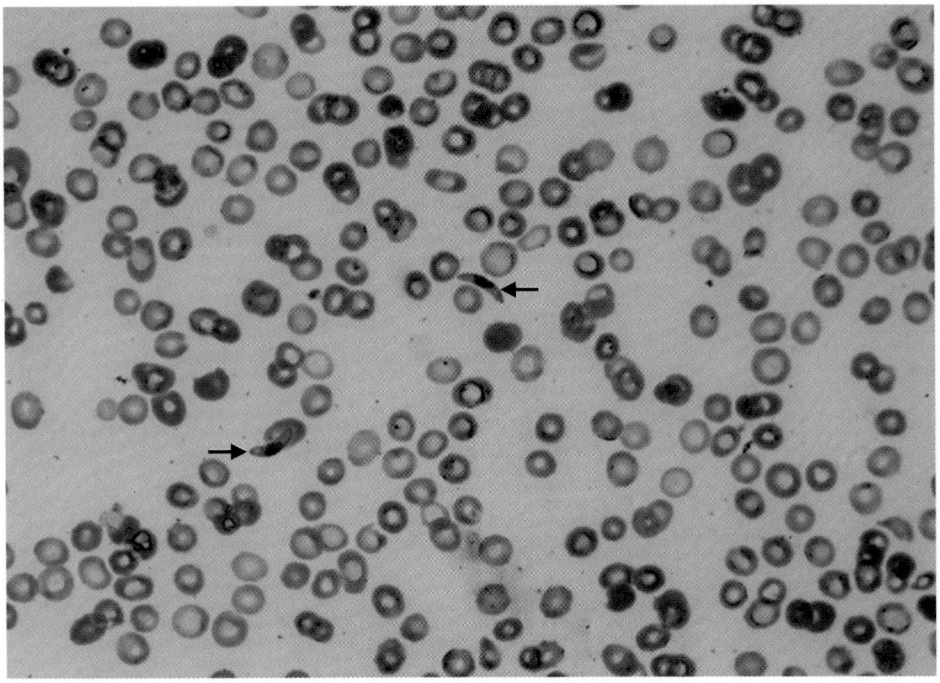

Fig. 1B: *Plasmodium falciparum.*

- *Plasmodium falciparum* infection is diagnosed on the peripheral smear by the identification of the classic banana-shaped or crescent-shaped gametocytes.
- The peripheral smear in *P. falciparum* infection shows only early ring forms and gametocytes with other stages of the parasite being absent (they undergo maturation in the blood vessels of the deeper organs).
- This is in contrast to *Plasmodium vivax* in which all stages of the parasite are seen to mature in the peripheral blood.

PLASMODIUM VIVAX (FIG. 2)

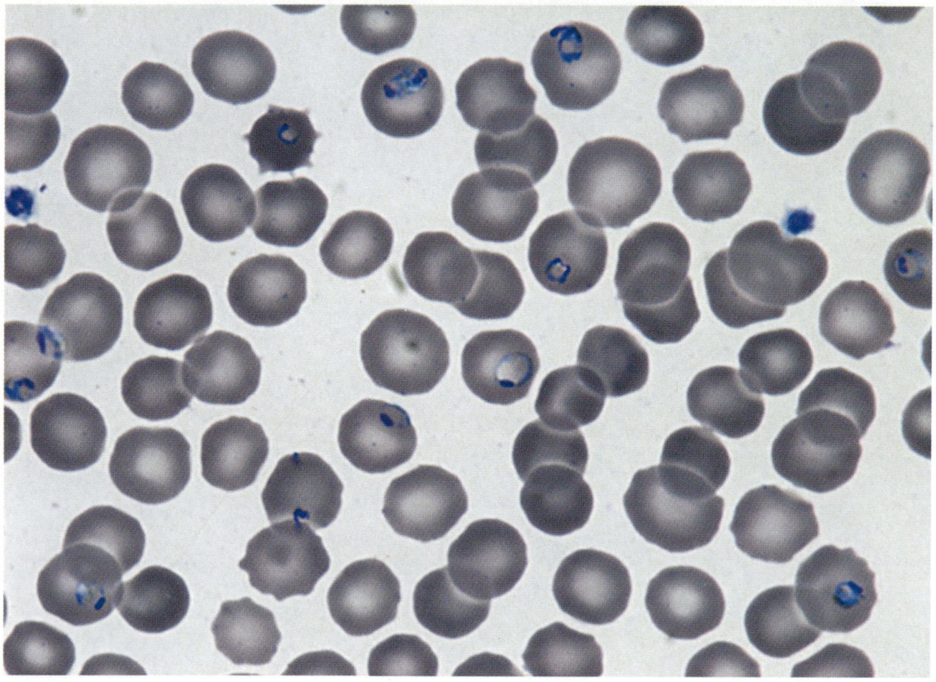

Fig. 2: *Plasmodium vivax.*

- *Plasmodium vivax* is characterized by the presence of various stages of the parasite like ring forms, early to late schizonts and gametocytes in the peripheral blood unlike *P. falciparum* in which only gametocytes are seen in the peripheral blood.
- The parasitized red blood cells show single rings in *P. vivax* as opposed to multiple rings in *P. falciparum.*
- The double rings seen at Nine O'Clock position in the image is due to overlapping red blood cells (RBCs).

ROULEAUX FORMATION (FIG. 3)

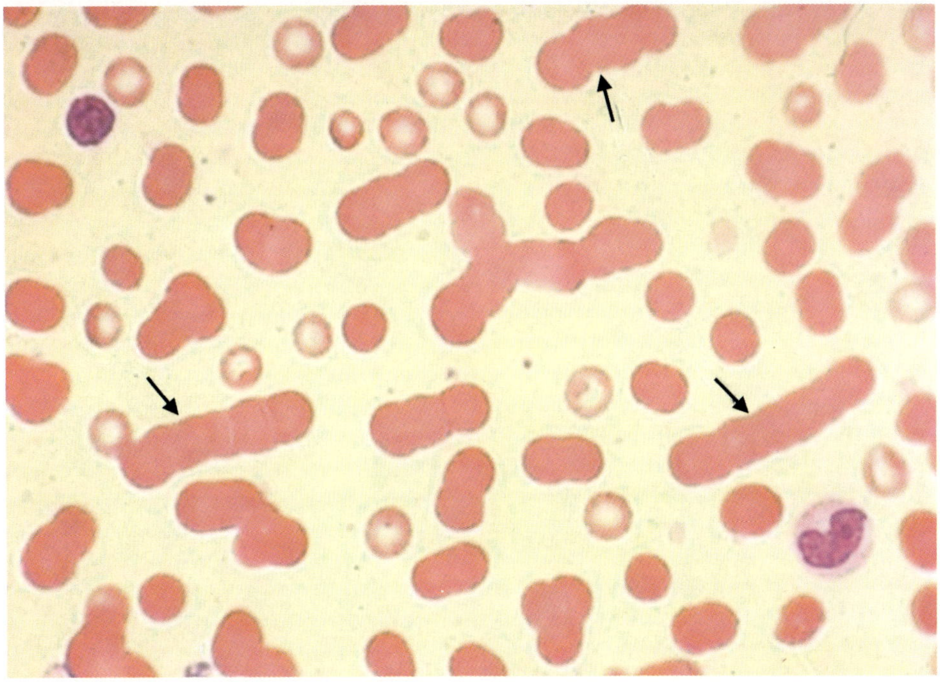

Fig. 3: Rouleaux are stacks or aggregations of red blood cells (RBCs).

- Common causes—Autoimmune hemolytic anemia (AIHA), myeloma chronic infections, connective tissue diseases, and chronic liver disease.

RED BLOOD CELL AGGLUTINATION (FIG. 4)

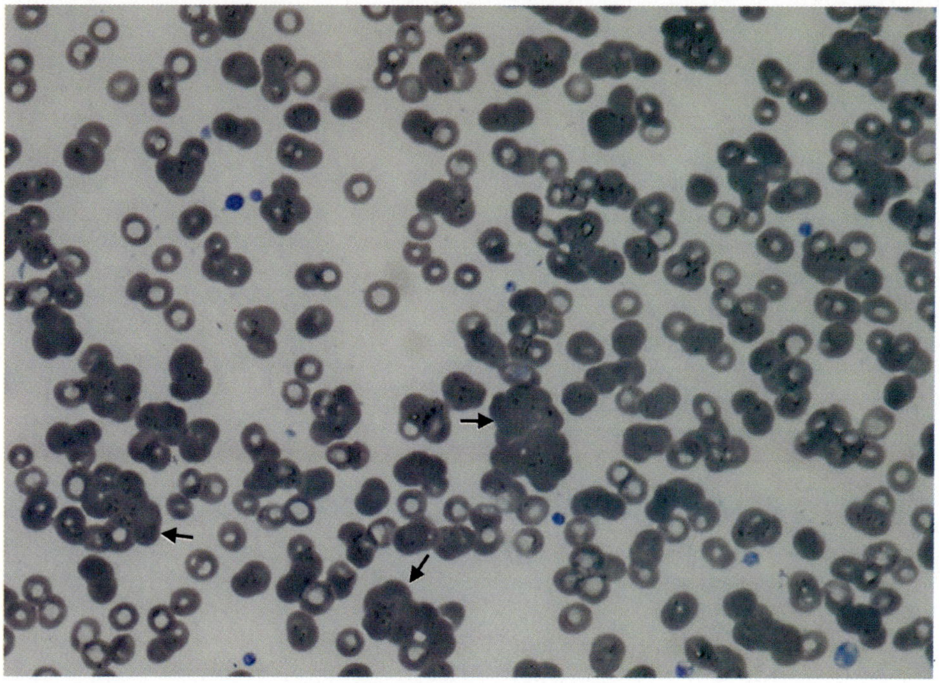

Fig. 4: Red blood cell agglutination.

- Clumping (agglutination) of red blood cells is commonly caused by cold agglutinins.
- Cold agglutinins are IgM antibodies that are seen in the setting of mycoplasma or viral infections, lymphoid neoplasms and plasma cell dyscrasias.
- The red blood cell count may be falsely low and the mean corpuscular volume (MCV) may be falsely elevated, as clumps of red cells are measured as single cell.

MICROCYTIC HYPOCHROMIC ANEMIA (FIGS. 5A AND B)

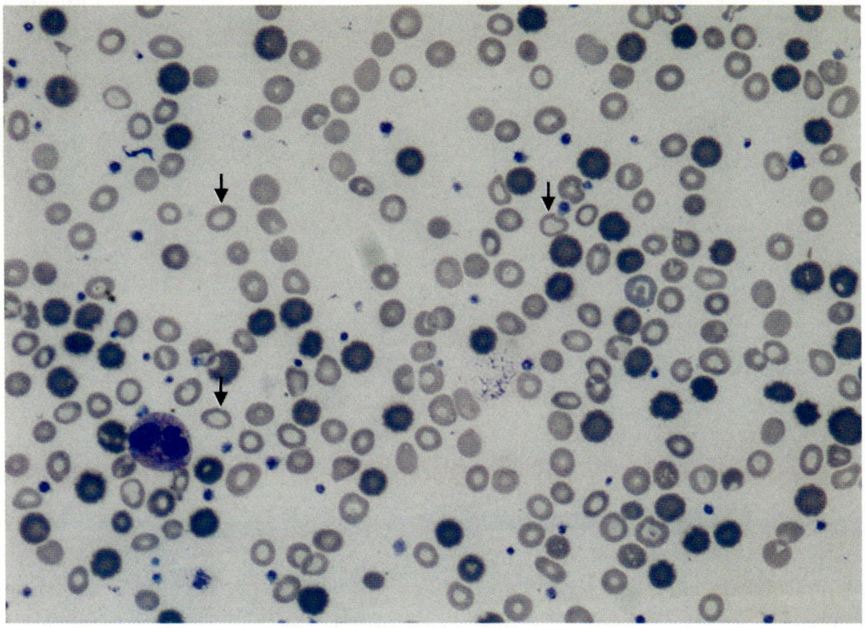

Fig. 5A: Microcytic hypochromic anemia.

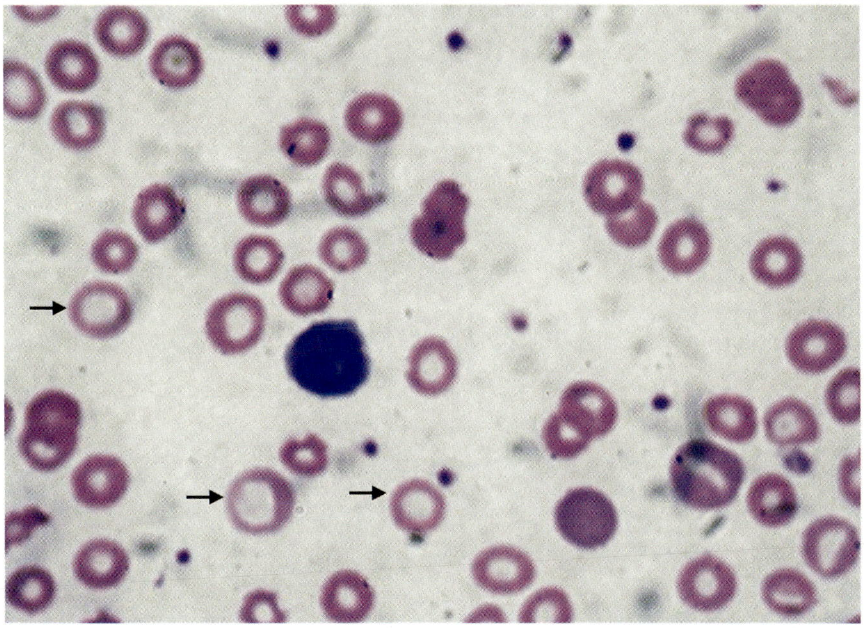

Fig. 5B: Microcytic hypochromic red cells.

- The size of a normal RBC is equal to the size of the nucleus of a small lymphocyte.
- Microcytes are red blood cells, smaller than the nucleus of a small lymphocyte and have a low MCV.
- Microcytic hypochromic red blood cells are smaller and fainter (less hemoglobinized) red blood cells.
- They are seen in iron deficiency anemia, thalassemic hemoglobinopathies, lead poisoning and sideroblastic anemia.
- Compare the size of the red blood cell to the nucleus of a small lymphocyte shown in the field for comparison.

SCHISTOCYTES HELMET CELLS (FIG. 6)

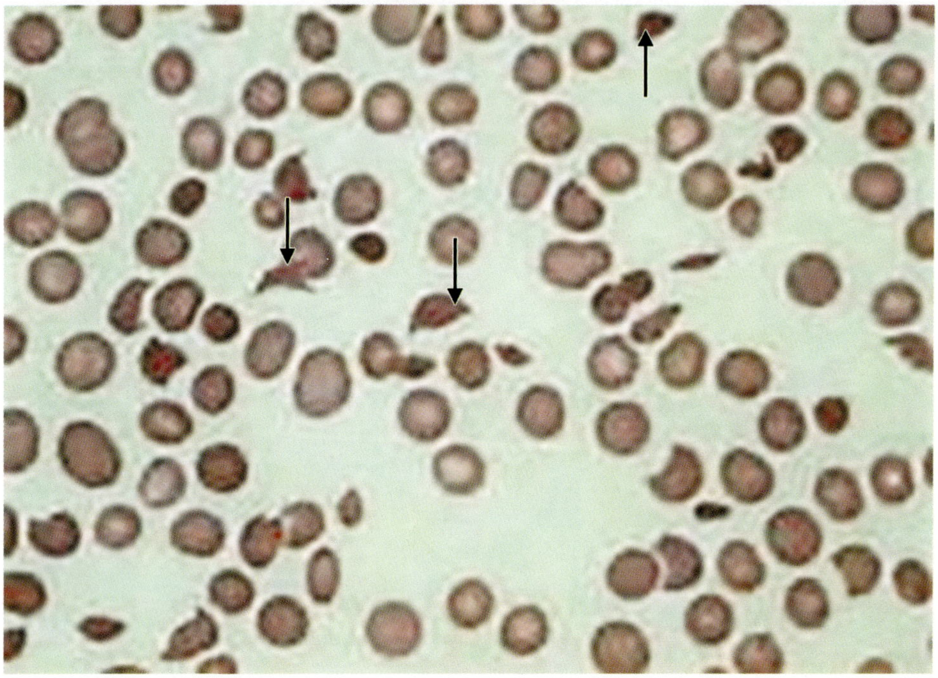

Fig. 6: Helmet-like cells in ICU.

- Fragmented red blood cells are also called schistocytes (helmet cells).
- Schistocytes are hallmark for microangiopathic hemolytic anemia.
- They are produced when red blood cells are fragmented on being subjected to excessive shear stress in the microcirculation.
- *Causes*: Sepsis, thrombotic thrombocytopenic purpura (TTP), defective valvular prosthesis and DIC and March hemoglobinuria.

SICKLE CELLS (FIG. 7)

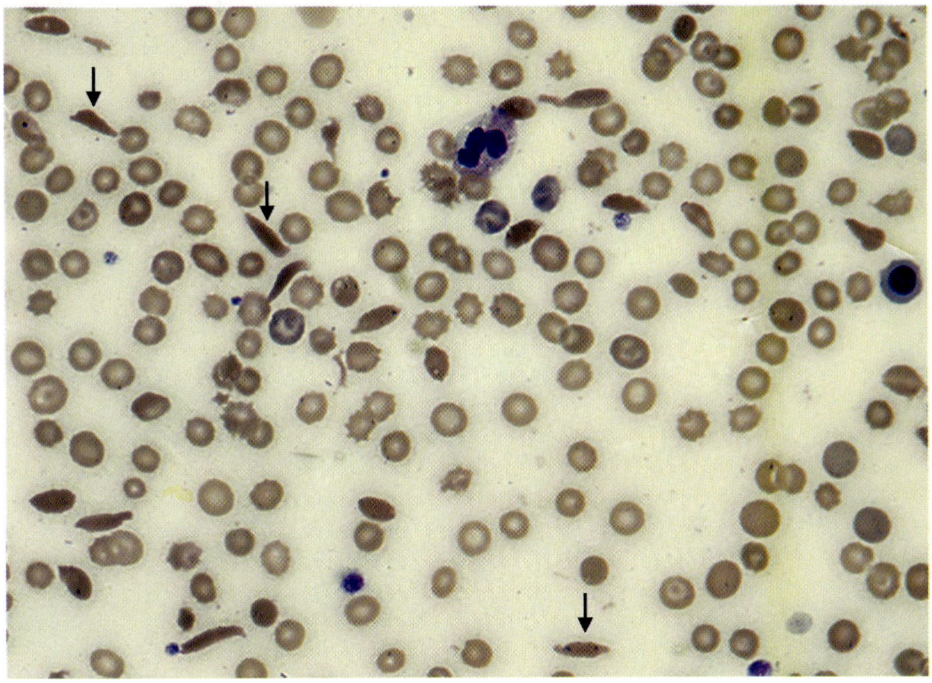

Fig. 7: Sickle cells.

- Sickle cells are so named because of their resemblance to the sickle. They are crescent shaped.
- Sickling is initially a reversible phenomenon when RBCs containing HbS are subjected to hypoxia. HbS polymerizes and damages the red cell membrane resulting in sickling. On oxygenation, sickled cells assume their normal shape.
- After repeated cycles of sickling and unsickling, the cells become irreversibly sickled.
- They are seen in sickle cell hemoglobinopathies.
- Sickling can be induced by exposure of the patient's blood sample to sodium metabisulfite which is a sickling agent.
- Common in Africa and tribals in Madhya Pradesh in India.

TOXIC GRANULES IN PERIPHERAL SMEAR (FIG. 8)

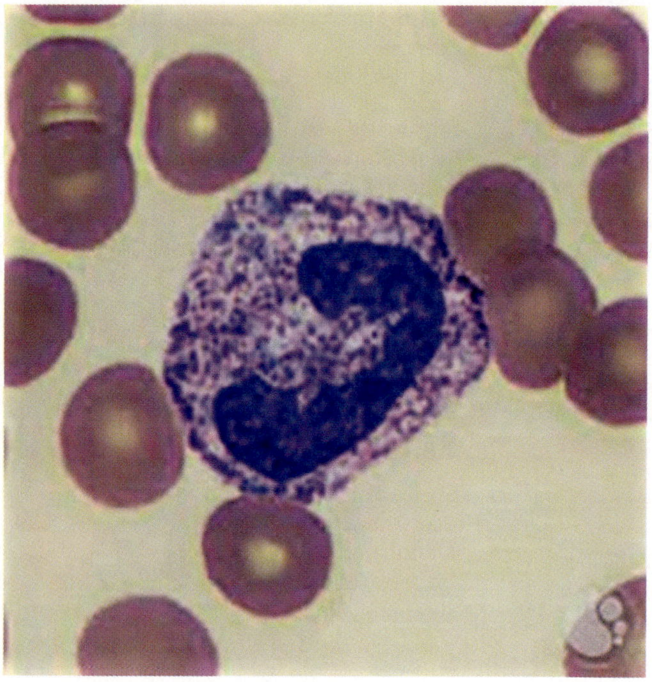

Fig. 8: Toxic granules are seen as presence of large granules in the cytoplasm neutrophils.

- Toxic granules are actually azurophilic granules, normally present in early myeloid forms, but are not normally seen at the band and segmented stages of neutrophil maturation (Fig. 8).
- Hallmark of sepsis.
- Other causes RA and autophagocytosis.

HYPERSEGMENTED NEUTROPHILS (FIG. 9)

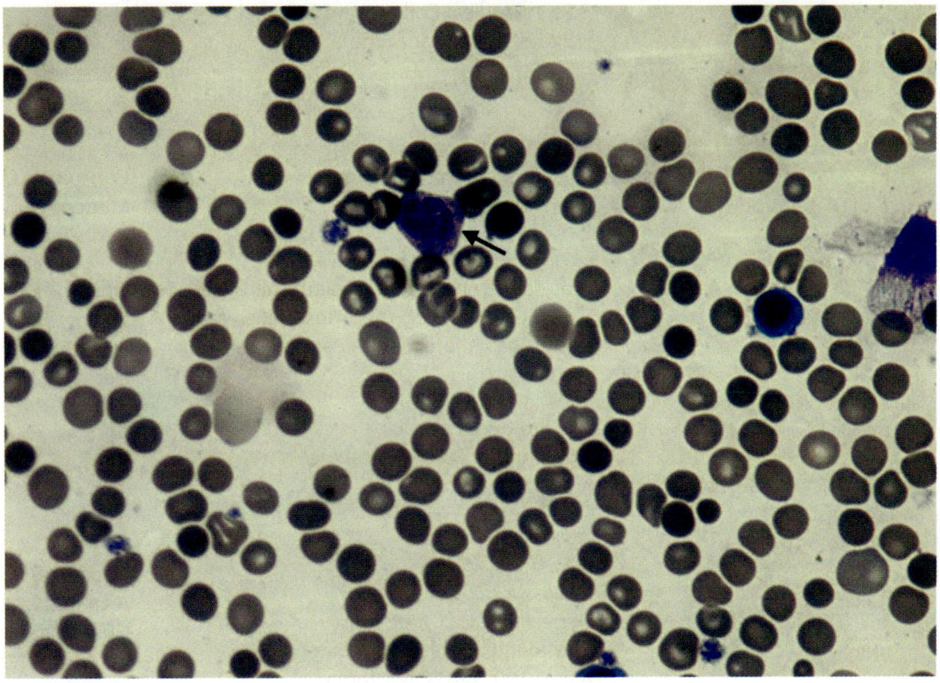

Fig. 9: Hypersegmented neutrophils.

- Normal neutrophils have three to four lobes.
- Neutrophils are said to be hypersegmented when there are at least 5% neutrophils showing 5 lobes or a single neutrophil with six lobes.
- Neutrophil hypersegmentation is seen in Vitamin B_{12} and folate deficiency, iron deficiency and myelodysplastic syndromes.
- Other features of Vitamin B_{12} deficiency are macro-ovalocytosis, tear drop cells, Cabot rings and basophilic stippling.

ACUTE PROMYELOCYTIC LEUKEMIA (FIGS. 10A AND B)

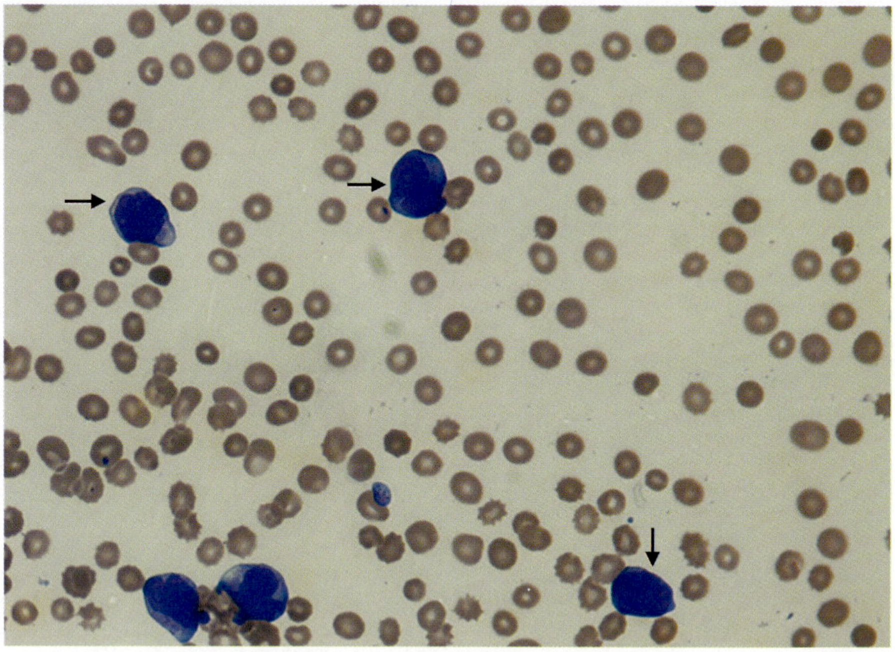

Fig. 10A: Acute promyelocytic leukemia.

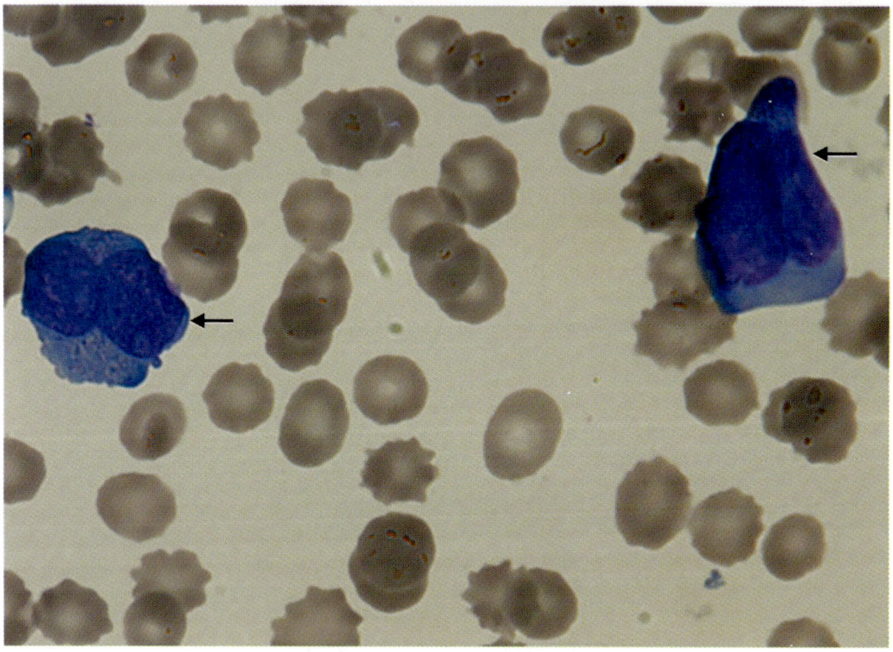

Fig. 10B: Acute promyelocytic leukemia.

- Acute promyelocytic leukemia is a variant of acute myeloid leukemia characterized by the presence of abnormal promyelocytes in the peripheral blood caused by differentiation arrest.
- The abnormal promyelocytes are characterized by the presence of abundant granules in the cytoplasm and the distinctive bilobed or buttock-shaped nucleus.
- It is an oncologic emergency as the patient is at a high risk of bleeding from DIC and hyperfibrinolysis.

CHRONIC MYELOID LEUKEMIA (FIG. 11)

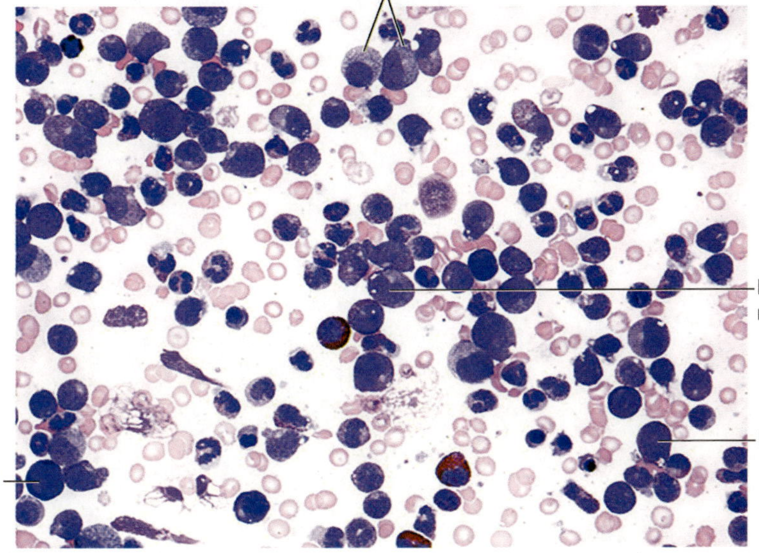

Fig. 11: Leukocytosis (2,30,000 cells per cubic mm).

- Most common cause of leukocytosis is sepsis however, other causes may be there without infection.
- Chronic myeloid leukemia (CML) is one of the causes.
- In the slide myelocyte, metamyelocytes and blast are seen, this is called left shift.

CHRONIC LYMPHOCYTIC LEUKEMIA (FIG. 12)

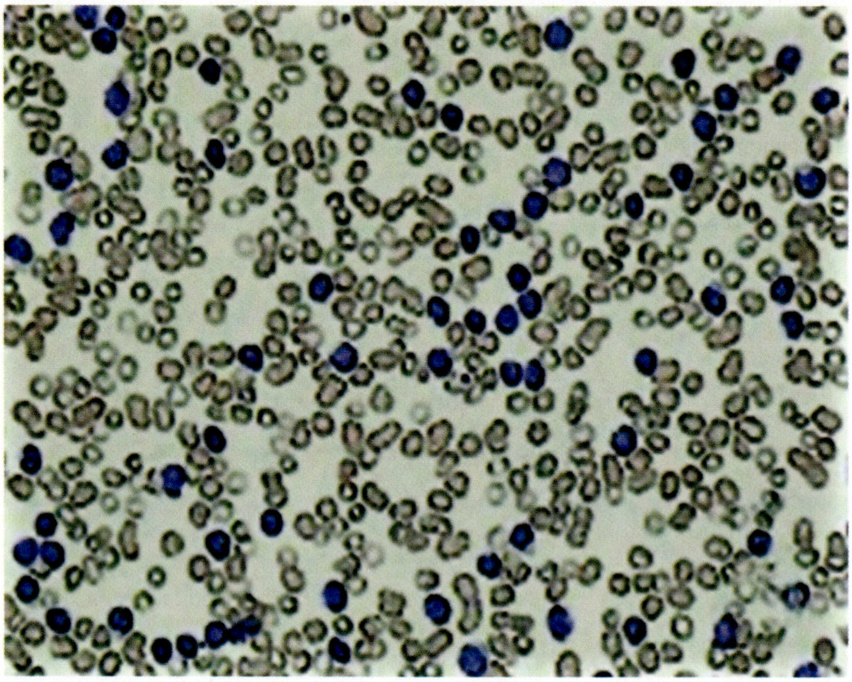

Fig. 12: Elderly gentleman with TLC count of 50,000 with normal Hb and platelet count.

- Small lymphocytes.
- Chronic lymphocytic leukemia needs more than 5,000/cumm clonal CD5 and CD23 positive cells to diagnose this disorder.
- 80% people do not require treatment.

BLAST AND MYELOBLAST CELLS (FIGS. 13A AND B)

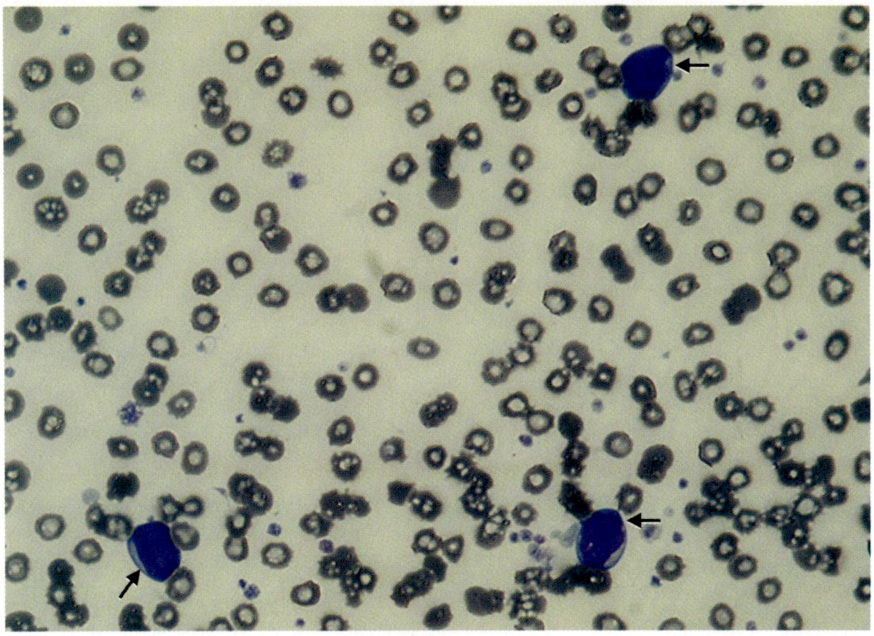

Fig. 13A: Blast cells.

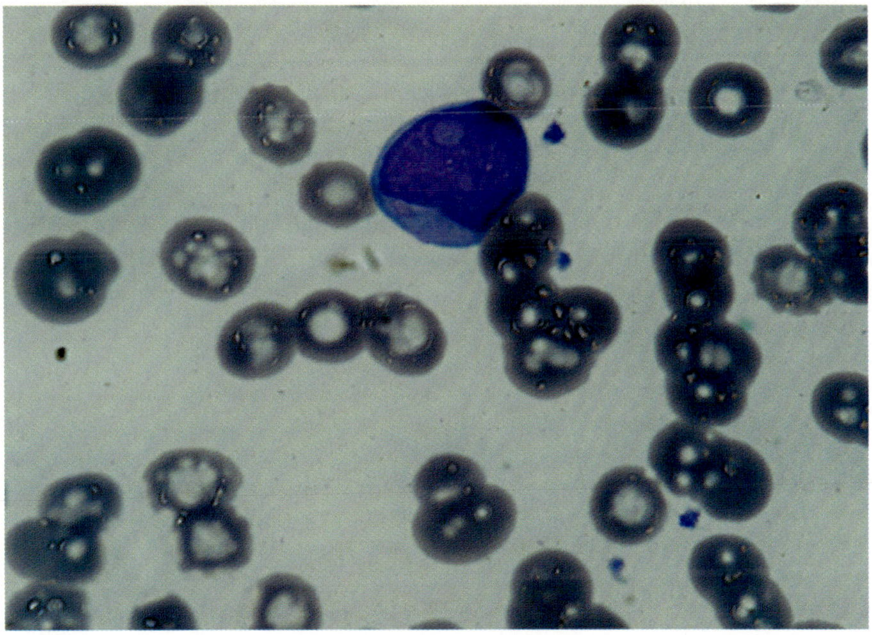

Fig. 13B: Myeloblast cells.

- Blasts are cells with an increased nuclear cytoplasmic ratio, opened up chromatin and one or more prominent nucleoli (The cytoplasm of the cell in the image shows an Auer rod which is classical of myeloid blasts).
- Blasts may be lymphoblasts seen in acute lymphoblastic leukemia (ALL) or myeloblasts seen in acute myeloid leukemia (AML) (≥20% in the blood or bone marrow).
- Blasts are also seen in the peripheral blood in chronic myeloproliferative neoplasms like chronic myeloid leukemia, primary myelofibrosis, myelodysplastic syndrome (MDS) and bone marrow infiltrative disorders.

HEMOPHAGOCYTIC LYMPHOHISTIOCYTOSIS—HEMOPHAGOCYTIC PHENOMENON (FIG. 14)

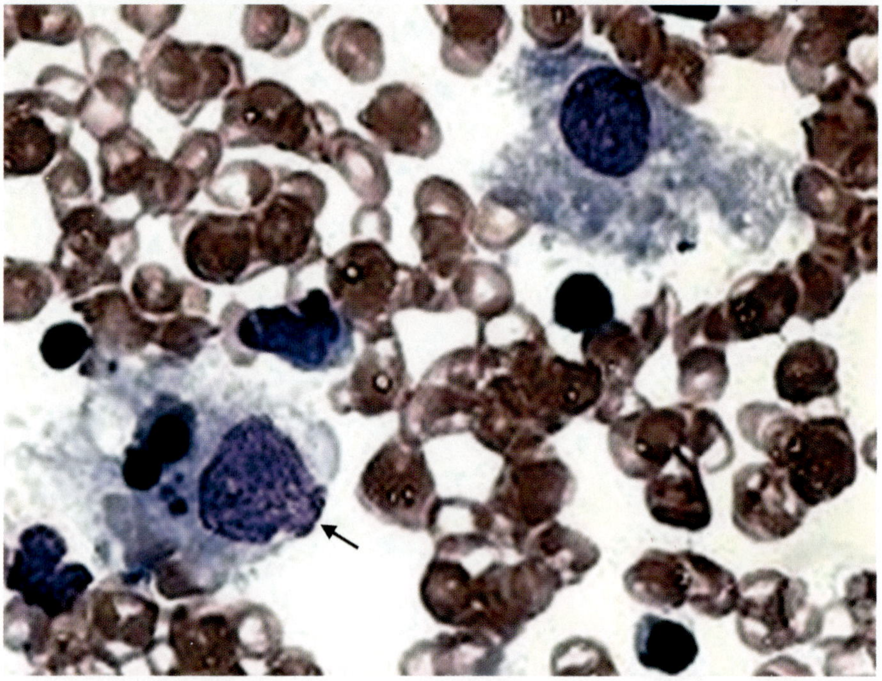

Fig. 14: Hemophagocytic phenomenon—macrophage engulfing the cells.

- Hemophagocytic lymphohistiocytosis (HLH) is inherited or acquired.
- Epstein-Barr virus (EBV) is the most common cause.
- Specified criteria are required to diagnose HLS.

EOSINOPHILS (FIG. 15)

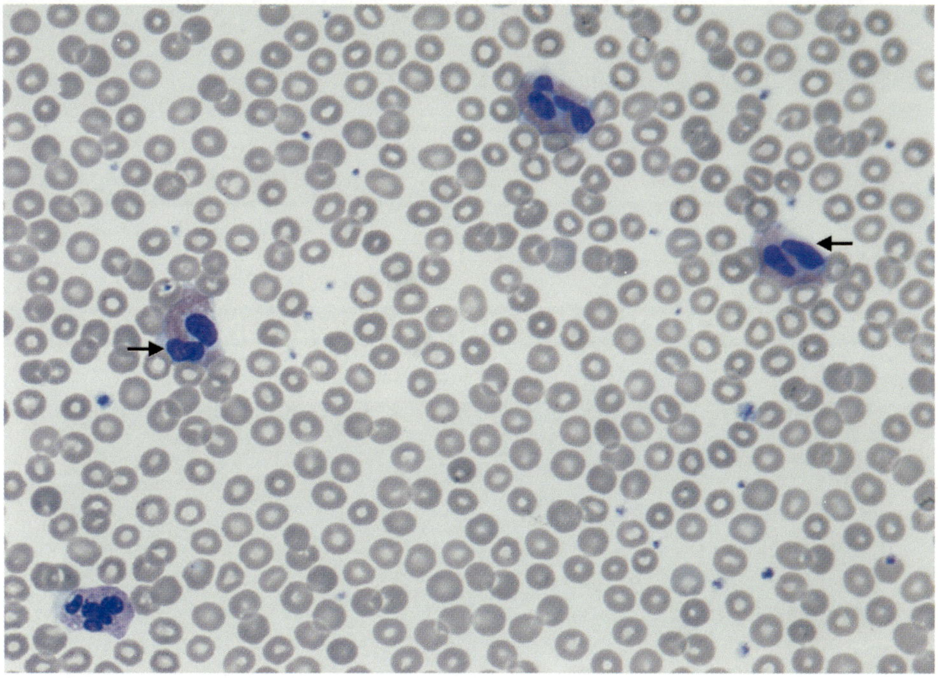

Fig. 15: Eosinophils.

- Eosinophils are granulocytes that are distinguished from other granulocytes like neutrophils and basophils by their distinctive granules.
- The eosinophil has characteristic coarse brick-red granules in the cytoplasm and a bilobed spectacle-shaped nucleus.
- They are increased in numbers in the peripheral blood in parasitic infections, allergic disorders like allergic bronchopulmonary aspergillosis (ABPA), autoimmune disorders like Churg-Strauss syndrome and in chronic eosinophilic leukemia.

CHAPTER 24

Lung Ultrasound in ICU

Deepak Govil, Jagadeesh KN, Rahul Harne

BRONCHIAL ASTHMA AND CHRONIC OBSTRUCTIVE PULMONARY DISEASE (FIG. 1)

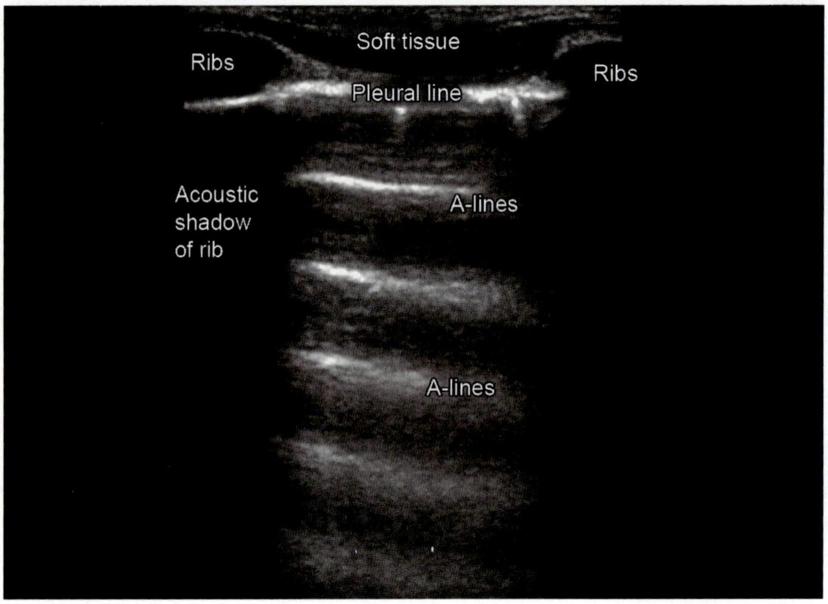

Fig. 1: Lung scan—A-lines.

Bronchial asthma and chronic obstructive pulmonary disease (COPD) patients will have hyperinflated, aerated lungs. Aerated lung will have A-pattern in lung ultrasound.

A pattern scan of lung in bronchial asthma and COPD:

- A-line scan in all the areas.
- B-lines absent.
- Lung sliding present (real time scan).

Image above, obtained with the help of Linear Probe, shows longitudinal scan, consists of upper and lower rib, intercostal muscle and skin, soft tissue. Bright line deeper to intercostal muscle and soft tissue is the 'Pleura', horizontal lines deeper to pleura are the reverberation artifacts of pleura and air interface.

Bronchial asthma and COPD, show A-pattern in aerated areas.

In real time scan we can appreciate slow to-and-fro movement of pleura with inspiration and expiration, called 'Lung Sliding' or 'Pleural Sliding'.

PNEUMOTHORAX (FIGS. 2A TO C)

A-lines (Fig. 2A)

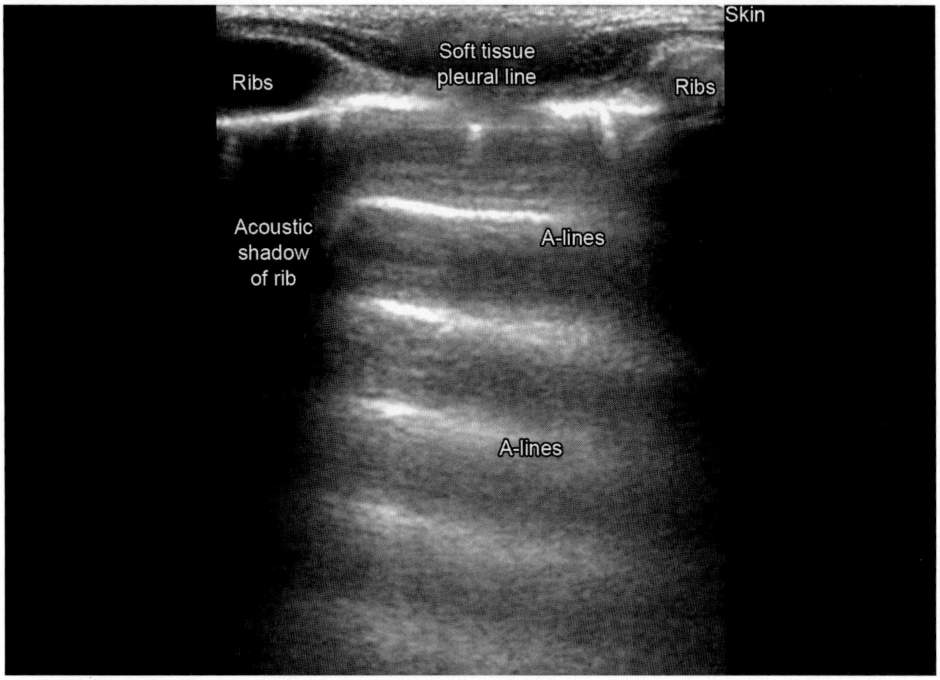

Fig. 2A: A-lines.

Pneumothorax on ultrasound examination have following features:

- *A-lines*: A pattern is represented by reverberation artefacts of pleural line, horizontal and deeper to pleura.
- *B-lines absent.*
- *Loss of lung sliding: In real-time scan.*
- *Lung point—in real-time scan. Presence of lung point confirms pneumothorax.*
- *Stratosphere sign on M mode.*

  Figure 2A is obtained by linear probe, perpendicular to ribs showing A-lines.

Lung Point (Fig. 2B)

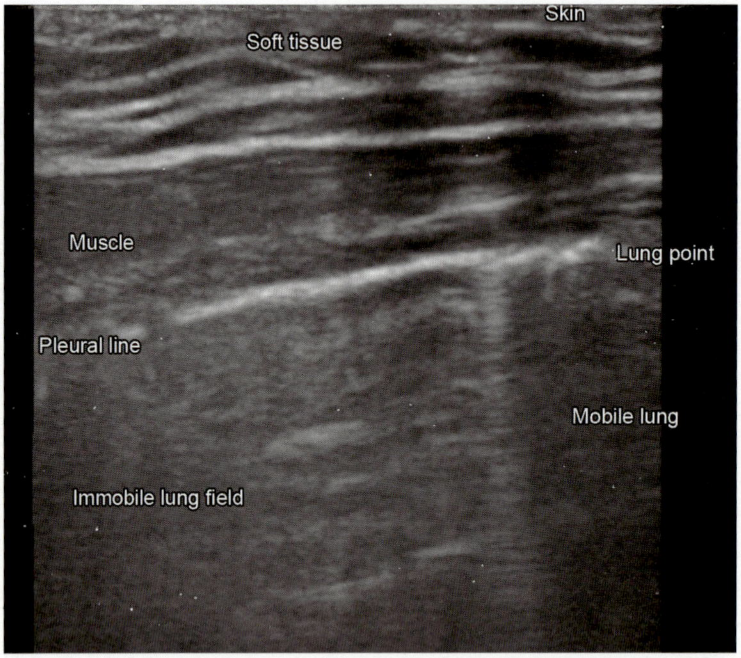

Fig. 2B: Lung point—pneumothorax separates visceral and parietal pleura. The point at which these surfaces meet is called lung point (seen on real time scan).

- Figure 2B is obtained by linear probe along the intercostal space, showing lung point (vertical line from pleural line represents where expanded and collapsed lung meet and move during respiration).

Barcode Sign (Fig. 2C)

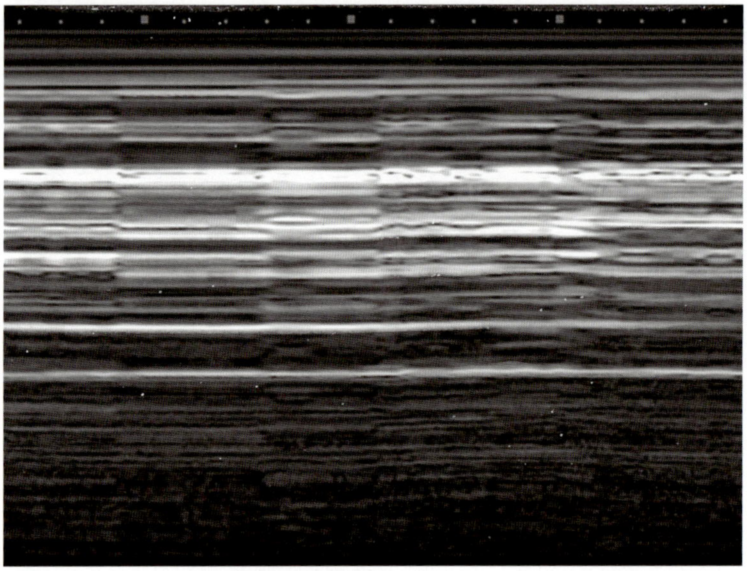

Fig. 2C: Stratosphere/Barcode sign.

- Figure 2C is obtained by linear probe along the intercostal space with M mode showing stratosphere sign (normal lung will show a sea shore sign with transition of lines differentiating movement at the pleural lines, whereas pneumothorax prevents detection of motion creating a single stratosphere sign).

PLEURAL EFFUSION (FIGS. 3A TO H)

Pleural Effusion—Sonology (Fig. 3A)

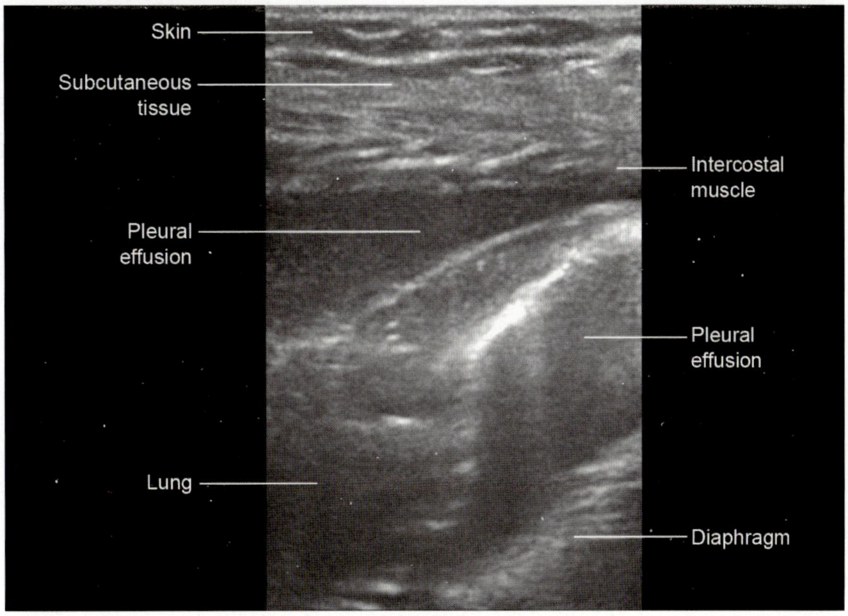

Fig. 3A: Pleural effusion—sonology.

- Image above is obtained by linear probe in longitudinal view shows anechoic pleural fluid surrounding collapsed lung.

Pleural Effusion with Fish Tail Lung (Fig. 3B)

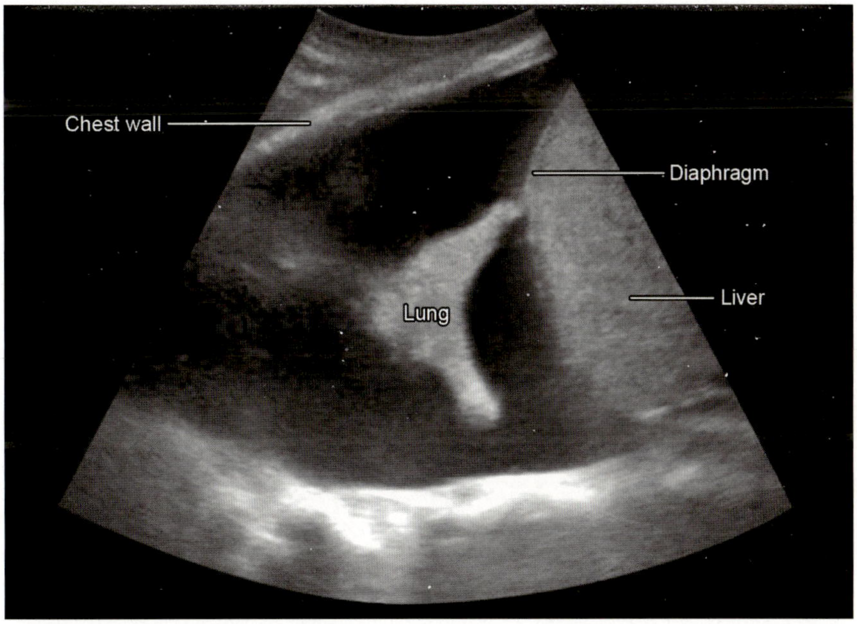

Fig. 3B: Pleural effusion with "fish tail" lung.

- Image above is obtained from curvilinear probe in longitudinal view, over anterior axillary line.
- Compressed lung has "fish tail" appearance and tips of tail show hyperechoic pattern due to obstructive atelectasis.

Pleurocentesis (Fig. 3C)

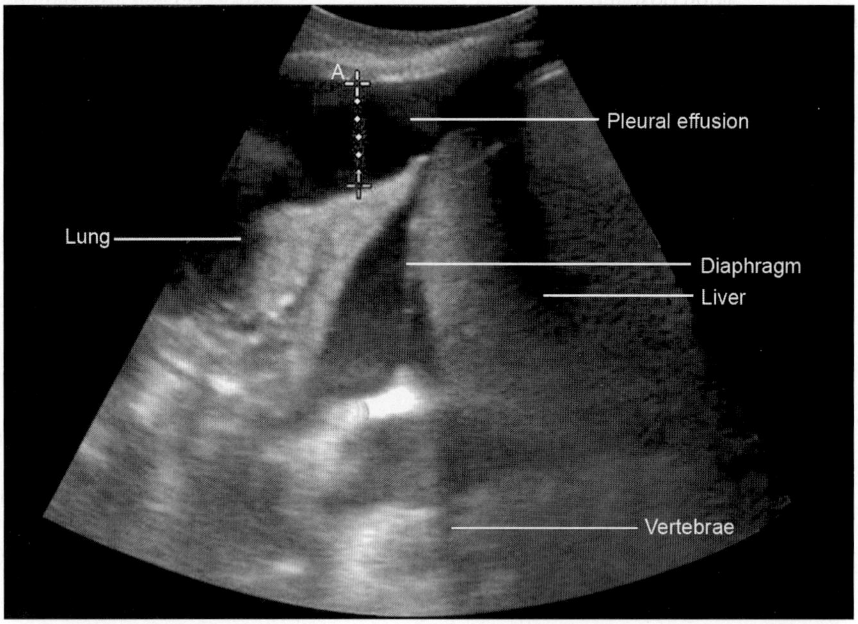

Fig. 3C: Pleurocentesis—safe aspiration.

- Image above is obtained with curvilinear probe in intercostal space.
- Shows chest wall in near field and compressed lung tissue, in the middle of the screen, and clearance (A +.....+) of more than 2 cm from lateral chest wall in inspiration.
- A space of 2 cm indicates safety in pleural fluid aspiration.

Massive Effusion/Hemothorax (Fig. 3D)

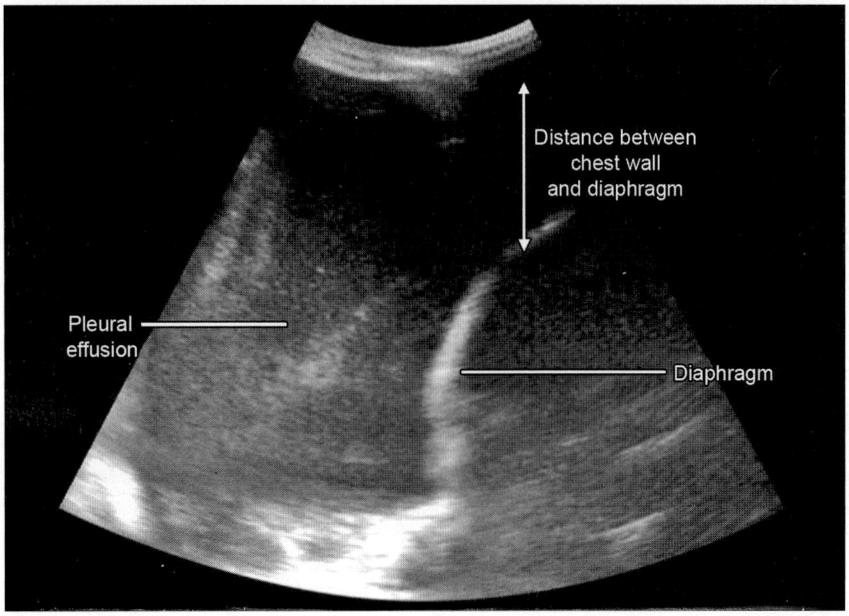

Fig. 3D: Massive effusion/hemothorax.

- Image above obtained by curvilinear probe in longitudinal view.
- Anechoic superficial half and hypoechoic lower half with spontaneous contrast. Spontaneous contrast represents exudative pleural effusion or hemothorax.
- Pleural effusion separating diaphragm and chest wall, about 4 cm, indicates effusion is massive, as lung is also not seen.

Pleural Effusion: Exudative (Fig. 3E.1)

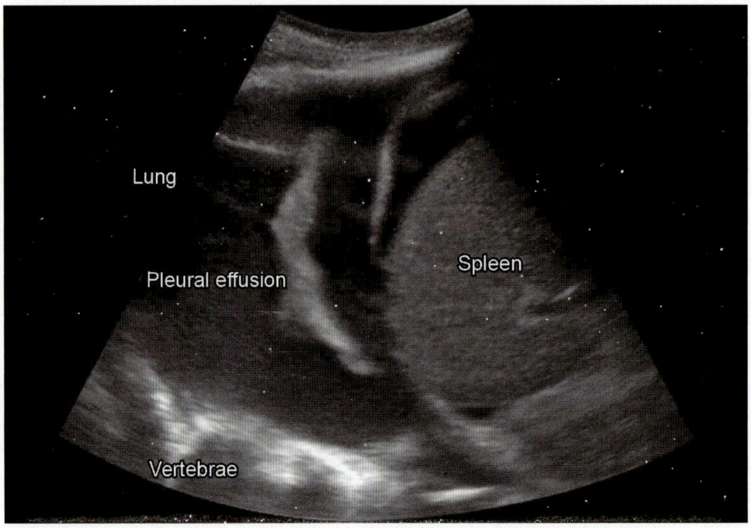

Fig. 3E.1: Pleural effusion—exudative.

- Image above is obtained by curvilinear probe in longitudinal view.
- Upper half of nondependent pleural effusion is thick black (hypoechoic), indicating probable transudative effusion and dependent effusion is gray (isoechoic), and representing possible exudative nature of effusion.

Pleural Effusion: Exudative (Fig. 3E.2)

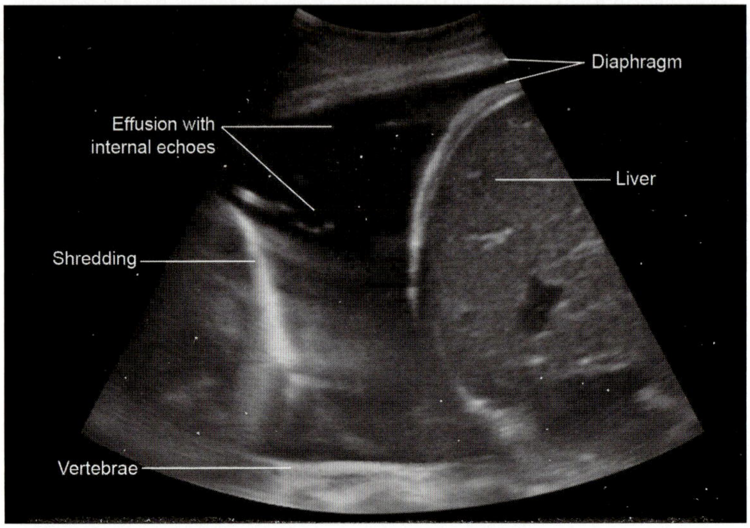

Fig. 3E.2: Pleural effusion—exudative.

- Image above is obtained by curvilinear probe in longitudinal view, and midaxillary line at the level of diaphragm.
- Hyperechoic line in the upper third of the field is separating deaerated and aerated lung and represents a possible infective pathology of lung.
- Hypoechoic area represents pleural effusion.
- Internal echoes within the effusion represent exudative effusion and probable chronicity of effusion.

Atelectatic Lung—M Mode (Fig. 3F)

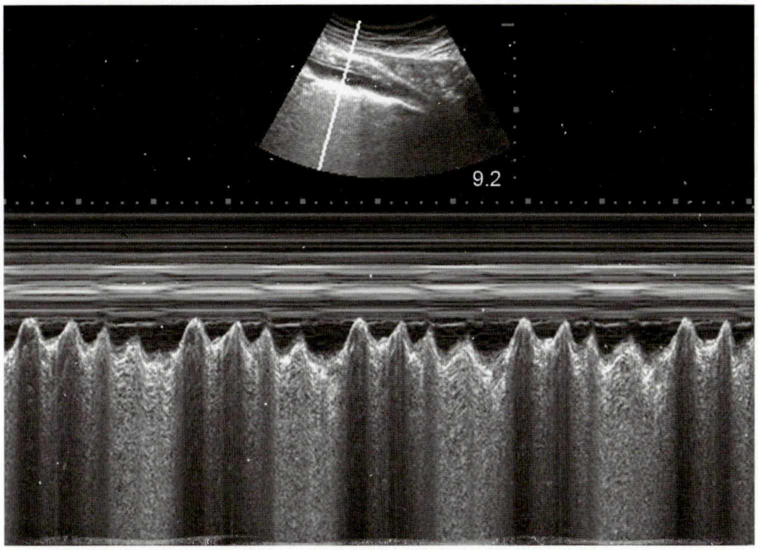

Fig. 3F: Atelectatic lung—M mode.

- Image above is obtained with curvilinear probe in longitudinal view with M mode.
- Wavy lower two-thirds is due to atelectasis but the lung is expandable. Cardiac contractions are transmitted through the atelectatic lung as 'lung pulse'.
- Upper one-third represents static chest wall.
- Nonexpansile lung due to pneumonia or obstructive atelectasis would show less pronounced "lung pulse".
- Nonatelectatic lung, would have shown sinusoidal pattern, in M mode.

Pleural Effusion—Complicated (Fig. 3G)

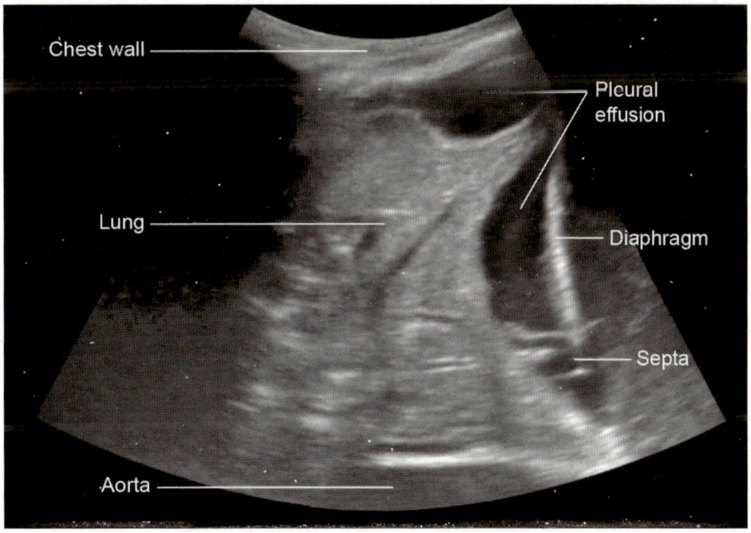

Fig. 3G: Pleural effusion—complicated.

- Image above is obtained with curvilinear probe, in longitudinal plane, via lateral chest wall.
- Hepatized lung shows tethering of lower border to diaphragm and producing "bird's beak" appearance.
- A few septa, can be seen in the lower end of scan, near the diaphragm.
- Exudative effusion, results in formation of septa and resultant tethering of lung to chest wall, diaphragm, and pericardium.

Pleural Effusion and Ascites (Fig. 3H)

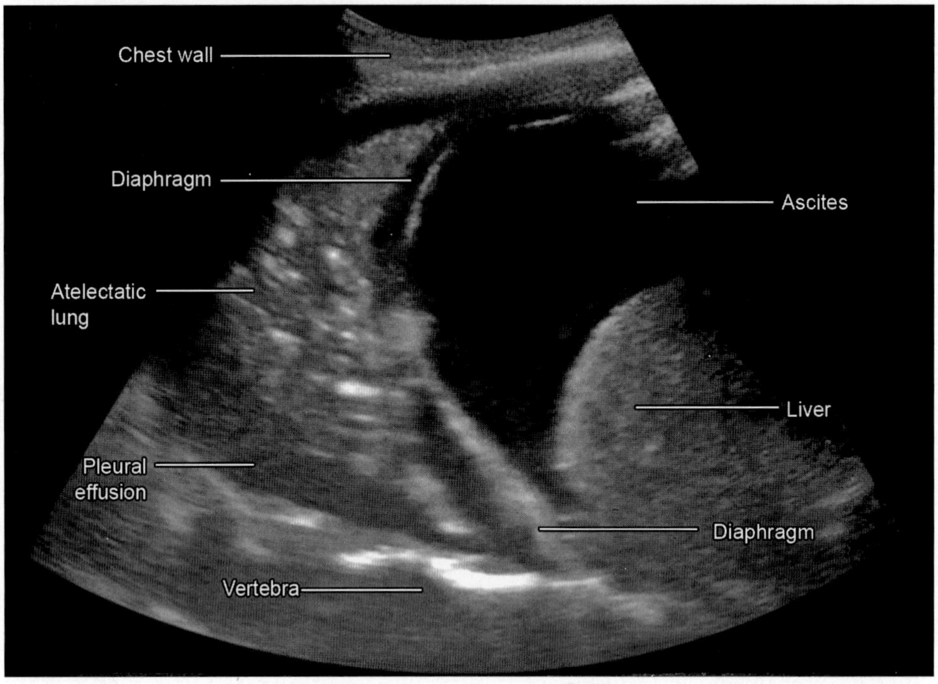

Fig. 3H: Pleural effusion and ascites.

- Image above is obtained by curvilinear probe in longitudinal view, depicting chest wall to vertebrae.
- Diaphragm separating pleural effusion surrounding atelectatic lung.
- Ascites and liver below the diaphragm.
- Compressed lung with hyperechoic bright spots representing—obstructive atelectasis.

ACUTE RESPIRATORY DISTRESS SYNDROME (FIGS. 4A TO C)

Multiple B-lines (Fig. 4A)

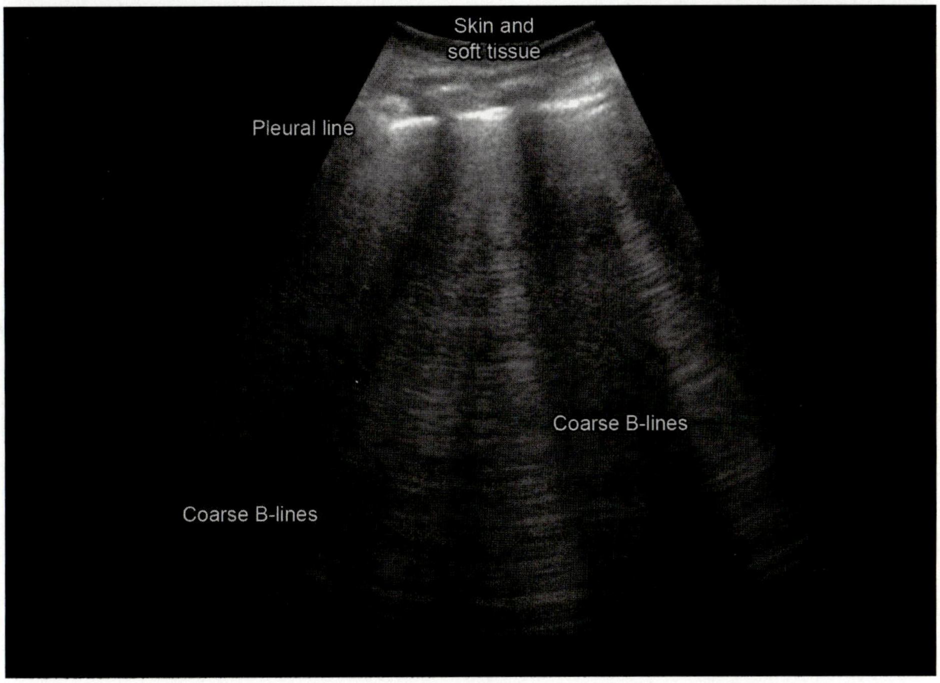

Fig. 4A: Acute respiratory distress syndrome (ARDS)—multiple B-lines.

Acute respiratory distress syndrome (ARDS) would have following features on lung sonography:

- Bilateral B-lines—diffuse to coarse.
- Pleural thickening with subpleural consolidations.
- Consolidation.
- Figure 4A above is obtained by curvilinear probe, perpendicular to ribs, shows multiple B-lines (Vertical echogenic reverberation artifacts originating—at pleural lines and extending to the deepest part of ultrasound image). More than three B-lines in any single view are pathological.

Subpleural Consolidation (Fig. 4B)

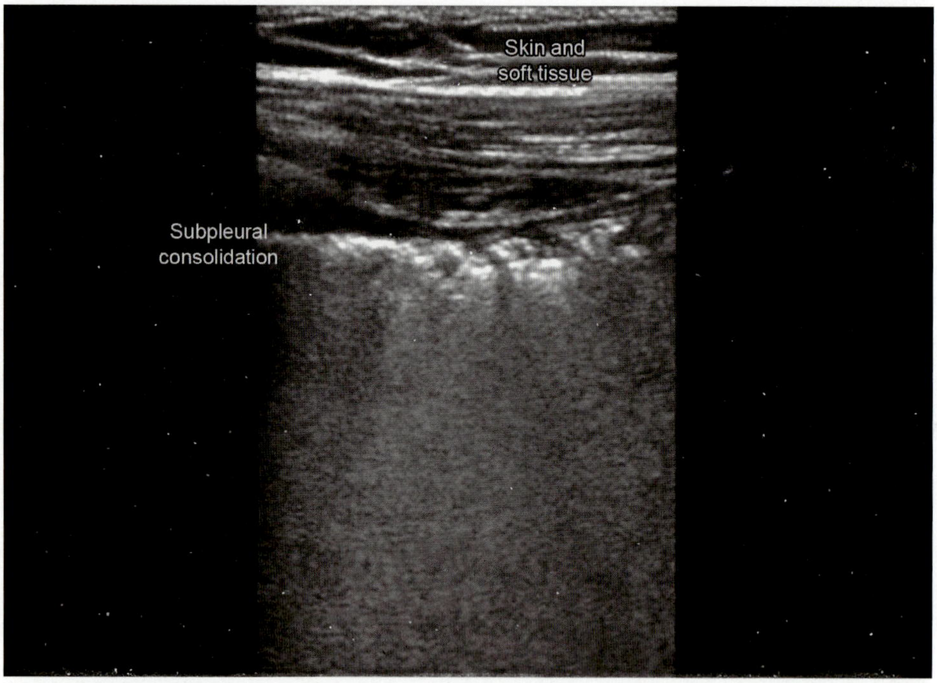

Fig. 4B: ARDS—subpleural consolidation, thickened and irregular pleura.

- Figure 4B above is obtained by linear probe in longitudinal view shows subpleural consolidation and thickened, irregular pleura.

Shred Sign (Fig. 4C)

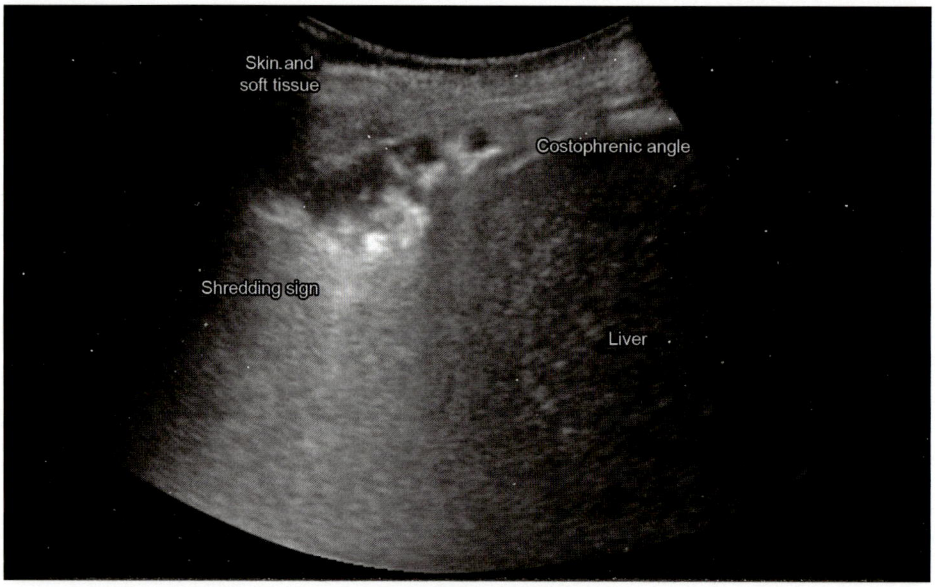

Fig. 4C: ARDS—shred sign.

- Figure 4C above is obtained by curvilinear probe in longitudinal view shows Shred sign (Irregular junction between the consolidated—lung and aerated lung).

PULMONARY EDEMA (FIG. 5)

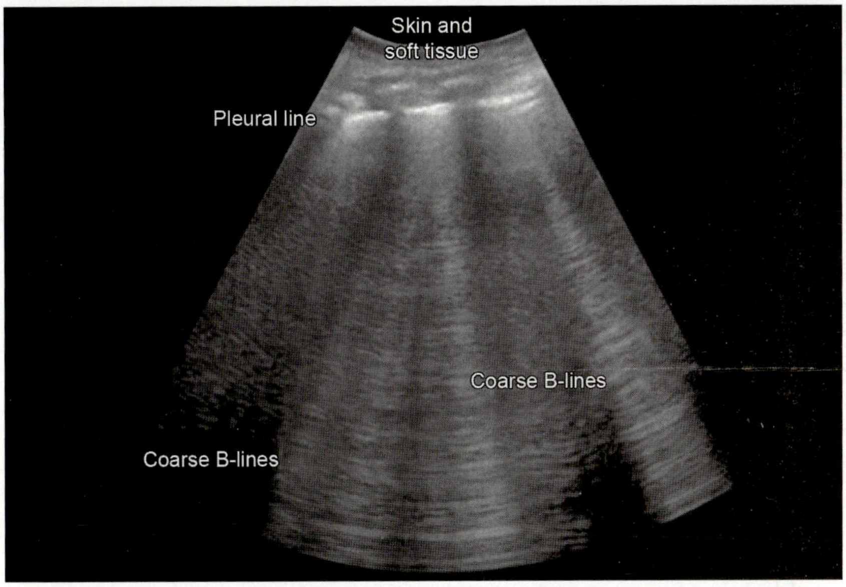

Fig. 5: Pulmonary edema: B-lines.

Patients with pulmonary edema would have bilateral diffuse B lines on lung ultrasonography.

- Symmetrical closely spaced, B-lines in all anterior zones is due to alveolar edema.
- Simultaneous cardiac scan is showing compromised systolic or diastolic function of the heart adds to the diagnosis. Figure 5 above is obtained by curvilinear probe, perpendicular to ribs show multiple diffuse B-lines.

PNEUMONIA (FIGS. 6A TO D)

Homogeneous opacity on the chest radiograph can be due to effusion, atelectasis or consolidation. Differentiation can be done with use of ultrasound at the bedside.

Subpleural Consolidation—Early Pneumonia (Fig. 6A)

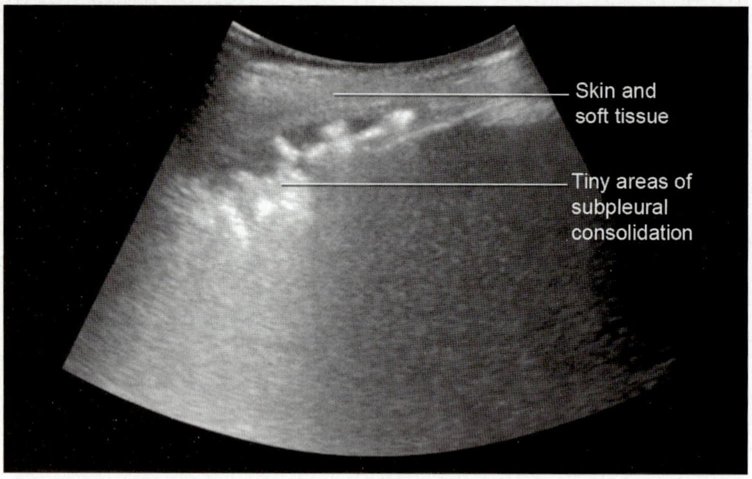

Fig. 6A: Subpleural consolidation—early pneumonia.

Image above is obtained by curvilinear probe in longitudinal axis, demonstrates the following:

- In early pneumonia, fluid fills only some of the alveoli. Whenever reactive fluid floods the alveoli, ultrasound produces B-lines, and form a short path of reverberation artifact.
- In the appropriate clinical setting, a localized patch of numerous B-lines, often with tiny area of subpleural consolidation, suggests early pneumonia.

Hepatization of Lung (Fig. 6B)

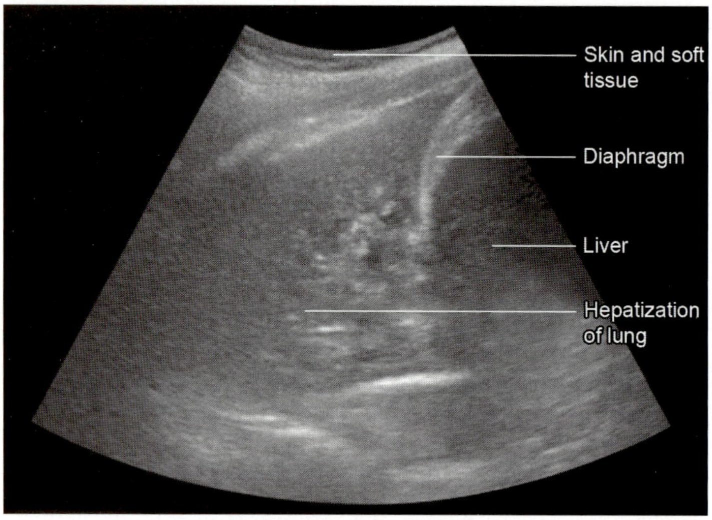

Fig. 6B: Hepatization of lung.

Image above is obtained by curvilinear probe in longitudinal axis, demonstrates the following:

- The tissue like texture of the consolidated lung appears isoechoic to liver.
- Multiple echogenic foci are seen within the consolidated—lung and correspond to air-filled airways.

Air Bronchogram (Fig. 6C)

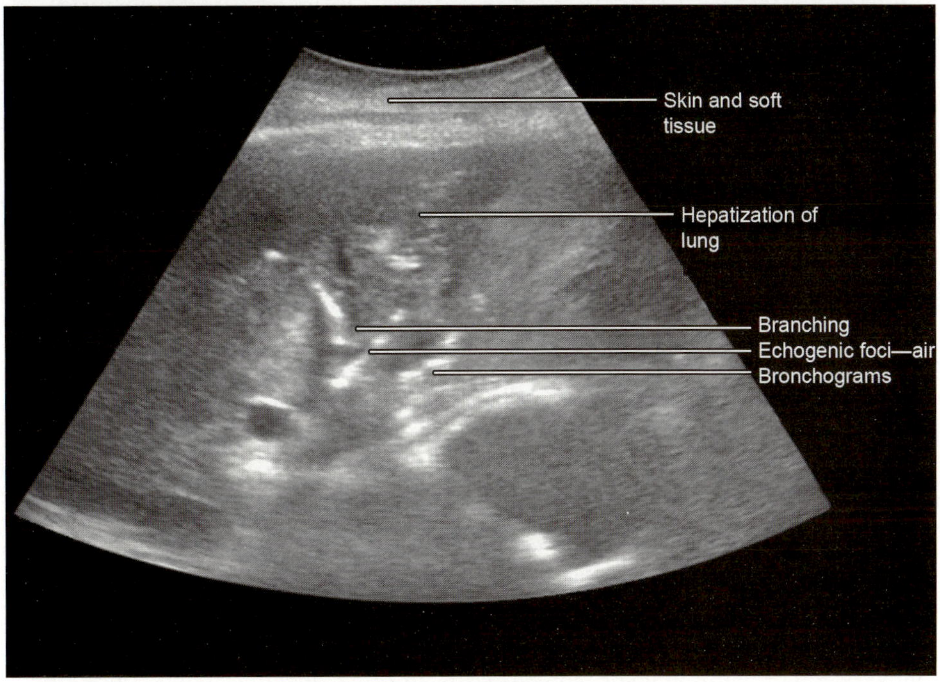

Fig. 6C: Pneumonia with air bronchogram.

Image above is obtained by curvilinear probe in longitudinal axis, demonstrates the following:

- The area of the solidified lung tissue appears wedge-shaped and appears uniformly hypoechoic.
- Sharp peripheral margins of the consolidated lung.
- Sonographic air and fluid bronchograms and air alveolograms.
- Movement of air and respiratory secretions within bronchioles during breathing show linear branching hyperechoic artifact, called 'Dynamic Air Bronchogram' during real time scan.

Dynamic air bronchogram is present in expansile lung. Lung collapse and atelectasis do not show dynamic air bronchograms.

Pneumonia—Vascular (Fig. 6D.1)

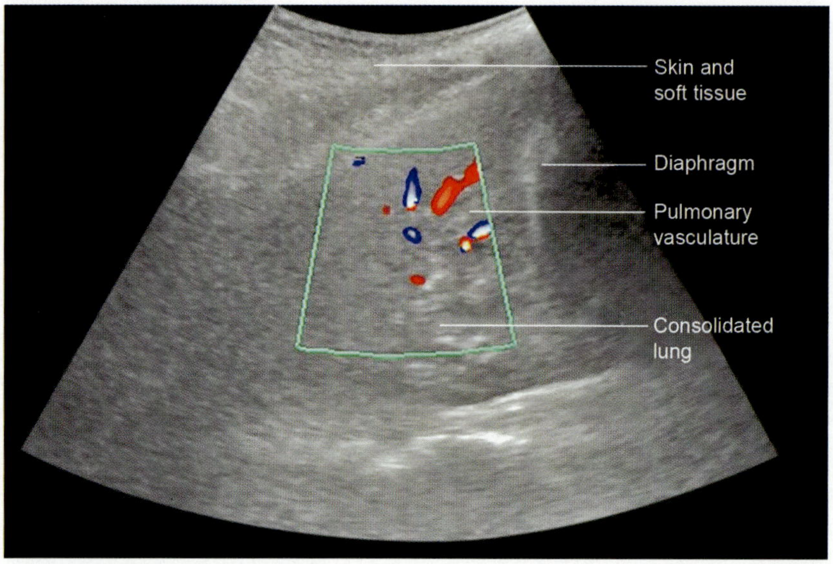

Fig. 6D.1: Pneumonia—vascular.

- Image above is obtained by curvilinear probe in longitudinal axis, *demonstrates* hepatization of lung with increased vascularity of lobar segment with the color Doppler scan. In other deaerated lung conditions like lung collapse, vascularity will be normal.

Pneumonia—Vascular (Fig. 6D.2)

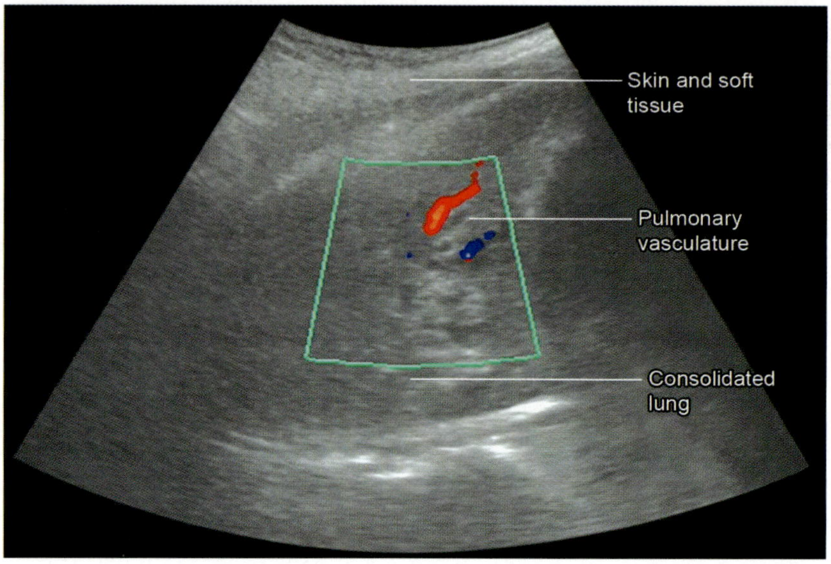

Fig. 6D.2: Pneumonia: color Doppler.

Image above is obtained by curvilinear probe in longitudinal axis, demonstrates the following:

- On the color Doppler scan, a pulmonary arterial and venous vasculature is well demonstrated in area of consolidation.
- Color Doppler demonstrates normal or increased flow in the vessels of the consolidated lung and may be helpful in distinguishing simple pneumonia from postobstructive pneumonia. The pulsatility index of blood flow in the consolidation is higher in cases of obstructive pneumonia.

CHAPTER

25

Interesting Images in ICU

Jeetendra Sharma, Mukesh K Gupta

NONINVASIVE VENTILATION MACHINE (FIG. 1)

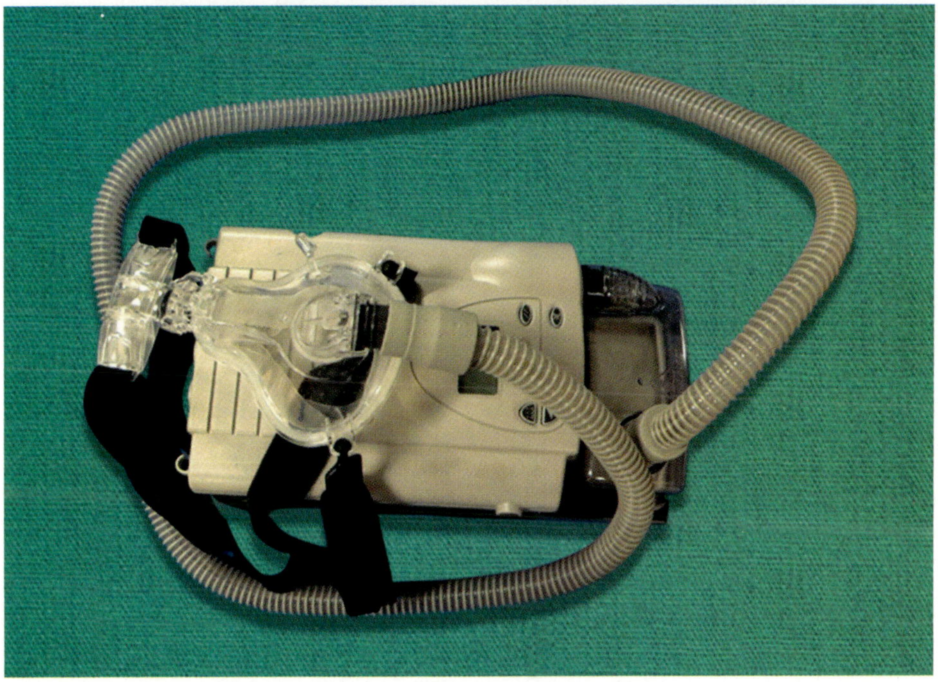

Fig. 1: Noninvasive ventilation machine.

- Noninvasive ventilation (NIV) machine commonly known as BiPAP machine.
- When ventilation is delivered through an interface without invasive artificial airway (endotracheal tube, tracheostomy tube, laryngeal mask airway, etc.) is known as noninvasive ventilation.
- The use of NIV has markedly increased over the past two decades for both acute and chronic respiratory failure. NIV not only used in ICU but more frequently out of the ICU.
- Cardiogenic pulmonary edema and chronic obstructive airway disease are most appropriate clinical condition.
- Absolute contraindications of NIV are unconsciousness, severe hemodynamic instability or cardiac arrest, respiratory arrest and requirement of endotracheal tube for airway protection.
- For the use of NIV require training and experience under supervision to avoid undesirable delay in endotracheal intubation.

MEDICAL DEVICE-RELATED PRESSURE INJURIES CAUSED BY NONINVASIVE VENTILATION ORONASAL MASK (FIG. 2)

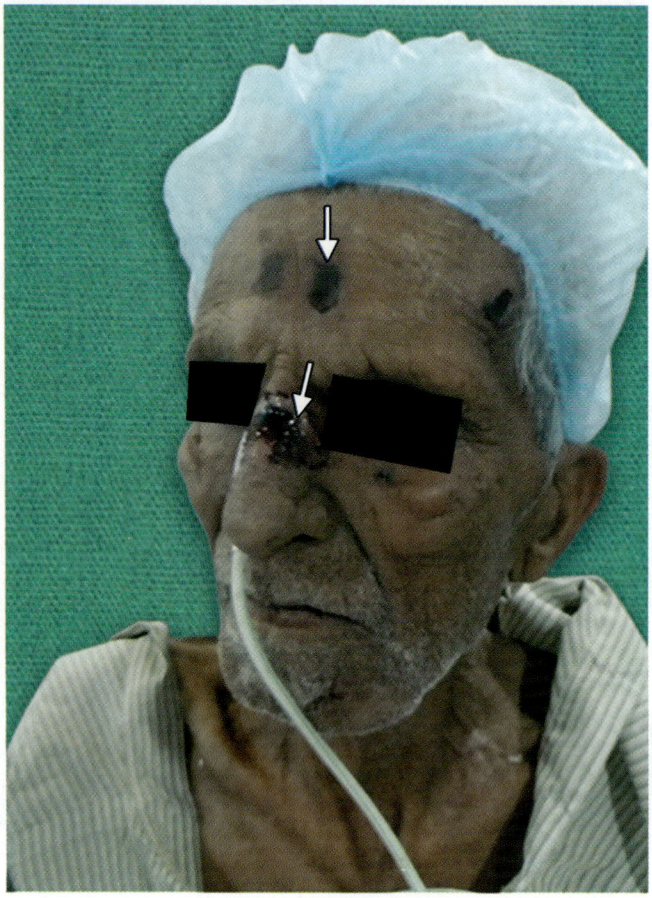

Fig. 2: Medical device-related pressure injuries caused by noninvasive ventilation oronasal mask.

- Noninvasive ventilation (NIV) routinely used in ICU for respiratory failure and most commonly used interface for NIV is oronasal mask.
- The face mask needs to be tight around the nose and mouth in order to create an effective seal that might cause pressure-related skin and tissue necrosis over the bridge of the nose.
- The most important cause is the pressure above the normal capillary filling pressure of the skin, along with contributing factors such as poor hydration, hypotension, and skin thinness due to anatomy and use of corticosteroids.
- Pressure injuries can be prevented or reduced by the use of thin hydrocolloids, film dressings, pressure-reducing dermal gel pads, or barrier products underneath the device to reduce moisture, friction, and shear.

HELMET INTERFACE FOR NONINVASIVE VENTILATION (FIG. 3)

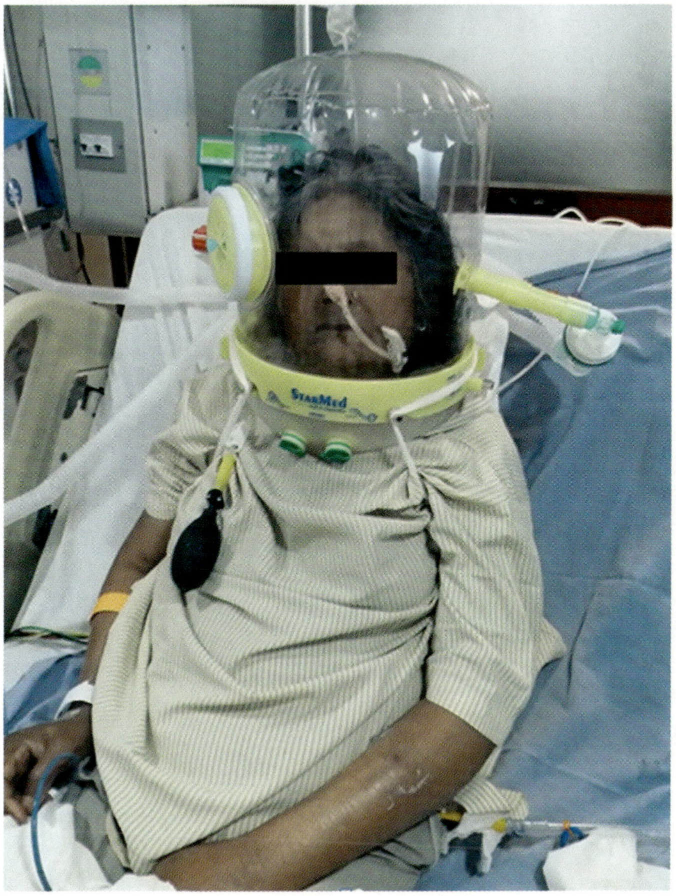

Fig. 3: Helmet interface for noninvasive ventilation.

- The helmet can be used as an alternative interface compared to face mask to improve performance of noninvasive ventilation (NIV).
- Advantages of helmet are less air leaks, no facial skin lesions, and no eye irritation, can be applied regardless of the facial contour, facial trauma, or edentulism, allows coughing and enteral nutrition can be take care in better way.
- Disadvantages of helmet are noise, large dead space, claustrophobia, vascular complications and skin lesions at the collar.

HIGH-FLOW NASAL CANNULA (FIG. 4)

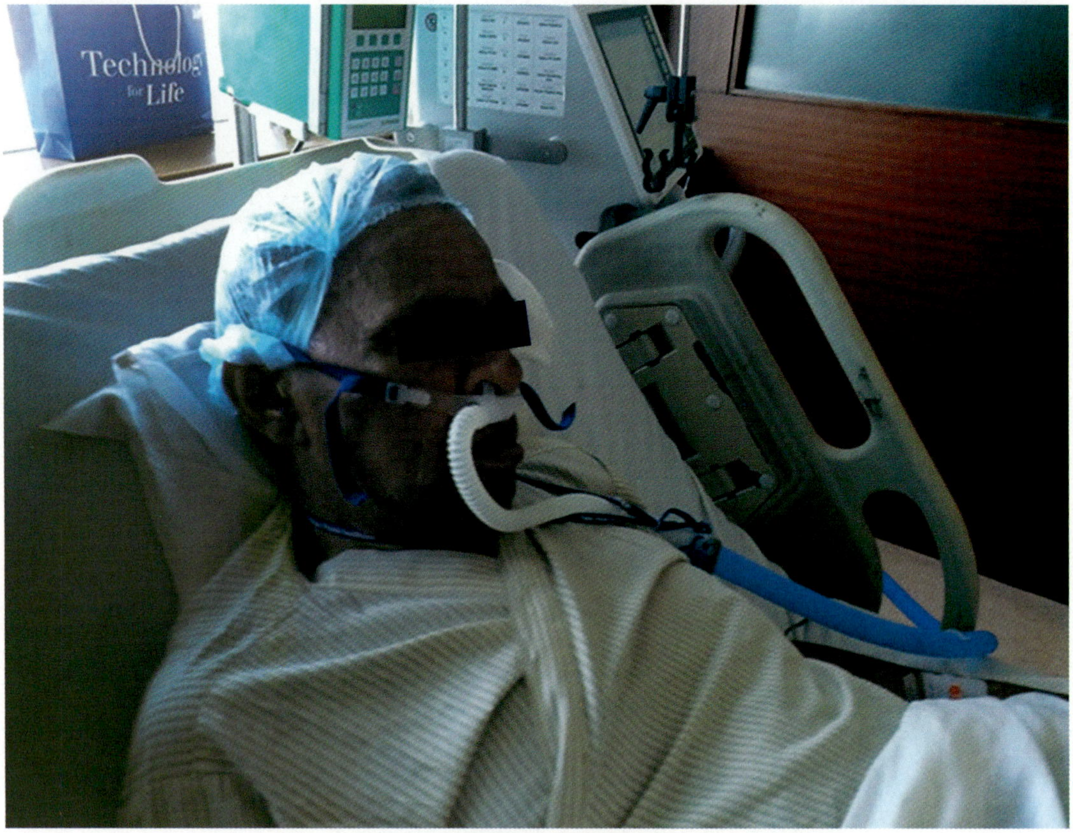

Fig. 4: High-flow nasal cannula.

- The high-flow nasal cannula (HFNC) is a relatively new oxygen delivery system.
- A conventional nasal cannula uses a low-flow system and at higher flow (> 6 L/min) can cause nasal dryness, epistaxis, and patient discomfort.
- The HFNC system is a novel device that combines oxygen, pressurized air, and warm humidification to deliver tolerable flow of up to 60 L/min through a nasal cannula.
- FiO_2 and flow rates can be adjusted. With higher flow, less room-air entrainment occurs, and the higher flow rates match the dyspneic patient's increased minute ventilation.
- Use of HFNC has emerged as an alternative to noninvasive positive pressure ventilation (NIPPV).

INVASIVE MECHANICAL VENTILATOR (FIG. 5)

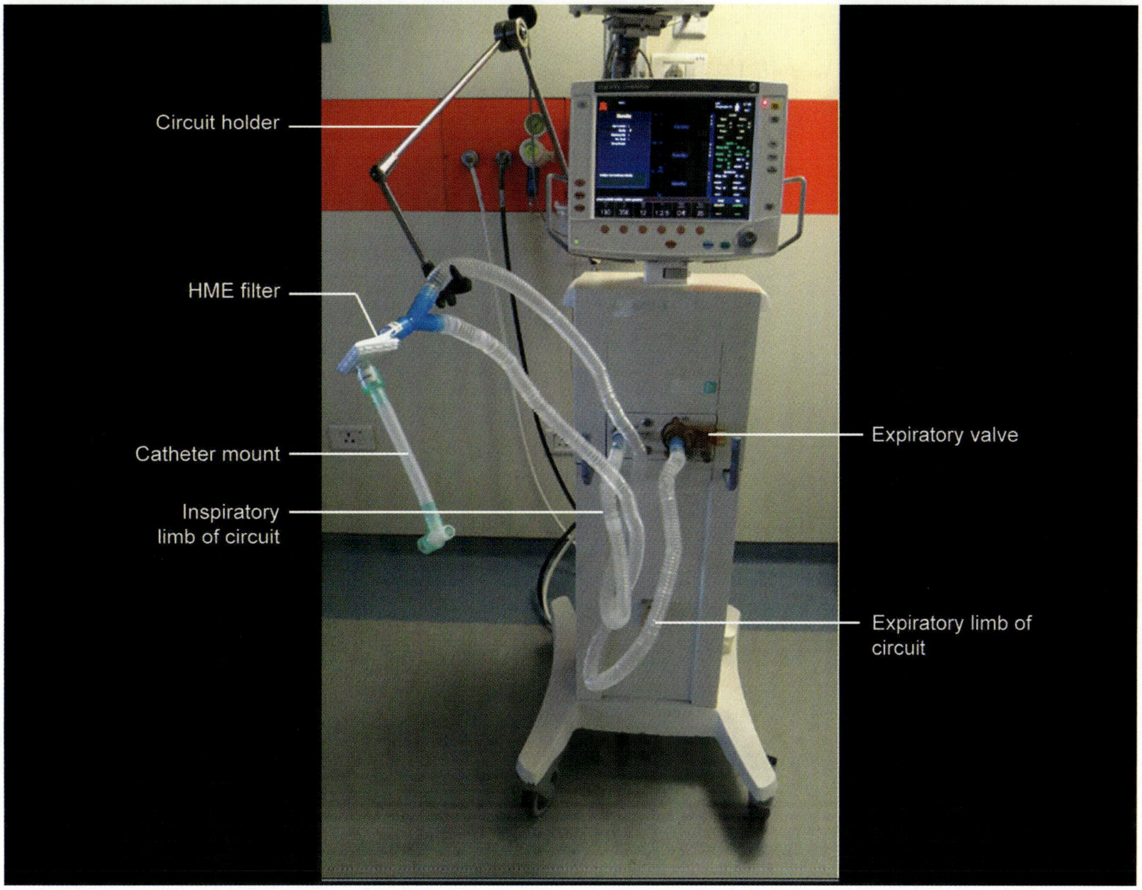

Fig. 5: Invasive mechanical ventilator. (HME: Heat and moisture exchange)

- Ventilator is a machine that generates the pressure necessary to cause flow of gas that increases the volume of the lung.
- Ventilator delivers breath is divided into four distinct phases:
  1. Changes from expiration to inspiration—triggering.
  2. Inspiration—limit or preset.
  3. Changes from inspiration to expiration—cycling.
  4. Expiration—passive.
- The main components of mechanical ventilator are gas source, control panel for various settings of breaths and a display.

HIGH PEAK AIRWAY PRESSURE WITH NORMAL PLATEAU PRESSURE (FIG. 6)

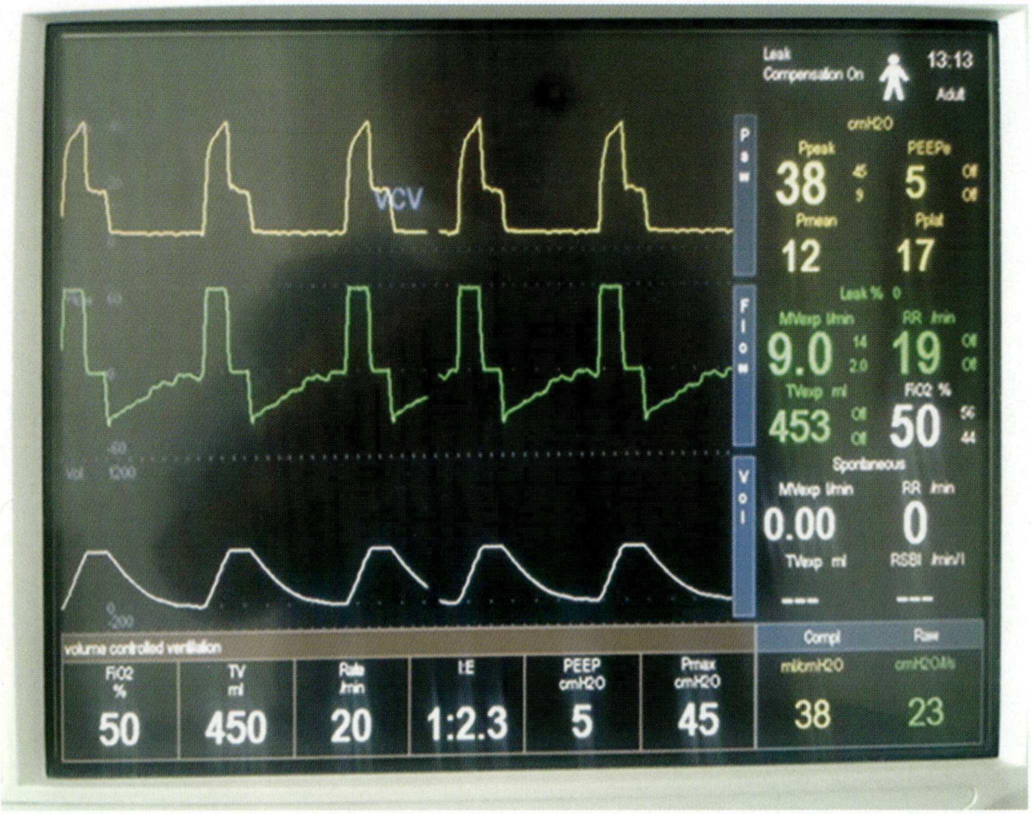

Fig. 6: High peak airway pressure with normal plateau pressure.

- High peak airway pressure with normal plateau pressure in the patient of endotracheal and bilateral endobronchial growth.
- Airway pressure = Flow × Resistance + Alveolar pressure.
- The total amount of airway pressure delivered by the ventilator to overcome resistive and elastic work is defined as the peak inspiratory pressure (Ppeak).
- During inspiratory pause when flow has stopped, the amount of resistive work is zero. Therefore, pressure measured at the end of inspiration represents elastic work is defined as plateau pressure (Pplat).
- If the difference between peak and plateau pressures is greater than about 5 cm/H_2O, increased airway pressure can likely be attributed to increased resistive work.
- Common causes are bronchospasm, anaphylaxis, endotracheal tube obstruction or ventilator circuit obstruction.

HIGH FREQUENCY OSCILLATORY VENTILATION (FIG. 7)

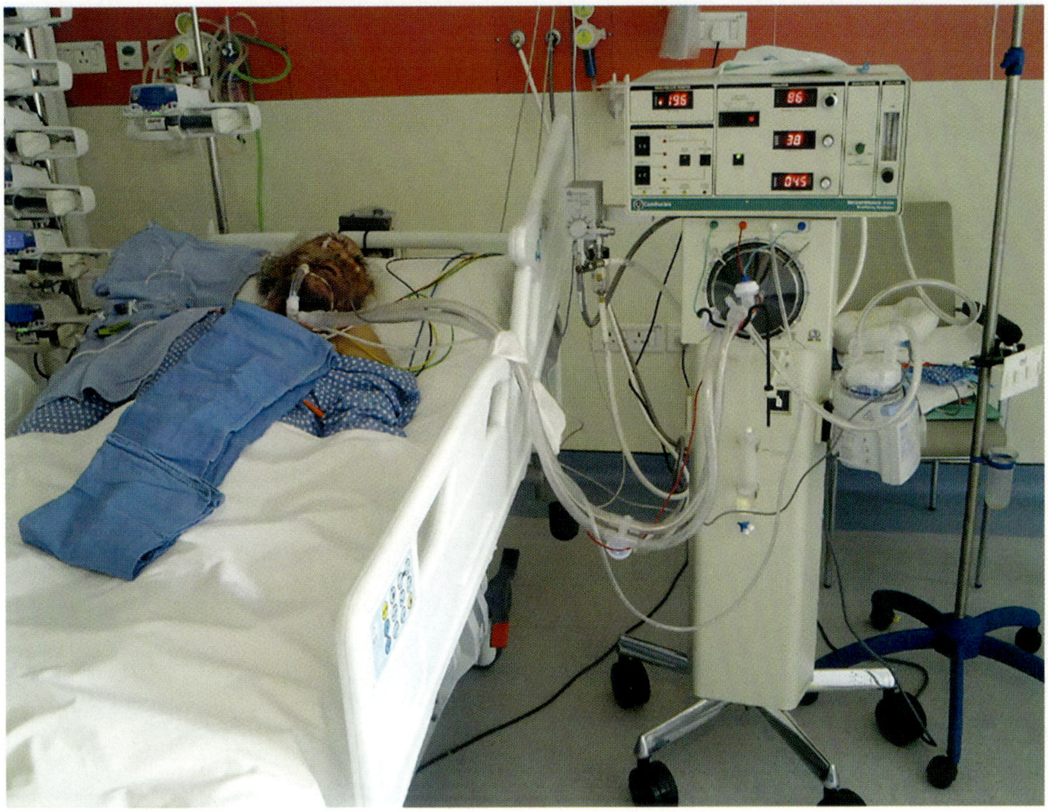

Fig. 7: High frequency oscillatory ventilation.

- High frequency oscillatory ventilation (HFOV) deliver small tidal volume of gas almost equal to anatomical dead space with a high frequency ranges from 120 to 1200 breath per minute at a constant high mean airway pressure. Expiration is also active in HFOV.
- HFOV oscillates the lung around a constant mean airway pressure higher than conventional ventilation.
- No mortality benefit yet demonstrated in randomized control trials in acute respiratory distress syndrome (ARDS), however it is useful to ventilate patient of bronchopleural fistula.

DOUBLE LUMEN TRACHEOSTOMY TUBE (FIG. 8)

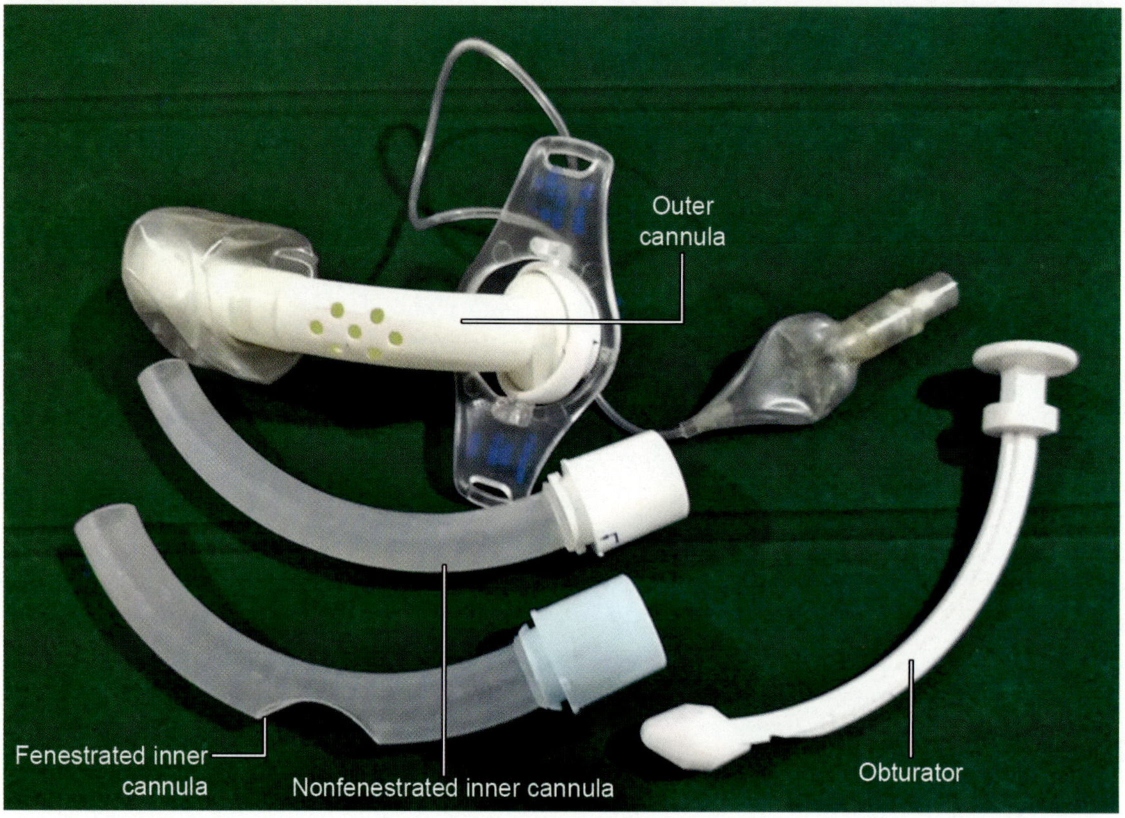

Fig. 8: Double lumen tracheostomy tube.

- Double lumen tracheostomy tube has a removable inner lumen.
- The inner lumen in double lumen tracheostomy tubes reduces the internal diameter by 1–1.5 mm.
- The inner lumen can be changed/cleaned frequently reducing the risk of occlusion.
- For ventilation, nonfenestrated inner cannula must be used.
- For the use of speaking valve, fenestrated inner cannula should be used however this may put the patient to aspiration if he does not has protective airway reflexes.

ADJUSTABLE FLANGE TRACHEOSTOMY TUBE (FIGS. 9A AND B)

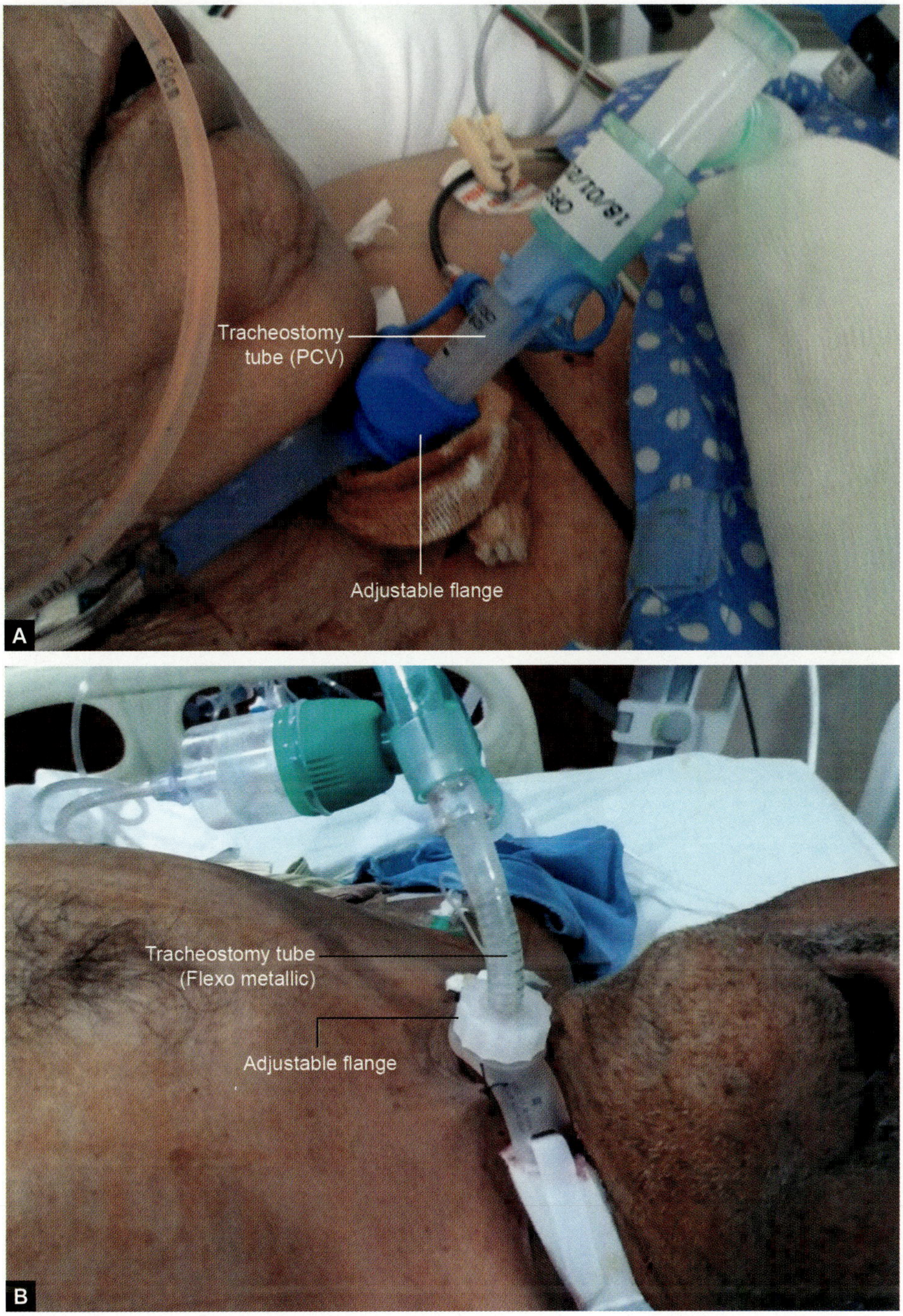

Figs. 9A and B: Adjustable flange tracheostomy tube.

- Tracheostomy tubes with adjustable flanges are specifically designed for patients who have deep set tracheas. These tubes are longer than usual tracheostomy tube.
- Flanges can be adjusted to desirable length of tube by simple locking system.
- Patients who might have deep-seated trachea are obese or have distorted anatomy within the neck due to inflammation, edema or tumor.
- Theses tubes can be used in patients with kyphosis.

HEIMLICH VALVE (FIG. 10)

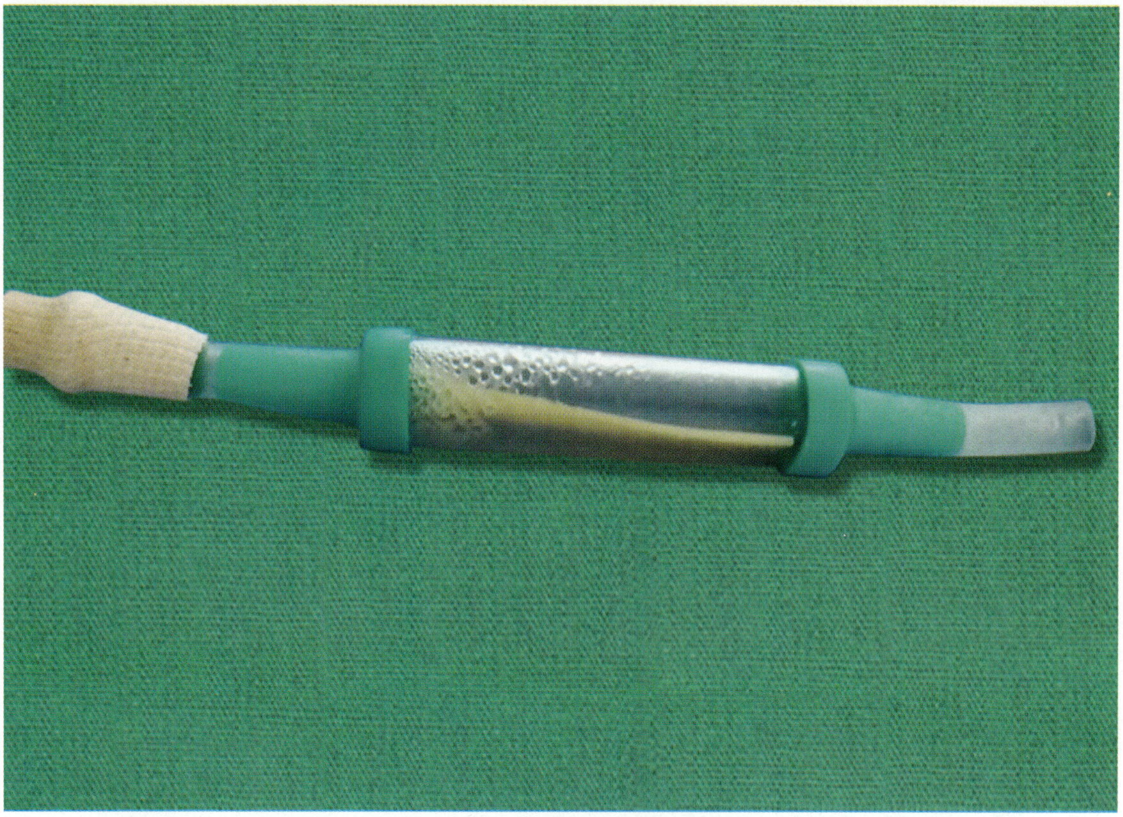

Fig. 10: Heimlich valve.

- The Heimlich valve is a small one-way valve used for chest drainage (in pnuemothorax) that empties into a flexible collection device and prevents return of gases or fluids into the pleural space.
- The Heimlich valve is about 5 inches long and facilitates patient ambulation.
- When air passes through the valve, a distinct "flutter" sound can be heard, ensuring that the device is working properly.
- Absence of the sound accompanied with no movement of the rubber sleeve during placement means that no air passes through the valve, which indicates either the resolution of pneumothorax or possible blockage of the intercostals drain.
- It is important to remember not to tape the end of the valve. The end must remain open to allow air out all the time.

VENOVENOUS EXTRACORPOREAL MEMBRANE OXYGENATION (FIGS. 11A AND B)

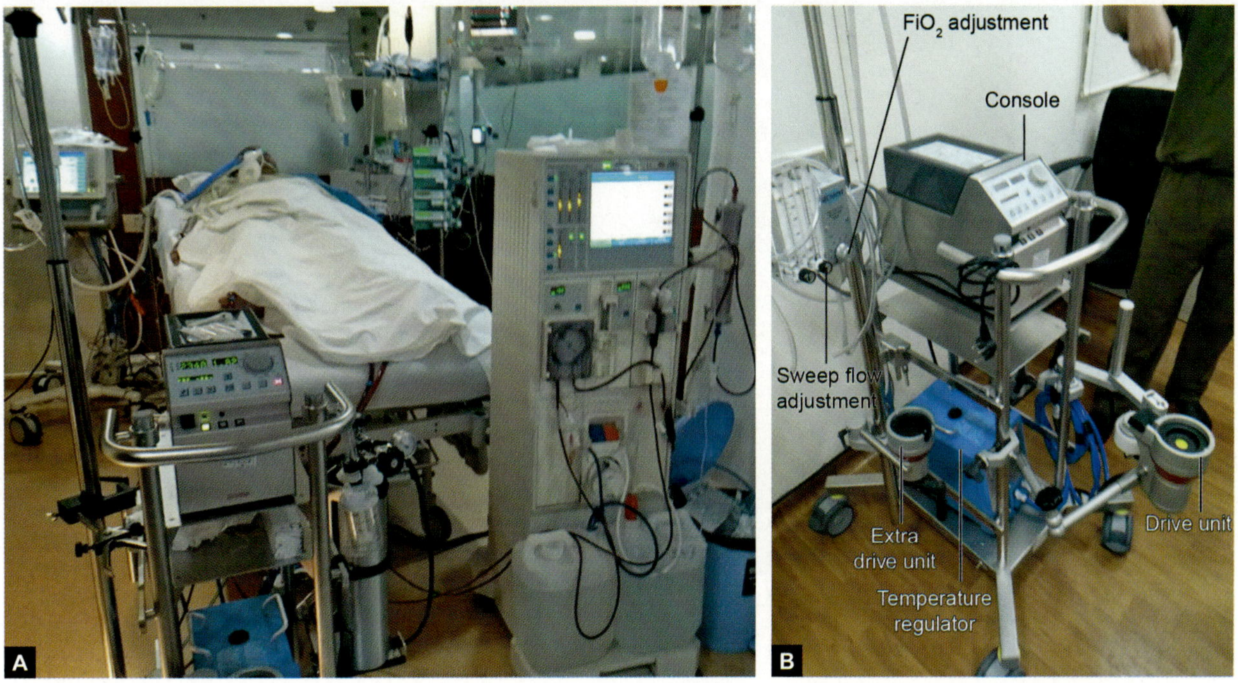

Figs. 11A and B: (A) Patient on venovenous (VV) extracorporeal membrane oxygenation (ECMO); (B) ECMO console.

- Venovenous (VV) extracorporeal membrane oxygenation (ECMO) and dialysis being done in the patient of severe viral pneumonia with acute kidney injury.
- In hypoxic respiratory failure due to any cause (primary or secondary), ECMO should be considered when the risk of mortality is 50% or greater, and is indicated when the risk of mortality is 80% or greater.
- Primary causes of respiratory failure: Infection—viral, bacterial, fungus, PCP; Primary lung disease—cystic fibrosis, hemorrhagic autoimmune diseases, idiopathic fibrosis, sickle cell crisis, primary pulmonary hypertension; Chest trauma, postpneumonectomy; Post-transplant—acute, chronic (Bronchiolitis obliterans); Chronic respiratory failure bridging to transplant.
- *Secondary causes of respiratory failure*: ARDS due to shock, trauma, sepsis, ischemic tissue, DIC, reinfusion reaction, anaphylaxis, cardiac failure with pulmonary edema, fluid over load.

VENOVENOUS BIFEMORAL ECMO CANNULAE (FIGS. 12A AND B)

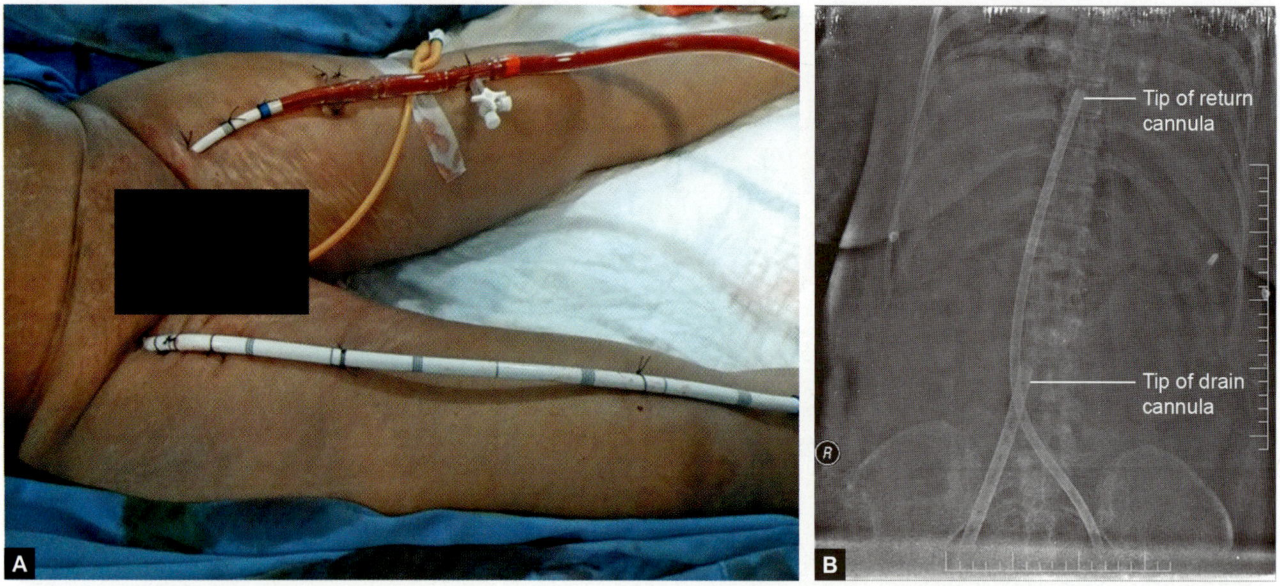

Figs. 12A and B: (A) Venovenous bifemoral ECMO cannulae insertion site; (B) Position of ECMO cannulae in abdominal X-ray.

- Most widely available cannulae are polyurethane cannula, which may be coated with heparin or nonheparin polymers that may reduce platelet activation and the inflammatory response at the blood-cannula interface.
- Flexibility and consistency of shape are influenced by the material of the cannula. Flexible cannulas are more difficult to insert but can adjust to the patient's anatomy and cause less tissue damage.
- Wire reinforcement of the cannula walls reinforce specific components and prevent kinking or collapse. These cannulae can be used to customize the angle of insertion and position within the heart when used during open-chest extracorporeal membrane oxygenation (ECMO).
- Potential complications of ECMO cannulation are vascular injury, hemorrhage (retroperitoneal hematoma, hemothorax, hemopericardium, etc.), cardiac arrhythmias, air embolism, compression of adjacent structures and pneumothorax.

EXTRACORPOREAL MEMBRANE OXYGENATION CENTRIFUGAL BLOOD PUMP (FIGS. 13A AND B)

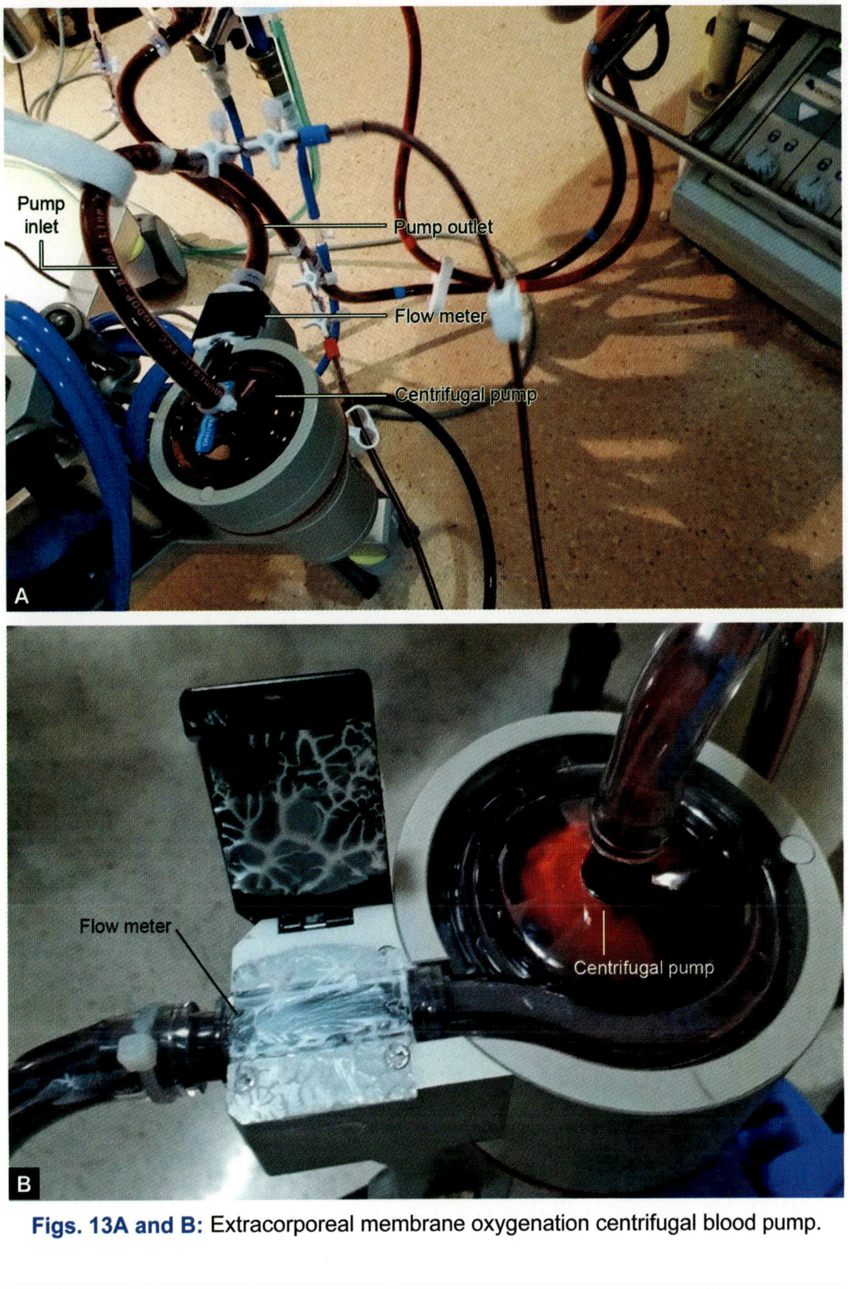

Figs. 13A and B: Extracorporeal membrane oxygenation centrifugal blood pump.

- Blood flow through the extracorporeal membrane oxygenation (ECMO) circuit is driven by a pump. Centrifugal pumps are increasingly used for ECMO rather than roller pumps as they cause less hemolysis and require less anticoagulation.
- Centrifugal pumps are light and small, the components do not wear out, and the perfusion pressure is limited by the revolutions per minute (RPM), so return line pressure is low and circuit rupture is extremely rare.
- The potential problems of a centrifugal pump head include stagnation and heating in the pump head, leading to thrombus at low flows or if the outlet line is occluded, and cavitation and hemolysis when the inlet line is occluded.
- Centrifugal pumps are preload dependent and after load sensitive, hence when the circuit is occluded, the pump will continue to spin.
- Blood flow through a circuit driven by a centrifugal pump must be continually monitored with an ultrasonic flow meter.
- Blood flow through a circuit driven by a centrifugal pump must be continuously monitored with an ultrasonic flow meter.

CERVICAL CORD INJURY (FIG. 14)

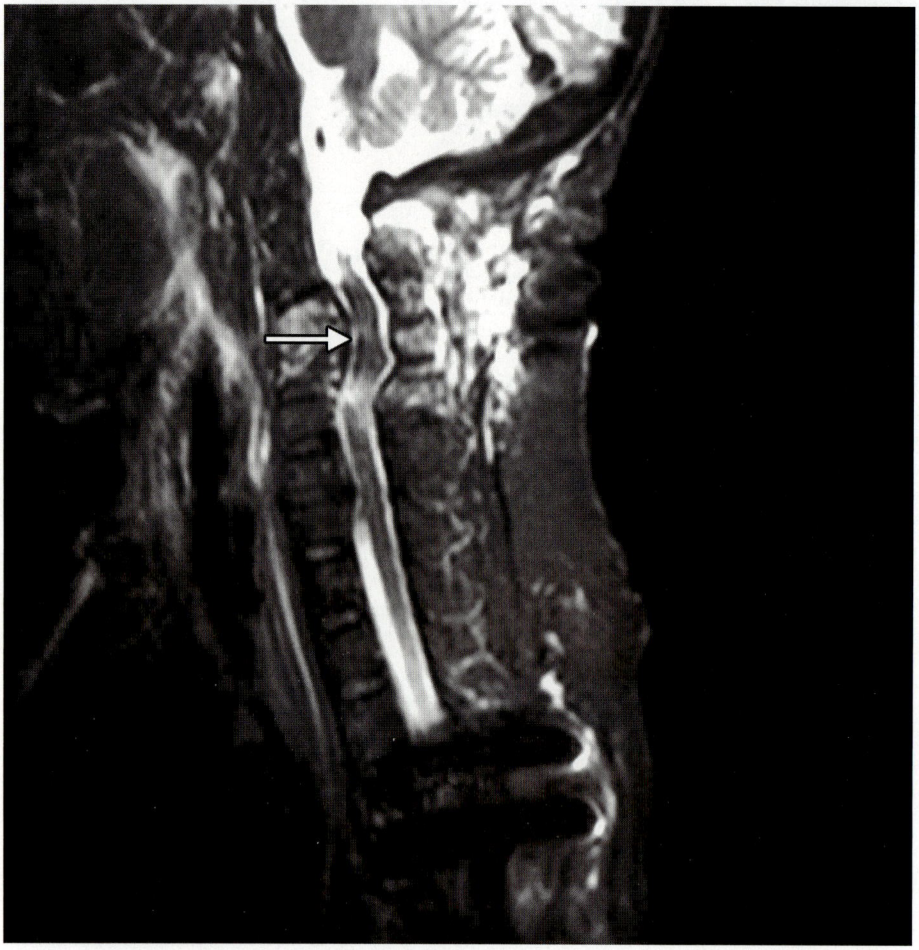

Fig. 14: Cervical cord injury.

- Patients with acute injury C3-C5 level or above usually require ventilatory assistance, because the phrenic nerve roots that supply the diaphragm arise from spinal segments C3 to C5.
- Patients with C1–C2 spinal injury levels are permanently ventilator dependent.
- Prognosis of spinal cord lesions is related to the level of the injury, development of pneumonia and other respiratory complications.

DIGITAL GANGRENE, A COMPLICATION OF RADIAL ARTERY CANNULATION (FIGS. 15A AND B)

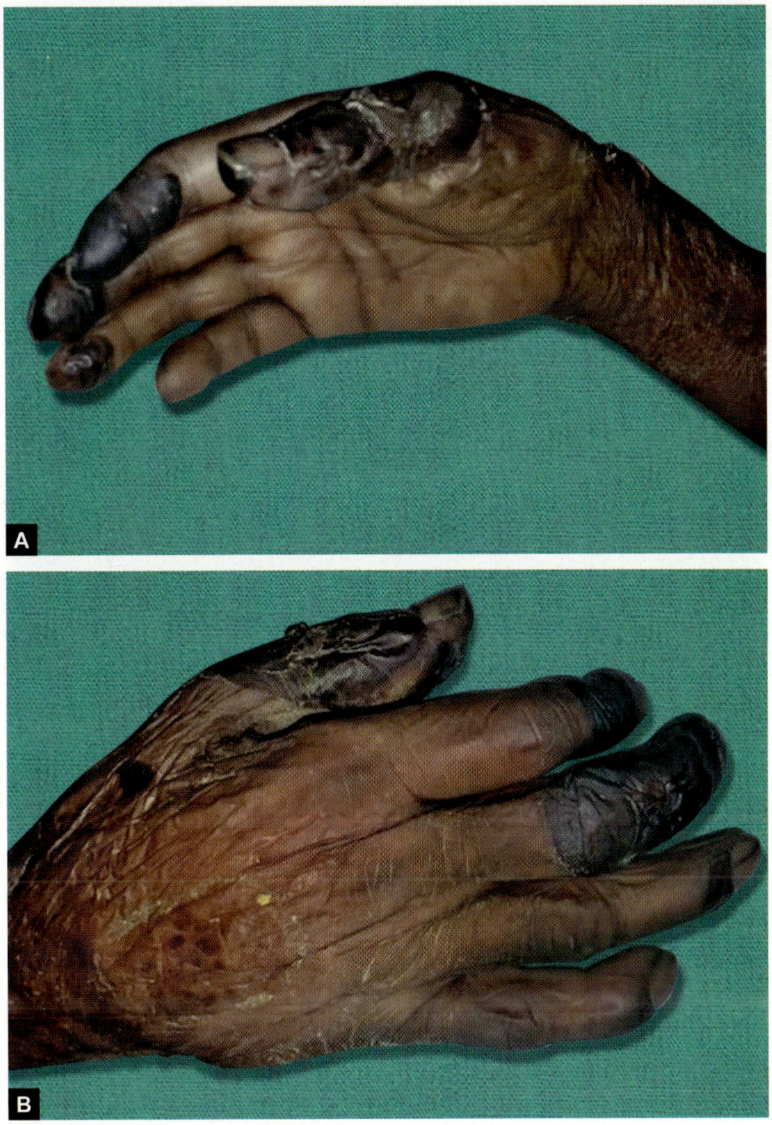

Figs. 15A and B: Digital gangrene, a complication of radial artery cannulation.

- Digital gangrene happened as a complication of radial artery cannulation due to thrombosis, images were taken about 20 days after removal of cannula.
- Arterial cannulation is the most common method of invasive blood pressure monitoring in ICU. The radial artery is often chosen, as it is superficial, allowing easy palpation with high successful cannulation rates, and is not an end artery.
- Although vascular insufficiency from radial artery catheterization is not very common, but it occurs frequently in those patients who are high risk for vascular insufficiency.
- Early recognition, intra-arterial papaverine injection through catheter and removal of catheter and can prevent ischemic compilations.
- Modified Allen's test is often used to assess of collateral circulation of the hand to predict vascular insufficiency after radial artery catheterization, however multiple studies proved modified Allen test does not have sufficient diagnostic validity to serve as a screening tool for collateral circulation deficits in the hand. Nor is it a good predictor of hand ischemia after arterial puncture.

ANCHOVY SAUCE APPEARANCE OF LIVER ABSCESS (FIG. 16)

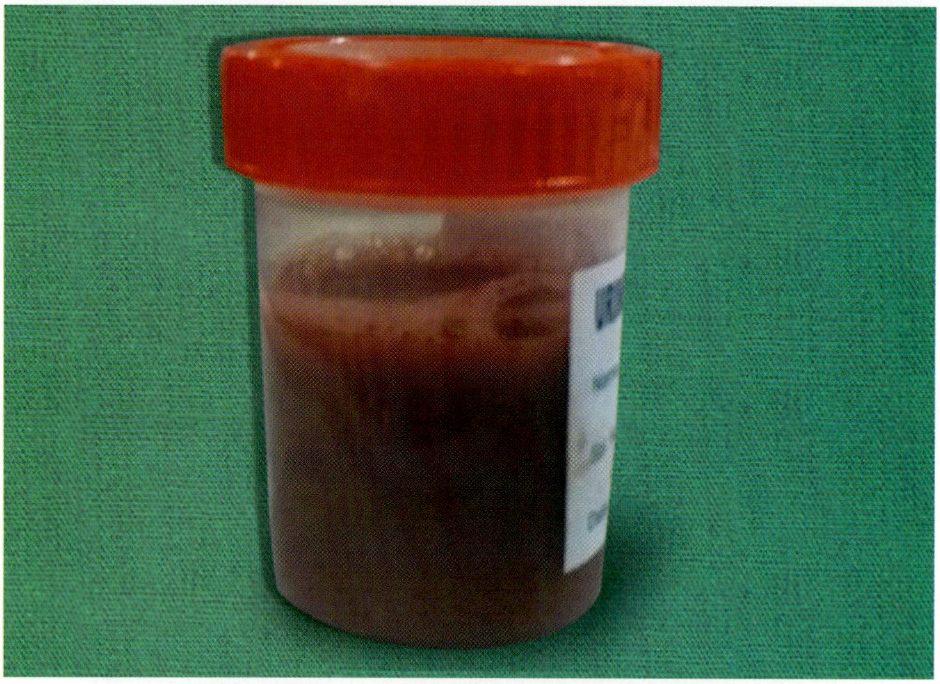

Fig. 16: Anchovy sauce appearance of liver abscess.

- Anchovy sauce like pus is typically seen in amebic liver abscess, composed of necrotic debris and blood.
- Amebiasis and cause brain abscess also with or without liver abscess.
- The liver is the most common extra-intestinal location of amebiasis, and amebic liver abscesses occur in 1% of patients with amebiasis.
- The presentation of amebic abscesses may be acute with fever and right upper quadrant pain or less specific with weight loss, fever, and abdominal pain.
- The majority of amebic liver abscesses in right lobe as single abscess.
- Drainage of abscess is only necessary in circumstances in which there are abscess complications, suspicion of bacterial coinfection, or diagnostic uncertainty.
- Most of the time antibiotic metrogyl 500–750 mg for 7–20 days treat abscess successfully.

PERIUMBILICAL HERNIA WITH GANGRENOUS BOWEL (FIGS. 17A AND B)

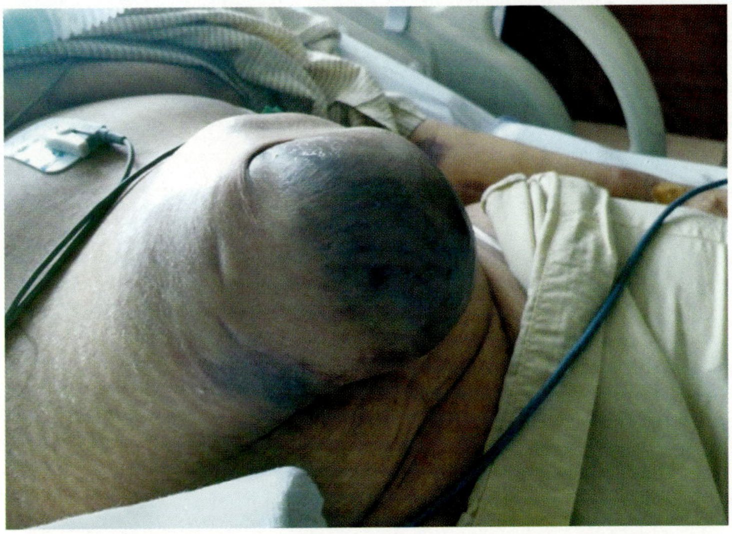

Fig. 17A: Bluish discoloration of skin over gangreous bowel.

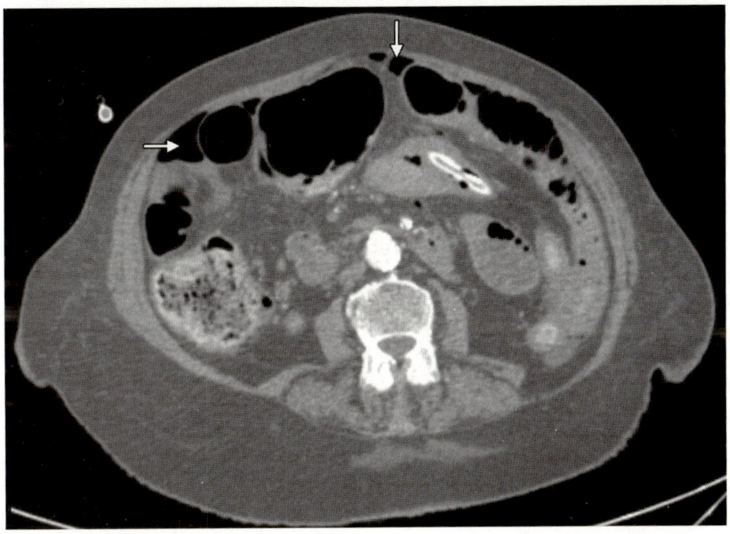

Fig. 17B: CT scan abdomen of same patient showing pneumoperitoneum.

- Patient was having long standing periumbilical hernia with underlying chronic atrial fibrillation for that she was on therapeutic oral anticoagulant dabigatran.
- Patient developed gut gangrene due to acute mesenteric ischemia that lead to perforation of bowel and pneumoperitoneum, seen in CT scan (Fig. 17B).
- Acute mesenteric ischemia is often a surgical emergency as a result of sudden onset of intestinal hypoperfusion, which can be due to occlusive or nonocclusive obstruction of arterial or venous blood flow.
- Occlusive arterial obstruction is most commonly due to emboli or thrombosis of mesenteric arteries.
- Mesenteric venous obstruction occurs when thrombosis one or more of the major veins that drain blood from your intestines.
- Nonocclusive arterial insufficiency is most commonly due to primary splanchnic vasoconstriction.

GANGRENOUS STOMA OF ILEOSTOMY (VASCULAR COMPROMISE) (FIG. 18)

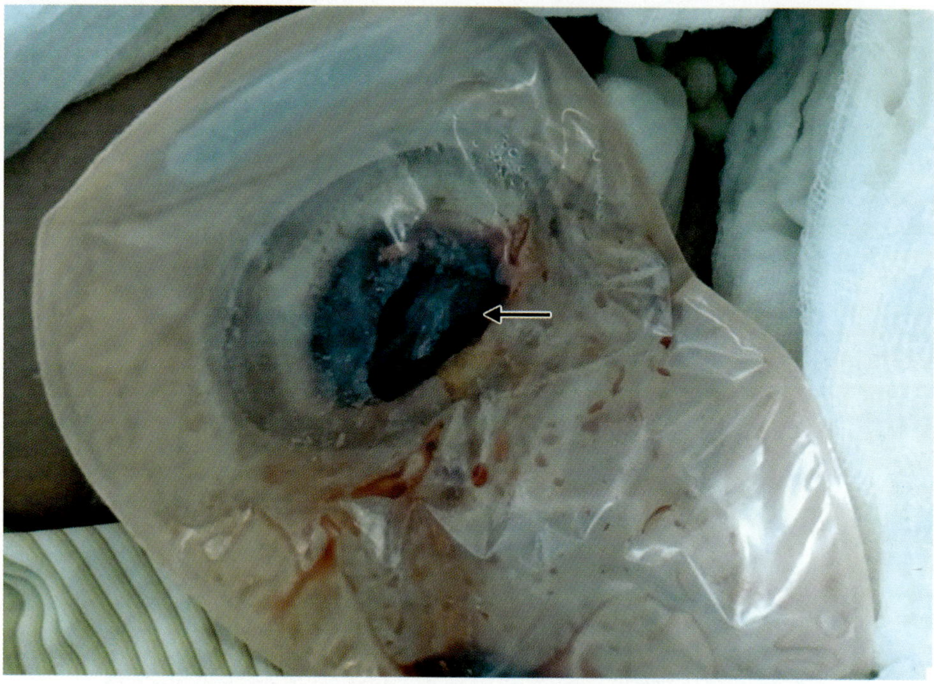

Fig. 18: Gangrenous stoma of ileostomy.

- The creation of intestinal stomas for diversion of enteric contents is a surgical intervention routinely done in ICU patients for several gastroenterologic disease processes.
- Commonly seen early postoperative stomal complications include improper stoma site selection, vascular compromise, retraction, peristomal skin irritation, peristomal infection/abscess/fistula, acute parastomal herniation and bowel obstruction.
- Vascular compromise represents the most serious early complication of stoma creation.
- Vascular compromise of intestinal stomas ranges from mild ischemia due to operative tissue trauma or vasospasm with mucosal sloughing to infarction and intestinal necrosis due to ligation of arterial supply or inadequate collateral arterial circulation.
- Vascular compromise of intestinal stomas ranges from mild ischemia due to operative tissue trauma or vasospasm with mucosal sloughing to infarction and intestinal necrosis due to ligation of arterial supply or inadequate collateral arterial circulation.
- Stomal ischemia can be recognized by dark or grayish appearance of stomal mucosa.
- Vascular compromised stoma requires revision surgery.

POSTLAPAROTOMY OPENED ABDOMINAL WALL (FIG. 19)

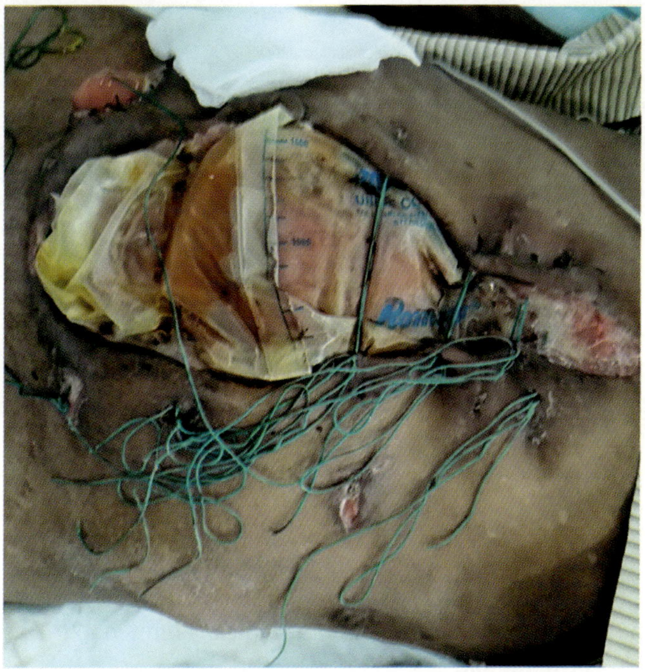

Fig. 19: Postlaparotomy opened abdominal wall.

- Postlaparotomy abdominal wall was kept open due to high intra-abdominal pressure to prevent 'abdominal compartment syndrome' (ACS).
- Inra-abdominal pressure > 12 mm Hg is labeled as intra-abdominal hypertension (IAH).
- Grading of IAH—Grade I = IAP 12–15 mm Hg; Grade II = IAP 16–20 mm Hg; Grade III = IAP 21–25 mm Hg; Grade IV = IAP > 25 mm Hg.
- ACS is defined as IAH-induced new organ dysfunction without a strict intra-abdominal pressure threshold.
- ACS affects commonly affects cardiovascular, renal and gastrointestinal system but it can affects hepatic, pulmonary and central nervous system also.
- Management initially consists of close observation and supportive care like reduction of intra-abdominal volume through evacuation of intraluminal contents, drainage of ascites, hematoma or collection, adequate pain control, use of muscle relaxants and avoidance of hypervolemia.
- In some cases, abdominal compartment decompression is required and an open abdomen is maintained using a variety of temporary abdominal closure techniques.

PALATAL HERPES (FIG. 20)

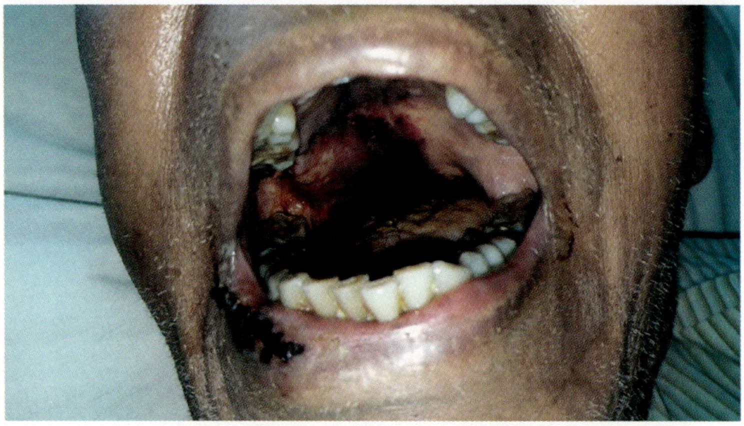

Fig. 20: Palatal herpes.

Oral and palatal lesions identified as herpetic lesions in immunocompetent.

- This is not a common site for herpes. This is more common in immunocompromised.
- Crop of vesicles usually rupture and leaves ulcers in keratinized and nonkeratinized oral mucosa.
- When it occurs in immunocompetent host, involvement is typically limited to the keratinized tissue, especially the hard palate and is almost always unilateral.

SUBCUTANEOUS PORT OF CHEMOPORT (FIG. 21)

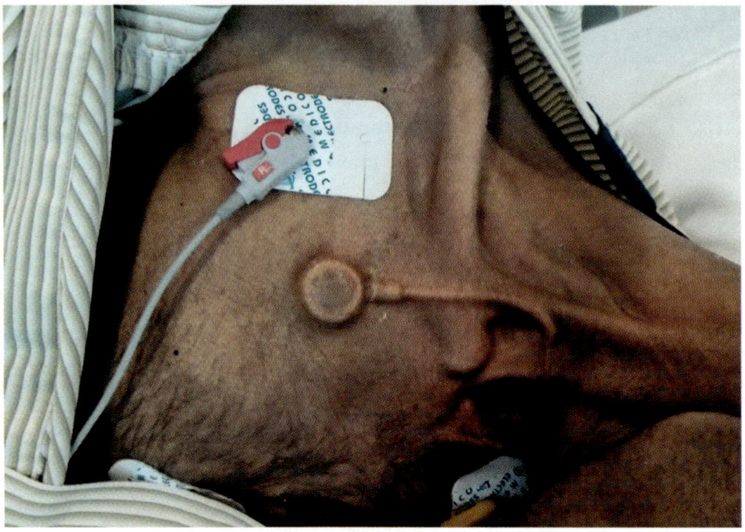

Fig. 21: Subcutaneous port of chemoport.

- Chemoport device is a catheter that is connected to a plastic and metal reservoir.
- Chemotherapy drugs are administered via the port with a needle that fits into the port.
- After completion of cycle of intravenous chemotherapy needle is removed.
- Port can also be used for drawing of blood sample for investigations.
- *Complications*: Bleeding, thrombosis, leaks, skin damage, insertion site infection, blood stream infection.
- A port can stay in place for months or even years, if needed.

POTASSIUM PERMANGANATE INGESTION (FIG. 22)

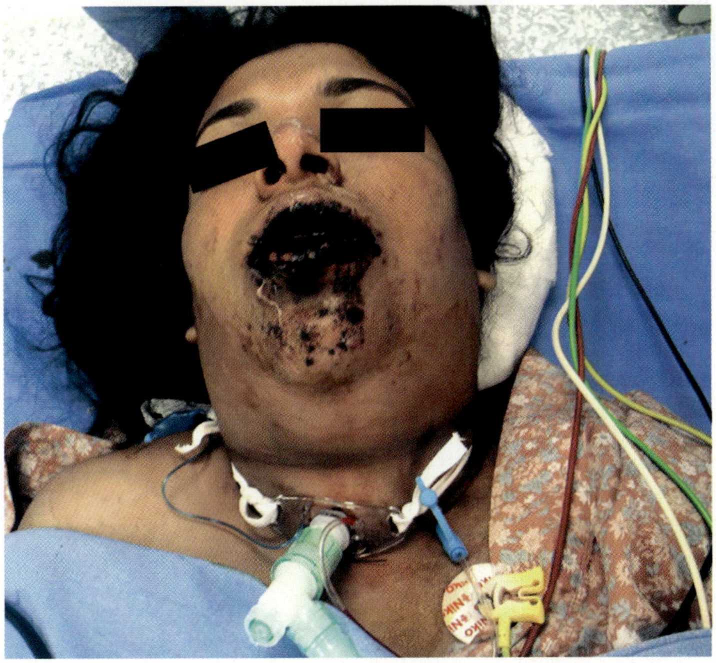

Fig. 22: Potassium permanganate ingestion.

- Swollen and black-brown stained lips and oral cavity of the patient with potassium permanganate ingestion.
- Formulations available are solutions, pellets, tablets, crystals, and powder. Patient shown in picture consumed potassium permanganate powder.
- The strong oxidizing action of potassium permanganate causes burns depending on the concentration and amount of local irritation and it causes liquefaction necrosis.
- Ingestion of concentrated solutions or dry crystals of potassium permanganate can cause swelling and bleeding of lips and tongue, pharyngeal edema, and swelling of the larynx.
- The immediate concern after the ingestion of potassium permanganate is the threat of acute laryngeal edema and this necessitates early endotracheal intubation or even emergency surgical airway.
- Emergency endoscopy has a significant role in diagnosis and management of potassium permanganate ingestion to determine the extent of upper gastrointestinal (GI) damage.

TERRY'S NAIL (FIG. 23)

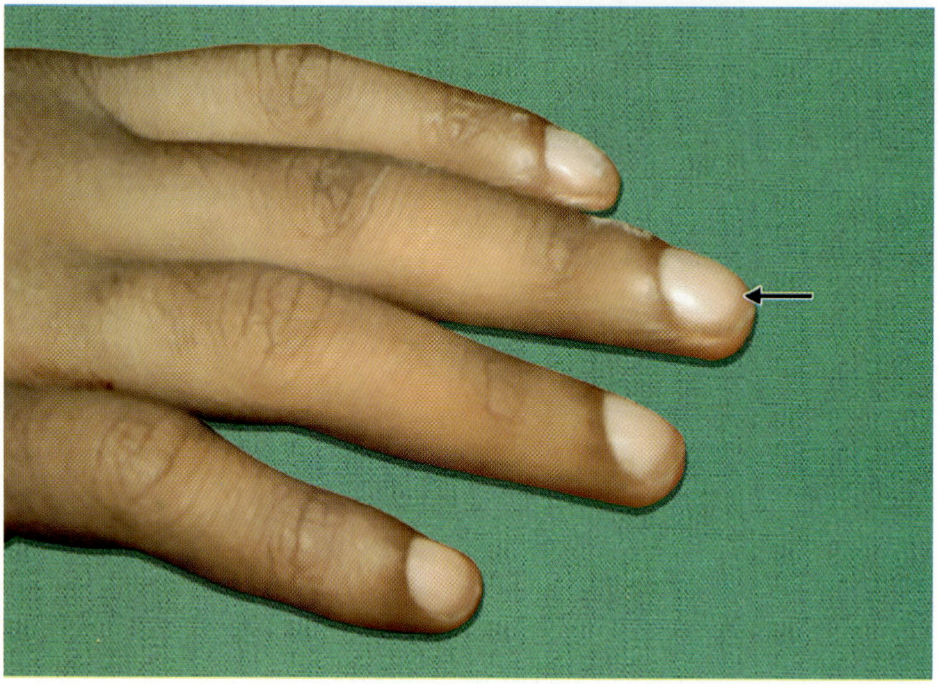

Fig. 23: Terry's nail.

- Patient of chronic liver failure showing white nail bed with a narrow zone of pink at the distal end, also known as "Terry's nail".
- The condition is thought to be due to a decrease in vascularity and an increase in connective tissue within the nail bed.
- Apart from liver failure and cirrhosis, it can also be seen in chronic kidney disease, congestive heart failure, diabetes, hyperthyroidism, malnutrition and advanced age.
- Terry's nails highlight the intimate connection between nail changes and systemic disease as well as the importance of thorough nail inspection with every physical examination.

STEVENS-JOHNSON SYNDROME AND TOXIC EPIDERMAL NECROLYSIS (FIG. 24)

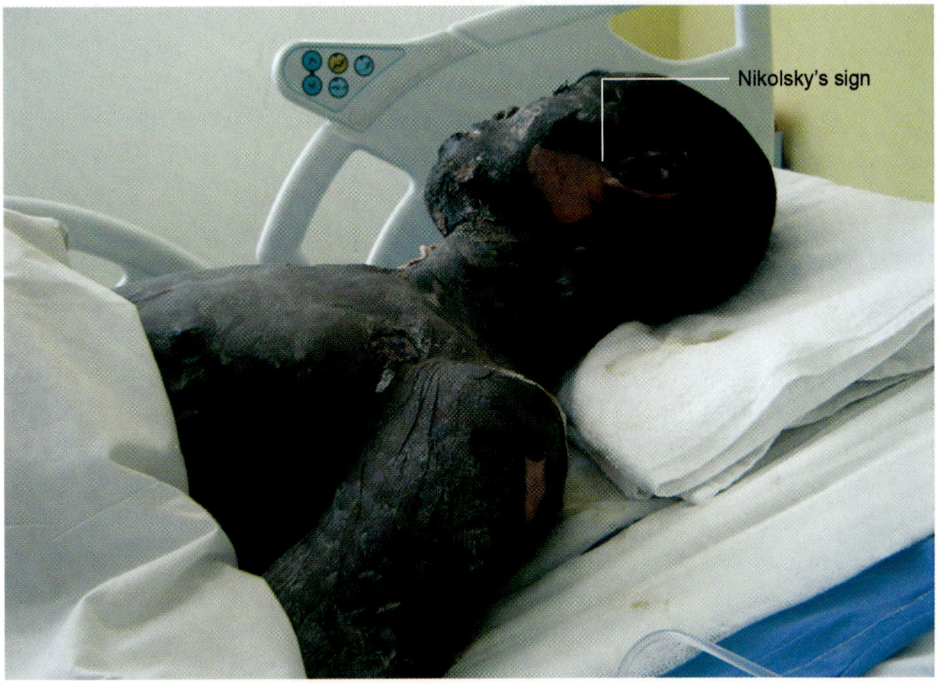

Fig. 24: Stevens-Johnson syndrome and toxic epidermal necrolysis.

- Patient suffered Stevens-Johnson syndrome (SJS) progressed to toxic epidermal necrolysis (TEN) after expose to intravenous vancomycin.
- SJS and toxic epidermal necrolysis, TEN are idiosyncratic reactions, most commonly triggered by drugs. Common drugs are anticonvulsants, antibiotics and nonsteroidal anti-inflammatory.
- Nikolsky's sign is sloughing off of epidermal layer when pressure is applied to the blistered or erythematous area.
- SJS has < 10% total body surface area involvement, TEN has > 30% total body surface area and SJS/TEN syndrome has 10–30% total body surface area.
- Identification and immediate removal of causative agent significantly affect the outcome.
- Multidisciplinary approach is required to treat such patients, that includes wound care, fluid and electrolyte management, nutritional support, ocular care, temperature management, pain control, and monitoring for of secondary infections.

FOLEY'S CATHETER USE TO STOP NASAL BLEEDING (FIG. 25)

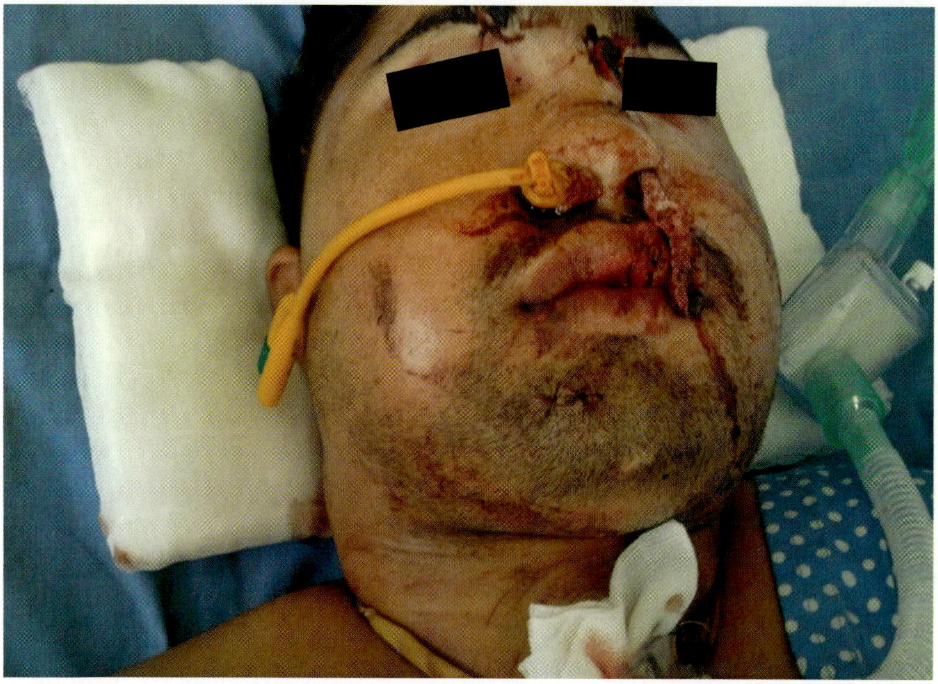

Fig. 25: Foley's catheter use to stop nasal bleeding.

- Foley catheter is an effective and rapid nonsurgical treatment alternative to surgical treatment options for refractory posterior epistaxis like endoscopic diathermy or endoscopic artery ligation.
- Normally nasal packing stops the nasal bleeding, however, if there is no nasal packing around or bleeding is refractory to nasal packing Foley's catheter can be used.
- Insert the Foley through the nose on the side that is bleeding just like a nasogastric tube. Once inserted so the catheter can be seen in the back of the mouth, inflate balloon with saline. After inflating the Foley balloon, pull the Foley catheter with enough pressure to equal the amount of pressure desired to stop the nosebleed.
- This is a temporary measure and should be replaced as soon as possible with definitive intervention.

FOOT DROP (FIGS. 26A AND B)

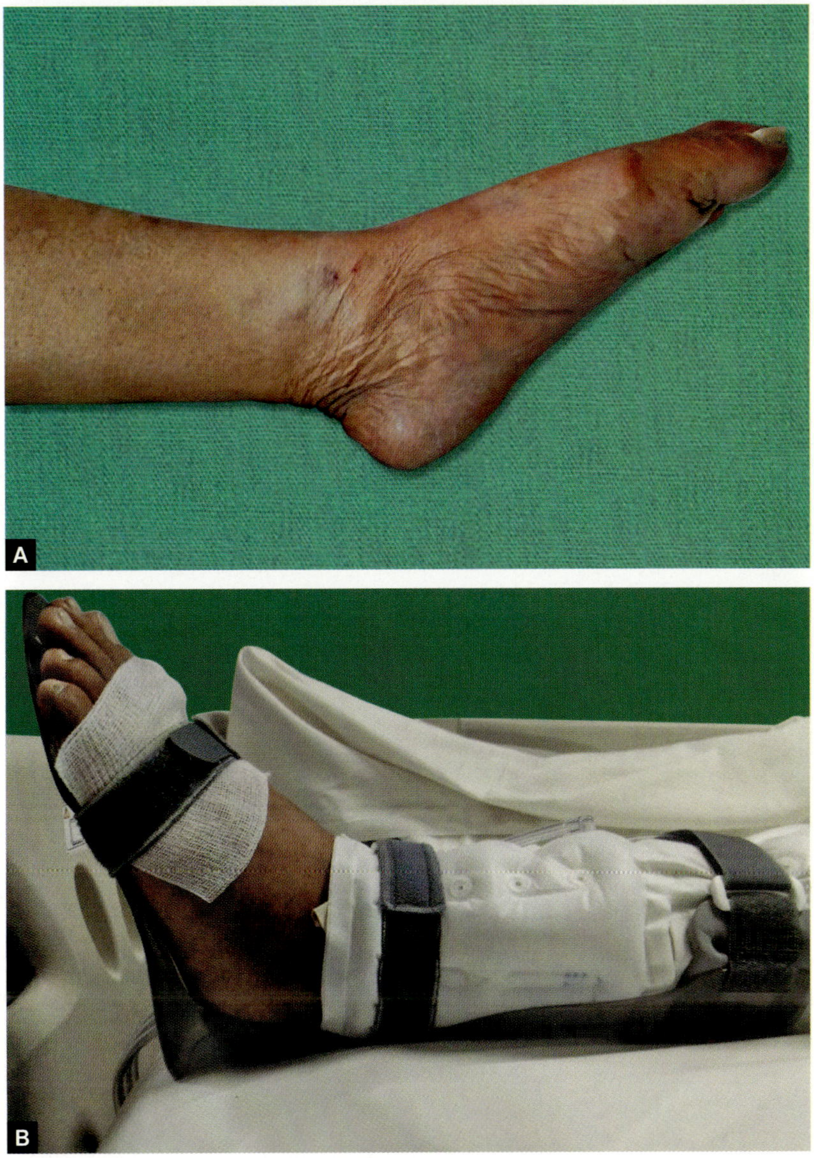

Figs. 26A and B: Foot drop.

- Critical illness-related muscular weakness typically have significant activity limitations, often requiring physical assistance for even the most basic activities.
- Foot drop is one of the manifestations of critical illness-related polyneuromyopathy, it is common even in those patients with apparent complete functional recovery.
- Early mobility and physical rehabilitation is an effective measure to prevent weakness.
- Foot drop splint should be used in the patient with foot drop. It helps to correct foot drop, and prevent more injury to the foot or ankle.
- A foot drop splint allows foot and ankle to be positioned neutrally (Fig. 26B).

SENGSTAKEN–BLAKEMORE TUBE (FIGS. 27A TO C)

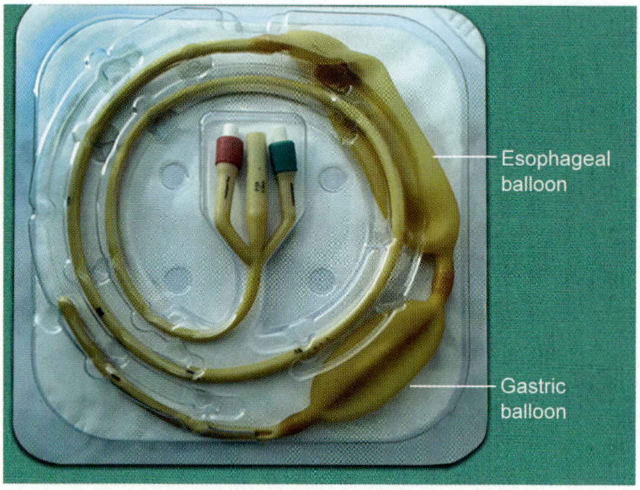

Fig. 27A: Sengstaken-Blakemore tube (SBT).

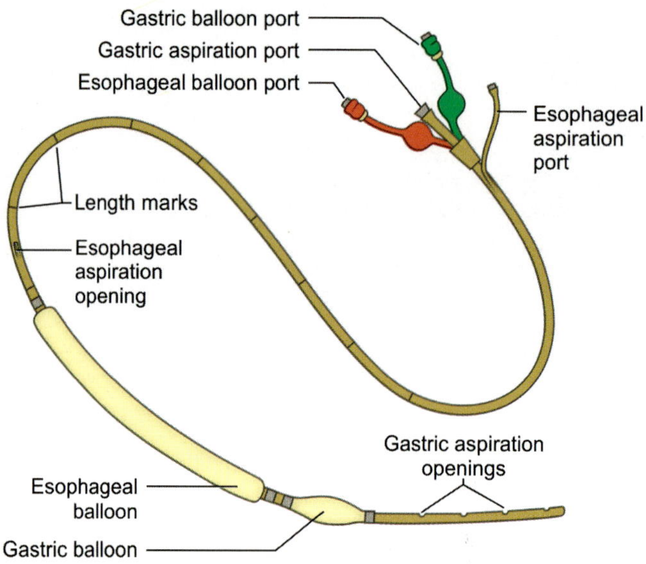

Fig. 27B: Illustration of parts of SBT.

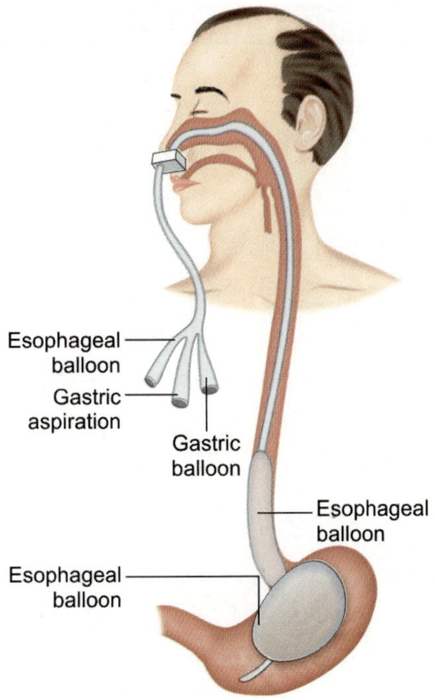

Fig. 27C: Illustration of SBT placement.

- Sengstaken-Blakemore tube is a tube inserted through the nose or mouth for control of upper gastrointestinal bleeding due to esophageal or gastric varices.
- After insertion gastric balloon should be inflated with 400–500 mL of air and esophageal balloon should be inflated with minimal air to achieve 30–45 mm Hg pressure; inflated gastric balloon requires 1–2 lbs of traction.
- Indications for placement of a Sengstaken-Blakemore tube:
  - Massive bleeding with failed endoscopic and medical management.
  - When endoscopic and medical management are unavailable, and bleeding is life threatening.
- Complications:
  - Tube can migrate proximal blocking the airway therefore endotracheal intubation is preferred.
  - Migration of gastric balloon into the esophagus causes tracheal compression and high peak airway pressure ventilator.
  - Aspiration.
  - Esophageal perforation or rupture.
  - Necrosis of nares, lips, tongue.
  - Pharyngeal and gastroesophageal erosions and ulcers caused by local pressure effects.
  - Hiccups.

PHYSICAL REHABILITATION BY MAKING PATIENT UPRIGHT ON TILT TABLE (FIG. 28)

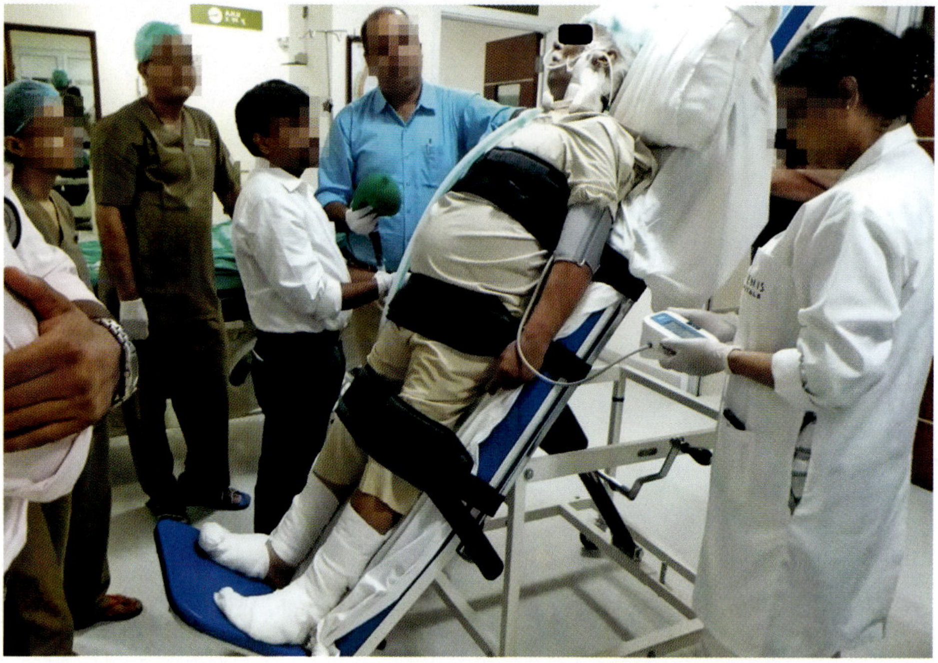

Fig. 28: Physical rehabilitation by making patient upright on tilt table.

- Muscle wasting and weakness commonly develops within days of ICU admission, with effects on survival and physical functioning lasting for years postdischarge.
- Early-onset physical rehabilitation is a safe intervention in ICU patients that, improves strength and physical functioning, and may improve delirium in the ICU as well as in-hospital and post-hospitalization care.
- Using tilt table for early rehabilitation of patients in ICU is a new trend of practice among the therapists.
- Tilt table can enhance the respiratory function of an ICU patients, and shortens the rate of his/her recovery.
- Inadequate multidisciplinary staffing and collaboration, deep sedation and a lack of knowledge regarding benefits to patients are among the most important potential barriers to successful implementation of early rehabilitation programs.

CHAPTER

26

Radiology Images in ICU

Nirad Mehta, Jalpa Bhandari, Isha Atre

CHEST X-RAY (FIG. 1)

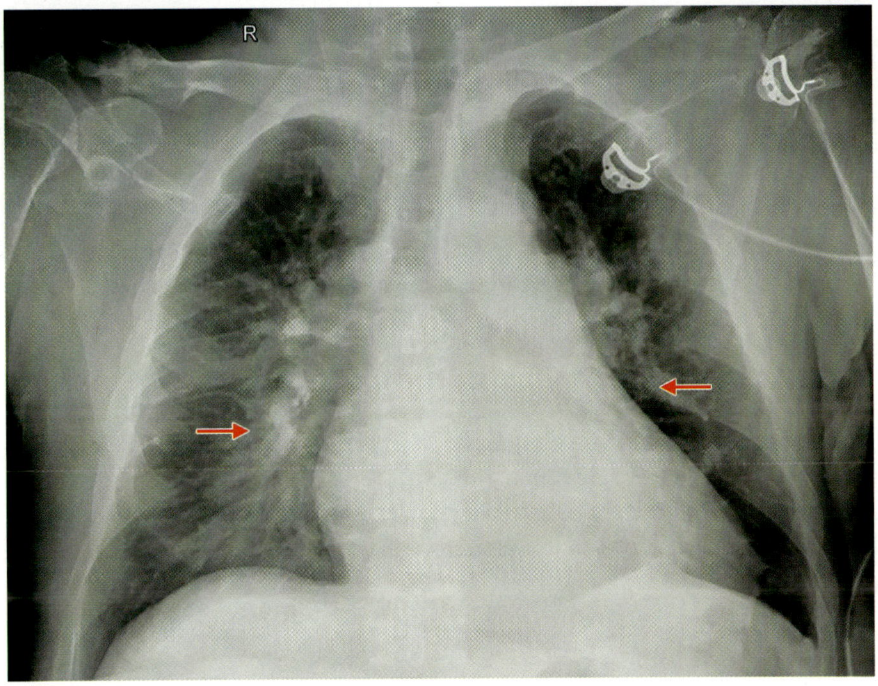

Fig. 1: Chest X-ray: Pulmonary edema (Arrows showing: bilateral perihilar haziness).

CHEST X-RAY AP VIEW: COPD WITH INFECTION (FIG. 2)

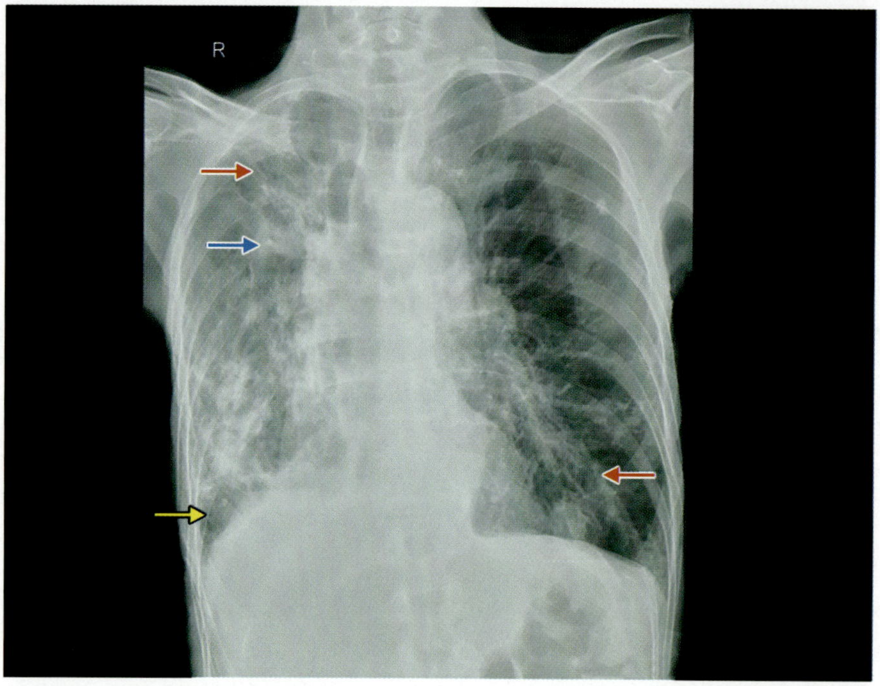

Fig. 2: Chest X-ray anteroposterior (AP) view: Chronic obstructive pulmonary disease (COPD) with infection.

- Loss of volume right lung, hyperinflation of left lung.
- *Blue arrow*: Patchy consolidates in the right upper zone.
- *Red arrows*: Reticular shadows in the right lung and left lower zone.
- *Yellow arrow*: Thin-walled cystic shadows in the right lower zone.

CHEST X-RAY: LEFT PLEURAL EFFUSION (FIG. 3)

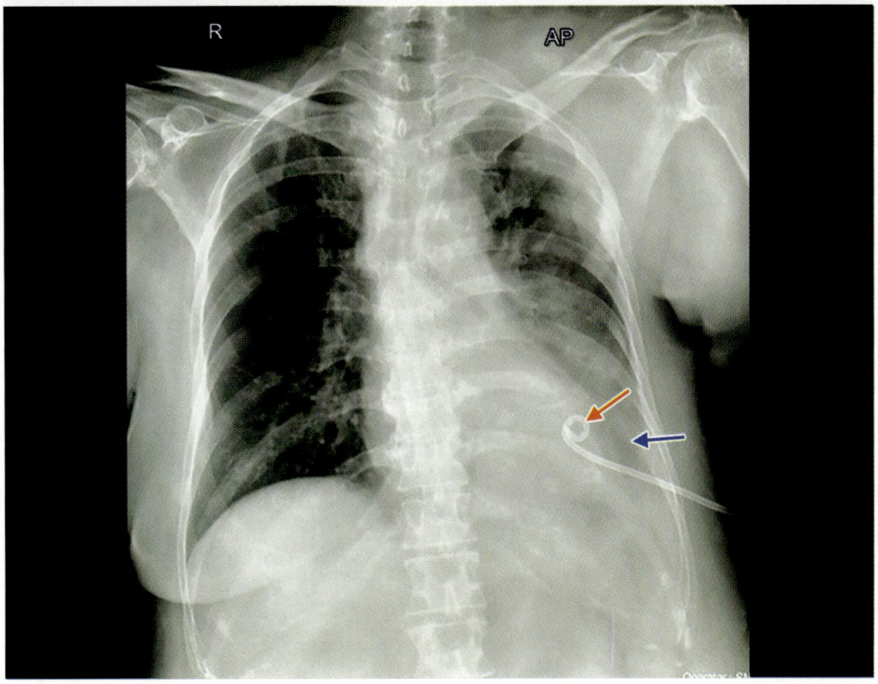

Fig. 3: Chest X-ray: Left pleural effusion. (AP: Anteroposterior)

- *Blue arrow*: Moderate left basal pleural effusion.
- *Red arrow*: Pigtail drainage catheter on the left side.

RIGHT LUNG LOBAR PNEUMONIA (FIG. 4)

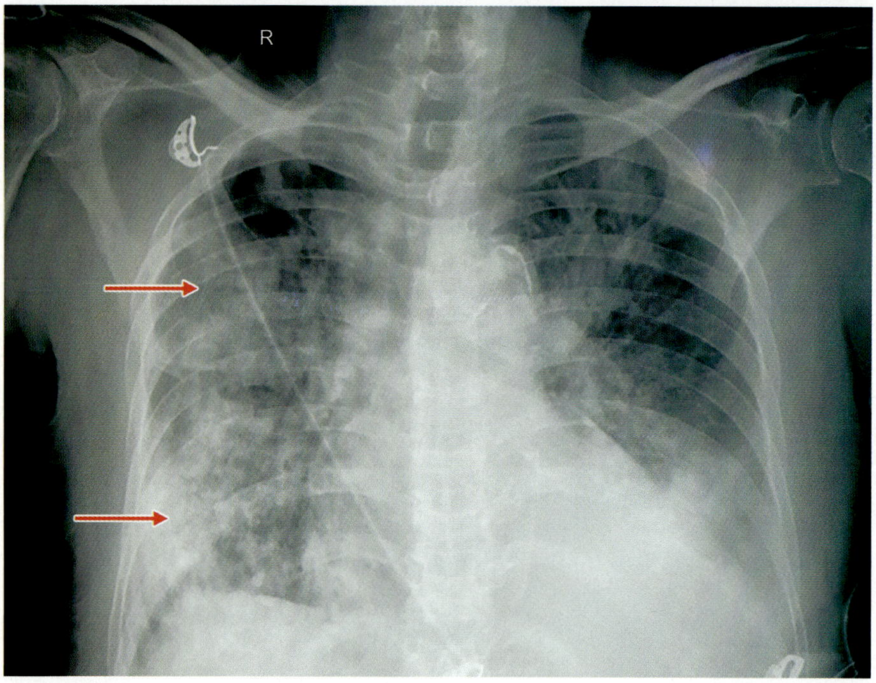

Fig. 4: Right lung lobar pneumonia.

- *Arrows*: Opacities of consolidations in right upper mid and lower zones, suggestive of consolidation of all lobes of right lung.

ACUTE RESPIRATORY DISTRESS SYNDROME: CHEST X-RAY (FIG. 5)

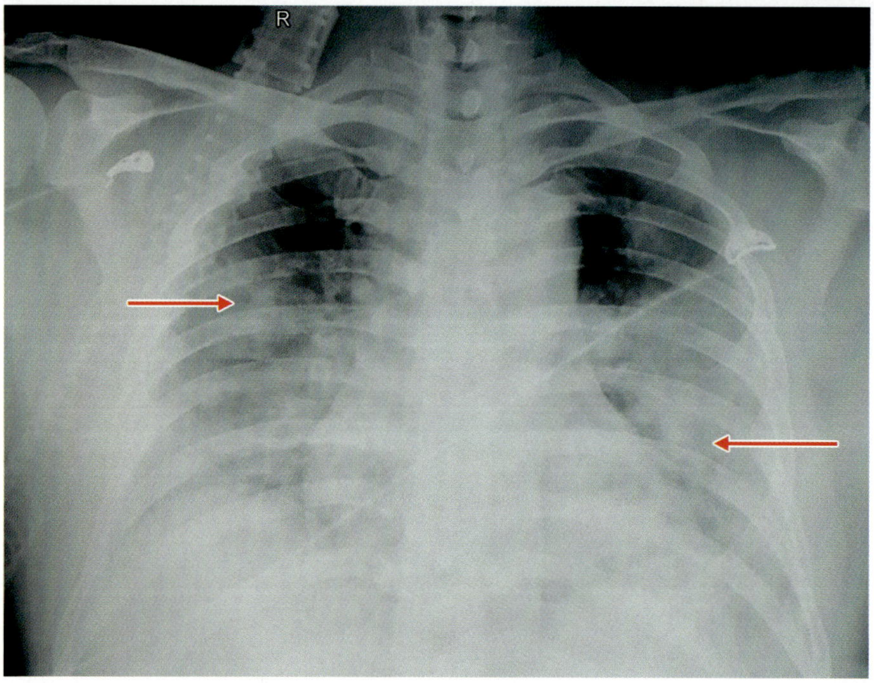

Fig. 5: Acute respiratory distress syndrome (ARDS): Chest X-ray.

- *Arrows*: Patchy consolidates are seen in the both mid and lower zones.

CHEST X-RAY: ASPIRATION PNEUMONIA (FIG. 6)

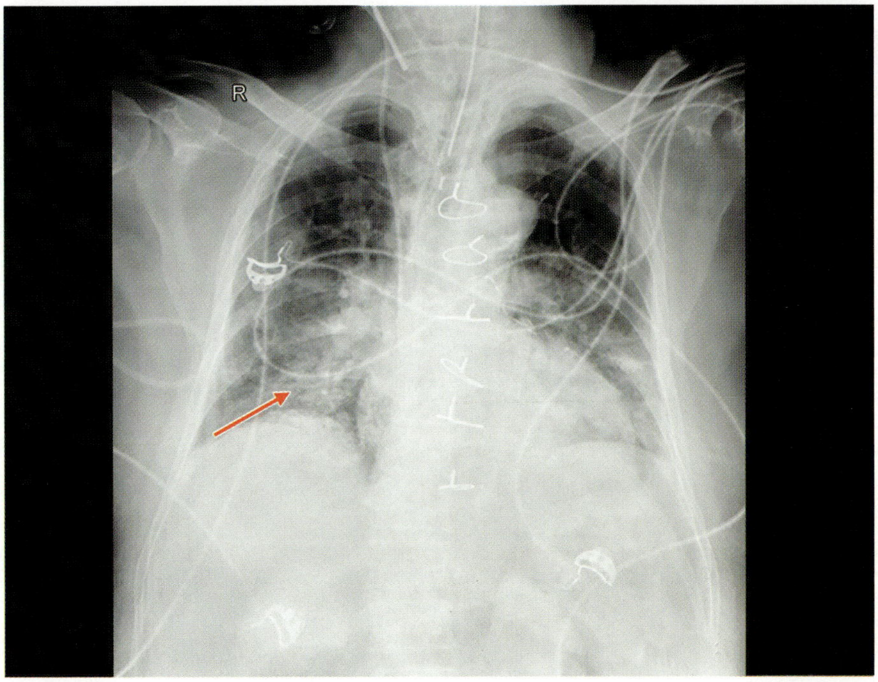

Fig. 6: Chest X-ray: Aspiration pneumonia.

ATYPICAL PNEUMONIA (FIG. 7)

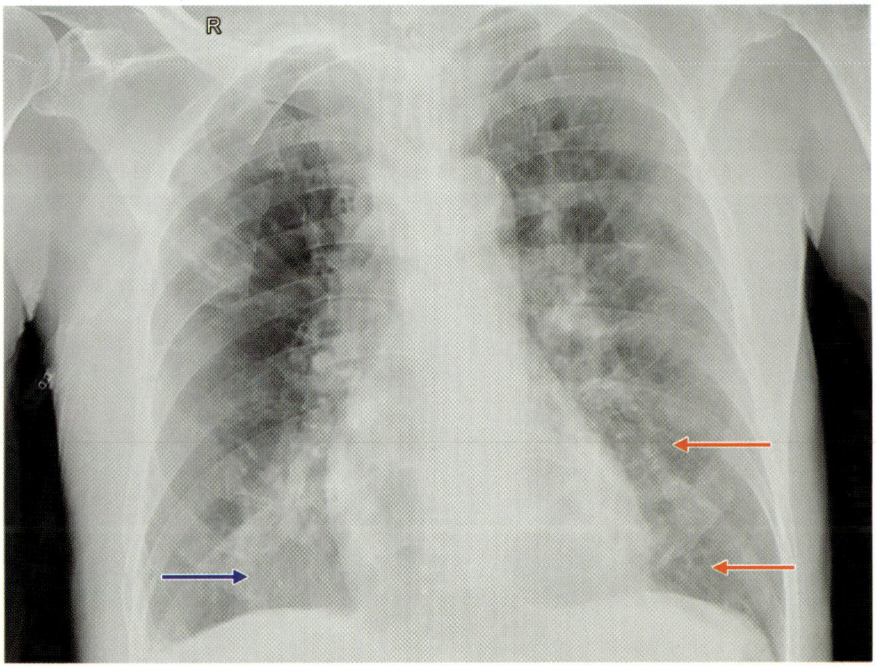

Fig. 7: Atypical pneumonia.

- *Red arrows*: Reticular shadows in left mid and both lower zones.
- *Blue arrow*: Patchy consolidates in right lower zone.

CHEST X-RAY OF PNEUMOMEDIASTINUM (FIG. 8)

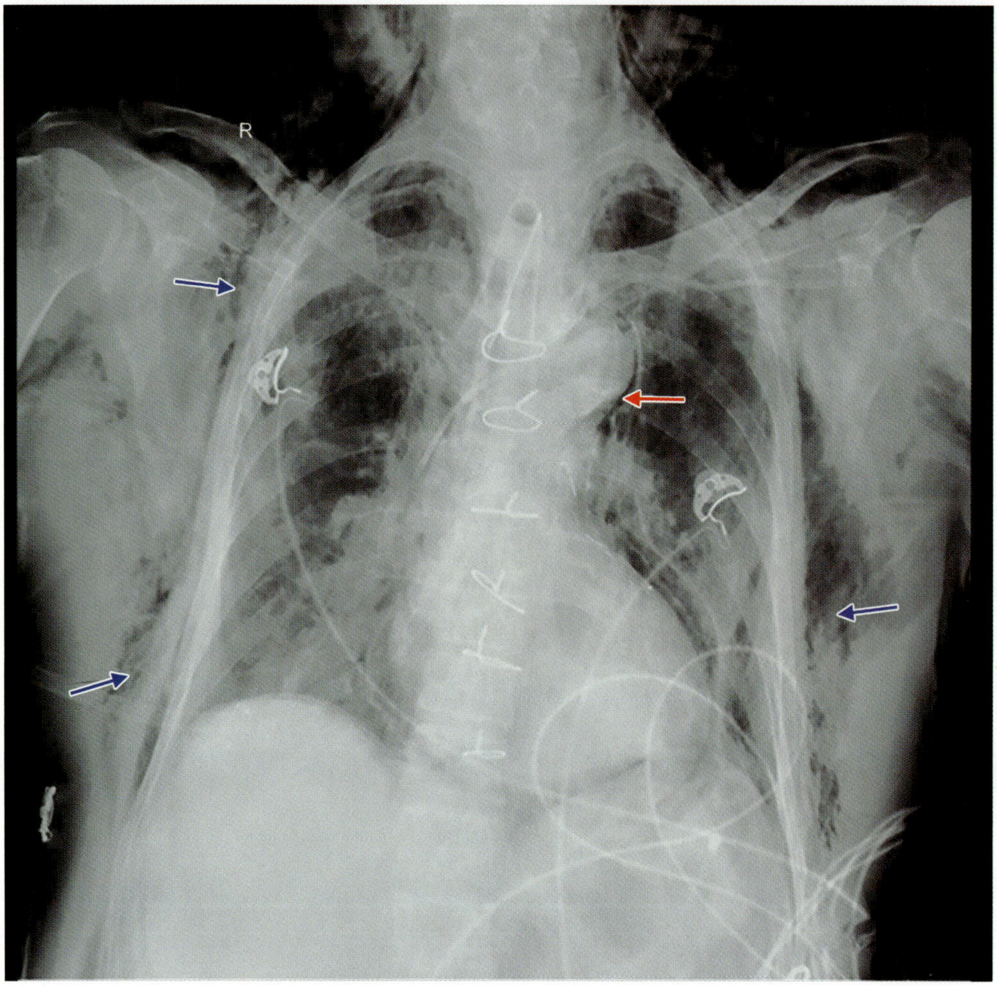

Fig. 8: Chest X-ray of pneumomediastinum.

- *Red arrow*: Free air in mediastinum around aortic knuckle; sign of pneumomediastinum.
- *Blue arrows*: Subcutaneous emphysema.

BOWEL OBSTRUCTION (FIG. 9)

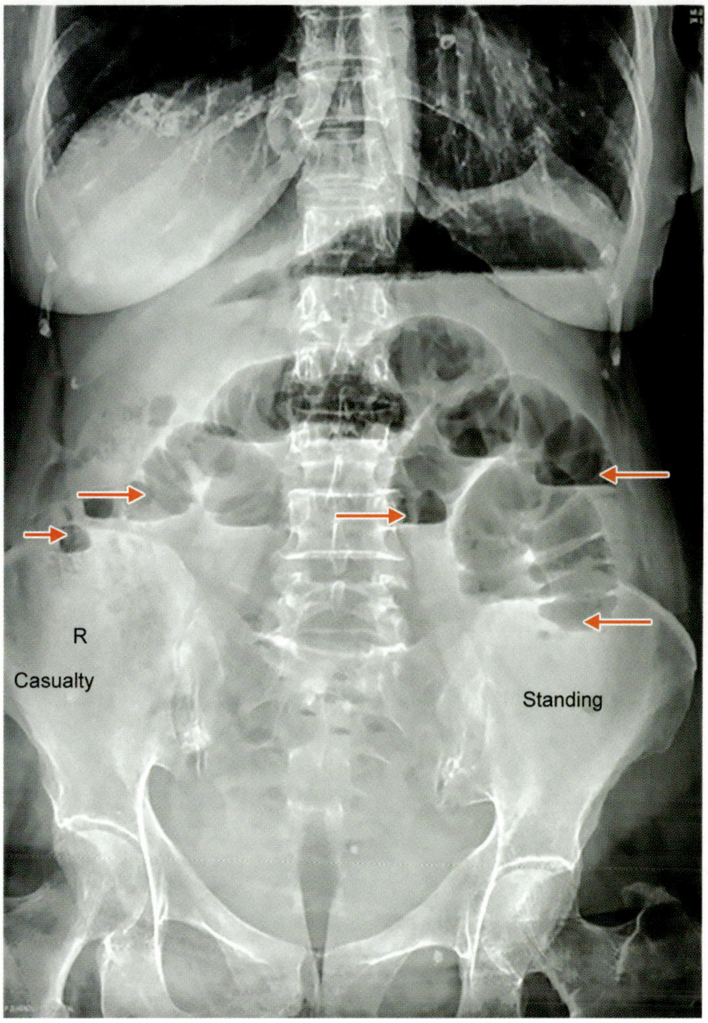

Fig. 9: Bowel obstruction—X-ray abdomen: Multiple dilated small bowel loops with air-fluid levels (arrows).

NORMAL ANATOMY: AXIAL SCANS CHEST AND ABDOMEN (FIGS. 10A TO I)

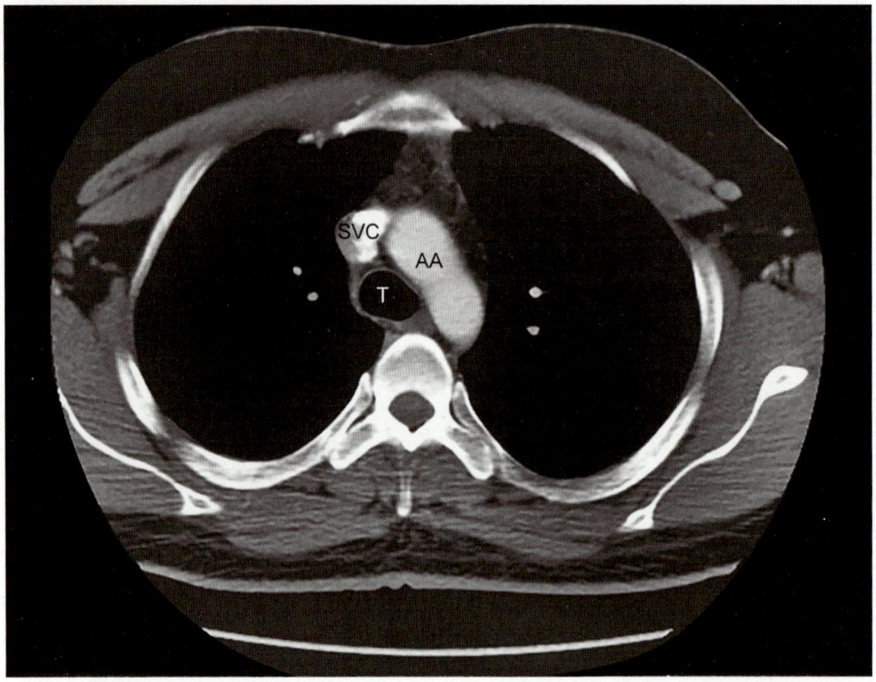

Fig. 10A: Contrast-enhanced computed tomography (CECT) axial: At the level of the arch of aorta. (AA: Arch of aorta; SVC: Superior vena cava; T: Trachea)

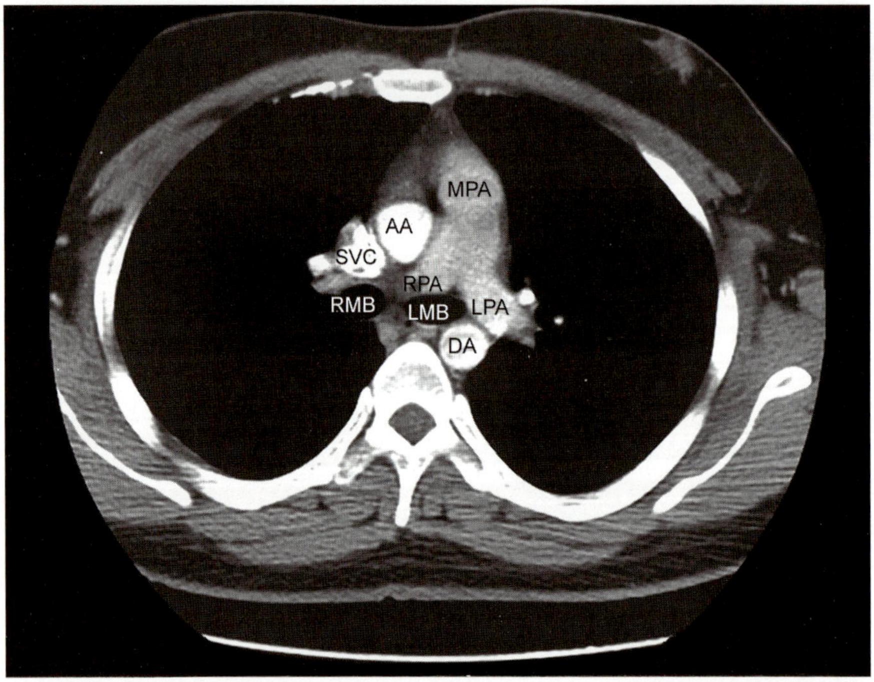

Fig. 10B: CECT axial: At the level of pulmonary bifurcation. (AA: Ascending aorta; DA: Descending aorta; LPA: Left pulmonary artery; MPA: Main pulmonary artery; RPA: Right pulmonary artery; SVC: Superior vena cava; RMB: Right main bronchus; LMB: Left main bronchus)

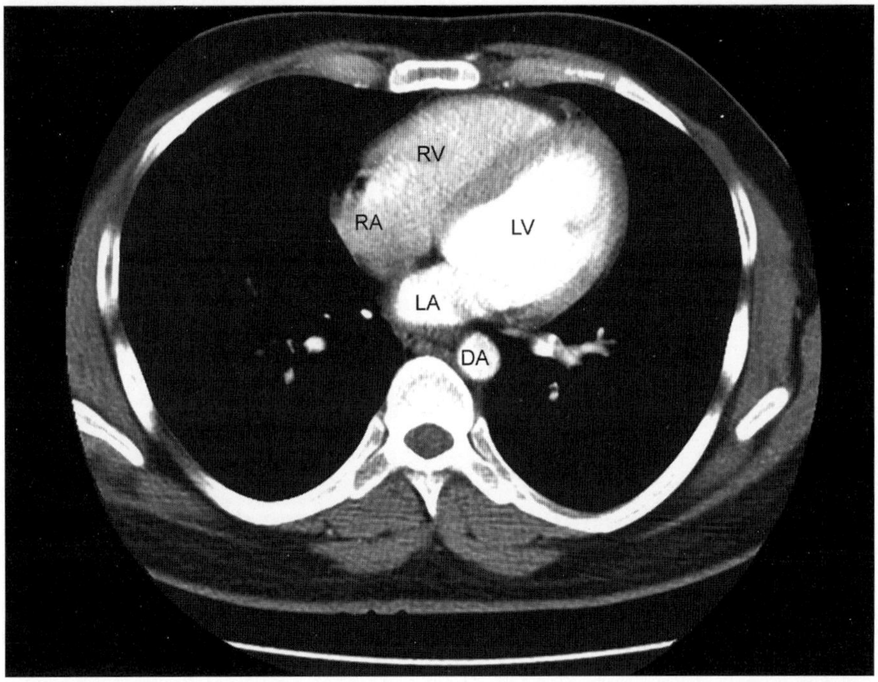

Fig. 10C: CECT axial: At the level of heart. (DA: Descending aorta; LA: Left atrium; LV: Left ventricle; RA: Right atrium; RV: Right ventricle)

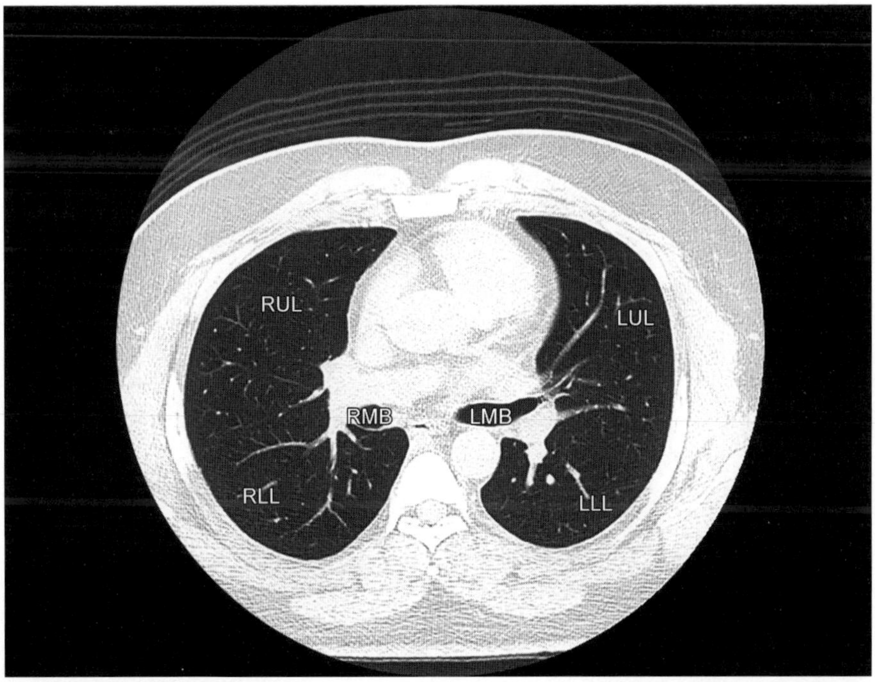

Fig. 10D: CECT axial: Lung window. (LMB: Left main bronchus; RMB: Right main bronchus; RUL: Right upper lobe; LUL: Left upper lobe; RLL: Right lower lobe; LLL: Left lower lobe)

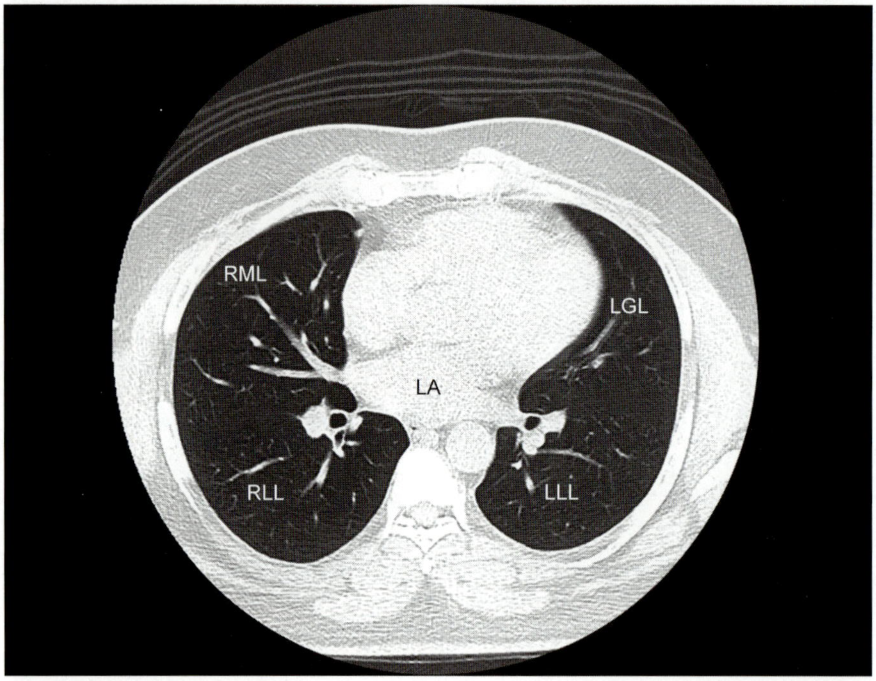

Fig. 10E: CECT axial: Lung window. (LA: Left atrium; LGL: Lingula; LLL: Left lower lobe; RLL: Right lower lobe; RML: Right middle lobe)

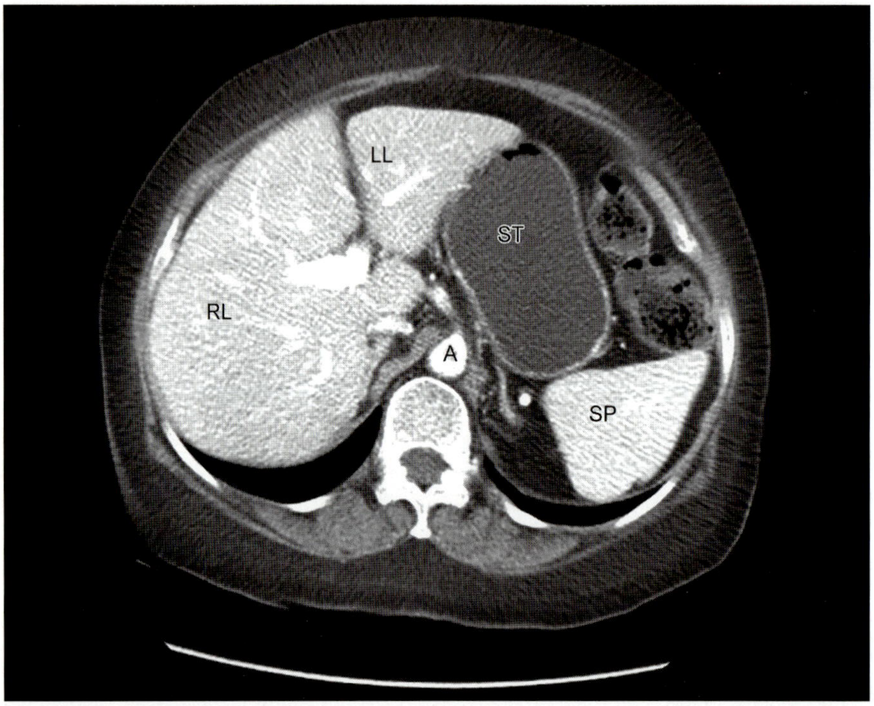

Fig. 10F: CECT upper abdomen. (A: Aorta; LL: Left lobe of liver; RL: Right lobe of liver; SP: Spleen; ST: Stomach)

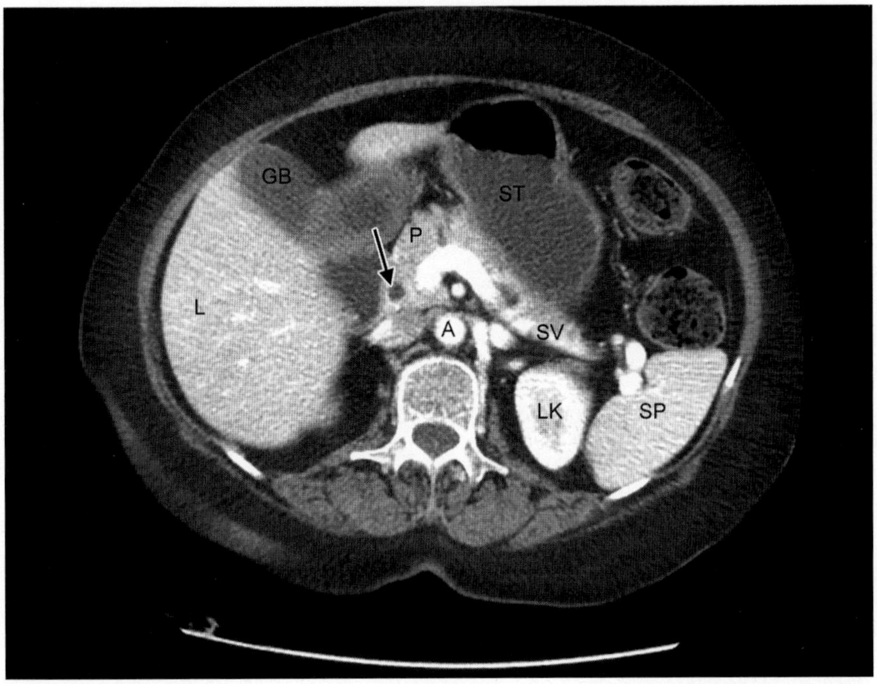

Fig. 10G: CECT upper abdomen. [A: Aorta; GB: Gallbladder; L: Liver; LK: Left kidney; P: Pancreas; SP: Spleen; ST: Stomach (black arrow); SV: Splenic vein]

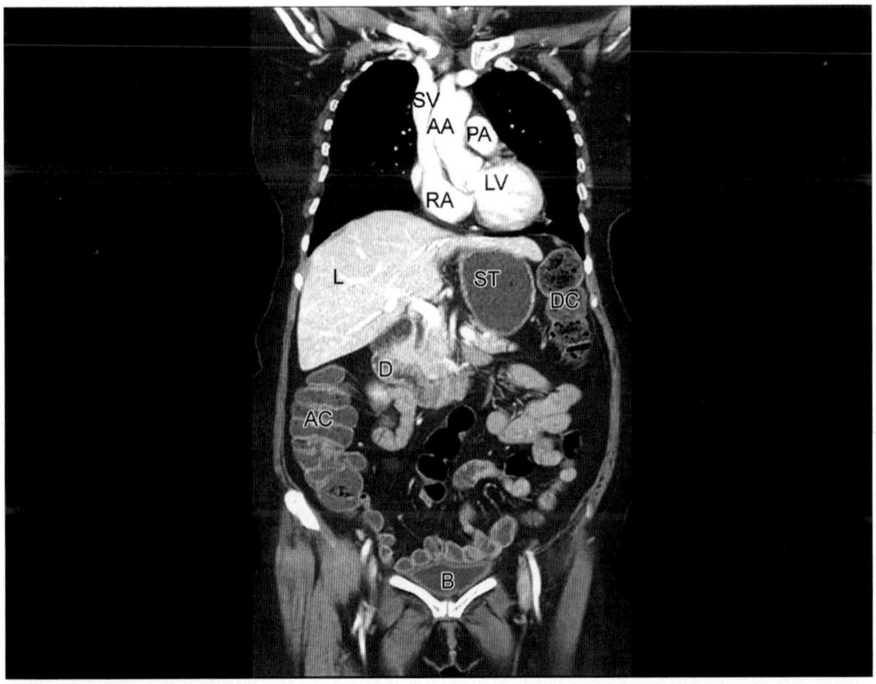

Fig. 10H: CCT abdomen—coronal image. (SV: Superior vena cava; AA: Ascending aorta; PA: Pulmonary artery; RA: Right atrium; LV: Left ventricular; L: Liver; ST: Stomach; DC: Descending colon; D: Duodenum; AC: Ascending colon; B: Urinary bladder)

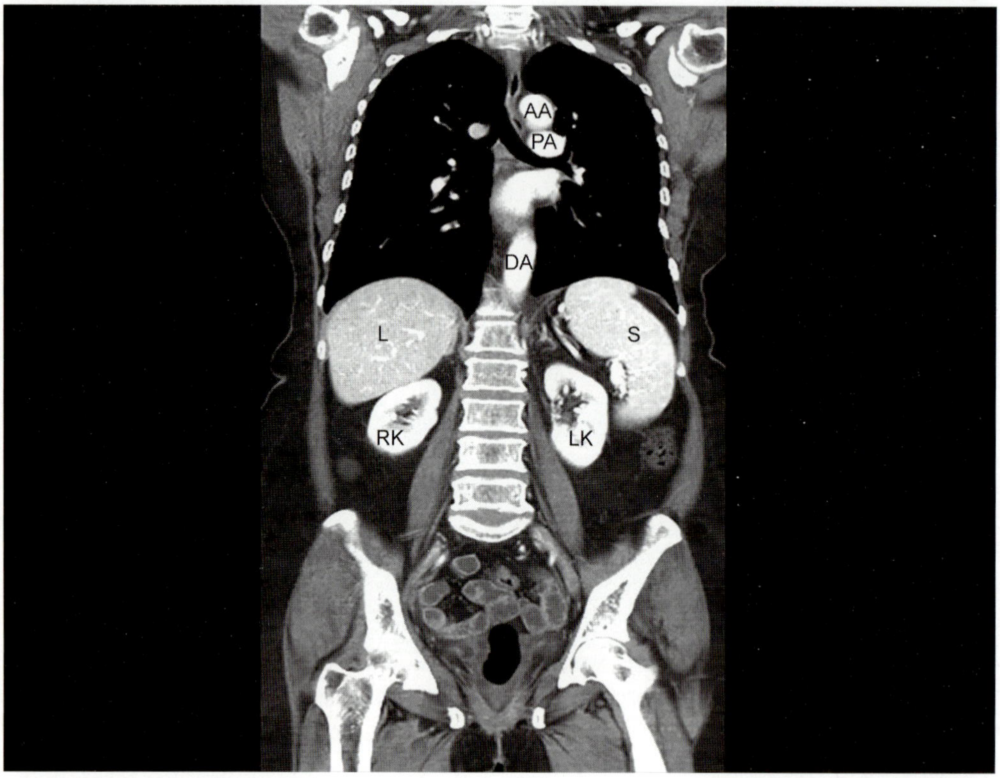

Fig. 10I: CECT coronal reformats at two levels. (AA: Ascending aorta; PA: Pulmonary artery; DA: Descending aorta; S: Spleen; LK: Left kidney; L: Liver; RK: Right kidney)

CECT: LUNG WINDOWS (FIG. 11)

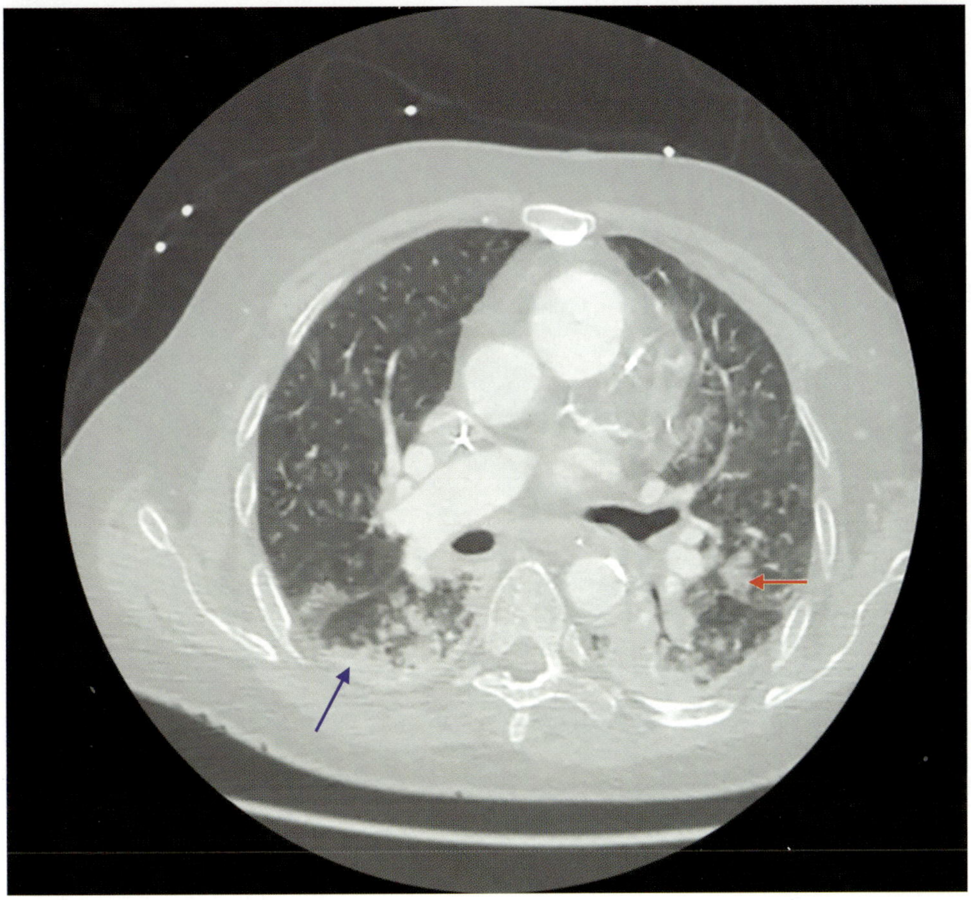

Fig. 11: CECT: Lung windows.

- *Blue arrow*: Basal patchy consolidations.
- *Red arrow*: Peribronchial nodular opacities.

CT CHEST (FIG. 12)

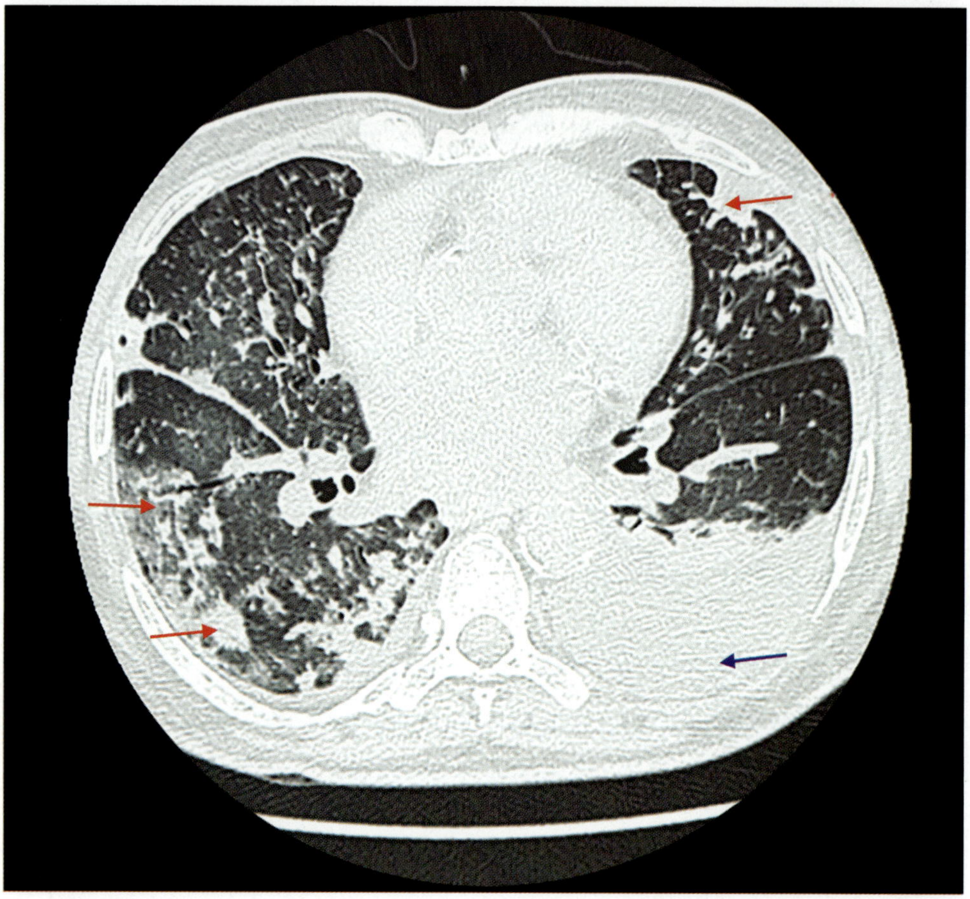

Fig. 12: CT chest.

- *Red arrows*: Bilateral patchy consolidations.
- *Blue arrow*: Left pleural effusion.

CECT CHEST: LYMPHOMA WITH MUCORMYCOSIS (FIGS. 13A AND B)

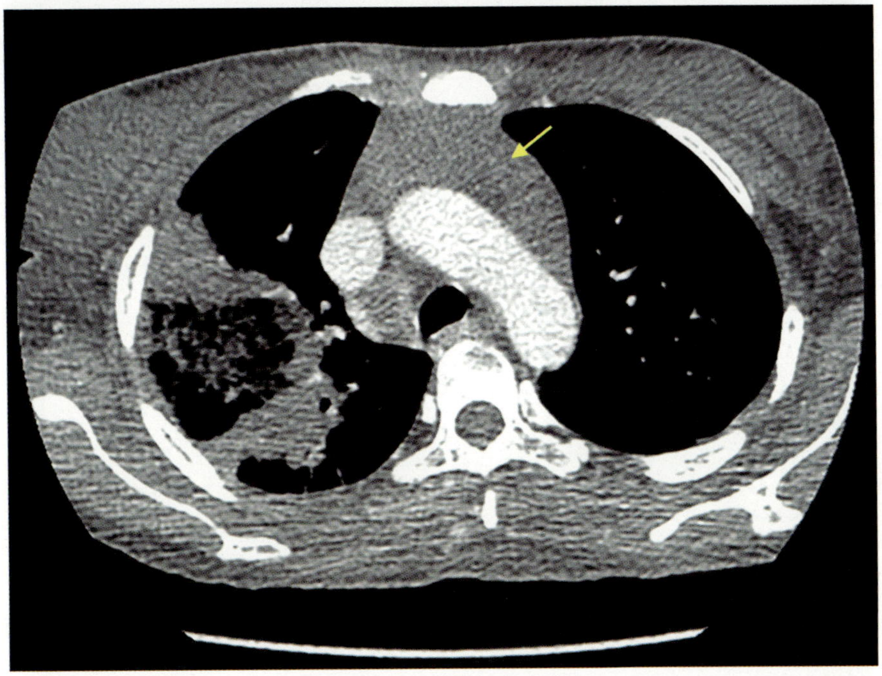

Fig. 13A: Mediastinal window.

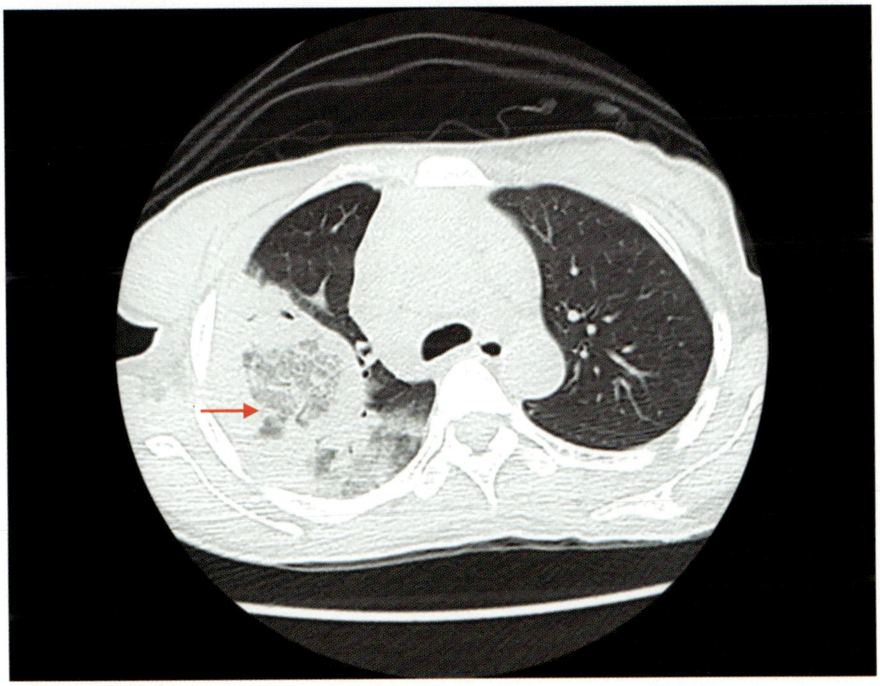

Fig. 13B: Lung window.

- *Mediastinal window*: Soft tissue in the anterior mediastinum (yellow arrow) (Fig. 13A).
- *Lung window*: Consolidation with reverse halo sign (central ground-glass opacity surrounded by consolidation) in right upper lobe (Fig. 13B). Red arrow shows anterior mediastinal soft tissue.

CECT CHEST (FIG. 14)

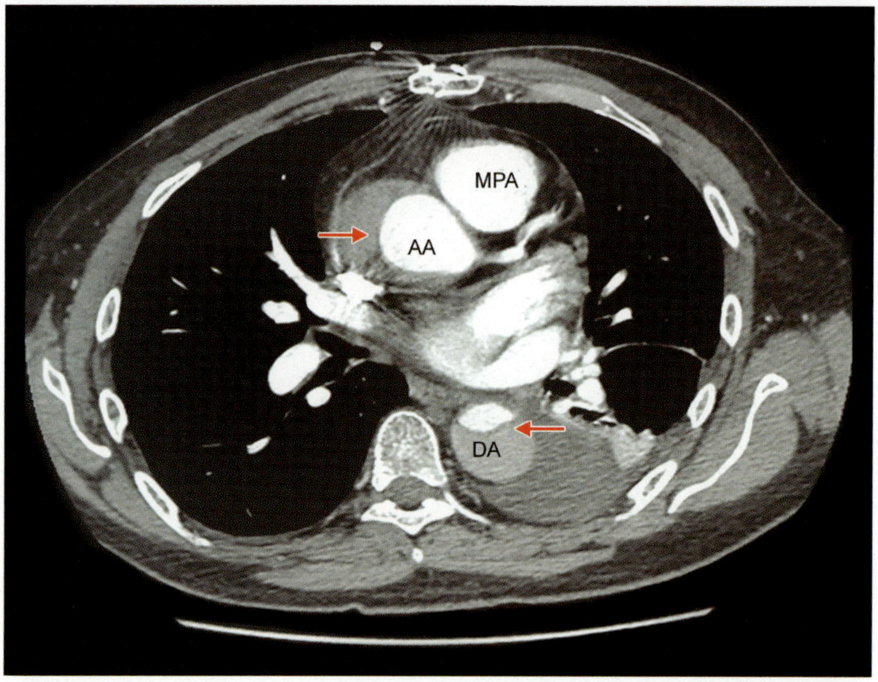

Fig. 14: CECT chest. (AA: Ascending aorta; MPA: Main pulmonary artery; DA: Descending aorta)

- Dissection flap suggestive of aortic dissection.

PULMONARY EDEMA (FIG. 15)

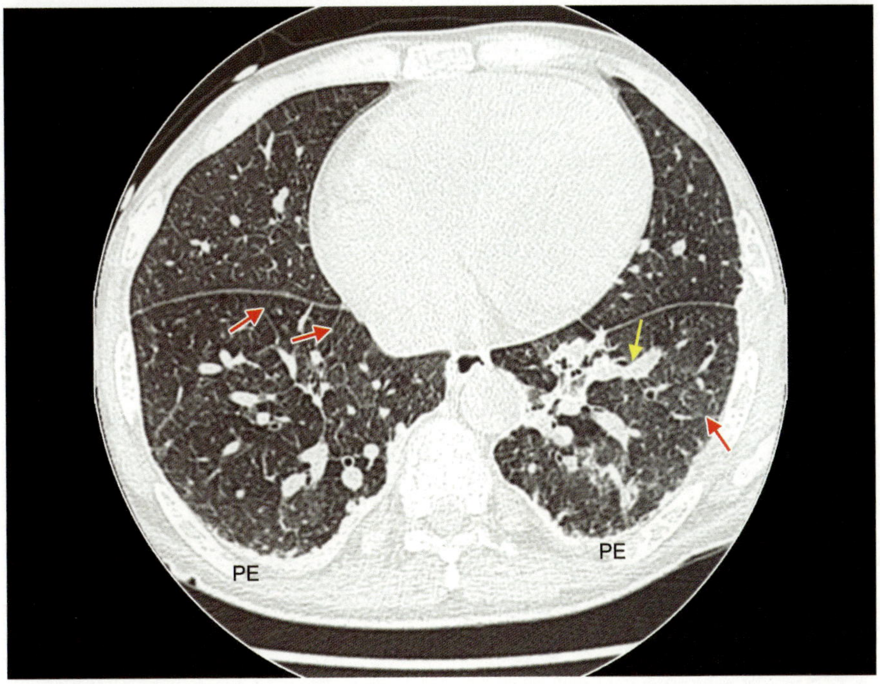

Fig. 15: Pulmonary edema (PE).

- *CT*: Lung window
- *Red arrows*: Smooth septal lines
- *Yellow arrow*: Peribronchial thickening.

CT CHEST: MEDIASTINAL AND LUNG WINDOW (FIGS. 16A AND B)

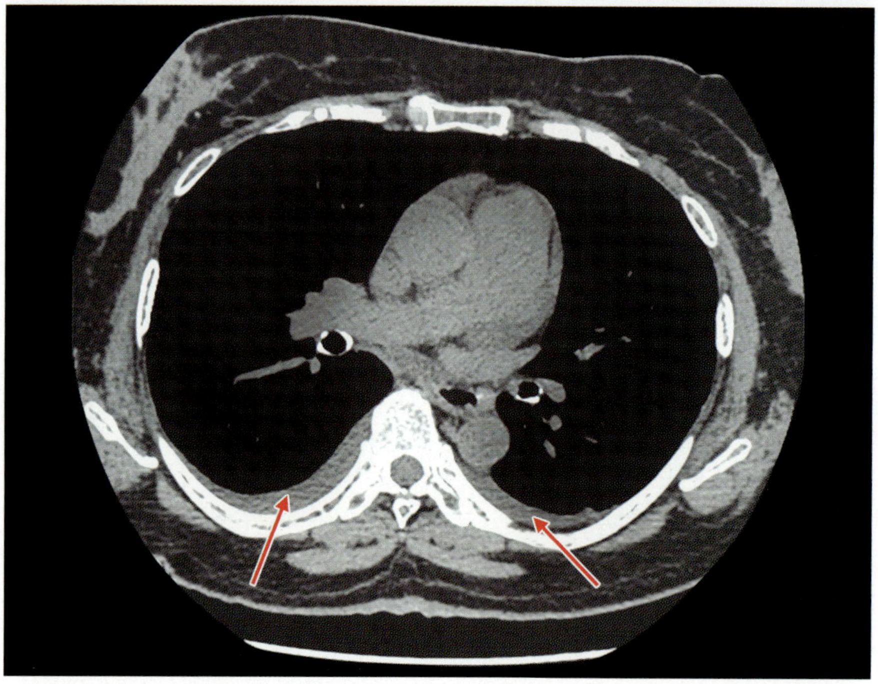

Fig. 16A: Plain CT chest: Mediastinal window.

- Bilateral patchy ground-glass opacities in the lower lobes, along with centriacinar nodular areas, more marked on the right.
- Bilateral mild pleural effusion.

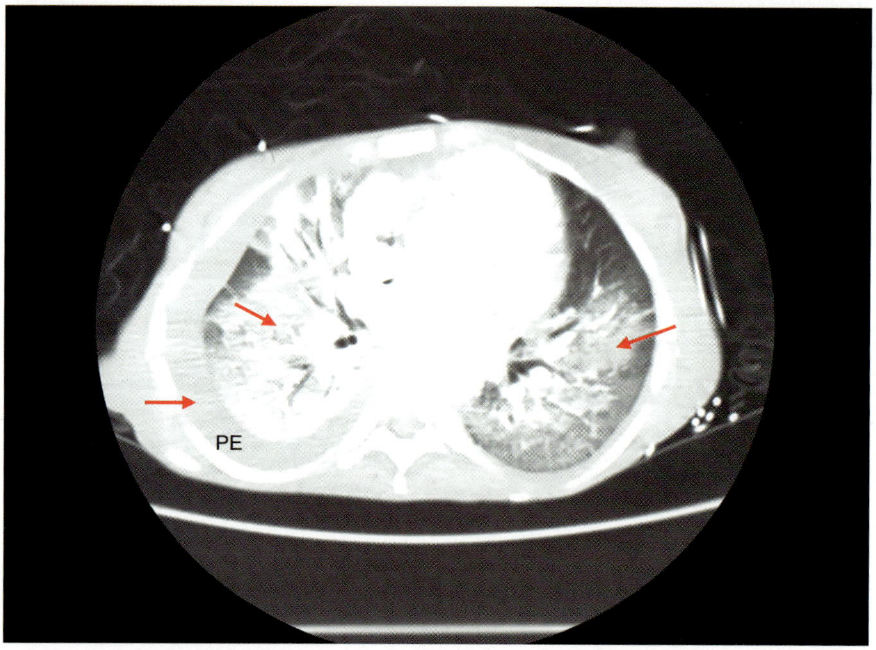

Fig. 16B: CT chest: Lung window. (PE: Pulmonary edema)

CT PULMONARY ANGIOGRAPHY (FIG. 17)

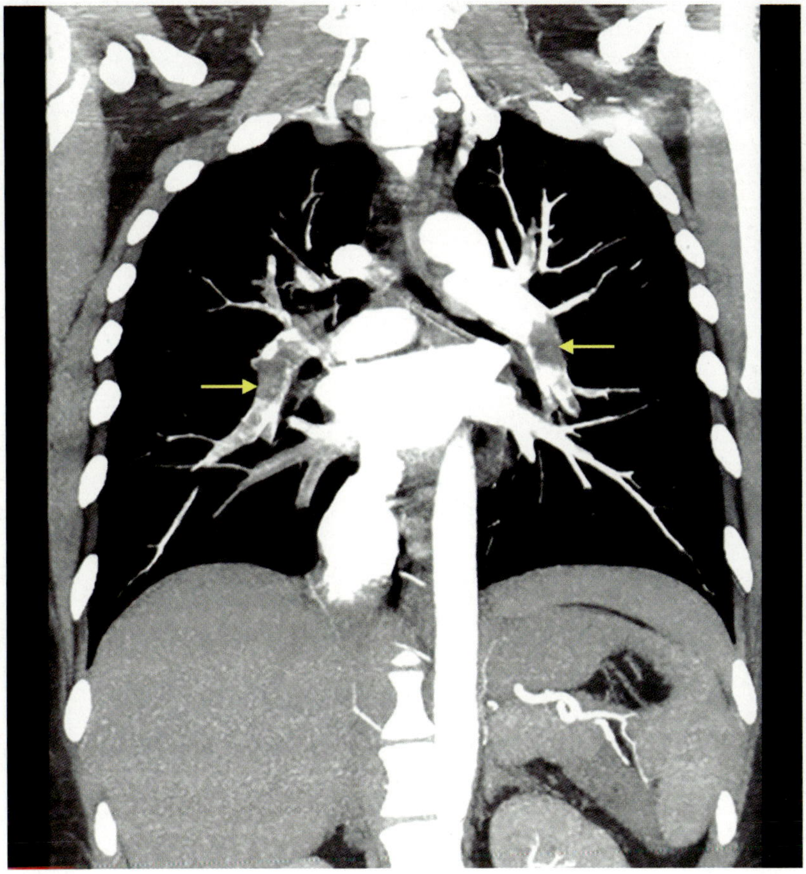

Fig. 17: CT pulmonary angiography: Coronal MIP (maximum intensity projection) reformation.

- Focal thrombus within the distal right pulmonary artery extending into the segmental branches of all the lobes.
- Thrombosis of the left upper lobar branches and inferior division of the left pulmonary artery extending into the segmental branches.

VARICEAL BLEEDING CECT (FIG. 18)

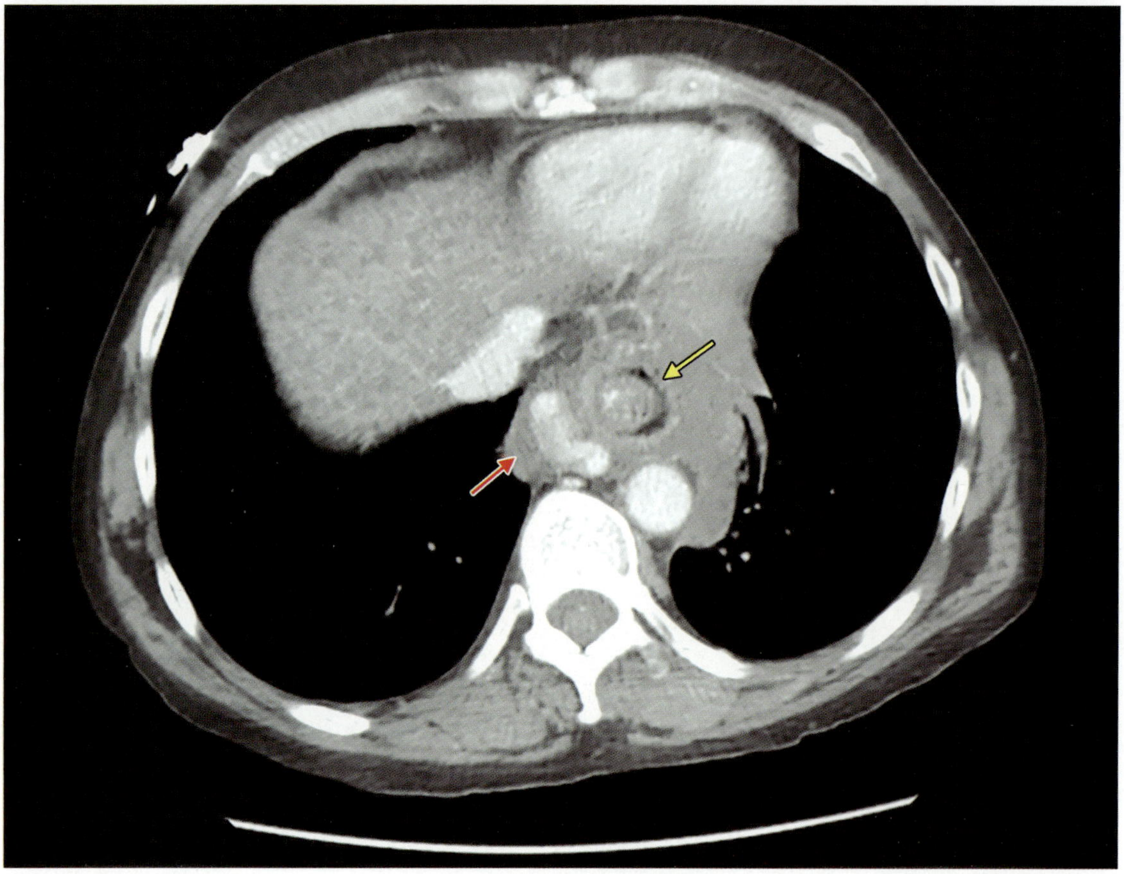

Fig. 18: Variceal bleeding CECT.

- *Red arrow*: Esophageal varices
- *Yellow arrow*: Esophagus with surrounding collection/hematoma.

ABDOMINAL WALL ABSCESS (FIG. 19)

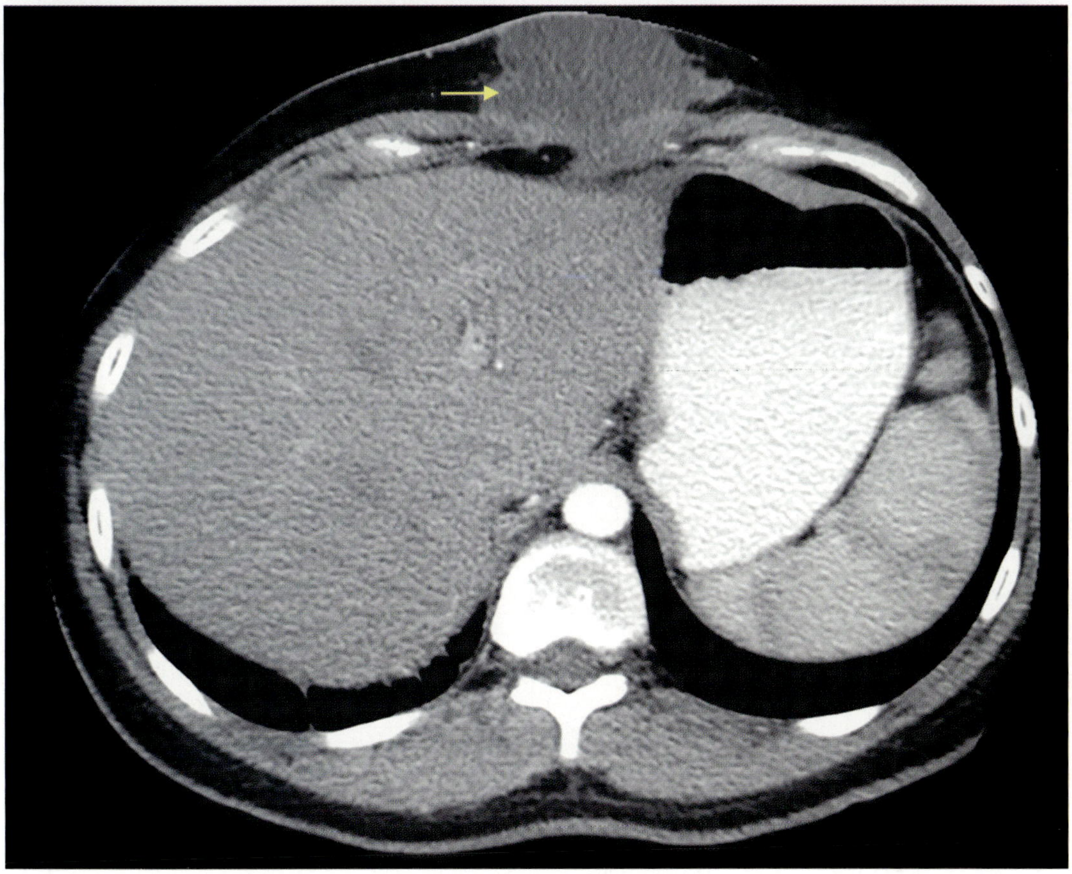

Fig. 19: Abdominal wall abscess.

- CECT abdomen at the level of aortic hiatus.
- *Yellow arrow*: Peripherally enhancing collection in anterior abdominal wall.

CECT ABDOMEN (FIG. 20)

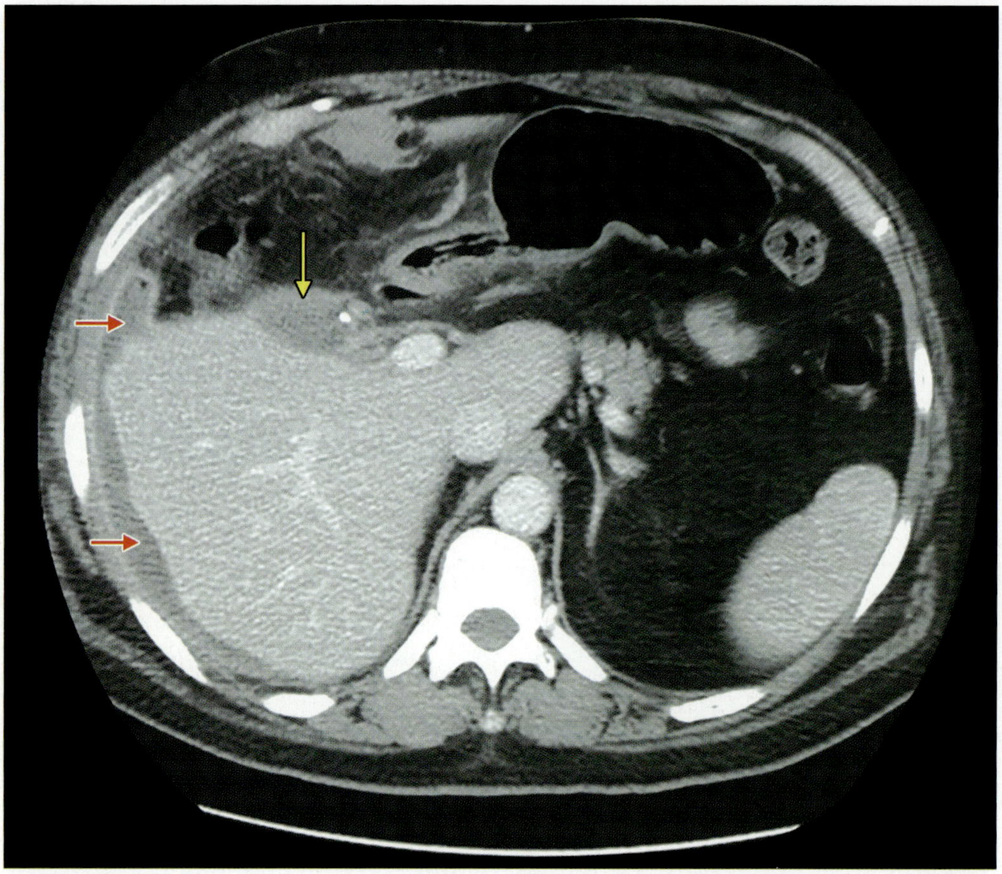

Fig. 20: CECT abdomen: Biliary leak following cholecystectomy.

- *Yellow arrow*: Fluid in gallbladder (GB) fossa.
- *Red arrows*: Biliary ascites, with enhancing peritoneum.

CECT ABDOMEN: ENTEROCUTANEOUS FISTULA (FIG. 21)

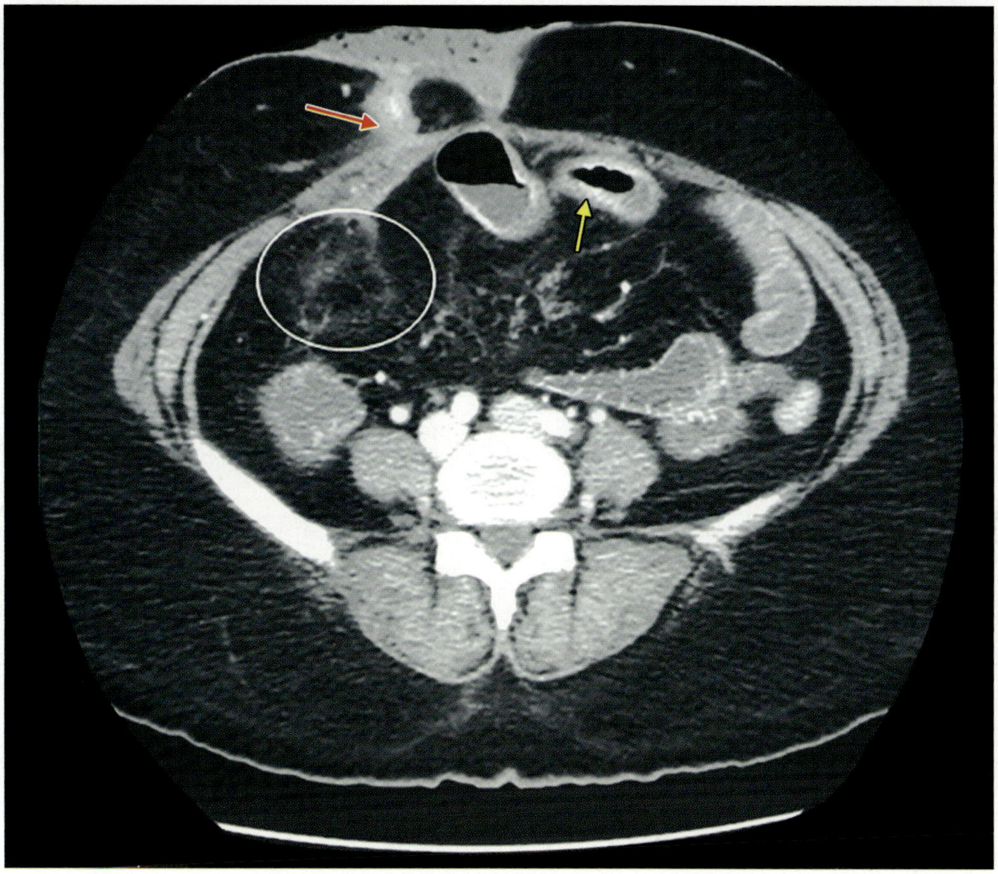

Fig. 21: CECT abdomen: Enterocutaneous fistula.

- *Red arrow*: Ileal loop.
- *Yellow arrow*: Thickened.
- *Circle*: Fat stranding in circle.

CECT ABDOMEN: INTESTINAL PERFORATION (FIG. 22)

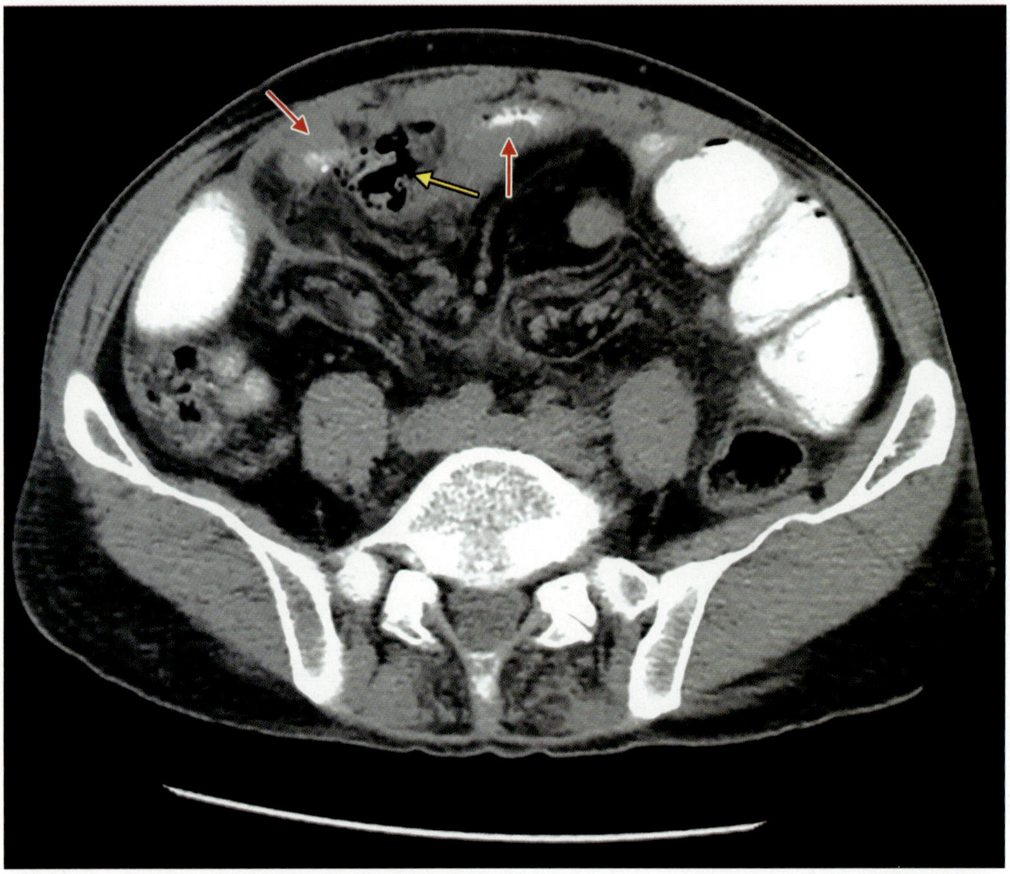

Fig. 22: CECT abdomen: Intestinal perforation.

- *Red arrows*: Thickened bowel loop.
- *Yellow arrow*: Leakage of contrast into air containing collection.

CECT ABDOMEN: LEFT PERINEPHRIC HEMATOMA (FIG. 23)

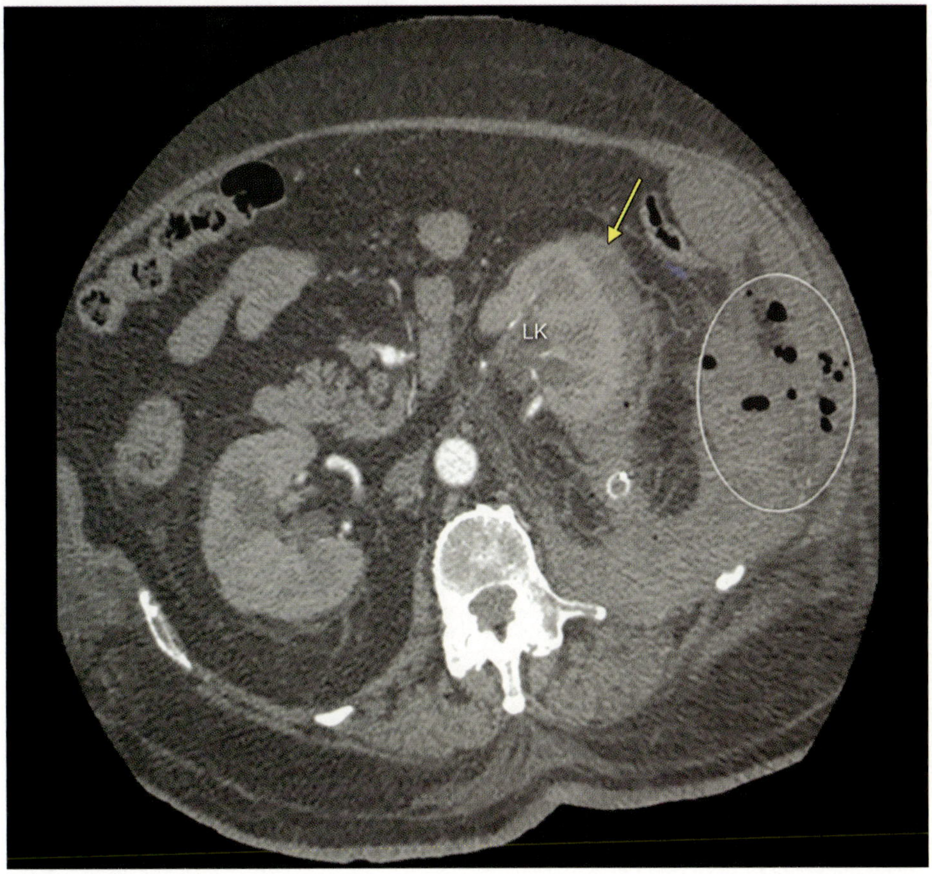

Fig. 23: CECT abdomen: Left perinephric hematoma (arrow) with retroperitoneal extension (circle). (LK: Left kidney)

CECT ABDOMEN: HYPODENSE LESION (FIG. 24)

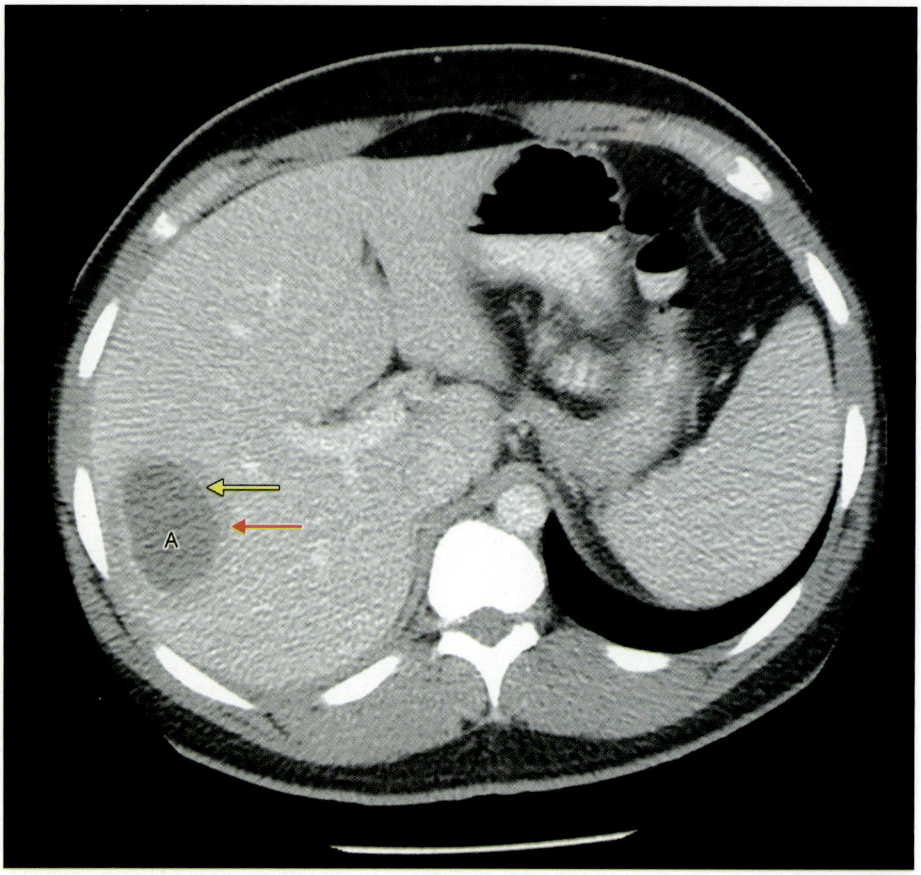

Fig. 24: CECT abdomen: Hypodense lesion (A) with enhancing wall (yellow arrow) and surrounding edema (red arrow).

CECT ABDOMEN: LIVER LACERATION (FIG. 25)

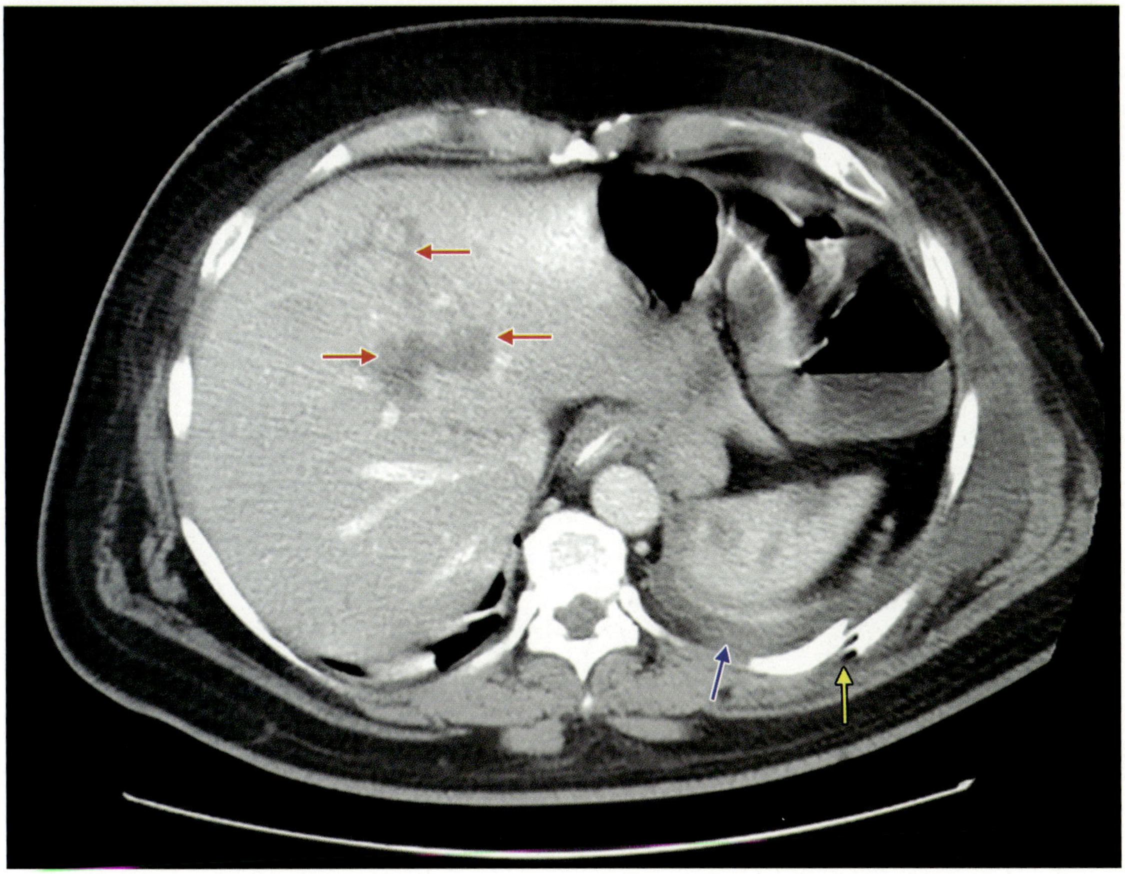

Fig. 25: CECT abdomen: Liver laceration (red arrows). Note the rib fractures (yellow arrow) and pleural effusion (blue arrow).

COLITIS (FIG. 26)

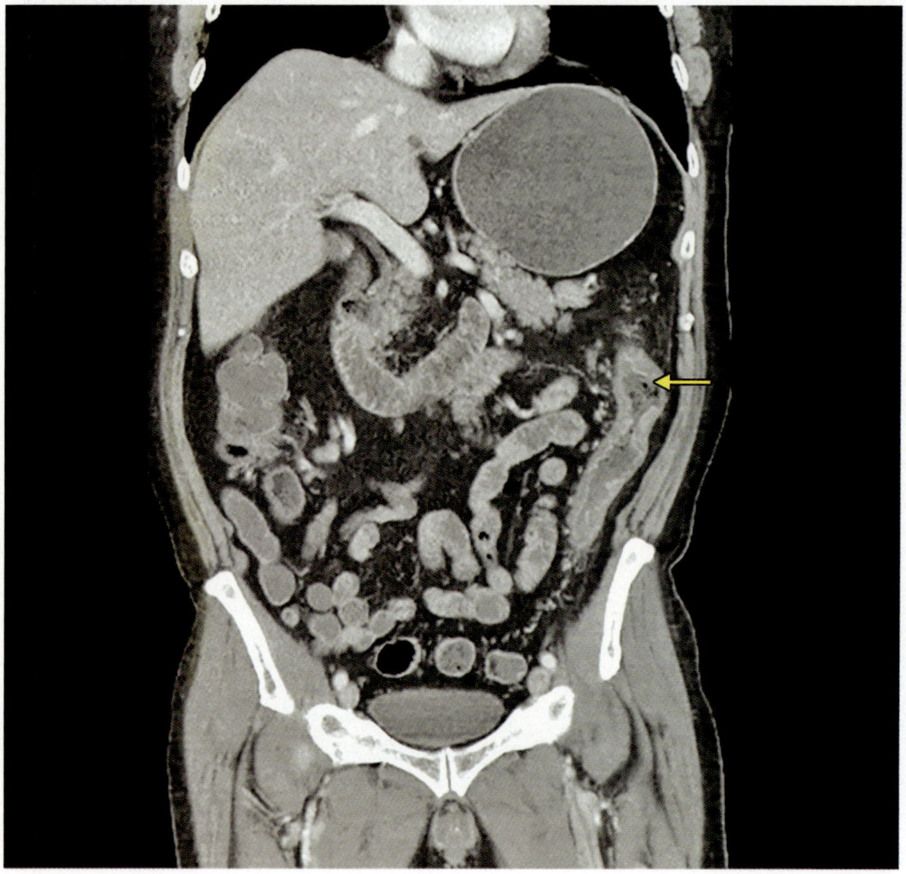

Fig. 26: Colitis.

- *CECT abdomen*: Coronal reformation.
- *Arrow*: Wall thickening of descending colon.

CECT CORONAL REFORMATION (FIG. 27)

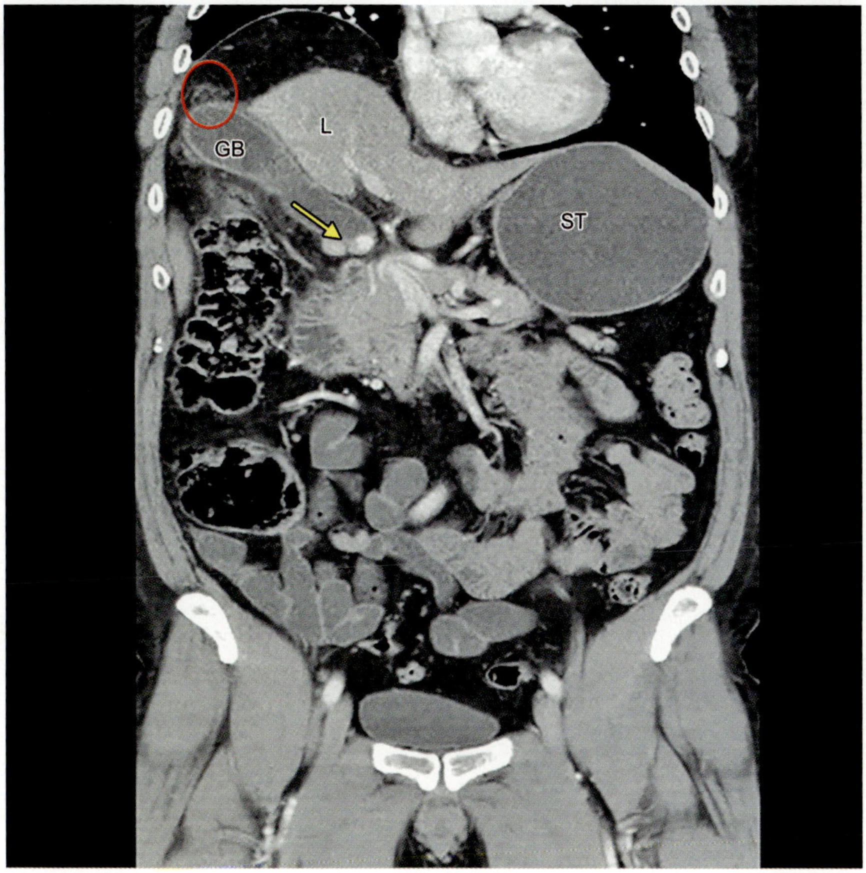

Fig. 27: CECT coronal reformation. (GB: Gallbladder; L: Liver; ST: Stomach)

- *Arrow*: Pericholecystic edema and fat stranding.
- *Circle*: Calculus in GB neck.

CECT ABDOMEN: CORONAL REFORMATION (FIG. 28)

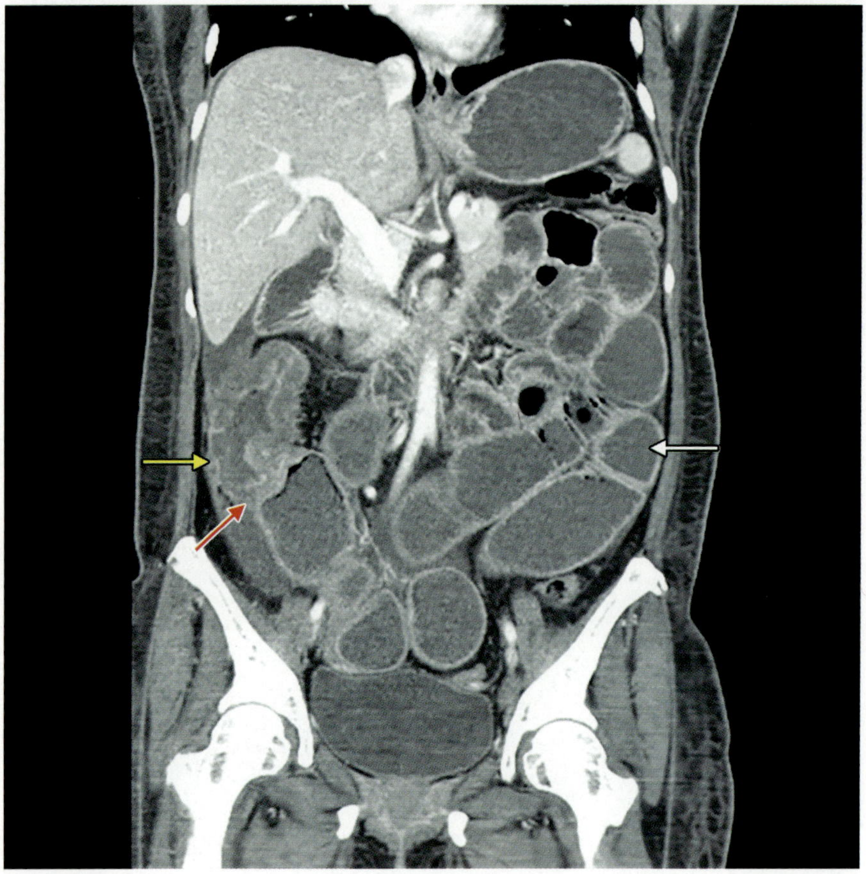

Fig. 28: CECT abdomen—coronal reformation.

- *Yellow arrow*: Thickened and pulled up cecum.
- *White arrow*: Dilated small bowel loops.
- *Red arrow*: Ileocecal (IC) junction.

OVARIAN VEIN THROMBOSIS (FIG. 29)

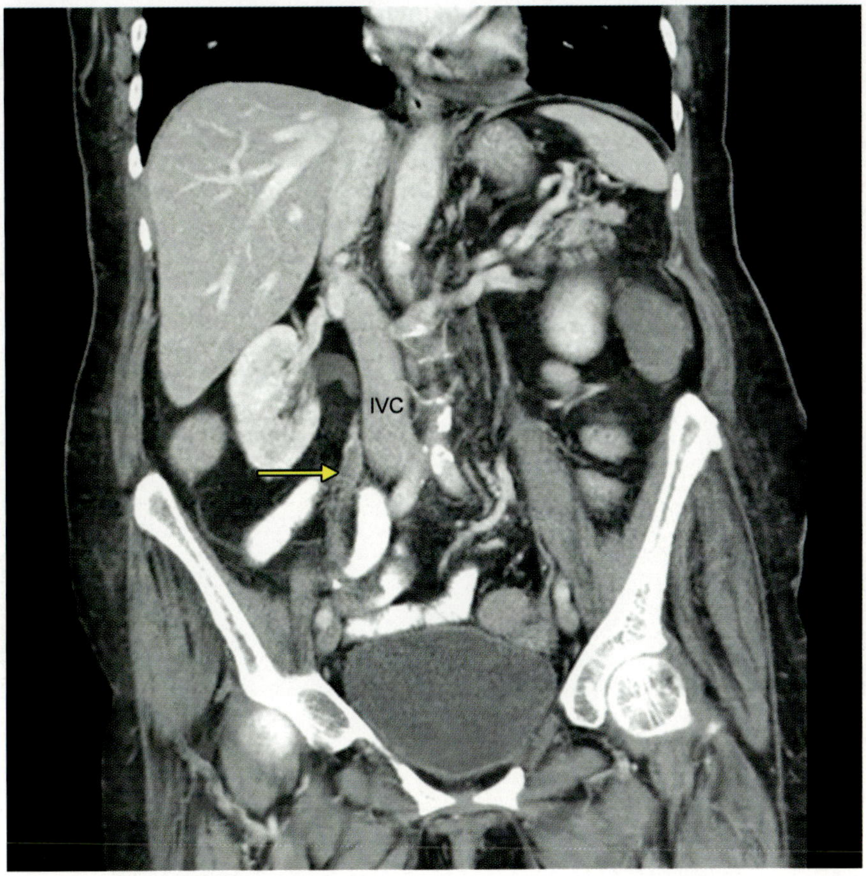

Fig. 29: Ovarian vein thrombosis. (IVC: Inferior vena cava)

- *CECT*: Coronal reformation. Dilated ovarian vein with filling defect.

CECT AXIAL AND CORONAL REFORMATION (FIGS. 30A AND B)

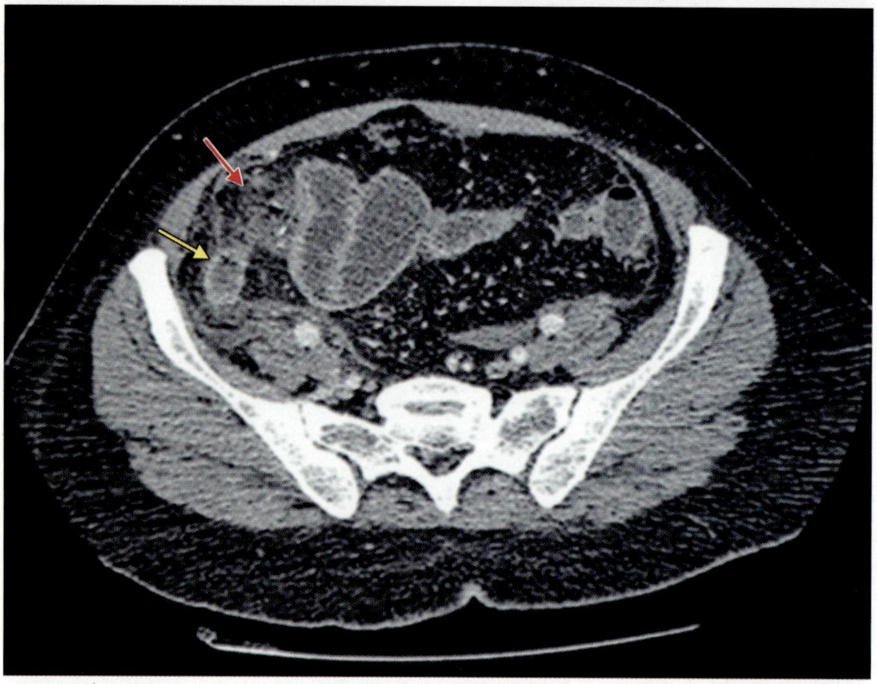

Fig. 30A: CECT axial reformation.

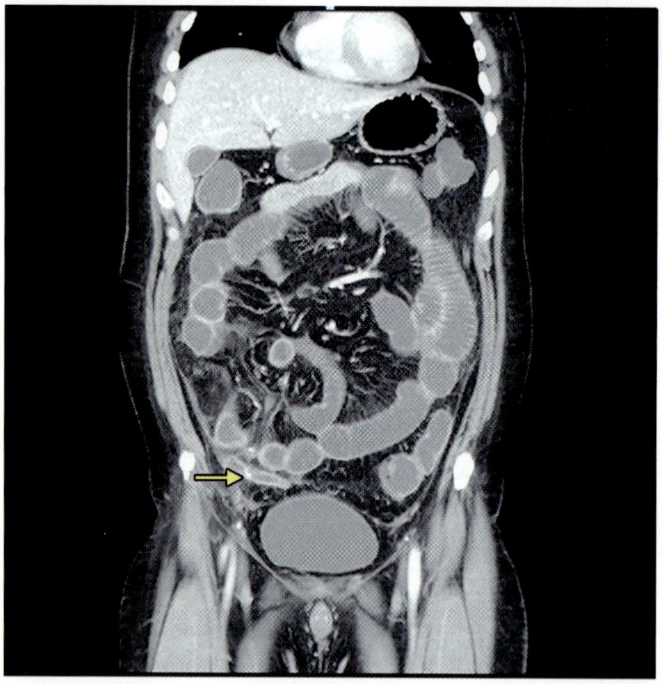

Fig. 30B: CECT coronal reformation.

- *Yellow arrows*: Appendix, containing appendicolith.
- *Red arrow*: Air filled collection, adjacent to appendix.

NECROTIZING PANCREATITIS (FIGS. 31A AND B)

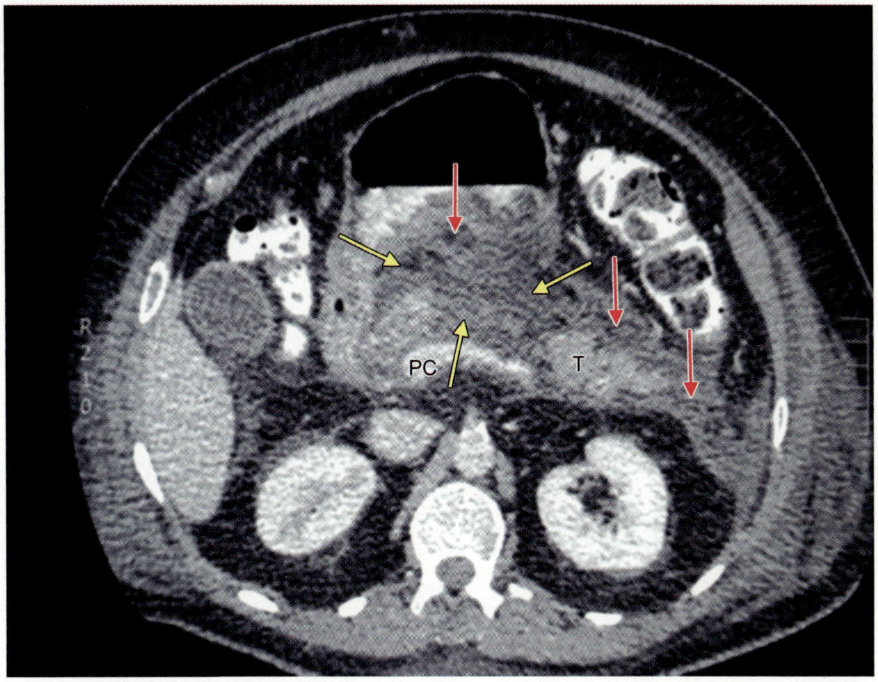

Fig. 31A: Necrotizing pancreatitis. (T: Tail of pancreas; PC: Pancreas)

- *CECT abdomen*: Most of pancreatic head and body does not enhance (yellow arrows). Pancreatic tail (T) reveals enhancement. Peripancreatic stranding and collection (red arrows).

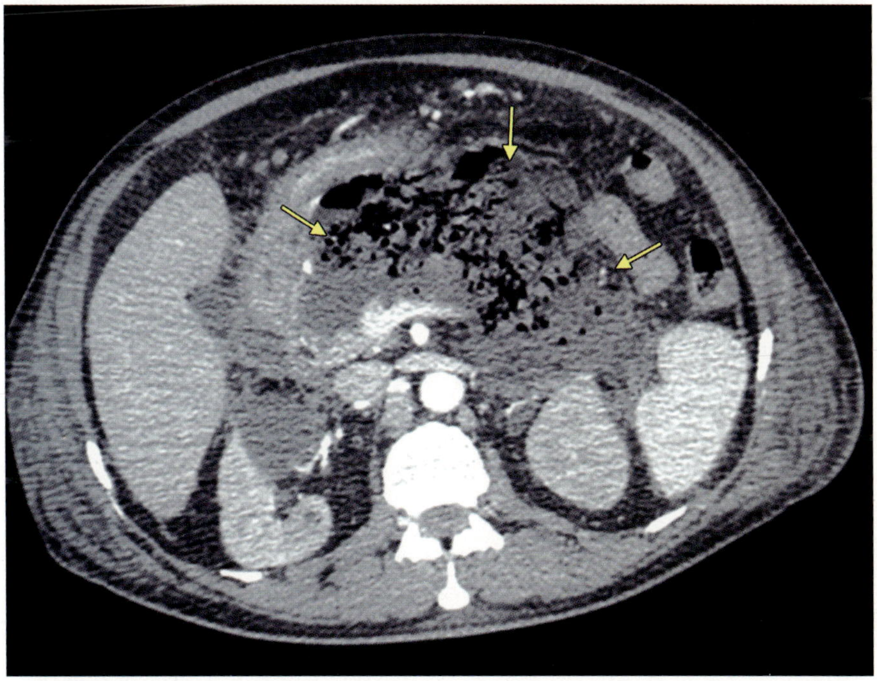

Fig. 31B: Emphysematous pancreatitis.

- *CECT abdomen*: Pancreatic/peripancreatic collection with air pockets.

SMALL BOWEL ISCHEMIA: CECT (FIG. 32)

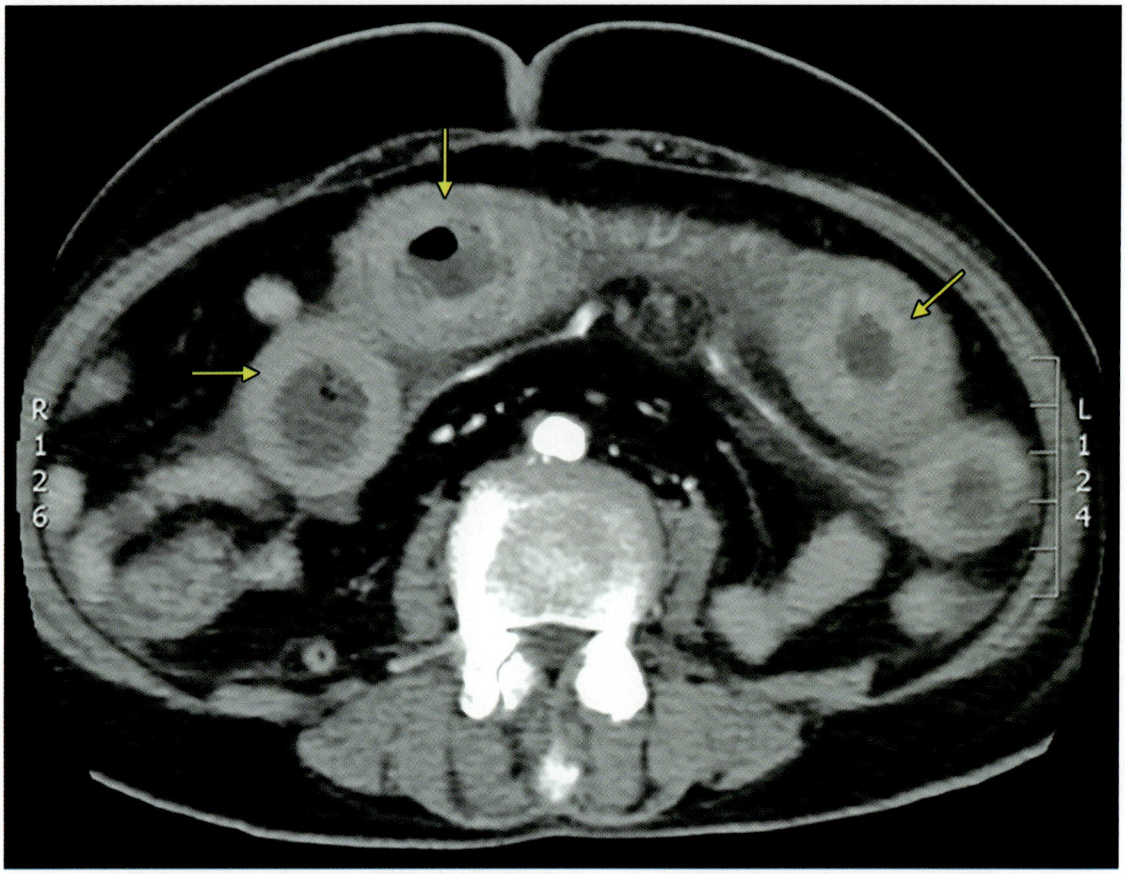

Fig. 32: Small bowel ischemia: CECT.

- *Arrows*: Thickened edematous bowel loops with "target appearance".

CECT: SPLENIC LACERATION (FIG. 33)

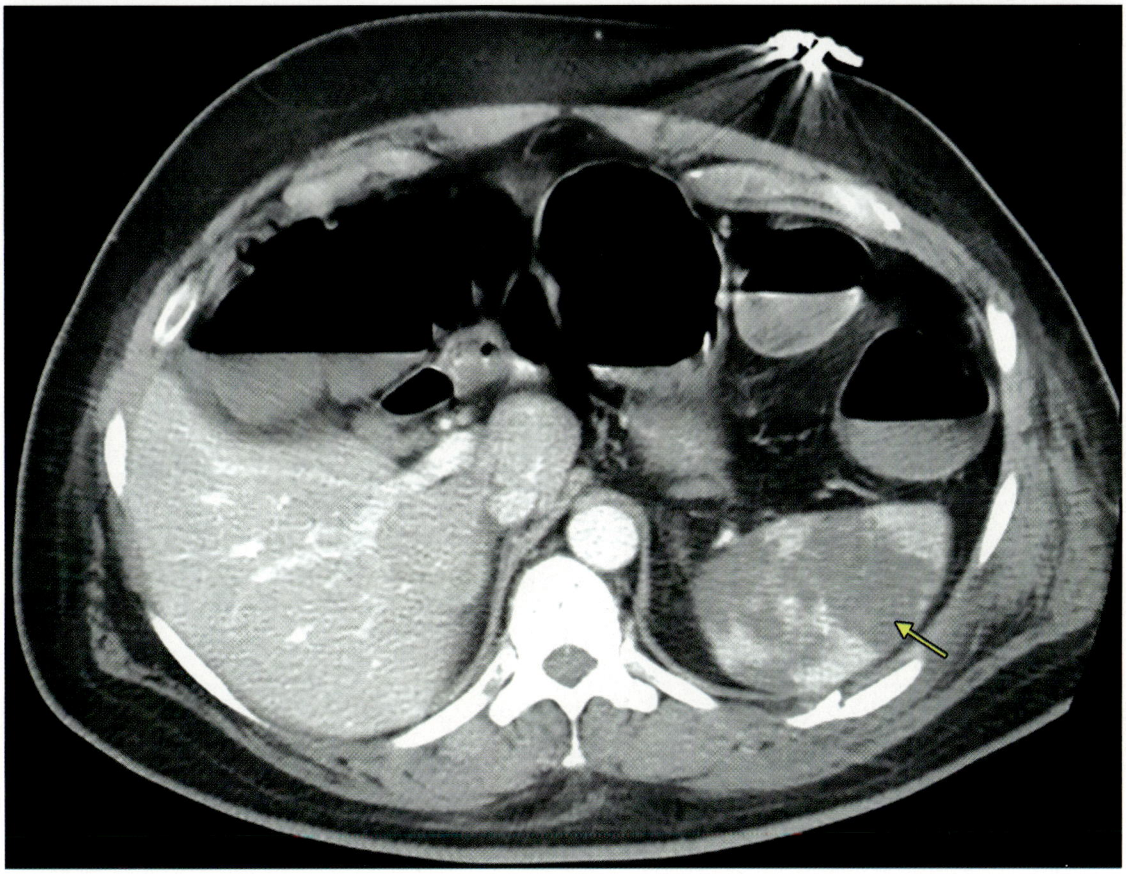

Fig. 33: CECT: Splenic laceration.

- *Arrow*: Hypodense nonenhancing areas in spleen.

CECT ABDOMEN (FIG. 34)

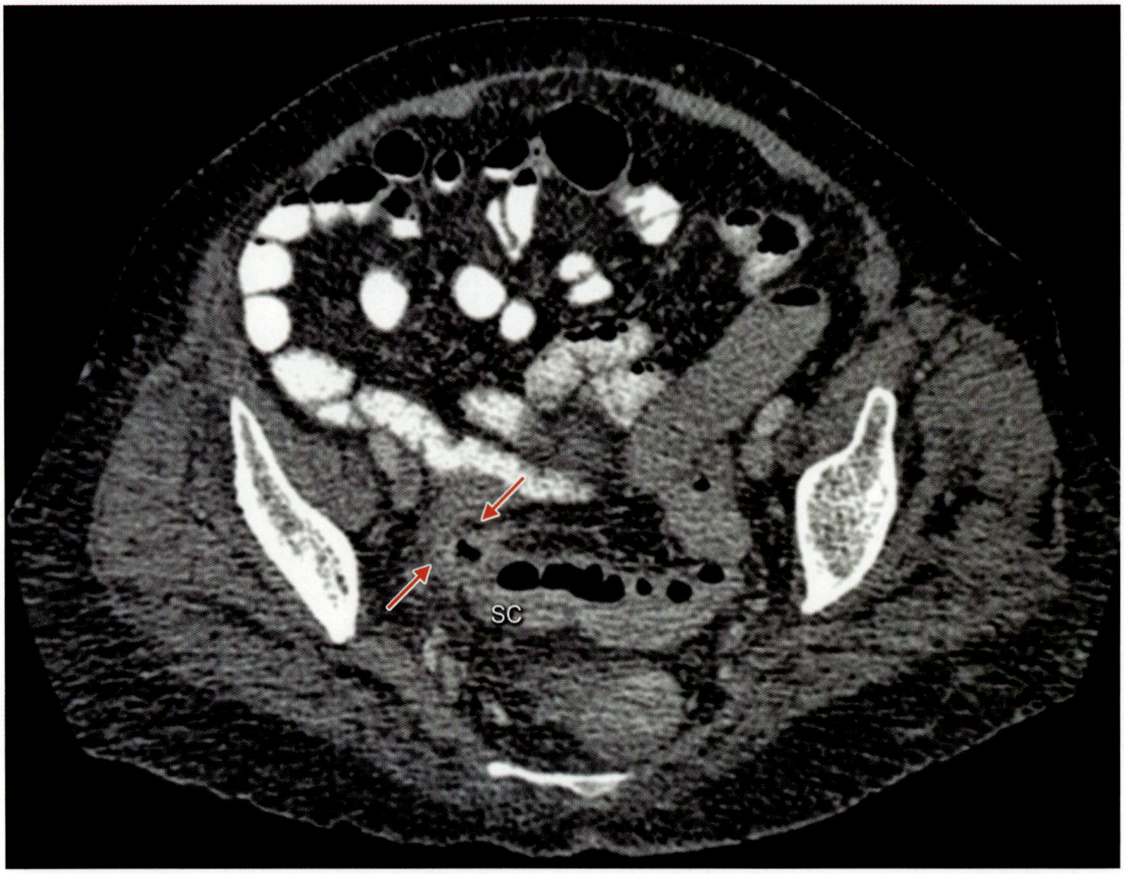

Fig. 34: CECT abdomen. (SC: Sigmoid colon)

- *Arrows*: Diverticulum with surrounding inflammation.

OGILVIE SYNDROME: COLONIC PSEUDO-OBSTRUCTION (FIG. 35)

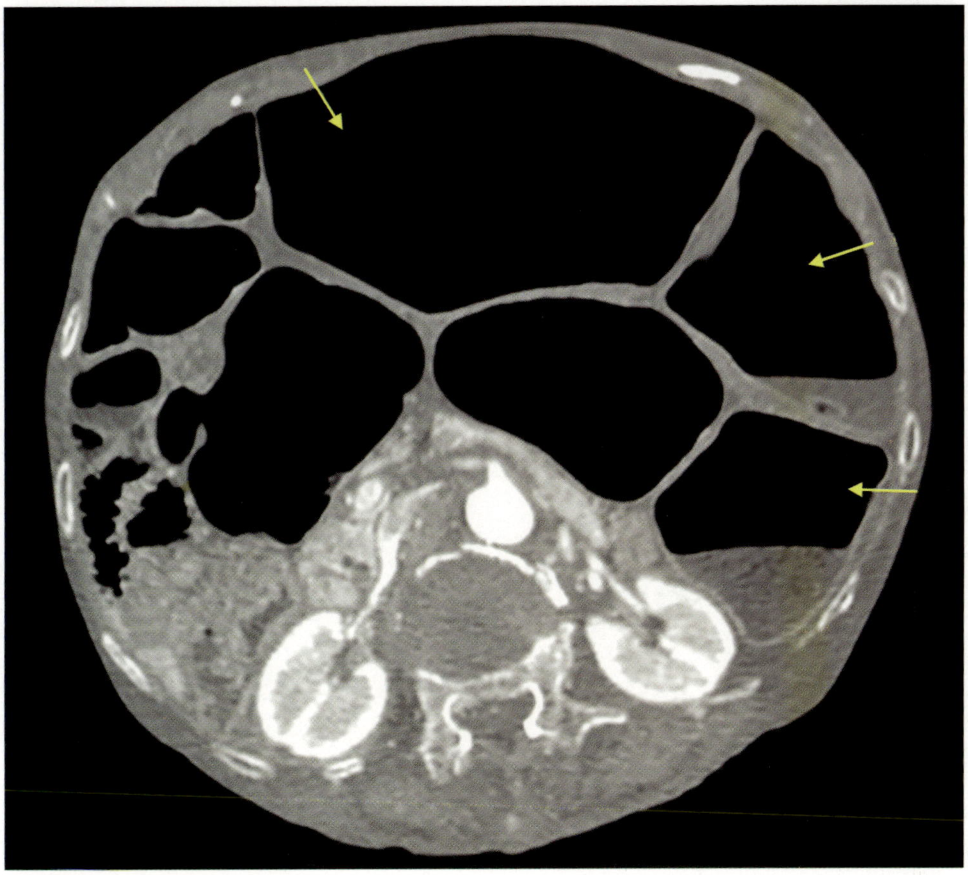

Fig. 35: Ogilvie syndrome: Colonic pseudo-obstruction. [CECT: Markedly dilated colonic loops (arrows)]

MECKEL'S DIVERTICULITIS: CECT ABDOMEN (FIG. 36)

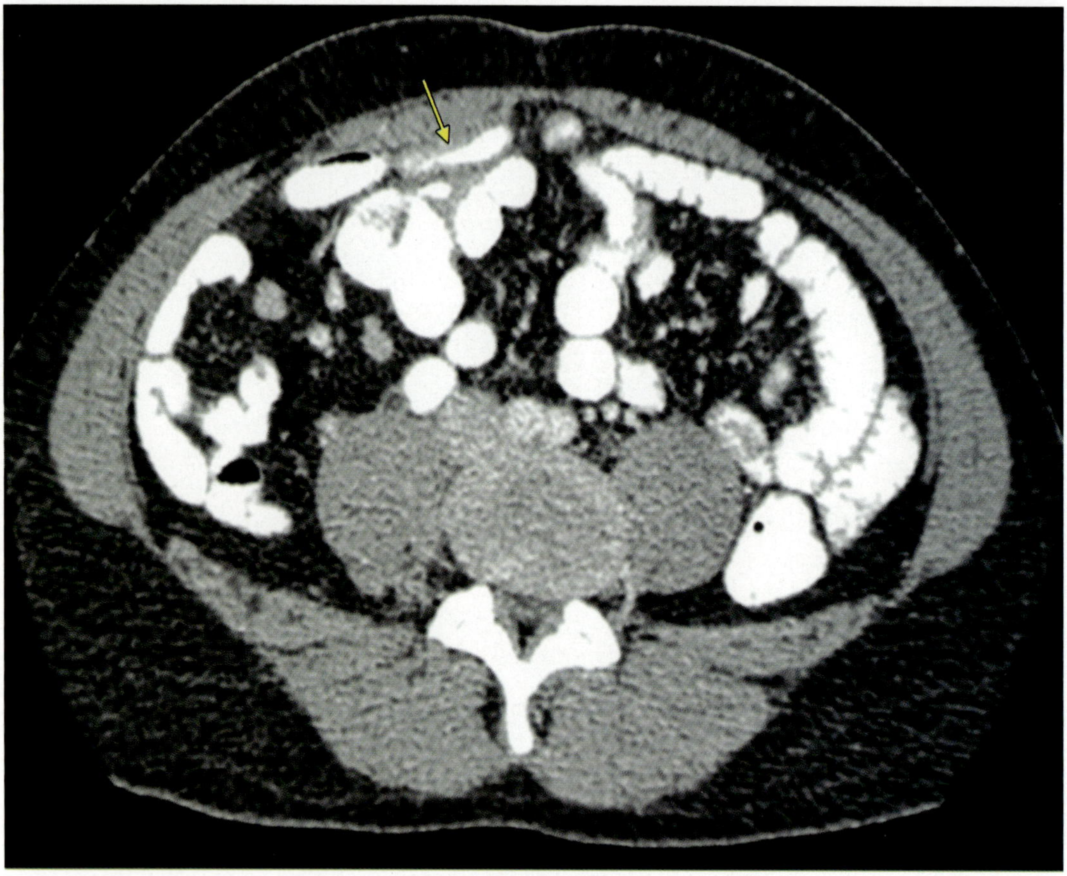

Fig. 36: Meckel's diverticulitis: CECT abdomen.

- *Arrow*: Meckel's diverticulum (arrow) with surrounding stranding.

CECT ABDOMEN SPLENIC VEIN AND SUPERIOR MESENTERIC VEIN (FIGS. 37A AND B)

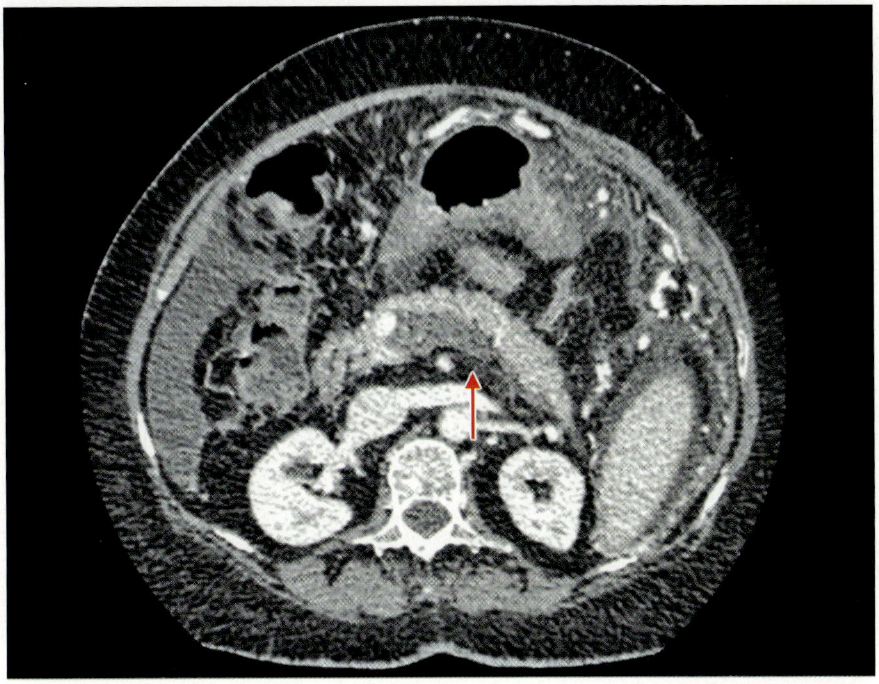

Fig. 37A: CECT abdomen—axial.

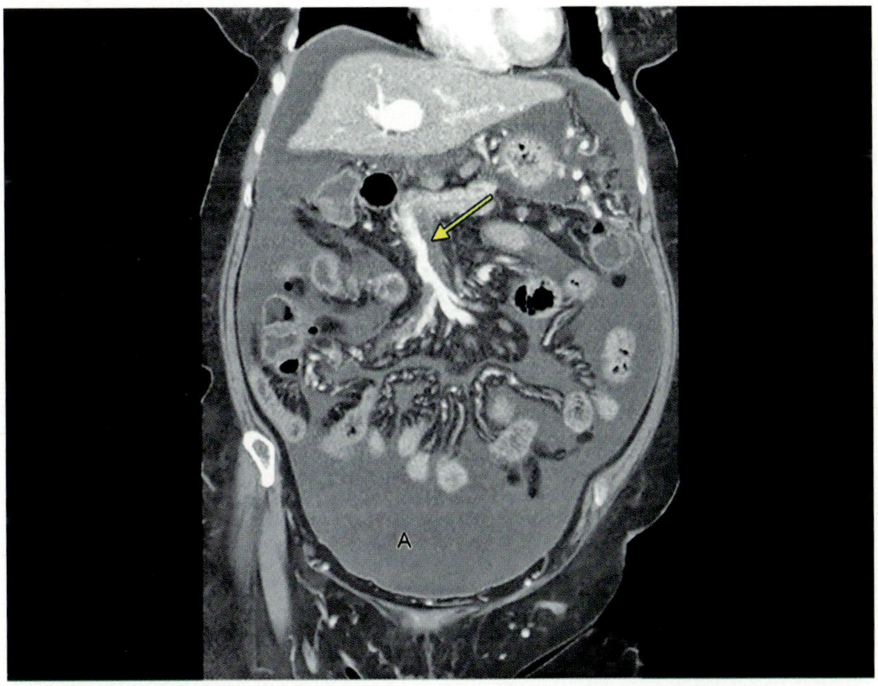

Fig. 37B: CECT abdomen—coronal reformation. (A: Ascitis)

- *Red arrow*: Splenic vein thrombosis.
- *Yellow arrow*: Thrombosis in superior mesenteric vein (SMV) and its tributaries.

NORMAL ULTRASOUND ANATOMY (FIGS. 38 TO 48)

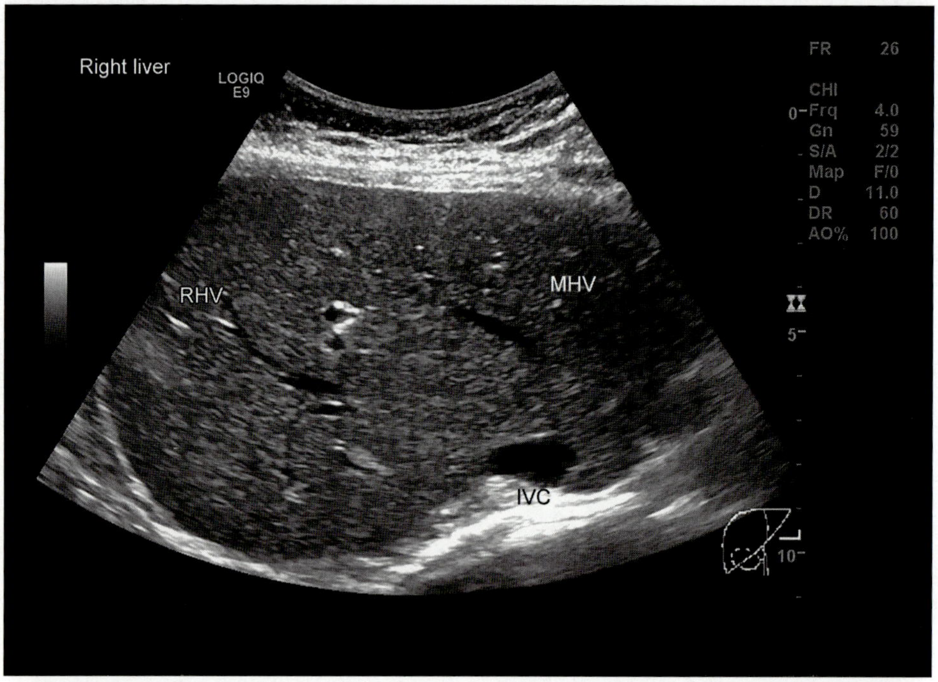

Fig. 38: Liver subcostal. (IVC: Inferior vena cava; MHV: Middle hepatic vein; RHV: Right hepatic vein)

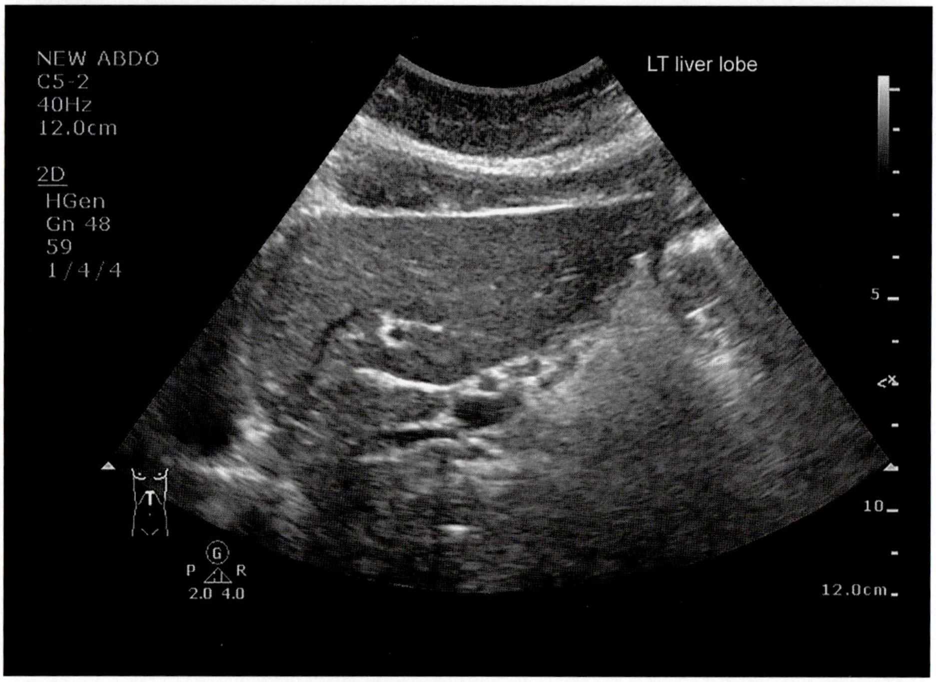

Fig. 39: Left (LT) liver lobe.

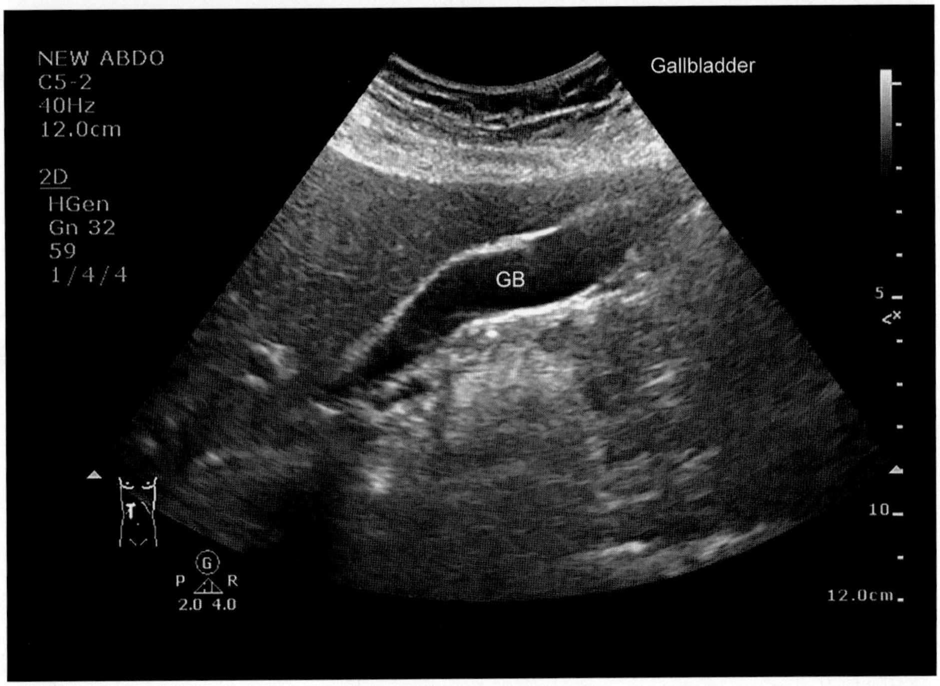

Fig. 40: Gallbladder (GB).

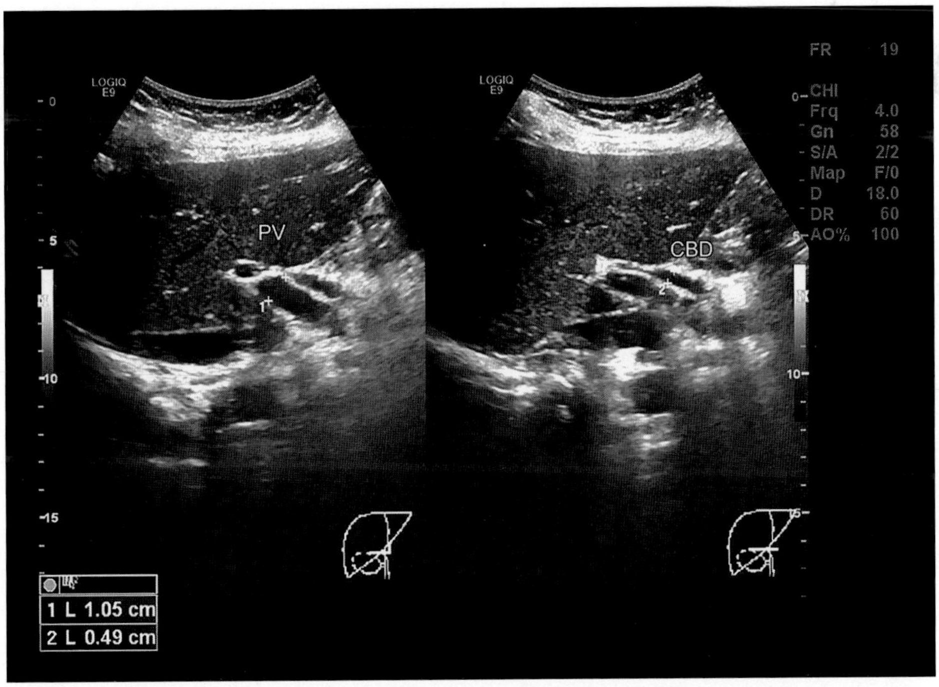

Fig. 41: Liver hilar region. (PV: Portal vein; CBD: Common bile duct)

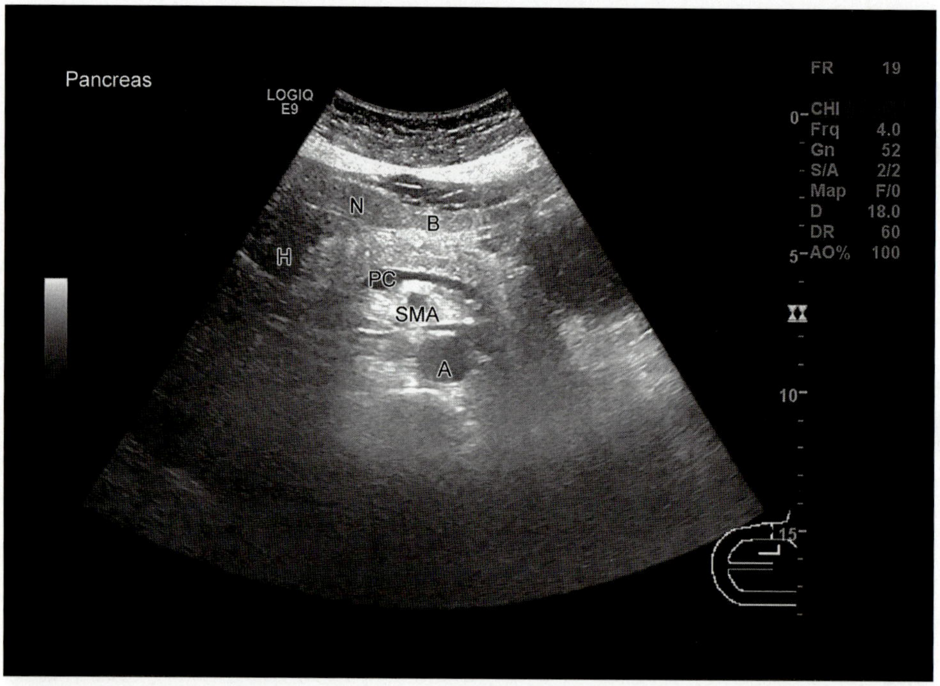

Fig. 42: Pancreas: Transverse. (A: Aorta; B: Body of pancreas; H: Head; N: Neck; PC: Portal confluence; SMA: Superior mesenteric artery).

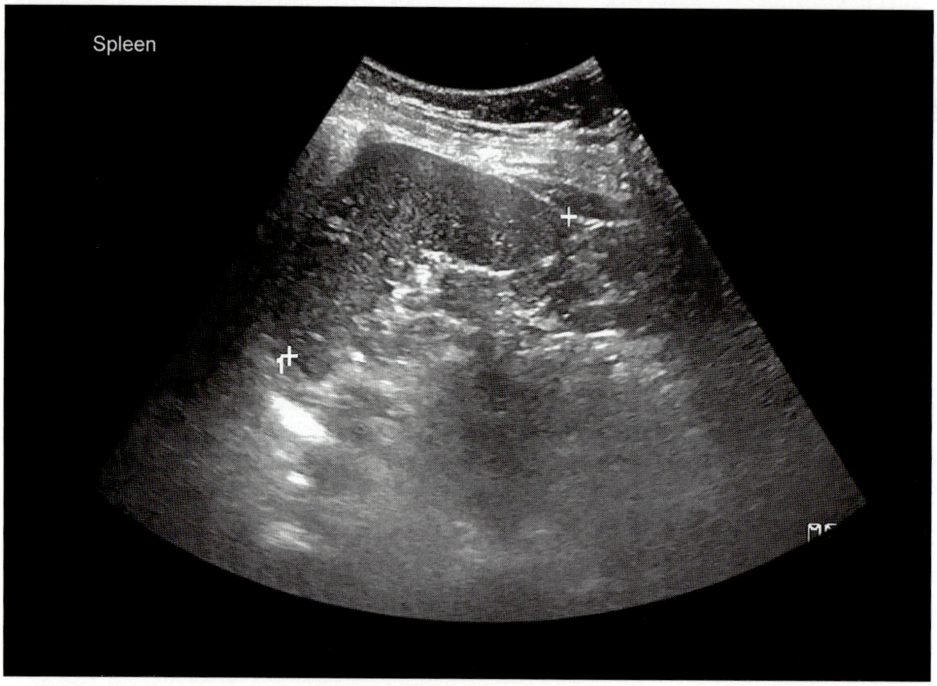

Fig. 43: Spleen (S): Long axis.

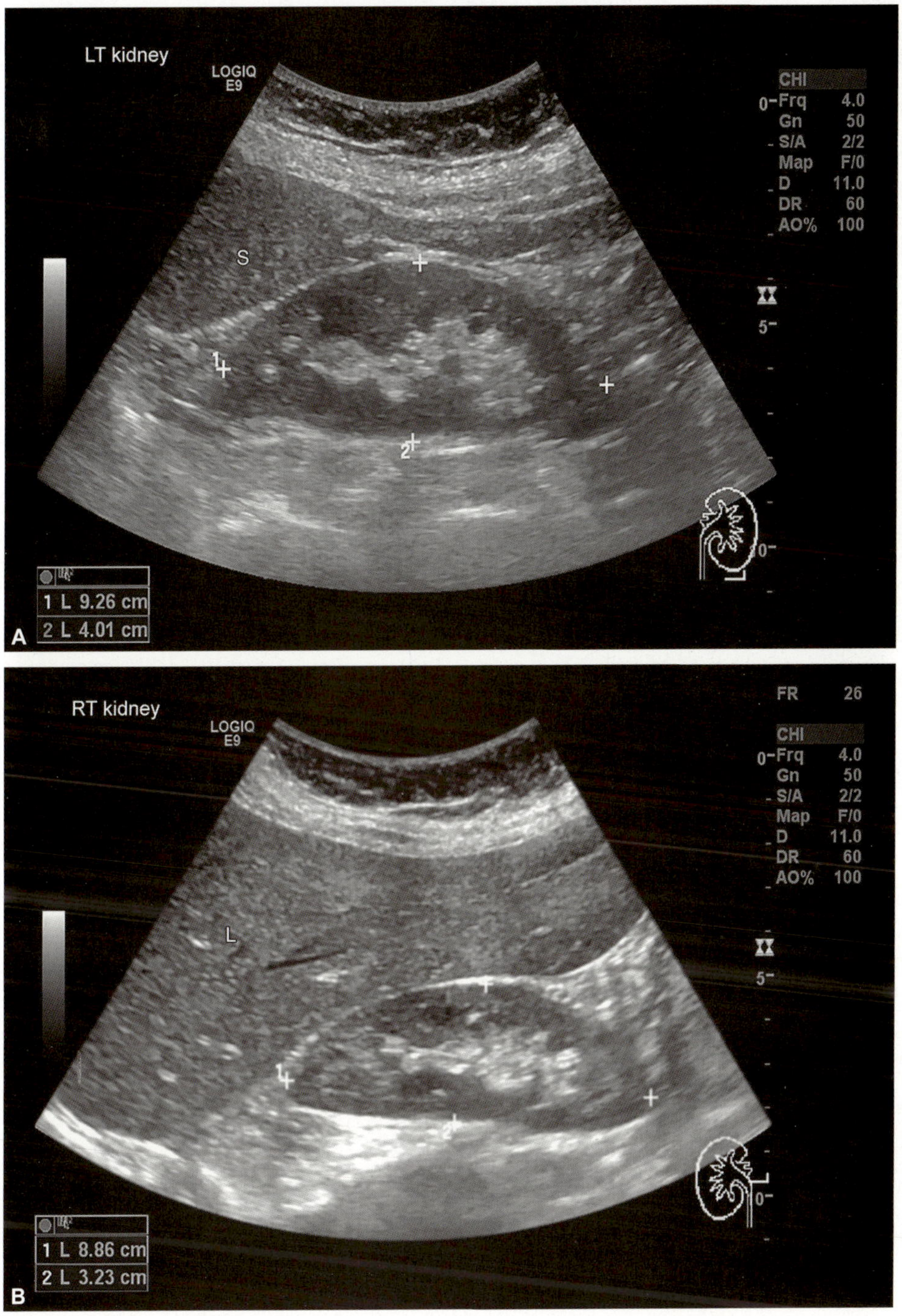

Figs. 44A and B: (A) Left kidney; and (B) Right kidney. (S: Spleen; L: Liver)

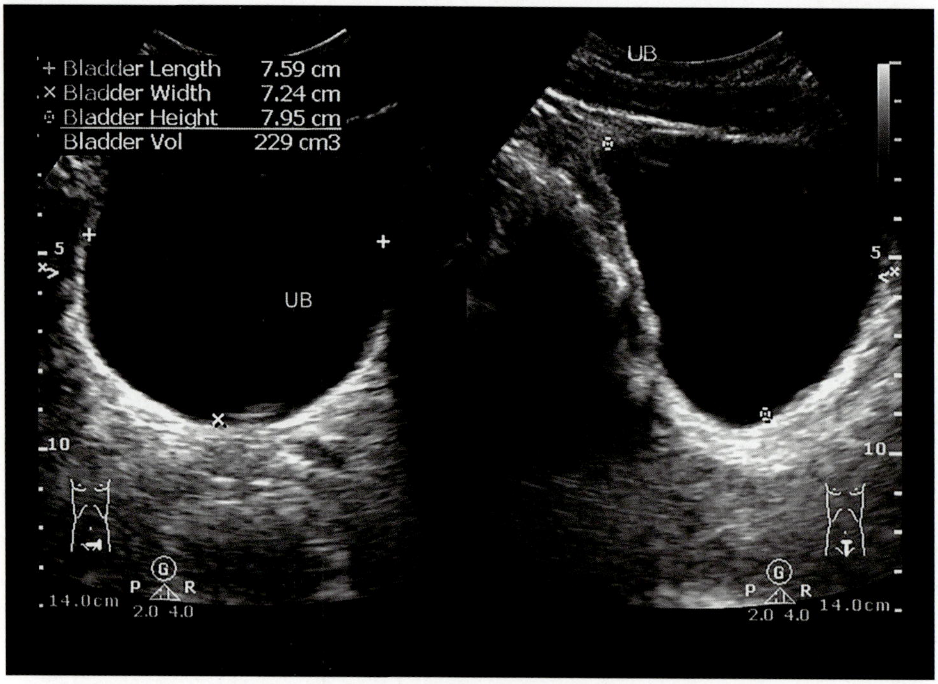

Fig. 45: Urinary bladder (UB).

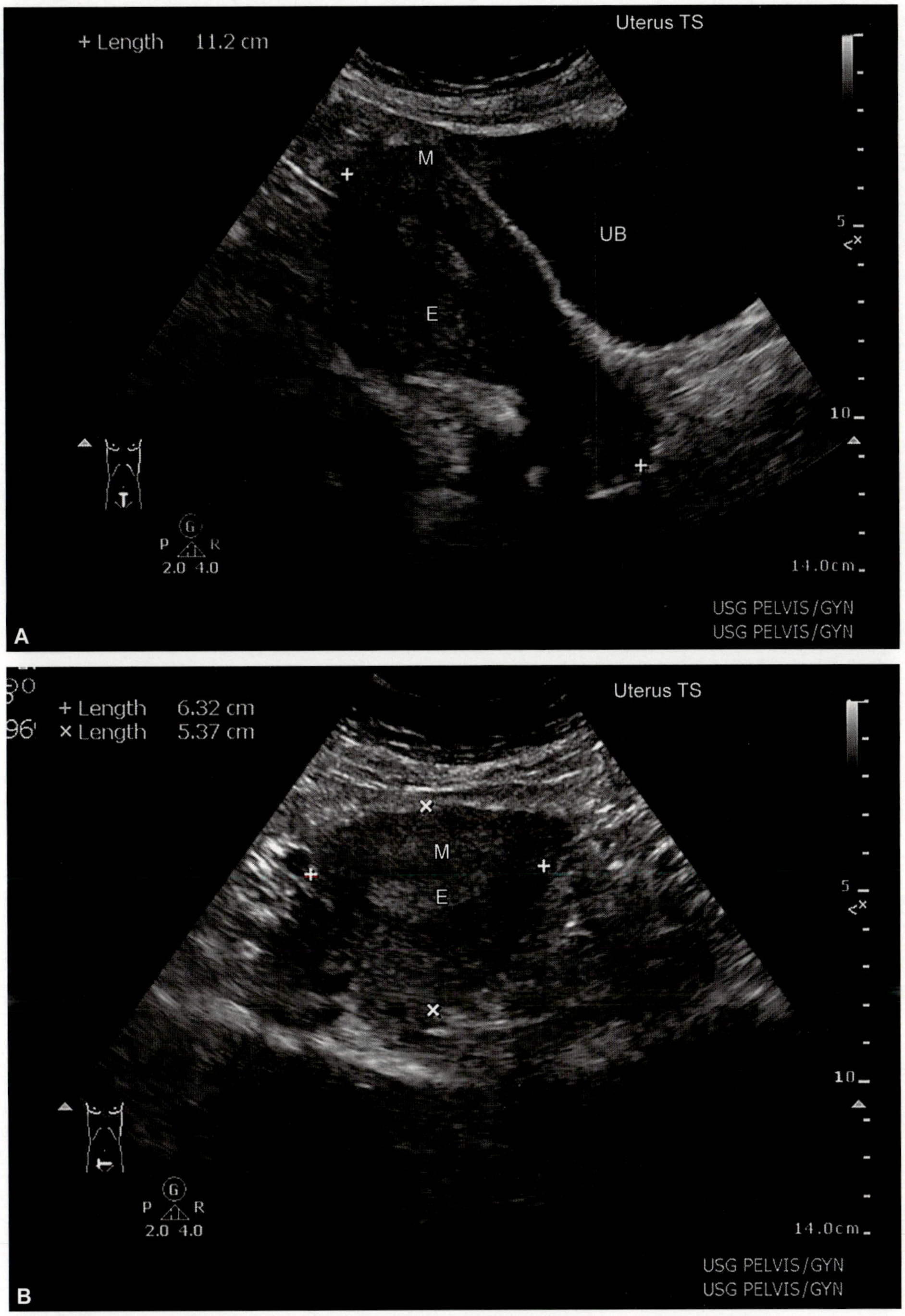

Figs. 46A and B: Uterus: Longitudinal and transverse. (E: Endometrium; M: Myometrium; UB: Urinary bladder)

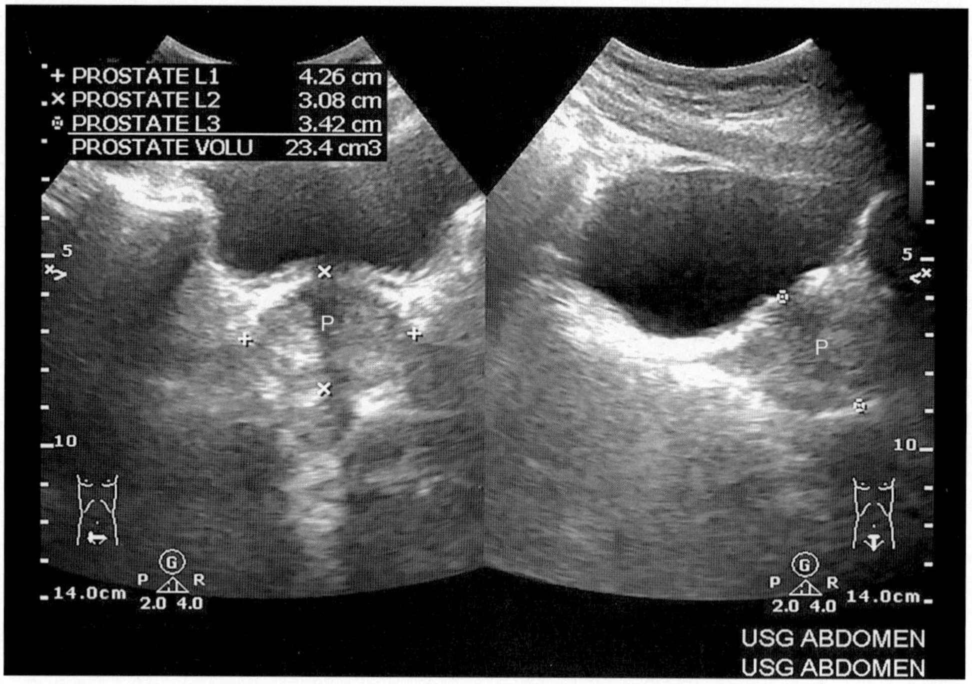

Fig. 47: Prostate: Transverse and longitudinal. (P: Prostate)

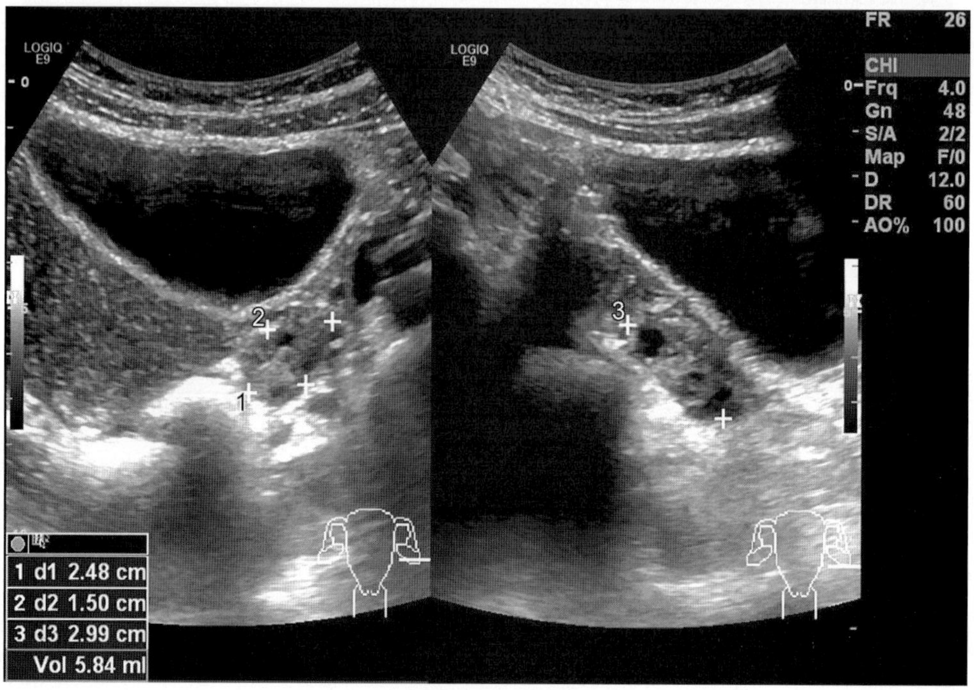

Fig. 48: Ovary transverse and longitudinal.

Index

Page numbers followed by f refer to figure.

A

Abdomen
 acute 279*f*
 contrast-enhanced computed tomography 595*f*, 605, 606, 606*f*, 612, 614, 617, 620, 623
Abdominal compartment syndrome 386, 386*f*
Abdominal wall
 abscess 605, 605*f*
 anterior 605
 postlaparotomy opened 575, 575*f*
Abscess 285
Acanthamoeba 479
Acapella 86
 device 86*f*
Acetazolamide 482
Acid-fast bacilli 414
 stain 414, 414*f*
Acid-fast stain 445*f*
 modified 424, 424*f*
Acquired immunodeficiency syndrome 471, 478
Actinomyces 346, 479
Actinomycetales 479
Air
 bronchogram 555
 containing collection 608
 embolism 568
Airway
 anatomy 7
 assessment 3, 6
 devices in ICU 20
 exchange catheter 55, 55*f*
 management 1
 pressure, high peak 562
Allen's test 184
 modified 571
Allergic bronchopulmonary aspergillosis 541
Allergic eye disease 478
Alpha coma 380, 380*f*
 demonstrative of 380
Alpha-hemolysis 413
Alpha-hemolytic streptococci 479
Alveolar hemorrhage, diffuse 501, 501*f*
Ambu auragain 42, 42*f*
Ambu aura-I laryngeal mask airway 41
Ambu auraonce 22*f*, 45, 45*f*
Ambu bag mask 20*f*
Ambu king vision 34*f*
American Heart Association Guidelines 343
American Stroke Association 343
Amikacin 447
Amoxicillin 447
Ampicillin 447
Amplatz left coronary catheter 146*f*
Ampullary orifice 252*f*
Amputed ischemic stump 388, 388*f*
Amyloidosis 105, 156
Anaerobic jar 450, 450*f*
Analgesia pumps, patient-controlled 361, 361*f*
Aneurysmal dilatation 468*f*
 and tortuosity 468
Aneurysms 232, 310
Angiography 143
 digital subtraction 344, 355, 355*f*, 399
Angioplasty 143
Ankylosing spondylitis 11
Anomalous pulmonary venous connection 119
Anterior chamber reaction 478, 487
Anterior wall
 motion index 193, 193*f*
  acute 193
 myocardial infarction 167*f*, 173*f*
Antiarrhythmics 156
Antibiotic 447
Antibody-mediated rejection
 acute 463
 severe 463*f*
Antineutrophil cytoplasmic antibody 494
 associated vasculitis 501*f*
Antiphospholipid antibody syndrome 501, 502*f*
Aorta 595*f*
 ascending 592*f*, 595*f*, 596*f*, 600*f*
 coarctation of 123, 150*f*
Aortic aneurysm 218, 232
Aortic cusps, thickened 121*f*
Aortic dissection 164, 523
 acute 223, 223*f*
 dissection flap suggestive of 600
Aortic hiatus, level of 605
Aortic regurgitation 121, 523
 severe 121*f*, 135, 135*f*
Aortic valve 151*f*
 aneurysm 135
 replacement 135, 136
  post-transcatheter 129*f*
 stenosis 523
Aortitis 135
Apophysomyces variabilis 439*f*
Arch of aorta 592*f*
Argon plasma coagulation 247, 268
Arrhythmias 154, 165
Arterial occlusion 310
Arteriovenous fistula, cannulation of 465
Arteriovenous malformation 355
 embolization 355
Artery
 aneurysm, anterior communicating 313
 anterior communicating 313*f*
Ascites 550
Aseptate fungal filaments 416, 416*f*
Aspergillosis 434, 443
 invasive 431
Aspergillus 416, 479
 fumigatus 436*f*
Aspiration
 pneumonia 589
 pneumonitis 398, 398*f*
Asymmetric septal hypertrophy 113*f*, 205
Atelectatic lung 549, 549*f*
Atherosclerosis 126
Atrial appendage
 left 107, 107*f*, 110
 right 108
Atrial fibrillation 108, 174*f*, 190, 190*f*, 195
 with fast ventricular response 195*f*
Atrial flutter 177*f*
Atrial myxoma, left 231, 231*f*
Atrial pressure, right 509
Atrial septal defect 117, 117*f*, 185, 228
 eisenmenger 185*f*
Atrial thrombus, left 227, 227*f*
Atrioventricular block, first-degree 154, 154*f*
Atropine 482
Autoimmune disorders 541
Autoimmune hemolytic anemia 529
Autologous lower extremity arteriovenous fistula 469
Autophagocytosis 534
Axonal injuries 285

B

Bacterial keratitis 478
Bag and mask 20
Bain circuit 57, 57*f*
Balloon
 catheter, inflation of 147*f*
 mitral valvotomy 149*f*, 222
Bamboo spine 11, 544
Barcode sign 544*f*
Barrett's esophagus 261, 261*f*
Basal ganglia bleed CT and MRI 295
Basal patchy consolidations 597

Basal pleural effusion, moderate left 587
Basal segmental openings, posterior 64
Basophilic stippling 535
Beer-Lambert's law, modification of 517
Bernoulli's principle 80, 81
Beta-hemolysis 413
Beta-hemolytic streptococci 479
Beta-lactamases, extended-spectrum 446*f*
Biatrial enlargement 105
Bicuspid aortic valve 123, 127
Bile duct, common 625*f*
Biliary ascites 606
Biliary cirrhosis 75
Bird's beak appearance 549
Bispectral index 360, 360*f*
Black necrotic patch 437*f*
Blast cells 539, 539*f*
Blastoconidia, size of 427*f*
Bleeding preargon photocoagulation, active 70*f*
Bleeding, ventricular extension of 344*f*
Blood
  collection 403*f*
    procedure 404
  count 484
  culture
    collection 403
    system, automated 447, 451*f*
  fluid level 288
  pressure 392
  pump, centrifugal 569, 569*f*
  serum fluid levels, classic 289*f*
  smear, thin 526*f*
  temperature 509
Blowout fracture of orbit 488
Blue rhino single dilator technique 51
Bougie 33*f*
Bowel ischemia, small 618, 618*f*
Bowel loop
  dilated small 614
  thickened 608
Bowel obstruction 591, 591*f*
Bowel perforation 399, 399*f*
Brachiocephalic arteriovenous fistula 468
Brachiocephalic trunk stenosis, left 475, 475*f*
Bradyarrhythmias 158
Brain
  abscess 346, 346*f*
  arterial
    blood supply of 338*f*
    supply of 338
  injuries, traumatic 285
  magnetic resonance imaging 484
  posterior fossa 285, 285*f*
Brimonidine 482
Bronchial asthma 452
Bronchial lumen 89*f*
Bronchiectasis 75, 91
  chest
    CT scan 91*f*
    X-ray 91*f*
Bronchiolitis obliterans 567
Bronchoalveolar lavage 505
Bronchopleural fistula, traumatic 389, 389*f*
Bronchoscope, flexible 88
Bronchoscopy airway 39, 39*f*
Bronchoscopy masks 40, 40*f*
Bronchus intermedius 63*f*
  lower 63
Bronchus, right main 592*f*, 593*f*
Bull's eye plot 115*f*
Bundle branch block
  complete left 166*f*
  left 142
  right 155, 155*f*, 172*f*, 178*f*, 191
Butterfly rash 491

C

Cabot rings 535
Calcinosis cutis 497*f*
Calcium-channel blocker 156
Calcofluor 423*f*
  mount 423
Calcofluor-potassium hydroxide 431*f*
Cameron ulcer 259, 260, 260*f*
Candida 479
  albicans 426, 426*f*
  auris 426, 427*f*
    on corn meal agar 426*f*
  glabrata 427
  invasive 425
  krusei 428, 428*f*
  meningoencephalitis 425
  parapsilosis 428, 428*f*
  pyelonephritis 422
  tropicalis 427
    morphology of 427*f*
Carbon dioxide, maximal concentration of 510*f*
Carbonic anhydrase inhibitors 482
Carcinoma 67*f*, 75
  esophagus 68, 262, 262*f*
Cardiac amyloidosis 105
Cardiac arrhythmias 568
Cardiac index 509, 510*f*
Cardiac interventions 143
Cardiac monitor 510*f*
Cardiac output 510*f*
  monitor 512*f*
  pulmonary artery catheter 512, 512*f*
Cardiac resynchronization therapy 163
  defibrillator 143
Cardiogenic shock 164, 537*f*
Cardiomegaly bilateral perihilar haze 100*f*
Cardiomyopathy 142, 155
  dilated 230
  idiopathic-dilated 166*f*
Cardiopulmonary bypass 519
Cardiovascular intervention 143
Cardioverter defibrillator
  automated implantable 160, 160*f*
  implantable 143
Carotid artery occlusion
  left internal 317
  right internal 316
Carotid stenting 341, 341*f*, 355
Carpentier classification, modification of 121
Cataract, intumescent white 481*f*
Catecholaminergic polymorphic
    ventricular tachycardia 175*f*
Catheter mount with port 56*f*
Ceftazidime 447
Ceftriaxone 447
Celiac disease 253, 253*f*
Center of bronchi 434*f*
Central ground-glass opacity 599
Central nervous system 199
Central retinal artery occlusion 485
Central thrombolysis 108*f*
Central venous catheters 412
Centriacinar nodular areas 602
Cerebral angiography 343
Cerebral arteriovenous malformation 344
Cerebral artery
  bilateral anterior 318*f*
  infarct, middle 303*f*
  left posterior 318*f*
  middle 342
  occlusion, bilateral anterior 318
  right
    anterior 303*f*
    posterior 305*f*
  thrombus, middle 342, 342*f*
Cerebral blood flow 364
Cerebral edema 285
  diffuse 298*f*
Cerebral hemorrhage 344*f*
Cerebral vessels 344*f*
Cerebritis 285
Cerebrospinal fluid 359, 412, 423
Cervical cord injury 570, 570*f*
Cervical meningomyelocele 16, 16*f*
Cervical spine
  fracture dislocation 400, 400*f*
  injury 366
Chamber pacemaker, dual 157
Chemosis 477
Cherry-red spot 485*f*
Chest
  computed tomography of 19, 501*f*, 598, 598*f*, 602
  contrast-enhanced computed tomography 599, 600
  drain, postintercostal 97*f*
  injury 392, 392*f*
  penetrating injury to 384*f*
  trauma 383*f*
  X-ray 18, 18*f*, 585, 585*f*, 586, 587*f*, 589
Chickenpox 407
  skin lesions 407*f*
Chigger borne typhus 409
Churg-Strauss syndrome 541

Ciaglia technique 51
Ciprofloxacin 447
Circle of Willis 338
Cladophialophora bantiana 440
Clavulanic acid 447
Cleft lip 16, 16*f*
Cleft palate 16, 16*f*
Clostridium difficile infection 241
Clotting time
Coagulase-negative *Staphylococcus* 487
Colitis 612, 612*f*
Collagen vascular disorders 126
Colon, ascending 595*f*
Colonic Crohn's: multiple colonic ulcers 243*f*
Colonic growth 239, 239*f*
Colonic lesions 239
Colonic loops, dilated 621*f*
Colonic mucosa, cobblestoning of 243*f*
Colonic pseudo-obstruction 621, 621*f*
Colonic stricture 240, 240*f*
Colonic ulcer 242, 242*f*
  large 241*f*
Colonoscopy 239
Color Doppler ultrasonography 500*f*
Common bile duct, dilated 277
Communicating artery aneurysm, right posterior 311
Computed tomography
  multiplanar imaging 283
  scan 392
Congenital deformity 73
Conjunctival defect 476*f*
  epithelial 477, 477*f*
Connective tissue
  diseases 529
  disorders 478
Consciousness, loss of 344
Constrictive pericarditis, chronic 106, 106*f*, 207*f*, 216
Contact lens 478
Contrast-enhanced computed tomography 393, 398, 592*f*
Contusion 285
Cor pulmonale, acute 155
Core valve 129
Cork screw devices 369
Corn meal agar 427*f*
Corneal edema 481, 482
Corneal epithelial defects 477
Corneal ulcer 478
Corneal ulceration
  with hypopyon 478*f*
  with infiltrate 478*f*
Coronal reformation 613, 614*f*, 615
Coronary angiogram 215
Coronary artery
  angiography
    left 144*f*
    right 144*f*
  bypass graft 120*f*
  disease 155, 179*f*
  mid-right 153*f*
  right 145*f*, 146*f*
Coronary cannulation, left 146*f*
Coronary predilation balloon catheter 148*f*
Coronary stent 148*f*
  expanded 148*f*
  infection 139
Corpuscular volume, mean 530
Cortical necrosis
  computed tomography of acute 458
  diffuse acute 458*f*, 459*f*
Cotton wool spots 490
Craniosynostosis 15, 15*f*
Cricothyrotomy 11
Crohn's disease 75, 243, 243*f*, 245, 246
Crohn's ileitis 245, 245*f*
Cryoglobulinemic vasculitis 501
Cryptococcosis CNS infection 441
Cryptococcosis lung infection 441
Cryptococcus 415, 423, 441*f*
  yeast cells 423*f*, 441*f*
Cuffed polyvinyl chloride endotracheal tube 25
Cutaneous polyarteritis nodosa 498, 498*f*
Cyclophosphamide 494
Cystic fibrosis 75
Cystic shadows, thin-walled 586
Cysts in Grocott stain 443*f*

D

Decerebrate posture 336
Decompressive craniectomy 349, 349*f*
Decorticate posture 336
Deep brain stimulation 362, 362*f*
Deep venous thrombosis 76, 183
Demyelinating disorders 285
Deoxyribonucleic acid 406
Descending aorta 592*f*, 593*f*, 596*f*, 600*f*
Descending colon 595*f*
  wall thickening of 612
Descending stent, left anterior 139, 139*f*
Diabetes mellitus 478
Diagnostic catheter
  Judkins left 144*f*
  Judkins right 144*f*
Diaphragmatic pinch 259*f*
Diastolic filling pattern, restrictive 105
Diastolic murmur 103*f*
Dimercaptosuccinic acid scan 472
Disc diffusion method 448
Discoid lupus erythematosus 492, 492*f*
Diverticulum 620
Dorzolamide 482
Dot sign 342
Double lumen tube 29, 30
  anterior position of left-sided 29*f*
  in situ 89*f*
Duke's criteria 133
Duodenal lesions 249
Duodenal nodule 249, 249*f*
Duodenal stricture, benign 250, 250*f*
Duodenal ulcer 2511*f*
  disease 251
  large 251, 251*f*
Duodenum 595*f*
  second part of 253*f*
Dynamic hyperinflation 385, 385*f*

E

Ebstein's anomaly 130, 212*f*
Echo-based Doppler methods 122
Echocardiography 103, 197, 208, 503*f*
  images, electrocardiography gated 104
Echogenic reverberation artifacts originating, vertical 551
Edematous bowel loops, thickened 618
Edwards SAPIEN valve 151*f*
Electrical cardiometry 523
Electrocardiogram 510*f*
Electrocardiography 154*f*, 155, 165, 190, 191, 192*f*
Electroencephalography 360, 372, 372*f*
  continuous 373
Emphysematous pancreatitis 617*f*
Emphysematous pyelonephritis 461*f*
  computed tomography of acute 461
Empyema 75
Encephalitis 285, 326
End-expiratory pressure, positive 384
Endobronchial lesion 70*f*
Endobronchial mass 66, 66*f*, 70
Endocarditis 135
Endogenous endophthalmitis 486
Endometrium 629*f*
Endophthalmitis 486, 487
  postoperative 486*f*
Endoscopic images 239, 274
Endoscopic ultrasound 249
Endotracheal intubation 5
Endotracheal tube 5*f*, 18, 19, 19*f*, 23, 25*f*, 27, 28, 511*f*
  before insertion of 5*f*
  double lumen 89
  malpositioned 19*f*
  obstructed 387, 387*f*
  position of 18, 18*f*
  preformed 27
Enterobacteriaceae 479
Enterocutaneous fistula 607, 607*f*
Enzyme-linked immunosorbent assay 409
Eosinophilic leukemia, chronic 541
Eosinophils 434*f*, 541, 541*f*
Epidural hematoma 337
Epidural hemorrhage 285
Episcleritis 504
Epithelial defect 478

Epstein-Barr virus 540
Ertapenem 447
Erythrocyte sedimentation rate 484, 500
Escherichia coli 448*f*, 487
Esophageal
- candidiasis 256, 256*f*
- carcinoma 67
- fistula 257, 257*f*
- lesions 254
- lumen 264*f*
- mucosa 256*f*
- self-expanding metal stent 263, 263*f*
- sphincter, lower 258
- stricture, benign 264, 264*f*
- variceal bleed 255
- varices 254, 604
  - large 254*f*, 275*f*
- wall with pus discharge, defect in 257*f*

Esophagus 67*f*, 604
- causing luminal narrowing 262*f*
- malignant lesions in 263*f*

Excessive daytime somnolence 72
Extracorporeal membrane oxygenation 519, 519*f*, 522, 567*f*, 568, 569, 569*f*
Extradural
- hematoma 337, 337*f*, 396, 396*f*
- hemorrhage 285

Extra-thoracic neck mass, anterior 10
Extravascular lung water 515
Eye injury, penetrating 483, 483*f*
Eyeball transverse diameter 350
Eyelid 437*f*

F

Face mask 78
- simple 78*f*

Fast ventricular rate 174*f*
Femoral artery 460*f*
- superficial 400, 469
- transection, distal superficial 400, 400*f*

Femoral sheath components 147*f*
Fever blisters 406
Fiberoptic bronchoscope 88*f*
Fiberscopy, flexible 40
Fibrin 487
Fibrosing *Aspergillus* mediastinitis 436
Filamentous fungi 479
Finger
- multiple gouty tophi in 466*f*
- pulse oximeter 87, 87*f*

Fish tail
- appearance 545
- lung 545, 545*f*

Fistula cannulation 465*f*
Fixed oxygen concentration delivery devices 82
Flail mitral leaflet 124
Flange tracheostomy tube, adjustable 565, 565*f*
FloTrac transducer 513*f*
Fluid-attenuated inversion recovery image 325
Fluoroscopic images 149, 163*f*, 214
Fogarty catheter 89, 89*f*
Folate deficiency 535
Foley's catheter 580, 580*f*
Foot drop 581, 581*f*
Foramen of Monro 353
Forceps technique 51
Forehead of child 437*f*
Foreign body 67*f*
Fracture 285
- white blow-out 488

Frontoparietal cortex, right 293*f*
Frontoparietal haemorrhage, left 294
Frontoparietal region, left 294*f*
Frontoparietal subdural hemorrhage 287
Fundal varices 266, 266*f*
Fundic gland polyp 269*f*
Fungal infection
- in critical care 421
- of surgical wound 391, 391*f*

Fungal rhinosinusitis, acute necrotizing 438*f*
Fungal stain 416
Fungal ulcer 478
- typical signs of 478

Fungi 479
Fusariosis 443
Fusarium 479
Fusiform aneurysms 232

G

Gallbladder 595*f*, 613*f*, 625*f*
- fossa 606

Gangrene, digital 571, 571*f*
Gangrenous bowel 573
Gastric antral vascular
- angioectasias 268, 268*f*
- ectasias 168*f*, 268

Gastric cancer 271, 271*f*
Gastric polyp 269, 269*f*
Gastric subepithelial lesion 270
Gastric ulcer 267
- benign 267, 267*f*

Gastroesophageal junction carcinoma 265, 265*f*
Gastrointestinal bleed 239
Gastrointestinal stromal tumor 270*f*
- subepithelial 273, 273*f*

Genital herpes infections 406
Gentamicin 447
Giant cell 434*f*
- arteritis 500, 500*f*
  - diagnosis of 500

Glasgow coma scale 336, 343, 397
Glaucoma
- acute angle-closure 480, 480*f*
- lens-induced 481

Glioma 328
Global end-diastolic volume 515
Global longitudinal strain 115
Glomerulonephritis 413
Glottis, anatomy of 5
Goodpasture syndrome 501
Gottron papules 497
Gout 466*f*
- arthritis 496
  - acute 496
- severe 466
- tophi 496*f*

Graduated dilator technique 51
Graft hydronephrosis, ultrasound image of 462
Graft kidney, hydronephrosis of 462
Graft nephrectomy 463*f*
Gram smear 410*f*
Gram stain 422
Gram-negative
- bacilli 411, 411*f*
- bacteremia 390
- bacteria 487

Gram-positive
- cocci 410
- lanceolate-shaped diplococci 410*f*

Granular myocardial texture, classical 105
Granulation tissue, proximal 71
Granulocytes 541
Granuloma, calcified 324
Granulomatosis 494
- with polyangiitis 494*f*

Graves' disease 75
Great saphenous vein 469*f*
Griggs technique 51
Grocott's methenamine silver 421

H

Haemorrhoids, large 275
Hallmark of sepsis 534
Halo sign 500*f*
Hanging drop
- preparation 420, 420*f*
- slide 420*f*

Headache 344
Heart
- block 154
  - complete 156, 156*f*, 194
- disease, congenital 75
- failure 82
  - acute decompensated 164

Heimlich valve 566, 566*f*
Helicobacter pylori 267
Heliotrope rash 497
Helmet-like cells 532*f*
Hematemesis 274
- recurrent 275

Hematoma 285, 604
- collection 337

Hematoxylin and eosin, histopathology 498*f*
Hemochron-activated clotting time 522
Hemodialysis 465
- procedure 464

Hemodynamic monitoring 506
- systems FloTrac, pulse contour-based 513

Hemopericardium 392, 392*f*
Hemophagocytic lymphohistiocytosis 540
Hemophagocytic phenomenon 540, 540*f*
Hemorrhage 293*f*, 294*f*, 477
 in left basal ganglia region 296*f*
 postpartum 459, 459*f*
 right frontoparietal 293
Hemorrhagic contusion 285, 291
Hemorrhoidectomy, stapled 276
Hemostatic endoscopic therapy 267
Hemothorax 547, 547*f*
Henoch-Schonlein purpura 499, 499*f*
Hepatic artery 399, 399*f*
Hepatic vein
 middle 624*f*
 right 624*f*
Hepatitis B infection, chronic 278*f*
Hepatocellular carcinoma, ruptured 278
Hernia sac 259*f*
Herniations 285
Herpes simplex 406*f*
 skin lesions 406
 virus 333*f*, 406
  encephalitis 333
Herpes zoster 408
 ophthalmicus 408
 skin lesions 408*f*
Hiatus hernia 259, 259*f*
Histoplasmosis 442
Hockey stick appearance 222
Hodgkin disease 156
Hollenhorst plaques 485
Homogeneous opacity 554
Hurwitz Robert classified 136
Hyperkalemia 156, 178*f*
Hypermature cataract 482
Hypersegmented neutrophils 535, 535*f*
Hypersensitivity pneumonitis 93*f*
Hypertrophic cardiomyopathy 113, 113*f*, 205
 with atrial flutter 177*f*
Hypertrophied gastric folds 272*f*
Hypoalbuminemia 76
 severe 76*f*
Hypodense cerebral hemisphere 303*f*
Hypodense lesion 610, 610*f*
Hypodense nonenhancing areas 619
Hypopyon 482, 487
Hypothyroidism 156
Hypoxemia
 chronic 75
 postoperative 82
 severe 92
Hypoxia 156
Hypoxic brain injuries 285

I

Ileal loop 607
Ileocecal junction 614
Ileostomy, gangrenous stoma of 574, 574*f*
Impetigo 413
Incentive spirometry 85, 85*f*
Incubator 451
India ink
 mount 423
 stain 415
Infarction, digital 474
Infection 285, 403
 mixed 479
Infective endocarditis 126, 132, 133*f*, 200, 200*f*, 226, 226*f*
Inflammatory bowel disease 243
Inflammatory disease 11
Infrared spectroscopy monitor, near 363*f*
Intensive care unit 4, 394, 478, 507
Interatrial septum 197
Intercostal chest drain 83
 with trocar 83*f*
Internal jugular vein, right 162
Internal mammary 146*f*
International Subarachnoid Aneurysm Trial 340
Interstitial lung disease 75, 92, 93*f*, 495, 505
Interstitial pneumonia 505
 nonspecific 505
 pattern 505*f*
Intervention devices 88
Interventricular septal hypertrophy 205
Interventricular septum 106*f*
Intestinal metaplasia 261*f*
Intestinal perforation 608, 608*f*
Intra-abdominal
 hypertension 575
 pressure, continuous monitoring of 386
Intra-alveolar hemorrhage 385, 385*f*
Intra-aortic balloon
 catheter 524*f*, 525*f*
  entry of 525*f*
 pump 164, 164*f*, 524, 524*f*, 525*f*
Intracranial aneurysm 343, 343*f*
 clipping of 340
 coiling 340, 340*f*, 341, 355
Intracranial pressure 337, 349, 352
 monitoring 351, 397
 probes 351*f*
 waveform 354, 354*f*
Intramural hematoma 218
 of aorta 218*f*
Intraocular pressure 482
 raised 480
Intraoral fibrous bands 8*f*
Intravascular ultrasound 217
Intraventricular hemorrhage 297
Invasive mechanical ventilator 561, 561*f*
Iron deficiency 535
Ischemia, digital 390
Ischemic heart disease 199
Ischemic pale retina 485*f*
Ischemic stroke 303

J

Jugular vein thrombus
 internal 320
 left internal 321
Junctional rhythm 178*f*
Juvenile dermatomyositis 497, 497*f*

K

Keratitis, exposure 478
Kidney
 disease, chronic 268*f*, 460, 466
 dysfunction 76
 enlarged right 458*f*
 injury, acute 459
 left 609*f*, 627*f*
 mucormycosis of 470, 470*f*
 primary hyperoxaluria 455*f*
 right 627*f*
 small left 458*f*
 transverse, mucor of 470*f*
Kimura spatula 479
Knee joint, magnetic resonance imaging 502*f*
Kyphoscoliosis 72
Kyphotic deformity 72

L

Lambl's excrescence 138, 138*f*
Large La clot 209*f*, 211*f*
Laryngeal axis 6
Laryngeal inlet 31*f*
Laryngeal mask airway 46, 46*f*, 47, 47*f*, 48, 49*f*
 intubating 44, 44*f*
Laryngeal tube suction 46, 46*f*
 intubating 44, 44*f*
Laryngoscope 24, 24*f*
Laryngoscopy, direct 5
Leadless pacemaker, fluoro image of 161
Leaflets, non-coaptation of 130*f*
Left lower lobe 65*f*
 basal segments 65
  anterior 65*f*
 bronchus 65
Left main bronchus 66*f*, 593*f*
 distal 64*f*
 mucous plug 66
Left midbrain, compression of 328*f*
Left upper lobe 68*f*
Left ventricle
 aneurysm 220, 220*f*
 hypertrophy 229, 229*f*
Left ventricular
 clot 140, 199, 199*f*
 ejection fraction 115, 160
 outflow tract 113, 121, 206*f*
 stroke work index 509
Leukocytoclastic vasculitis 498*f*
Leukocytosis 537*f*

Lid speculum 479
Limb
ischemia 164, 477
leads, low voltage complexes in 195*f*
Linitis plastica 272
stomach 272, 272*f*
Liquefying hematoma 312
Lithium dilution cardiac output 516
Liver 595*f*, 613*f*, 627*f*
abscess 572, 572*f*
ruptured large 278
disease, chronic 529
secondary to 268*f*
hilar region 625*f*
laceration 393, 393*f*, 611, 611*f*
lobe, left 624*f*
right lobe of 594*f*
subcostal 624*f*
Loeffler's endocarditis 111, 111*f*
Loeffler's endomyocarditis 111
Lower esophagus, food bolus in 276
Lower lobe
apical segment bronchus, right 63
basal segment, right 67
bronchus 64*f*
right 63
numerous cysts in 443*f*
right 63*f*, 64*f*
Lumbar drain 359, 359*f*
Lundberg intracranial pressure waves 354
Lundberg waveforms 354*f*
Lung
biopsy
mount preparation of 423*f*
wet-mount preparation of 422*f*
collapse, underlying 96*f*
disease, suppurative 75
hepatization of 554, 554*f*
injury, ventilator induced 384
lobar pneumonia, right 587, 588, 588*f*
numerous gray nodules in 442*f*
parenchyma indicating invasion 434*f*
point 543, 544, 544*f*
pulse 549
scan 542*f*
sliding, loss of 543
ultrasound in ICU 542
window 593*f*, 594*f*, 597, 597*f*, 599, 599*f*
Lymphoblastic leukemia, acute 539
Lymphocytic leukemia, chronic 538
Lymphoma 75, 599

M

MacIntosh blade 24
Macrogametocytes 418
Macrophage engulfing cells 540*f*
Macular edema 490
Magill forceps 23, 23*f*
Magnetic resonance imaging 502
Malar rash 491, 497
Malaria 409
Malarial parasite 417, 526
Mallampati score 6
modified 6, 6*f*
Malt extract agar 435*f*
Mandibular hypoplasia 9
Mapleson-C circuit 58, 58*f*
March hemoglobinuria 532
Marfan syndrome 126
Mask ventilation 22
Massive effusion 547, 547*f*
Massive pericardial calcification 216
McCoy laryngoscope 33, 33*f*
Mechanical thrombectomy 370, 370*f*
penumbra suction aspirator for 369, 369*f*
Meckel's diverticulitis 622, 622*f*
Mediastinal soft tissue, anterior 599
Mediastinal window 599, 599*f*
Medical therapy 479
Membranous posterior wall 61
Meningioma 327
Meningiomatosis, multiple 331, 331*f*
Meningitis 285, 325
Mentohyoid three fingers 3*f*
Mesenteric artery, superior 626*f*
Mesenteric vein, superior 623, 623
Metabolic disorders 285
Metabolic syndrome 376, 376*f*
Metallic tracheal stent, tracheal self-expanding 70*f*
Metatarsophalangeal joint 496
Methicillin-resistant *Staphylococcus aureus* 412, 446*f*
Microaneurysms 490
Microbial keratitis 479
Microcytic hypochromic
anemia 531, 531*f*
red cells 531*f*
Microgametocytes 418
Micrognathia 9
Microscopy 445
Microsporidia 479
Middle lobe
bronchus, right 63
right 63*f*
Midesophageal aortic valve 123*f*, 126*f*
Mini-tracheostomy
set 52, 52*f*
tube 52
Mitral commissural fusion 110
Mitral leaflet, anterior 204, 222
Mitral prosthesis, multiple vegetations on 137*f*
Mitral regurgitation 103, 104, 128, 201, 201*f*, 221, 221*f*
severe 124*f*, 128
central 128*f*
Mitral stenosis 109, 110, 172*f*, 188, 222, 222*f*
chest X-ray of severe 188, 188*f*
Mitral valve 116, 221, 227*f*, 231*f*
area 110
in severe rheumatic 212*f*
leaflets 109*f*
thickened 109*f*
prolapse 201
vegetation 503*f*
Molecular diagnostic technique 449
Monckeberg's medial sclerosis 460
Moraxella 479
Motor and sensory evoked potential 371, 371*f*
Mouth opening, restricted 8
Mt Fuji sign 348
Mucopurulent discharge 478
Mucormycosis 437, 599
Mucosa, normal overlying 273*f*
Multifocal avascular necrosis 502*f*
Multiparameter hemodynamic monitor 510*f*
Mycobacteria
culture 445*f*
detection of 445*f*
Mycobacterium 450
tuberculosis 450
infection 242
Mycotic aneurysm 346, 346*f*
Myeloblast cells 539, 539*f*
Myelodysplastic syndrome 535, 539
Myeloid leukemia
acute 539
chronic 537
Myeloma
chronic infections 529
multiple 156
Myocardial infarction 160
inferior wall 169*f*, 174*f*
Myocarditis 156
Myocardium 105
Myometrium 629*f*

N

Nalidixic acid 447
Narrow band imaging 270
Nasal bleeding, stop 580*f*
Nasal bridge 437*f*
Nasal cannula 81*f*
high flow 81, 560, 560*f*
system, high flow 81*f*
Nasal mask with noninvasive ventilation 82*f*
Nasal oxygen cannula, high flow 50
Nasal prongs 77, 77*f*
Nasopharyngeal airway 22
Neck
fat deposition around 72
injury 391, 391*f*
short 12, 12*f*
X-ray 17, 17*f*
Neoplastic disease 75
Nephrocalcinosis 455
Nephrology 455
Neuroimaging 283, 335
Neuromonitoring 335

Neurotrauma and stroke imaging 285
Nikolsky's sign 579
Nitrofurantoin 447
Nocardia 479
 filaments of 424
Nodular episcleritis of eye 504*f*
Nodular hemorrhagic areas, multiple 432*f*
Nodular lesion, subepithelial 273, 273*f*
Noncontrast computed tomography 396
Nonhemorrhagic contusions 285
Noninvasive cardiac system 523
Noninvasive cardiometry 523
Noninvasive positive pressure ventilation 560
Noninvasive ventilation 557-559
 device 82
 helmet interface for 559, 559*f*
 machine 557, 557*f*
 oronasal mask 558, 558*f*
Nonischemic dilated cardiomyopathy 160
Non-rebreather mask 79
Non-ST elevation myocardial infarction 166*f*
Nonsteroidal anti-inflammatory drugs 496
Nonsustained ventricular tachycardia 181*f*
Nontunneled hemodialysis catheter 467, 467*f*

O

O-arm 358, 358*f*
Obstructive cardiomyopathy, hypertrophic 204*f*, 205*f*, 229
Obstructive hydrocephalus 334
Obstructive pulmonary disease
 chronic 76, 82, 155, 385, 542
 with infection, chronic 586*f*
Ocular chemical burns 476
Ocular emergencies 476
Ocular surgery 478
Odontoid fracture 397, 397*f*
Ogilvie syndrome 621, 621*f*
Olecranon bursa 496*f*
Oncotic pressure 76
Optic disc edema 490
Optic neuritis 484
Optical nerve sheath diameter 350, 350*f*
Oral fiberscopy 39, 39*f*
Oral mucositis 491*f*
Oral ulcers 491
Orbital cellulitis 489, 489*f*
Orientia tsutsugamushi 409
Oropharyngeal airway 21, 21*f*
Orotracheal intubation 5
Oscillatory ventilation, high frequency 563, 563*f*
Ostium secundum
 atrial septal defect 117*f*, 197, 197*f*
  aortic rims of 118*f*
 large 118*f*
 rims of 117*f*
Ovarian vein
 thrombosis 615, 615*f*
 with filling defect, dilated 615
Ovary transverse and longitudinal 630*f*
Oxygen
 delivery devices 77
 therapy, high flow 50*f*

P

P waves, multiple 170*f*
Pacemaker 143
 implantation, temporary 156
 temporary external 518
 with cable, external 518*f*
Pain 481, 482
Palatal herpes 576, 576*f*
Palliative biliary stenting 252
Pancreas 595*f*, 626*f*
 body of 626*f*
 laceration 393, 393*f*
 pancreatitis necrosis of 279
 tail of 617*f*
Pancreatic tail 617
Pancreatitis, necrotizing 617, 617*f*
Papillary muscles 116
Papillopathy 490, 490*f*
Paradoxical bouncing motion 106*f*
Parameters measured 509
Parenchymal contusion 397, 397*f*
Parietal pericardium 122*f*
Partial pressure 510*f*
Patchy consolidations, bilateral 598
Patchy ground-glass opacities, bilateral 602
Patent ductus arteriosus 150*f*
Pectus carinatum 73
Pedal edema 76
Pediatric endotracheal tube 25*f*
Pelvic fractures 395, 395*f*
Penicilliosis 442
Peptic ulcer disease 250*f*
Percutaneous coronary intervention 193, 214
Percutaneous endoscopic gastrostomy 277
Percutaneous tracheostomy 51, 51*f*, 69
Percutaneous transluminal coronary angioplasty 217
Periampullary carcinoma 252, 252*f*
Perianal fistula 246, 246*f*
 formation 246
Peribronchial nodular opacities 597
Peribronchial thickening 601
Pericardial effusion 120, 122*f*, 203, 203*f*, 224, 224*f*
 large 186, 186*f*
Pericarditis, effusive-constrictive 122
Pericholecystic edema 613
Perihilar ground-glass, bilateral 100*f*
Perihilar haziness, bilateral 585*f*
Perinephric hematoma, left 609, 609*f*
Periodic acid-Schiff stain 434*f*
Periodic lateralized epileptiform discharges 378
Peripheral capillary oxygen saturation 510*f*
Peripheral vascular diseases 523
Periumbilical hernia 573
Phacolytic glaucoma 482, 482*f*
Phacomorphic glaucoma 481, 481*f*
Phaeohyphomycosis 440
Pharyngeal axis 6
Pharyngitis 413
Phlegmasia cerulea dolens 183, 183*f*
Photophobia 478, 481, 482
Phrenic nerve stimulator 366, 366*f*
Physical rehabilitation 584*f*
Picco system 515
Pierre Robin syndrome 14, 14*f*
Pig tail
 catheter 83*f*
 in situ 84*f*
Pigeon chest 73
 anterior view 73*f*
 lateral view 73*f*
Pigtail catheter 145*f*
Pigtail drainage catheter 587
Pinna, inflammation of 493*f*
Piperacillin 447
Pitting pedal edema 76*f*
Pituitary macroadenoma 332, 332*f*
Plasmodium falciparum 526, 527*f*
 gametocytes of 418, 418*f*, 526*f*
 infection 527
 ring-form trophozoites of 417, 417*f*
Plasmodium vivax 527, 528, 528*f*
 developing schizonts of 420*f*
 ring-form trophozoites of 419*f*
 Schizonts of 420
Plateau pressure, normal 562, 562*f*
Pleural effusion 96, 219, 219*f*, 545, 545*f*, 548*f*, 549, 550, 611*f*
 and ascites 550*f*
 bilateral mild 602
 complicated 549*f*
 left 587*f*, 598
 left-sided 96*f*
Pleuritic chest pain, right-sided 99*f*
Pleuritis 429*f*
Pleurocentesis 546, 546*f*
Pneumocystis jiroveci infections 443
Pneumocystosis 443
Pneumoencephalus 348, 348*f*
Pneumomediastinum
 chest X-ray of 590, 590*f*
 sign of 590
Pneumonia 90, 90*f*, 554, 556, 556*f*
 atypical 589*f*
 early 554*f*
 ventilator associated 28
 with air bronchogram 555*f*
Pneumonitis, probably hypersensitivity 93*f*
Pneumoperitoneum 399, 399*f*, 573*f*
Pneumothorax 95, 394, 394*f*, 543, 544*f*
Point-of-care testing 521
Polyangiitis 494
Polymerase chain
 reaction 406, 449*f*
  real-time 449*f*

Polymorphic ventricular premature contraction 175*f*
Polyvinyl chloride 25
Pontine hemorrhage 300, 301
Port for procedures, catheter mount with 56
Portal vein 625*f*
Postcardiac surgery 155
Post-percutaneous coronary intervention 155
Postpuncture site 184
Potassium
  hydroxide 422, 422*f*, 423*f*, 431*f*
    wet mount 422
  permanganate ingestion 577, 577*f*
Prednisolone 482
Promyelocytic leukemia, acute 536, 536*f*
Prostate 630*f*
Prosthetic valve endocarditis 137
Proteus
  mirabilis 409
  vulgaris 409
Proton pump inhibitor 251
Pseudoaneurysm 232
  of inferior wall 141*f*
  of left ventricle 141
Pseudodiverticulum formation 250*f*
Pseudohyphae 428, 428*f*
  of candida 425*f*
Pseudomembranous colitis 241, 241*f*
Pseudomonas 479, 487
Ptosis 335, 335*f*
Pulmonary angiography, computed tomography 603, 603*f*
Pulmonary artery 510*f*, 595*f*, 596*f*
  catheter 508, 511*f*
  dilated 187*f*, 188*f*
    main 208*f*
  filament on 512
  hypertension, severe 172*f*
  left 592*f*
  lower lobar branches of 99*f*
  main 185*f*, 225, 225*f*, 592*f*, 600*f*
  occlusion pressure 509
  pressure 509
  right 225, 225*f*, 592*f*
Pulmonary bifurcation 592*f*
Pulmonary capillary wedge pressure, wedge tracing 511*f*
Pulmonary edema 100, 100*f*, 553, 553*f*, 585*f*, 601, 601*f*, 602*f*
Pulmonary embolism 99, 155, 225, 225*f*
Pulmonary hypertension 191, 191*f*
  chest X-ray 187, 187*f*
  severe 187
Pulmonary necrotizing aspergillosis, chronic 433*f*
Pulmonary rehabilitation device 85
Pulmonary vascular
  resistance 509
Pulse
  contour cardiac output monitor 515*f*
  wave Doppler 507
Pupil, mid-dilated 481
Pupillary defect, relative afferent 484
Pyogenic infection 413

Q

QT syndrome, congenital long 176*f*, 179*f*, 180*f*
Quadricuspid aortic valve 136

R

Radial artery
  calcification of 460*f*
  cannulation, complication of 571, 571*f*
Radiation proctitis 247, 247*f*
Rashes 497
Raynaud's phenomenon 495
  severe 495
Red blood cell 417, 528
  agglutination 530, 530*f*
  aggregations of 529*f*
  clumping of 530
Reflux esophagitis 258, 258*f*
Relapsing polychondritis 493, 493*f*
Renal abscess 461*f*
Renal biopsy 471*f*
Renal infarction 470*f*
Renal replacement therapy, continuous 473
Renal transplant recipient 472, 442*f*
Renal vein thrombosis 457
  right 457*f*, 458*f*
  transverse, right 457*f*
Reservoir face mask 79, 79*f*
Respiration
  accessory muscles of 74*f*
  prominent accessory muscles of 74
Respiratory distress 74
  syndrome
    acute 94, 94*f*, 384, 384*f*, 551, 551*f*, 563, 588, 588*f*
    mild acute 82
Respiratory failure, secondary causes of 567
Resuscitation 392
Reticulonodular opacities, bilateral diffuse 93*f*
Reticulonodular shadow, bilateral diffuse 94*f*
Retinal hemorrhages 490, 490*f*
Retrognathia 15
Retroperitoneal hematoma 568
Rheumatic disease 131
Rheumatic fever 413
Rheumatic heart disease 110, 130, 131*f*, 172*f*, 188, 201
Rheumatoid arthritis 504*f*
Rheumatology 491
Rhizopus arrhizus 439*f*
Rhizopus homothallicus 440*f*
Rib fractures 395, 395*f*, 611*f*
Right atrium, dilated 130*f*
Right axis deviation 191
Right eye, alkali injury in 476*f*
Right foot, arterial insufficiency in 389, 389*f*
Right tibia, fracture of 99*f*
Right ventricle
  inflow 131*f*
  myxoma 134
Right ventricular
  dysfunction 76
  dysplasia, arrhythmogenic 142, 142*f*
  hypertrophy 191*f*
  outflow tract 142, 192
Rituximab 494
Rouleaux formation 529
Ryle's tube 388
  inadvertent placement of 388, 388*f*

S

Sabouraud's dextrose agar 435*f*
Saddle nose deformity 494*f*
Saphenofemoral loop arteriovenous fistula 469*f*
Saphenofemoral vein loop arteriovenous fistula cannulation 469*f*
Saphenous vein graft 145*f*
Sarcoidosis 156
Savary-Gilliard dilators 264
Saw tooth, typical inverted 177*f*
Scarlet fever 413
Scedosporiosis 443
Schamroth's test 75*f*
Schamroth's window, obliteration of 75*f*
Schistocytes helmet cells 532
Schüffner's dots 419
Scleroderma 495, 495*f*
Scoliosis 371
Scrub typhus 409
  eschar 409*f*
Seizure 344
  disorders 285
Sengstaken-Blakemore tube 582, 582*f*, 583
Senile systemic amyloidosis 450
Sepsis 164, 532
Septal bounce 106
Septate fungal filaments 416, 416*f*
Septic emboli 390, 390*f*
Serratia 479
Shallow anterior chamber 481
Shawl sign 497
Shield ulcer 478
Shock 274
Shred sign 552
Shunt, left to right 119*f*
Sickle cells 533, 533*f*
Sigmoid colon 620*f*
Sigmoidoscopy 275
Single chamber
  implantable cardioverter defibrillator 159, 159*f*
  temporary pacing 158
Single dilator technique 51, 51*f*
Sinus bradycardia 181*f*

Sinus
left transverse 319
of Valsalva, aneurysm of 126
P wave 196*f*
rhythm 166*f*, 168*f*-172*f*, 178*f*, 179*f*, 181*f*
normal 165*f*
with ventricular couplets 180*f*
right sigmoid 319*f*
right transverse 320
sclerodegenerative 178*f*
thrombus, left sigmoid 319
venosus atrial septal defect 119
type of 119*f*
Situs inversus with dextrocardia 190, 190*f*
Skin
disinfectants 403
lesions 406
over gangreous bowel, bluish discoloration of 573*f*
Skull fracture 347, 347*f*
Sleep apnea syndrome, obstructive 72
Speckle tracking echocardiography 115, 115*f*
Spectroscopy
monitor, near-infrared 363, 517*f*
near-infrared 517
Spinal AV fistula 345, 345*f*
Spine, abnormal lateral curvature of 72
Spleen 594*f*, 595*f*, 596*f*, 619, 626*f*, 627*f*
Splenic injury 394, 394*f*
Splenic laceration 619, 619*f*
Splenic vein 595*f*, 623
thrombosis 623
Spontaneous echo contrast 222
Squamous cell epithelium, normal 261*f*
Staphylococci 412, 412*f*
Staphylococcus
aureus 346, 412, 479, 487
epidermidis 412, 479, 487
haemolyticus 412
saprophyticus 412
Stent upper-edge dissection 214, 214*f*
Stent with inflated balloon 148*f*
Stercoral rectal ulcers 244, 244*f*
Stereotactic frame in-situ 362
Stereotactic-guided electrode, insertion of 362
Sternocleidomastoid and scalene muscles, prominent 74
Stevens-Johnson syndrome 478, 579, 579*f*
Stiff neck 11
Stomach 594*f*, 595*f*, 613*f*
lesions 266
Stratosphere sign 543, 544*f*
Streptococci 413, 413*f*
Streptococcus pneumoniae 479
Streptococcus viridans 346
Stroke 285, 355
volume
maximum 514*f*
mean 514*f*
minimum 514*f*
variation 514*f*
Stromal edema 478
Stuck mitral valve 202, 202*f*
Subaortic membrane 208, 208*f*
Subarachnoid haemorrhage, bilateral 292*f*
Subarachnoid hemorrhage 343, 365
Subcutaneous emphysema 98, 590
bilateral 98*f*
Subcutaneous port of chemoport 576, 576*f*
Subdural collection, bilateral 288
Subdural hematoma 396, 396*f*
acute 347, 347*f*
chronic 347, 347*f*
Subdural hemorrhage 285
Subglottic suction 28
Subglottic tracheal stenosis 69*f*
Submucosal venous channel in stomach 266*f*
Subpleural consolidation 552, 552*f*, 554*f*
Sudden cardiac death 113
Sulfamethoxazole 447
Supraglottic airway device 49
insertion 20
Surgical therapy 479
Swan-Ganz catheter 509*f*
in packing 508*f*
Swan-Ganz pulmonary artery catheter 509
Swan-Ganz X-ray position 511*f*
Swedish nose 56, 56*f*
Swelling, subepithelial 249*f*
Syphilis 126
Systemic inflammatory response syndrome 279*f*
Systemic lupus erythematosus 491, 501, 502*f*
malar rash of 491*f*
Systemic vascular resistance 509
index 509
Systolic anterior motion 204*f*
Systolic murmur 103*f*

T

Tachycardia
AV nodal re-entrant 171*f*
narrow complex 171*f*, 175*f*, 182*f*
Talaromyces marneffei 442
Target controlled infusion pump 367, 367*f*
Tazobactam 447
Temporal hemorrhagic contusions, left 290
Tension pneumothorax, right-sided 95*f*
Terminal chlamydoconidia 426*f*
Terry's nail 578, 578*f*
Tetralogy of Fallot 192*f*
chest X-ray 189*f*
electrocardiography of 192
Thoracic aorta short axis 218
Thoracic aortic aneurysm
chest X-ray of 234*f*
postendovascular stent, chest X-ray of 235*f*
Thoracic bioimpedance 523
Thorax 19
Thrombectomy 355
Thrombocytopenia 164
Thromboelastography 368, 368*f*, 520
graph, normal 520*f*
machine 520*f*
Thrombotic microangiopathy, severe 459
Thrombotic thrombocytopenic purpura 532
Thyrohyoid two fingers 3*f*
Ticarcillin 447
Tiger diagnostic catheter 145*f*
Timolol 482
Tissue
diastolic velocities 114*f*
Doppler imaging 114
Doppler waveforms 114*f*
systolic velocity 114*f*
transglutaminase antibodies 253
Tongue hematoma 387, 387*f*
Tonic-clonic seizures 375, 375*f*
Total trismus 8*f*
Toxic epidermal necrolysis 579, 579*f*
Toxic granules 534*f*
in peripheral smear 534
Toxins 156
T-piece 54, 54*f*
Trachea 592*f*
lower 62
normal 61*f*
Tracheal carcinoma 70
Tracheal compression, posterior 67*f*
Tracheal injury 386, 386*f*, 398, 398*f*
Tracheal separation, complete 391*f*
Tracheal silicon stent 71*f*
in situ 71
Tracheal stenosis, postintubation 71
Tracheal stoma 51
Tracheal tube introducer 33
Tracheal wall, extrinsic compression of posterior 67
Tracheoesophageal fistula 68*f*
near carina 68
Tracheostomy 11
dilator bronchoscopic view 69*f*
tube 53, 53*f*
double lumen 564, 564*f*
Transcatheter aortic valve replacement 129, 151*f*
Transcranial Doppler 364, 364*f*
Transesophageal echocardiography 107, 107*f*, 218, 506, 507
probe 507*f*
Transgastric two-chamber view 116
Transmitral variation 207*f*
Transplant kidney 455, 462*f*, 463
primary hyperoxaluria 455*f*
Transpulmonary thermodilution 515
Transthoracic echocardiography 105*f*, 110, 197*f*
Transthoracic right ventricle 134*f*, 142*f*
Transthyretin amyloidosis 105, 450
Trauma 126, 285, 478

Treacher Collins syndrome 14, 14*f*
Trichosporon in Grocott's stain,
  septate hyphae of 429
Trichosporosis, acute invasive 429
Tricuspid regurgitation 130
Tricuspid valve 131, 226
Trifascicular block 172*f*
Trimethoprim 447
Triphasic waves, evidence of 378
Truncal obesity 72
Tuberculoma 322, 322*f*, 323, 323*f*
Tuberculosis 409
  liquid culture of 450, 450*f*
Tumors 156
  benign 285
  neoplastic 285
Typhoid 409

U

Ulcer
  circumferential 242
  nonhealing 498*f*
Ulcerated lesion in right coronary artery 215*f*
Ulcerative colitis 75, 248, 248*f*
Ulceroproliferative growth 239*f*, 252*f*
Ulceroproliferative tumor 265*f*
  in gastric body 271*f*
Ultrafiltration, slow continuous 473
Ultrasound anatomy, normal 624
Univent tube 31, 31*f*
Upper limb, cellulitis of 390, 390*f*
Upper lobe
  bronchus, normal right 62*f*
  bronchus, right 62
  right 30
Urinary bladder 595*f*, 628*f*, 629*f*
Urine
  collection through catheter port 405*f*
  sample through urinary catheter port 405
Urobag 405*f*
Uterus 629*f*

V

Valvular prosthesis, defective 532
Valvular thickening 105
Vancomycin-resistant enterococci 446*f*
Variceal bleeding 604, 604*f*
Varicella 407, 407*f*
Vascular calcification 460
Vascular injury 164
Vascular pathology 310
Vascular steal phenomenon 474, 474*f*
Vasculitis, ANCA-associated 501
Vena cava
  inferior 117*f*, 615*f*, 624*f*
    noncollapsing dilated 207*f*
  superior 108, 117*f*, 118*f*, 119, 119*f*, 225*f*,
    592*f*, 595*f*
Venous capillary pressure 76
Venous drainage of brain 339, 339*f*
Venous oxygen saturation, mixed 509
Venous sinus thrombosis 310
Venovenous
  extracorporeal membrane oxygenation 567
  hemodiafiltration, continuous 473
  hemodialysis, continuous 473
  hemofiltration, continuous 473
Ventilator circuit 57, 57*f*
Ventilatory defect, restrictive 72
Ventricular drain, external 353, 353*f*
Ventricular fibrillation 160
Ventricular premature complexes 191, 191*f*
Ventricular septal defect 192
Ventricular tachycardia 142, 158, 158*f*, 160
Venturi mask 80, 80*f*
Verrucous endocarditis 503
Vertebral artery dissection 314
Vertebral fixation 371
Vessel wall edema 500*f*
Vestibular schwannoma 330
Vibrio cholera 420
Video electroencephalography 373, 373*f*
Videoendoscope, flexible 37, 38, 38*f*
Videolaryngoscope 34, 34*f*, 35, 35*f*, 36, 36*f*
Vision, blurring of 481, 482
Vitamin B_{12} 535
  deficiency 535
Vitreous cells 487

W

Waist hip ratio, high 72
Warden procedure 119
Wave Doppler, continuous 507
Wegener's granulomatosis 494, 494*f*
Wilkins' score 222
World Federation of Neurological Surgeons 343
Wrist, X-ray 460

X

X-ray pelvis 460
  vascular calcification, 460*f*

Y

Yeast cell 425*f*
  budding 415*f*
  numerous 442*f*
  oval 422*f*

Z

Ziehl-Neelsen stain, modified 424, 424*f*